PEDIATRIC

SECRETS

PEDIATRIC SECRETS

Fourth Edition

Richard A. Polin, MD
Professor of Pediatrics
Columbia University College of Physicians and Surgeons
Director, Division of Neonatology
Children's Hospital of New York-Presbyterian
New York, New York

Mark F. Ditmar, MD
Director, AtlantiCare/duPont Pediatric Hospitalist Program
AtlantiCare Regional Medical Center
Pomona, New Jersey
Clinical Assistant Professor of Pediatrics
Jefferson Medical College
Philadelphia, Pennsylvania

ELSEVIER
MOSBY

ELSEVIER
MOSBY

1600 John F. Kennedy Boulevard, Suite 1800
Philadelphia, PA 19103-2899

Pediatric Secrets
Fourth Edition

NOTICE

Knowledge and best practice in this field are constantly changing. As new research and experience broaden our knowledge, changes in practice, treatment, and drug therapy may become necessary or appropriate. Readers are advised to check the most current information provided (i) on procedures featured or (ii) by the manufacturer of each product to be administered, to verify the recommended dose or formula, the method and duration of administration, and contraindications. It is the responsibility of the practitioner, relying on his or her own experience and knowledge of the patient, to make diagnoses, to determine dosages and the best treatment for each individual patient, and to take all appropriate safety precautions. To the fullest extent of the law, neither the Publisher nor the Editors assume any liability for any injury and/or damage to persons or property arising out or related to any use of the material contained in this book.

Previous editions copyrighted 2001, 1997, 1989.

Library of Congress Cataloging-in-Publication Data
Pediatric secrets / [edited by] Richard A. Polin, Mark F. Ditmar.—4th ed.
    p. ;   cm.
    Includes index.
    ISBN-13: 978-1-56053-627-7   ISBN-10: 1-56053-627-6
    1. Pediatrics–Examinations, questions, etc. I. Polin, Richard A. (Richard Alan), 1945-
II. Ditmar, Mark F.
    [DNLM: 1. Pediatrics–Examination Questions. WS 18.2 P3702 2005]
RJ48.2.P347 2005
618.92'0076–dc22   2005047892

Vice President, Medical Education: Linda Belfus
Developmental Editor: Stan Ward
Senior Project Manager: Cecelia Bayruns
Marketing Manager: Kate Rubin

ISBN-13: 978-1-56053-627-7
ISBN-10: 1-56053-627-6

Working together to grow
libraries in developing countries

www.elsevier.com | www.bookaid.org | www.sabre.org

ELSEVIER   BOOK AID International   Sabre Foundation

Printed in the United States of America.
Last digit is the print number: 9 8 7 6 5 4 3 2

CONTENTS

CONTRIBUTORS

Peter C. Adamson, MD
Chief, Division of Clinical Pharmacology and Therapeutics, Children's Hospital of Philadelphia, Philadelphia, Pennsylvania

Kwame Anyane-Yeboa, MD
Associate Professor of Pediatrics, Columbia University College of Physicians and Surgeons; Division of Genetics, Children's Hospital of New York-Presbyterian, New York, New York

Richard Aplenc, MD, MSCE
Pediatric Oncology/Stem Cell Transplant, Children's Hospital of Philadelphia; Center for Clinical Epidemiology and Biostatistics, University of Pennsylvania, Philadelphia, Pennsylvania

Balu H. Athreya, MD
Department of Pediatrics, Division of Rheumatology, Alfred I. duPont Hospital for Children, Wilmington, Delaware; Department of Pediatrics, Jefferson Medical College, Philadelphia, Pennsylvania

Joan Bregstein, MD
Assistant Professor of Clinical Pediatrics, Columbia University College of Physicians and Surgeons; Attending, Pediatrics, Children's Hospital of New York-Presbyterian, New York, New York

Elizabeth Candell Chalom, MD
Clinical Assistant Professor of Pediatrics, University of Medicine and Dentistry of New Jersey, Newark, New Jersey; Director, Pediatric Rheumatology, Saint Barnabas Medical Center, Livingston, New Jersey

Mark F. Ditmar, MD
Director, AtlantiCare/duPont Pediatric Hospitalist Program, AtlantiCare Regional Medical Center, Pomona, New Jersey; Clinical Assistant Professor of Pediatrics, Jefferson Medical College, Philadelphia, Pennsylvania

Andrew H. Eichenfield, MD
Chief, Division of Pediatric Rheumatology, Mount Sinai Medical Center, New York, New York

Alexis M. Elward, MD
Assistant Professor of Pediatrics, Washington University School of Medicine; Division of Infectious Disease, St. Louis Children's Hospital, St. Louis, Missouri

Anders Fasth, MD, PhD
Professor of Pediatric Immunology; Division of Immunology, The Queen Silvia Children's Hospital, Göteborg, Sweden

Maria C. Garzon, MD
Associate Professor of Clinical Dermatology and Clinical Pediatrics, Columbia University College of Physicians and Surgeons; Director, Pediatric Dermatology, Children's Hospital of New York-Presbyterian, New York, New York

Daniel E. Hale, MD
Professor of Pediatrics; Division Chief of Pediatric Endocrinology and Diabetes, University of Texas
Health Science Center at San Antonio, San Antonio, Texas

Constance J. Hayes, MD
Professor of Clinical Pediatrics, Columbia University College of Physicians and Surgeons;
Division of Pediatric Cardiology, Children's Hospital of New York-Presbyterian, New York, New York

Georg A. Holländer, MD
Professor in Pediatrics, Department of Research, University of Basel; The University Children's
Hospital, Basel, Switzerland

Allan J. Hordof, MD
Professor of Clinical Pediatrics, Columbia University College of Physicians and Surgeons; Division of
Pediatric Cardiology, Children's Hospital of New York-Presbyterian, New York, New York

David A. Hunstad, MD
Instructor in Pediatrics, Washington University School of Medicine; Division of Infectious Disease,
St. Louis Children's Hospital, St. Louis, Missouri

Joshua E. Hyman, MD
Assistant Professor of Orthopedics, Columbia University College of Physicians and Surgeons;
Children's Hospital of New York-Presbyterian, New York, New York

Douglas Jacobstein, MD
Division of Gastroenterology and Nutrition, Children's Hospital of Philadelphia, Philadelphia,
Pennsylvania

Kent R. Kelley, MD
Assistant Professor of Clinical Neurology and Clinical Pediatrics, Feinberg School of Medicine,
Northwestern University; Attending Physician, Neurology, Children's Memorial Hospital,
Chicago, Illinois

Chris A. Liacouras, MD
Associate Professor of Pediatrics, University of Pennsylvania School of Medicine; Division of
Gastroenterology and Nutrition, Children's Hospital of Philadelphia, Philadelphia, Pennsylvania

Peter Mamula, MD
Assistant Professor of Pediatrics, University of Pennsylvania School of Medicine; Division of
Gastroenterology and Nutrition, Children's Hospital of Philadelphia, Philadelphia, Pennsylvania

Jonathan E. Markowitz, MD, MSCE
Assistant Professor of Pediatrics, University of Pennsylvania School of Medicine; Director, Inpatient
Gastroenterology, Division of Gastroenterology and Nutrition, Children's Hospital of Philadelphia,
Philadelphia, Pennsylvania

Steven E. McKenzie, MD, PhD
Cardeza Professor of Medicine, Professor of Pediatrics, Jefferson Medical College, Philadelphia,
Pennsylvania

Steve Miller, MD[†]
AP Gold Associate Professor of Clinical Pediatrics, Columbia University College of Physicians
and Surgeons; Director, Division of Pediatric Emergency Medicine, Children's Hospital of
New York-Presbyterian, New York, New York

†Deceased.

Kimberly D. Morel, MD
Assistant Professor of Clinical Dermatology and Clinical Pediatrics, Columbia University College of Physicians and Surgeons, New York, New York

Michael E. Norman, MD
Pediatric Nephrologist, Charlotte, North Carolina

Sharon E. Oberfield, MD
Professor of Pediatrics, Columbia University College of Physicians and Surgeons; Director, Pediatric Endocrinology, Children's Hospital of New York-Presbyterian, New York, New York

Carlos D. Rosé, MD
Associate Professor of Pediatrics, Jefferson Medical College, Philadelphia, Pennsylvania; Chief, Division of Rheumatology, Alfred I. duPont Hospital for Children, Wilmington, Delaware

Cindy Ganis Roskind, MD
Assistant Professor of Clinical Pediatrics, Columbia University College of Physicians and Surgeons; Attending, Pediatrics, Children's Hospital of New York-Presbyterian, New York, New York

Philip Roth, MD, PhD
Associate Professor of Pediatrics, State University of New York-Downstate Medical Center, Brooklyn, New York; Associate Chairman, Department of Pediatrics and Director of Neonatology, Staten Island University Hospital, Staten Island, New York

Jeffrey Skolnik, MD
Division of Hematology and Oncology, Children's Hospital of Philadelphia, Philadelphia, Pennsylvania

Thomas J. Starc, MD, MPH
Professor of Clinical Pediatrics, Columbia University College of Physicians and Surgeons; Division of Pediatric Cardiology, Children's Hospital of New York-Presbyterian, New York, New York

Joseph W. St. Geme, III, MD
Professor of Pediatrics and Molecular Microbiology, Washington University School of Medicine; Director, Division of Infectious Disease, St. Louis Children's Hospital, St. Louis, Missouri

Robert Wilmott, MD
IMMUNO Professor and Chairman, Department of Pediatrics, Saint Louis University School of Medicine; Cardinal Glennon Children's Hospital, St. Louis, Missouri

PREFACE

As a Chinese proverb states, "One who asks a question may be a fool for 5 minutes, but one who does not ask a question remains a fool forever." It is through a process of constant questioning and reappraisal that thoughtful education is maximized and, in the field of medicine, that patient care is ultimately improved.

The purpose of *Pediatric Secrets* is to pose and answer questions about the care of children that are typically addressed in a variety of settings: the office, the hospital, at school, or at home. The scope of the questions is broad; it ranges from basic pathophysiology to general pediatric principles to practical management issues. Some of the questions have no right or wrong answer and may involve areas of clinical controversy or uncertainty. We hope that the points discussed will stimulate efforts on the part of the reader to develop an ongoing appreciation of and interest in changing approaches to pediatric medicine.

We are grateful to the chapter authors for their diligence and adaptability; to Linda Belfus for her vision and grace; to Stan Ward for his editorial assistance; to Trevor MacDougall for his editorial dexterity with both a microscope and a telescope; to Heidi Kleinbart for her organizational wizardry; to the newest members of our households, Lindsey Steinbrenner and Grace Ditmar, for the newborn refresher courses; and to the holdover members of our households—Helene, Allison, Mitchell, Jessica, and Gregory Polin and Nina, Erin, and Cara Ditmar—for continuing to leave the light on for us.

Dr. Steve Miller, who was involved with this and previous editions of *Pediatric Secrets* as an author of the Emergency Medicine chapter, died tragically during the preparation of this manuscript. He was a physician of enormous intelligence, innovation, and compassion, and he is missed terribly. We dedicate this edition to his memory.

Richard A. Polin, MD
Mark F. Ditmar, MD

TOP 100 SECRETS

These secrets are 100 of the top board alerts. They summarize the concepts, principles, and most salient details of pediatric practice.

1. Methods to increase compliance by adolescents with medical regimens include the following: simplifying the regimen, making the patient responsible, discussing potential side effects, using praise liberally, and educating the patient.

2. A pelvic examination is not required before prescribing oral contraceptives for teenagers without risk factors. Appropriate screening for sexually transmitted diseases and possible cervical dysplasia can be scheduled, but delaying oral contraception unnecessarily increases the risk of pregnancy.

3. Emergency contraception should be discussed with all sexually active adolescents; 90% of teenage pregnancies are unintended.

4. Teenagers with attention deficit hyperactivity disorder (ADHD) and conduct disorders are at high risk for substance abuse disorders. Substance abuse is often associated with comorbid psychiatric disorders.

5. Calluses over the metacarpophalangeal joints of the index and/or middle fingers (Russell sign) may indicate repetitive trauma from self-induced attempts at vomiting in patients with eating disorders.

6. Appreciating that ADHD is a *chronic* condition (like asthma or diabetes) is useful for management strategies, follow up, and ongoing patient/parental education and involvement.

7. Although colic is common and resolves spontaneously by 3 months, do not underestimate the physical and psychological impact of the condition on a family.

8. Bilingual children develop speech milestones normally; two-language households should not be presumed as a cause of speech delay.

9. Most amblyopia is unilateral; vision testing solely with both eyes open is inadequate.

10. Congenitally missing or misshapen teeth can be markers for hereditary syndromes.

11. Syncope in a deaf child should lead one to suspect prolongation of the QT wave on the electrocardiogram.

12. Bounding pulses in an infant with congestive heart failure should cause one to consider a large patient ductus arteriosus.

13. If a bruit is heard over the anterior fontanel in a newborn with congestive heart failure, suspect a systemic arteriovenous fistula.

14. The chief complaint in a child with congestive heart failure may be nonspecific abdominal pain.

15. Diastolic murmurs are *never* innocent and deserve further cardiac evaluation.

16. Patients with atypical Kawasaki disease (documented by coronary artery abnormalities despite not fulfilling classic criteria) are usually younger (<1 year old) and most commonly lack cervical adenopathy and extremity changes.

17. Neonates with midline lumbosacral lesions (e.g., sacral pits, hypertrichosis, lipomas) should have screening imaging of the spine performed to search for occult spinal dysraphism.

18. Hemangiomas in the "beard distribution" may be associated with internal airway hemangiomas.

19. Infantile acne necessitates an endocrine workup to rule out precocious puberty.

20. If a child develops psoriasis for the first time or has a flare of existing disease, look for streptococcal pharyngitis.

21. Look for associated autoimmune thyroiditis in children who present with a family history of thyroid disease and extensive alopecia areata or vitiligo.

22. Most cardiac arrests in children are secondary to respiratory arrest. Therefore, early recognition of respiratory distress and failure in children is crucial.

23. Because children are much more elastic than adults, beware of internal injuries after trauma; these can occur *without* obvious skeletal injuries.

24. Because children get colder faster than adults as the result of a higher ratio of body surface area to body mass, be sure that hypothermia is not compounding hemodynamic instability in a pediatric trauma patient in shock.

25. Hypotension and excessive fluid restriction should be avoided at all costs in the child in shock with severe head injury because such a patient is highly sensitive to secondary brain injury from hypotension.

26. The most common finding upon the examination of a child's genitalia after suspected sexual abuse is a normal examination.

27. Because the size of a normal hymenal opening in a prepubertal child can vary significantly, the quality and smoothness of the contours of the hymenal opening, including tears and scarring, are more sensitive indicators of sexual abuse.

28. Palpation for an enlarged or nodular thyroid is one of the most overlooked parts of the pediatric physical examination in all age groups.

29. Because 20–40% of solitary thyroid nodules in adolescents are malignant, an expedited evaluation is needed if a nodule is discovered.

30. Unless a blood sugar level is checked, the diagnosis of new-onset diabetic ketoacidosis can be delayed because abdominal pain can mimic appendicitis, and hyperventilation can mimic pneumonia.

31. Beware of syndrome of inappropriate antidiuretic hormone secretion and possible cerebral edema if a normal or low sodium level begins to fall with fluid replenishment during the treatment of diabetic ketoacidosis.

32. Acanthosis nigricans is found in 90% of youth diagnosed with type 2 diabetes.

33. Growth hormone deficiency present during the first year of life is associated with hypoglycemia; after the age of 5 years, it is associated with short stature.

34. Fecal soiling is associated with severe functional constipation.

35. More than 40% of infants regurgitate effortlessly more than once a day.

36. Nasogastric lavage is a simple method for differentiating upper gastrointestinal bleeding from lower gastrointestinal bleeding.

37. Conjugated hyperbilirubinemia in any child is abnormal and deserves further investigation.

38. Potential long-term complications of pediatric inflammatory bowel disease include chronic growth failure, abscesses, fistulas, nephrolithiasis, and toxic megacolon.

39. Bilious emesis in a newborn represents a sign of potential obstruction and is a true gastrointestinal emergency.

40. In patients with Down syndrome and behavioral problems, do not overlook hearing loss (both sensorineural and conductive); it occurs in up to two thirds of patients with this condition, and it can be a possible contributor to those types of problems.

41. Fluorescence in situ hybridization (FISH) is indicated for the rapid diagnosis of trisomies 13 and 18 and multiple syndromes in children with moderate to severe mental retardation and apparently normal chromosomes (subtelomeric FISH probes).

42. Three or more minor malformations should raise concern about the presence of a major malformation.

43. The diagnosis of fetal alcohol syndrome is problematic in infants because facial growth and development can modify previously diagnostic features over a 4- to 6-year period.

44. Diabetes mellitus is the most common teratogenic state; insulin-dependent diabetic mothers have infants with an eight-fold increase in structural anomalies.

45. An infant with nonsyndromic sensorineural hearing loss should be tested for mutations in the connexin 26 gene. Mutations in that gene contribute to at least about 50% of autosomal recessive hearing loss and about 10–20% of all prelingual hearing loss.

46. In children <12 years old, the lower limit of normal for the mean corpuscular volume (MCV) can be estimated as $70 + (\text{the child's age in years})/\text{mm}^3$. For a patient that is more than 12 years old, the lower limit for a normal MCV is $82/\text{mm}^3$.

47. In the setting of microcytosis, an elevated red blood cell distribution width index suggests a diagnosis of iron deficiency rather than thalassemia.

48. After iron supplementation for iron-deficiency anemia, the reticulocyte count should double in 1–2 weeks, and hemoglobin should increase by 1 gm/dL in 2–4 weeks. The most common reason for persistence of iron deficiency anemia is poor compliance with supplementation.

49. Children with elevated lead levels are at increased risk for iron deficiency anemia because lead competitively inhibits the absorption of iron.

50. Chronic transfusion therapy to reduce sickle hemoglobin levels to 30–40% of the total lowers the likelihood of stroke.

51. Because 30% of patients with hemophilia have no family history of the disorder, clinical suspicion is important in the presence of excessive and frequent ecchymoses.

52. Marked neutropenia (<500/mm^3 absolute neutrophil count) in a previously healthy child often heralds the onset of overwhelming sepsis.

53. The determination of immunoglobulin G subclass concentrations is meaningless in children who are less than 4 years old.

54. Neutrophil deficiency should be considered in a newborn with a delayed separation of the umbilical cord (>3 weeks).

55. Clinical features of autoimmunity do not exclude the diagnosis of a primary immunodeficiency.

56. A male child with a liver abscess should be considered to have chronic granulomatous disease until it is proven otherwise.

57. The most common congenital infection is cytomegalovirus, which in some large screening studies occurs in up to 1.3% of newborns, although most of these infants remain asymptomatic.

58. Up to 25% of infants <28 days old with bacterial sepsis and positive blood cultures will have culture-confirmed meningitis.

59. Erythematous papules with a pale center ("doughnut lesions") located on the hard and soft palates are pathognomonic for streptococcal pharyngitis.

60. The *red man syndrome*, which is a complication of vancomycin administration, can usually be avoided by slowing the rate of drug infusion or by premedicating with diphenhydramine.

61. A petechial-purpuric rash in a glove-and-stocking distribution should raise the possibility of infection with parvovirus B19.

62. Perinatal asphyxia accounts for less than 15% of cases of cerebral palsy.

63. Because primary and secondary apnea are indistinguishable in newborns, the initial clinical response should be identical in the delivery room.

64. Hyperbilirubinemia is generally not an indication for the cessation of breast feeding but rather for increasing its frequency.

65. Sepsis is in the differential diagnosis of virtually every neonatal sign and symptom.

66. Breast feeding lowers the risks of necrotizing enterocolitis and nosocomial sepsis.

67. Ten percent of febrile infants with documented urinary tract infections have normal urinalyses; this emphasizes the importance of obtaining a urine culture if clinical risk factors are present.

68. Vigorous correction of constipation has been shown to diminish both enuresis and the frequency of urinary tract infections.

69. Chromosomal and endocrinologic evaluation should be done if testes are bilaterally undescended and nonpalpable or one or two testicles are undescended with hypospadias present.

70. In patients with acute renal failure, the measurement of urinary indices (urine sodium concentration, fractional excretion of sodium, urine specific gravity, and osmolality) should be done *before initiating any therapy* to help distinguish between prerenal, renal, and postrenal etiologies.

71. The two most productive facets of patient evaluation to explain renal disease as a possible cause of symptoms are as follows: (1) the measurement of blood pressure and (2) the examination of the first morning void after the bladder is emptied of urine stored overnight (when a specimen is most likely to be concentrated).

72. The most common cause of persistent seizures is an inadequate serum antiepileptic level.

73. Antiepileptic drugs in tablet and capsule form produce less variation in blood concentrations than liquid preparations, particularly suspensions, do.

74. Resist polypharmacy: three or more medications have not been shown to improve seizure control as compared with one or two drugs, and side effects and compliance become much more problematic.

75. The diagnosis of cerebral palsy is rarely made at <1 year old because neurologic findings in infancy are subject to significant change.

76. Migraine headaches are usually bilateral in children but unilateral (75%) in adults.

77. Seizures with fever in patients older than 6 years of age should not be considered febrile seizures.

78. Children with fever and neutropenia must continue to receive broad-spectrum antibiotics until definitive signs of marrow recovery are documented, typically with the presence of a peripheral monocytosis and an absolute neutrophil count >200/mm^3 and rising.

79. Empiric antifungal agents are administered to children with neutropenia who remain febrile or develop new fever within 3 to 7 days of starting broad-spectrum antibiotics because the risk of invasive fungal infection increases with the duration and depth of neutropenia.

80. After age and white blood cell count, *early response to therapy* is the most important prognostic feature for children with acute lymphoblastic leukemia.

81. Leukemias and lymphomas that have a high proliferation and cell turnover rate (e.g., Burkitt's lymphoma, T-cell lymphoblastic leukemia) place patients at the highest risk of complications from tumor lysis syndrome.

82. Eighty percent or more of patients who present with acute lymphoblastic leukemia have a normochromic, normocytic anemia with reticulocytopenia.

83. Because it changes more quickly as inflammation changes, C-reactive protein is better than sedimentation rate for monitoring the response to therapy in patients with osteomyelitis.

84. Pseudoparalysis (with decreased arm or leg movement) with no systemic illness may be a presenting sign in an infant with osteomyelitis.

85. Back pain is atypical for scoliosis and may point to another diagnosis.

86. Consider magnetic resonance imaging for patients with scoliosis and the less common *left-sided* thoracic curves because 5–7% of these patients can have intraspinal abnormalities (e.g., hydromelia).

87. A plain x-ray is unreliable in the diagnosis of developmental dysplasia of the hip in infants less than 6 months of age because ossification of the femoral head is incomplete.

88. Older children with unexplained *unilateral* deformities (e.g., pes cavus) of an extremity should have screening magnetic resonance imaging to evaluate for intraspinal disease.

89. Asthma rarely causes clubbing in children. Consider other diseases, particularly cystic fibrosis.

90. Most children with recurrent pneumonia or persistent right middle lobe atelectasis have asthma. But . . . all that wheezes is not asthma.

91. Home peak flow monitoring is most helpful in those asthmatic patients with very labile disease or poor symptom recognition.

92. A normal respiratory rate strongly argues against a bacterial pneumonia.

93. Upper lobe pneumonias with radiation of pain to the neck can cause meningismus and mimic appendicitis; lower lobe pneumonias can present with abdominal pain.

94. Nasal polyps or rectal prolapse in children suggests cystic fibrosis.

95. The three most common causes of anaphylaxis in pediatric hospitals and emergency departments are latex, food, and drugs. Suspected allergies to shellfish, peanuts, and nuts warrant a prescription for an epinephrine pen because of the increased risk of future anaphylaxis.

96. Up to 10% of normal, healthy children may have low-level (1:10) positive–antinuclear antibody (ANA) testing that will remain positive. Without clinical or laboratory features of disease, it is of no significance.

97. The daily spiking fevers of systemic juvenile rheumatoid arthritis can precede the development of arthritis by weeks to months.

98. Antistreptolysin O antibodies are positive in only 80% of patients with acute rheumatic fever. Test for anti-DNase B antibodies to increase the likelihood to more than 95% when diagnosing a recent group A beta-hemolytic infection.

99. Because up to 10% of patients can have asymptomatic *Borrelia burgdorferi* infection and because both immunoglobulin M and immunoglobulin G antibodies to *B. burgdorferi* can persist for 10–20 years, the diagnosis of Lyme disease in older children and adolescents can be tricky in patients with atypical clinical presentations.

100. Abdominal pain (mimicking an acute abdomen) and arthritis can frequently precede the rash in Henoch-Schönlein purpura disease and thus confuse the diagnosis.

CHAPTER 1

ADOLESCENT MEDICINE

Mark F. Ditmar, MD

CLINICAL ISSUES

1. What are the major health risks for adolescents?
- **Unintentional injury:** Particularly alcohol-related automobile accidents.
- **Violence:** Suicide and homicide account for about 80–85% of deaths in 15- to 19-year-old adolescents and 60–70% of deaths in 10- to 14-year-old adolescents in the United States.
- **Substance abuse:** In surveys, nearly 10% of 12- to 17-year-old adolescents admit to illicit drug use during the previous 30 days.
- **Sexually transmitted diseases (STDs):** Up to 30% of all STDs reported annually to the Centers for Disease Control and Prevention (CDC) involve adolescents. Adolescents between 15 and 19 years of age have the highest age-specific rates of chlamydial and gonorrheal infections of any population group.
- **Teen pregnancy:** 90% are unintended.
- **Obesity:** 15% of U.S. teenagers are obese (body mass index [BMI] ≥ 95% for age), and 15% are at risk for obesity (BMI between 85–95% for age).

2. Name the major risk factors that are associated with injuries to adolescents.
- **Use of alcohol while engaged in activities** (e.g., driving, swimming, boating)**:** 20% of all adolescent deaths are alcohol-related car crashes.
- **Failure to use safety devices** (e.g., seat belts, motorcycle or bicycle helmets)**:** Seat belt use among adolescents is the lowest of any age group (30–50%), and fewer than 10% use bicycle helmets.
- **Access to firearms:** 50% of deaths among black male teenagers and 20% of deaths among white male teenagers are due to firearms, primarily handguns.
- **Athletic participation:** Most injuries are reinjuries, which highlights the importance of proper rehabilitation.

  Elster AB, Kuznets NJ (eds): AMA Guidelines for Adolescent Preventive Services (GAPS). Baltimore, Williams & Wilkins, 1994, pp 29–40.

3. What diagnoses require mandatory disclosure regardless of confidentiality?
In most states . . .
- Notification of child welfare authorities under state **child-abuse** (physical and sexual) reporting laws
- Notification of law enforcement officials of **gunshot** and **stab wounds**
- Warning from a psychotherapist to a reasonably identifiable victim of a patient's **threat of violence**
- Notification to parents or other authorities if a patient represents a reasonable threat to himself or herself (i.e., **suicidal ideation**)

4. When can teenagers give their own consent for medical care or procedures?
Teenagers who are married, who are parents themselves, who are members of the armed forces, who are living apart from their parents, or who are high school graduates may fit the definition of an "emancipated" or "mature" minor. However, the definition varies from state to

state. For certain services, many states waive the legal requirement of emancipation, and any individual under age 18 may obtain services without parental permission. These include care for sexually transmitted diseases, contraception services, pregnancy-related care, substance abuse treatment, mental health services, and treatment for rape or sexual assault.

5. **How does the "HEADS FIRST" system assist in adolescent interviewing?**
   This mnemonic, which was originally devised at State University of New York Upstate Medical University, allows for a systematic approach to multiple health issues and risk factors that affect teenagers:

   H — **H**ome: living arrangements, family relationships, support
   E — **E**ducation: school issues, study habits, achievement, employment, expectations
   A — **A**buse: physical, sexual, emotional, verbal
   D — **D**rugs: peer and personal use, alcohol, tobacco, marijuana, cocaine, others
   S — **S**afety: injury prevention, safety equipment, seat belts, helmets, hazardous activities
   F — **F**riends: peer pressure, interaction, confidants
   I — **I**mage: self-esteem, body image, weight management
   R — **R**ecreation: exercise, relaxation, television/media time
   S — **S**exuality: changes, feelings, experiences, orientation, contraception
   T — **T**hreats: depressed or upset easily, suicidal ideation or attempts, harm to others

   Cavanaugh RM: Evaluating adolescents with fatigue. Pediatr Rev 23:337–347, 2002.

EATING DISORDERS

6. **What types of dieting raise concern for the development of an eating disorder?**
   Dieting that is associated with . . .
   - Decreasing weight goals
   - Increasing criticism of body image
   - Increasing social isolation
   - Amenorrhea or oligomenorrhea

7. **How is the diagnosis of anorexia made?**
   Anorexia nervosa consists of a spectrum of psychological, behavioral, and medical abnormalities. The *1996 Diagnostic and Statistical Manual for Primary Care: Child and Adolescent Version* criteria list five components:
   - **Refusal to maintain body weight** or BMI at or above minimal norms for age and height (less than 85% of expected weight for height or a BMI of less than 17.5 in an older adolescent)
   - **Intense fear of gaining weight** or becoming fat
   - **Disturbances of perception** of body shape and size
   - **Denial of seriousness** of weight loss or low body weight
   - In postmenarchal girls, **amenorrhea** (i.e., the absence of at least three consecutive menstrual cycles)

8. **What are good and bad prognosticators for recovery from anorexia?**
   Good: Early age at onset, high educational achievement, improvement in body image after weight gain, emotionally well-adjusted, supportive family
   Bad: Late age at onset, continued overestimation of body size, self-induced vomiting or bulimia, laxative abuse, family dysfunction, male

9. **What hormonal abnormalities may be seen in anorexia nervosa?**
    Amenorrhea is seen in most cases due to hypothalamic/pituitary dysfunction with very low levels of luteinizing hormone (LH) and follicle-stimulating hormone (FSH). Twenty-five percent of affected girls experience amenorrhea before significant weight loss occurs, which suggests that there is a psychological effect on physiology. Symptoms that are suggestive of **hypothyroidism**—constipation, cold intolerance, dry skin, bradycardia, and hair or nail changes—are common. Thyroid studies, however, have relatively normal results, except for a low triiodothyronine (T_3) and an increased reverse T_3 (rT_3), which is a less-active isomer.

    The T_3/rT_3 reversal is also seen in conditions that are associated with weight loss, possibly indicating that it is a physiologic means of adapting to a lower energy state. Other abnormalities include a loss of diurnal variation in **cortisol**, diminished plasma **catecholamine** levels, normal or increased **growth hormone** levels, and flattened glucose tolerance curve.

10. **How common is laxative abuse in anorexia nervosa?**
    Self-reported use is approximately 10%, but when urine screening is done, it has been found to be 20–30%. Biochemical urine screening can be done using high-performance thin-layer chromatography, especially if laxatives have been ingested within 36 hours. Direct toxicity of laxatives can lead to steatorrhea and occasionally to fat-soluble vitamin malabsorption. Fat globules in stool suggest laxative abuse.

    Turner J, Batik M, Palmer LJ, et al: Detection and importance of laxative use in adolescents with anorexia nervosa. J Am Acad Child Adolesc Psychiatry 39:378–385, 2000.

11. **What are the indications that a pediatric patient with anorexia nervosa should be admitted to a hospital?**
    - <75% of ideal body weight or ongoing weight loss despite intensive management
    - Refusal to eat
    - Body fat <10%
    - Heart rate <50/min daytime; <45/min nighttime
    - Systolic blood pressure <90 mmHg
    - Orthostatic changes in pulse (>20 beats per minute) or blood pressure (>10 mmHg)
    - Temperature <96°F
    - Arrhythmia

    American Academy of Pediatrics, Committee on Adolescence: Identifying and tolerating eating disorders. Pediatrics 111:204–211, 2003.

12. **What causes sudden death in anorectics?**
    Chronic emaciation affects the myocardium. Anorectics develop depressed cardiovascular function and an altered conduction system. Electrocardiogram (ECG) changes are common. Patients with anorexia have significantly lower heart rates (averaging 20 beats/min less than peers), lower R values in V6, and longer QRS intervals. These ECG changes often occur without underlying electrolyte abnormalities. The arrhythmogenic potential is heightened if electrolytes (specifically potassium) are distorted by excessive vomiting or laxative abuse. Sudden death is likely as a result of the culmination of chronic myocardial injury in emaciated patients (>35–40% below ideal weight) with resultant heart failure and dysrhythmia.

    Panagiotopoulos C, McCrindle BW, Hick K, Katzman DK: Electrocardiographic findings in adolescents with eating disorders. Pediatrics 105:1100–1105, 2000.

13. **Do males and females with anorexia nervosa have a similar clinical profile?**
    It is estimated that less than 5% of anorexia nervosa involves boys. Males are more likely to . . .
    - Have been obese before the onset of symptoms.
    - Be ambivalent regarding the desire to gain or lose weight.
    - Have more issues about gender and sexual identity.

- Involve dieting with sports participation.
- Engage in "defensive dieting" (avoiding weight gain after an athletic injury).

Rosen DS: Eating disorders in adolescent males. Adolesc Med 14:677–689, 2003.

KEY POINTS: ANOREXIA NERVOSA

1. Hallmark: A compulsive and unrelenting drive to be thin and then thinner.

2. BMI <17.5 in older adolescents strongly suggests anorexia.

3. 95% female, but evidence suggests increasing prevalence among males.

4. Inquire about the possibility of an eating disorder with a *direct* question: "How do you feel about your weight?"

5. Sedimentation rates: Usually normal in eating disorders; elevation suggests other diagnoses, such as inflammatory bowel disease.

6. Most common causes of death: Cardiac dysfunction and suicide.

14. **How is the diagnosis of bulimia nervosa made?**
    Bulimia nervosa is a syndrome of voracious, high-caloric overeating and subsequent forced vomiting (by gagging or ipecac) and/or other purging methods (e.g., laxatives, diuretics). This often occurs during periods of frustration or psychological stress. Its incidence is felt to be higher than that of anorexia nervosa, and males are rarely involved. The diagnosis is made using a patient's **history**.

15. **List the medical complications of bulimia nervosa.**
    Electrolyte abnormalities: Hypokalemia, hypochloremia, and metabolic alkalosis may occur. The hypokalemia can cause a prolonged QT interval and T-wave abnormalities.
    Esophageal: Acid reflux with esophagitis and (rarely) Mallory-Weiss tear may be found
    Cardiac: Ipecac use can result in cardiomyopathy due to a toxic effect of one of its principal components, the alkaloid emetine.
    Central nervous system: Neurotransmitters can be affected, thereby causing changes in the patient's perceptions of satiety.
    Miscellaneous: Enamel erosion, salivary gland enlargement, cheilosis, and knuckle calluses are signs of recurrent vomiting.

Mehler PS: Bulimia nervosa. N Engl J Med 349:875–81, 2003.

16. **How do anorexia nervosa and bulimia nervosa differ?**
    See Table 1-1.

17. **What modalities are used to treat eating disorders?**
    - **Nutritional rehabilitation:** Very large caloric intakes (e.g., 3000–4000 kcal/day) may be needed to achieve adequate gain. Controversy exists regarding strict versus lenient inpatient protocols. Routine use of appetite stimulants, nasogastric feedings, or hyperalimentation is not recommended.
    - **Medication:** Prokinetic agents (e.g., domperidone) are used to minimize postprandial bloating. Antidepressants, including serotonin-specific reuptake inhibitors, are more commonly used in bulimia nervosa.
    - **Psychotherapy:** Individual and family therapy may both be useful.

Woodside DB: A review of anorexia nervosa and bulimia nervosa. Curr Probl Pediatr 25:67–89, 1995.

TABLE 1-1. COMPARISON OF ANOREXIA NERVOSA AND BULIMIA NERVOSA	
Anorexia nervosa	**Bulimia nervosa**
Vomiting or diuretic/laxative abuse uncommon	Vomiting or diuretic/laxative abuse
Severe weight loss	Less weight loss; avoidance of obesity
Slightly younger	Slightly older
More introverted	More extroverted
Hunger denied	Hunger pronounced
Eating behavior may be considered normal and a source of self-esteem	Eating behavior is egodystonic
Sexually inactive	Sexually active
Obsessional fears with paranoid features	Histrionic features
Amenorrhea	Menses irregular or absent
Death from starvation/suicide	Death from hypokalemia/suicide

From Shenker IR, Bunnell DW: Bulimia nervosa. In McAnarmey ER, Kreipe RE, Orr DP, Comerci, GD (eds): Textbook of Adolescent Medicine. Philadelphia, W.B. Saunders, 1992, p 545.

18. **Name the three features that constitute the "female athletic triad."**

Disordered eating, amenorrhea, and **osteoporosis.** These three distinct yet interrelated disorders are often seen in active girls and young women. All female athletes are at risk for developing this triad, with 15–60% of female athletes demonstrating abnormal weight-control behaviors. Diagnosis is based on history, physical examination, and laboratory evaluation. The basic laboratory workup should include urine human chorionic gonadotropin, thyroid-stimulating hormone, prolactin, FSH, LH, testosterone, dehydroepiandrosterone sulfate (DHEA-S), and progesterone challenge test. Ongoing counseling is often indicated, as are nutritional and hormonal interventions. Treatment commonly includes calcium supplements and oral contraceptives.

   Greydanus DE, Patel DR: The female athlete: before and beyond puberty. Pediatr Clin North Am 49:553–580, 2002.
   American Academy of Pediatrics. Committee on Sports Medicine and Fitness: Medical concerns in the female athlete. Pediatrics 106:610–613, 2000.

MENSTRUAL DISORDERS

19. **What is the difference between primary and secondary amenorrhea?**

Primary amenorrhea: No onset of menses by age 16 *or* within 3 years of onset of secondary sex characteristics *or* within 1 year of Tanner V breast/pubic hair development
Secondary amenorrhea: No menses for 3 months after previous establishment of regular menstrual periods

20. **What causes primary amenorrhea?**

The key feature in the differential diagnosis is whether the amenorrhea is associated with the development of secondary sex characteristics.

Amenorrhea *without* secondary sex characteristics
- Chromosomal or enzymatic defects (e.g., Turner syndrome, chromosomal mosaics, 17α-hydroxylase deficiency)
- Congenital absence of uterus

- Gonadal dysgenesis (with elevated gonadotropins)
- Hypothalamic-pituitary abnormalities (with diminished gonadotropins)

Amenorrhea *with* secondary sex characteristics
- Dysfunction of hypothalamic release of gonadotropin-releasing hormone (GnRH) (e.g., stress, excessive exercise, weight loss, chronic illness, polycystic ovary disease, medications, hypothyroidism)
- Abnormalities of pituitary gland (e.g., tumor, empty sella syndrome)
- Ovarian dysfunction (e.g., irradiation, chemotherapy, trauma, viral infection, autoimmune inflammation)
- Abnormalities of genital tract (e.g., cervical agenesis, imperforate hymen, testicular feminization with absent uterus)
- Pregnancy

21. **How can estrogen influence be evaluated on vaginal or cervical smears?**
    Vaginal smear: In patients with normal estrogen, 15–30% of cells are superficial (small pyknotic nuclei with large cytoplasm), and the remainder are intermediate (larger nuclei with visible nucleolus but still with cytoplasm predominant). If parabasal cells are noted (nuclear:cytoplasmic ratio of ≥50:50), relative estrogen deficiency should be suspected.
    Cervical smear: Cervical mucus is smeared onto a glass slide and allowed to dry. If a fern pattern appears, estrogen is normal (i.e., because salts crystallize only if estrogen is unopposed by progesterone). No fern pattern occurs during the second half of menses, after ovulation, because of the presence of progesterone. Absence of ferning during pregnancy is also a result of higher progesterone levels.

22. **What is the value of a progesterone challenge test in a patient with amenorrhea?**
    If bleeding ensues within 2 weeks after the administration of oral medroxyprogesterone (10 mg daily for 5 days) or intramuscular progesterone in oil (50–100 mg), the test is positive. This indicates that the endometrium has been primed by estrogen and that the pituitary-hypothalamic-ovarian axis and outflow tract are functioning.

23. **A 14-year-old girl has Tanner III features and monthly abdominal pain but no onset of menstrual flow. What is the likely diagnosis?**
    An **anatomic abnormality of the vagina** (e.g., imperforate hymen or transverse vaginal septum) or **cervix** (e.g., agenesis).

24. **An obese 16-year-old girl has oligomenorrhea, hirsutism, acne, and an elevated LH/FSH ratio. What condition is likely?**
    Polycystic ovary syndrome. This disorder is characterized by the triad of *menstrual irregularities* (amenorrhea/oligomenorrhea), *hirsutism,* and *acne* that begins during puberty. Obesity is common. In these individuals, there is an apparent gonadotropin-dependent, functional ovarian hyperandrogenism with elevated LH (or LH:FSH ratio >3:1) and insulin resistance. A dysregulation of ovarian synthesis of androgens and estrogen is likely. Studies of mainly white, European females have found that 60% of teens with oligomenorrhea have endocrine signs that are compatible with polycystic ovary syndrome. Endocrine evaluation should strongly be considered in oligomenorrheic adolescents before reassurance is given or before prescriptions are written for oral contraceptives.

    Richardson MR: Current perspectives in polycystic ovary syndrome. Am Fam Physician 68:697–704, 2003.

25. **What are the range of complications of polycystic ovary syndrome?**
    - Infertility
    - Abnormal lipid metabolism

- Type 2 diabetes
- Endometrial cancer
- Cardiovascular disease

Ehrmann DA: Polycystic ovary syndrome. N Eng J Med 352:1223–1236, 2005.

26. **What constitutes excessive menstrual bleeding in an adolescent?**

As a rule, most menstrual periods do not last >8 days, do not occur more frequently than every 21–40 days, and are not associated with >80 mL of blood loss. The quantitation can be difficult because pad or tampon numbers correlate poorly with total blood loss. Blood clots or a change in pad numbers appears to have more reliability. Suspicion of excessive loss should prompt an evaluation of hematocrit and/or reticulocyte count.

27. **How common are anovulatory menstrual periods in adolescents?**

Anovulatory cycles (and with them, an increased likelihood of irregular periods) occur in 50% of adolescents for up to 2 years after menarche and in up to 20% after 5 years (the rate in adults). Anovulatory cycles result in unopposed estradiol production, which can cause the following: (1) breakthrough bleeding at varying intervals due to insufficient hormone to support a thickened endothelium, and (2) heavy and prolonged menstrual flow due to lack of progesterone. However, most anovulatory menstrual cycles are normal because the intact negative feedback loop (i.e., rising estradiol lowers FH and LSH, which, in turn, lower estradiol) does not allow for prolonged elevated estrogen with endometrial proliferation.

28. **Describe the evaluation for a patient with dysfunctional uterine bleeding.**

Dysfunctional uterine bleeding is abnormal bleeding in the absence of structural pelvic pathology. It remains a diagnosis of exclusion. Depending on the age of the patient and her history of sexual activity, the following studies should be considered:

- Speculum examination for evidence of trauma, vaginal foreign body, and diethylstilbestrol-induced adenosis
- Bimanual examination for ovarian mass, uterine fibroid, and signs of pregnancy or pelvic inflammatory disease
- Pap smear for cervical dysplasia
- Pregnancy test
- Serum prolactin
- Thyroid function tests
- Coagulation studies (especially for von Willebrand disease)

Albers JR, Hull SK, Wesley RM: Abnormal uterine bleeding. Am Fam Physician 69:1915–1932, 2004.

29. **How can the *timing* of abnormal uterine bleeding help identify the most likely cause?**

Abnormal bleeding at the normal time of cyclic shedding
- Blood dyscrasia (especially von Willebrand disease)
- Endometrial pathology (e.g., submucous myoma, intrauterine device)

Abnormal bleeding at any time during the cycle, but normal cycles
- Vaginal foreign body
- Trauma
- Endometriosis
- Infection
- Uterine polyps
- Cervical abnormality (e.g., hemangioma)

Noncyclic bleeding or abnormal cyclic bleeding (<21 days or >45 days, usually associated with anovulatory cycles)
- Physiologic (especially during early adolescence)
- Polycystic ovary disease
- Psychosocial pathology
- Excessive exercise
- Endocrine disorders
- Adrenal/ovarian tumors
- Ovarian failure

  Adapted from Kozlowski K, Gottlieb A, Graham CJ, Cleveland ER: Adolescent gynecologic conditions presenting in emergency settings. Adolesc Med 4:63–76, 1993.

30. **What are the two key clinical features that determine the management of dysfunctional uterine bleeding?**
    Hemoglobin concentration (i.e., anemia) and signs of orthostatic hypotension. The more severe the clinical feature, the more urgent and aggressive the management must be, particularly in the setting of acute hemorrhage.

31. **How should a very anemic teenager with positive orthostatic signs be managed?**
    If there are orthostatic changes and the hemoglobin is low (<10 mg/dL) . . .
    - Hospitalize for high-dose intravenous conjugated estrogen therapy (e.g., 25 mg every 4 hours for up to 24 hours)
    - Consider transfusion (usually not required)
    - Unresponsive bleeding may require dilatation and curettage (also rarely required in adolescents)
    - Coagulation studies (due to a higher likelihood of underlying coagulopathy)

      Rimsza ME: Dysfunctional uterine bleeding. Pediatr Rev 23:227–232, 2002.

KEY POINTS: MENSTRUAL DISORDERS

1. Abnormally heavy bleeding at menarche or unusually long menstrual periods: Consider von Willebrand disease.

2. Irregular menstrual bleeding patterns: Common in early adolescence, because regular ovulatory menstrual cycles typically do not develop for 1–1½ years after the onset of menarche.

3. Always consider pregnancy in a patient with secondary amenorrhea.

4. Signs of androgen excess (hirsutism and/or acne) in the setting of menstrual irregularities suggest polycystic ovary syndrome.

5. Progressively worsening dysmenorrhea suggests endometriosis as a cause of chronic pelvic pain in adolescents.

6. Ask about dysmenorrhea: It affects >50% of teenage girls and causes considerable school absence.

32. **Why is dysmenorrhea more common in *late* rather than *early* adolescence?**
    Dysmenorrhea occurs almost entirely with ovulatory cycles. Menses shortly after the onset of menarche is usually anovulatory. With the establishment of more regular ovulatory cycles after 2–4 years, primary dysmenorrhea becomes more likely.

33. **In a teenager with dysmenorrhea, what factors suggest an underlying identifiable pathologic problem rather than primary dysmenorrhea?**
    Primary dysmenorrhea is painful menses without identifiable pelvic pathology and accounts for the vast majority of cases in teenagers. However, underlying pathology is more likely if any of the following conditions are present: **menorrhagia** (excessive volume or duration of menses); **intermenstrual bleeding**; **pain at times other than menses** (suggesting outflow obstruction); or **abnormal uterine shape** on examination (suggesting uterine malformation).

34. **What classes of medications are used for dysmenorrhea?**
    Prostaglandin inhibitors: Evidence strongly suggests a key role for prostaglandins in pain production (especially prostaglandin $F_{2\alpha}$ and prostaglandin $E_{2\alpha}$). Nonsteroidal anti-inflammatory agents can limit local production. Naproxen, ibuprofen, and mefenamic acid are all effective. If side effects of indomethacin and phenylbutazone are present (particularly gastric irritation), limit their use. Aspirin is no more effective than placebo.
    Oral contraceptives: Oral contraceptives act by reducing endometrial growth, which limits the total production of endometrial prostaglandin. Ovulation is suppressed, which also minimizes pain. A 30–35 μg combined estrogen-progestin pill is preferred. After 4–6 months, oral contraceptives may be stopped and symptoms reassessed if the need for contraception is not an issue.
    Central-acting analgesic: Tramadol acts by binding to m-opioid receptors and inhibiting the reuptake of norepinephrine and serotonin. It is neither an NSAID nor a narcotic, and it appears to be nonaddictive.
    Alternative medicines: Herbal teas, fruits, and vegetables may be beneficial.

    Laufer MR, Goldstein DP: Dysmenorrhea, pelvic pain and the premenstrual syndrome. In Emans SJ, Laufer MR, Goldstein DP (eds): Pediatric and Adolescent Gynecology, 4th ed. Philadelphia, Lippincott-Raven, 1998, pp 363–410.

OBESITY

35. **What is the body mass index (BMI)?**
    BMI = (weight [kg]/height [m^2]). As an indicator of body fat, it is recommended by the CDC as the main screening tool for obesity. When plotted on standard charts, a BMI from 85–95% for age and sex indicates "at risk for overweight," and a BMI above the 95th percentile indicates "overweight." It is estimated that about 30% of U.S. adolescents are overweight or at risk of being overweight. BMI growth charts are available at:

    http://www.cdc.gov/nchs/about/major/nhanes/growthcharts/clinical/charts/htm

36. **What are the risk factors for obesity in teenagers?**
    - **Positive family history:** With one obese parent, probability of obesity is 40%; with two obese parents, this increases to 70–80%.
    - **Degree of obesity as a child:** More severe obesity is likely to persist.
    - **Socioeconomic status:** Generally, higher socioeconomic status confers a higher likelihood of obesity. This trend is maintained in adulthood for boys, but it reverses in late adolescence for girls.
    - **Television viewing:** Increased television viewing appears to correlate with a higher likelihood of obesity.
    - **Race:** Obesity is more common among whites than blacks.
    - **Family size:** Obesity decreases as family size increases; it has the greatest prevalence among single children.

    Strauss RS: Childhood obesity. Pediatr Clin North Am 49:175–197, 2002.

37. **Are boys or girls more likely to remain obese teenagers throughout puberty?**
    Girls. During puberty, body fat *decreases* by 40% in boys and *increases* by 40% in girls. Puberty leads to the normalization of body weight in 70% of obese males but in only 20% of

obese females. Girls who have early menarche (age, ≤11 years) are twice as likely to become obese adults as are late maturers (age, ≥14 years). Girls also have significant declines in physical activity during adolescence.

Kimm SY, Glynn NW, Kriska AM, et al: Decline in physical activity in black girls and white girls during adolescence. N Engl J Med 347:709–715, 2002.

38. What morbidities can be associated with adolescent obesity?
- Hypertension
- Lipid abnormalities
- Apnea
- Orthopedic problems (e.g., slipped epiphyses, Blount disease)
- Gallstones
- Steatohepatitis
- Intracranial hypertension
- Accelerated pubertal and skeletal development
- Diabetes mellitus, type 2
- Polycystic ovary syndrome

Dietz WH, Robinson TN: Overweight children and adolescents. N Engl J Med 352:2100–2109, 2005.

39. What features constitute the *metabolic syndrome*?
- Central obesity (excessive fat around the abdomen)
- Lipid abnormalities
- Hypertension
- Insulin resistance and/or glucose intolerance
- Prothrombotic state
- Proinflammatory state (elevated C-reactive protein)

Well-described in adults with obesity, this constellation of biomarkers and risk factors for adverse cardiovascular outcomes has been increasingly recognized in adolescents.

Weiss R, Dziura J, Burgert TS, et al: Obesity and the metabolic syndrome in children and adolescents. N Engl J Med 350:2362–2374, 2004.

40. What features on physical examination are particularly important in the evaluation of the obese patient?
- Blood pressure (hypertension)
- Facial dysmorphic features (evidence of genetic syndrome)
- Tonsils (hypertrophy; potential for obstructive apnea)
- Thyroid (goiter, possible hypothyroidism)
- Acanthosis nigricans (type II diabetes)
- Hirsutism (polycystic ovary syndrome)
- Striae (Cushing syndrome)
- Right upper quadrant (RUQ) tenderness (gallbladder disease)
- Small hands/feet, cryptorchidism (Prader-Willi syndrome)
- Limited hip range of motion (slipped capital femoral epiphysis)
- Lower-leg bowing (Blount disease)

Eissa MAH: Overview of pediatric obesity: Key points in the evaluation and therapy. Consultant Pediatr 2:293–296, 2003.

41. Do obese children and adolescents become obese adults?

In most tracking studies, only 25–50% have become obese adults. However, in some studies it has ranged as high as 75%. The most important risk factors for persistence of obesity are later age of onset and increased severity of obesity at any age.

Gauthier BM, Hickner JM, Ornstein S: High prevalence of overweight children and adolescents in the Practice Partner Research Network. Arch Pediatr Adolesc Med 154:625–628, 2000.

KEY POINTS: OBESITY

1. Younger children: Main impact of obesity is social and emotional rather than medical.

2. Obesity: Most common chronic condition in children.

3. Keep weight reduction or stabilization goals *reasonable*—if too unrealistic, discouragement and weight cycling are more likely.

4. Obesity and short stature—think *thyroid abnormalities* and evaluate thyroid-stimulating hormone and T_4 levels.

5. Big three calorie culprits: (1) High-fat fast food, (2) large portions, and (3) sugar-containing soft drinks.

6. If a child is at risk as a result of family history, the earlier the modifications (e.g., limiting TV time), the better.

---

42. **What is the long-term outlook for the obese teenager?**
Obesity in adolescence is associated with medical, economic, and social consequences. Obese teenagers, especially females, have lower rates of school completion, lower rates of marriage, lower household incomes, and higher rates of poverty. Even if weight corrections occur later, the early obesity is associated with increased atherosclerotic heart disease in men and women, with colorectal cancer and gout in men, and with arthritis in women.

    Schwimmer JB, Burwinkle TM, Varni JW: Health-related quality of life of severely obese children and adolescents. JAMA 289:1813–1819, 2003.

43. **How effective are intervention and treatment for obesity in adolescents?**
Weight-reduction regimens involving behavior modification and dietary therapy are modestly effective with regard to short-term results, but they are notoriously ineffective for the achievement of long-term weight loss. Expert committee recommendations for evaluation and treatment are available at:

    http://www.pediatrics.org/cgi/content/full/102/3/e29
    Fowler-Brown A, Kahawati LC: Prevention and treatment of overweight in children and adolescents. Am Fam Physician 69:2591–2598, 2004.

SEXUAL DEVELOPMENT

44. **What is Tanner staging for boys?**
In 1969 and 1970, Dr. James Tanner categorized the progression of stages of puberty, dividing pubertal development in boys into pubic and genital development (Table 1-2).

45. **What is the normal progression of sexual development and growth for boys during puberty?**
Nearly all boys begin puberty with testicular enlargement. This is followed in about 6 months by pubic hair and then about 6–12 months later by phallic enlargement. For boys, puberty lasts an average of 3.5 years and begins an average of 2 years later than it does in girls (Fig. 1-1).

46. **What are the ranges of normal in the stages of pubertal development in girls?**
Tanner divided pubertal development in girls according to pubic hair and breast development (Table 1-3).

TABLE 1-2.	TANNER STAGING FOR BOYS
Stage	**Description**
Pubic hair	
I	None
II	Countable; straight; increased pigmentation and length; primarily at base of penis
III	Darker; begins to curl; increased quantity
IV	Increased quantity; coarser texture; covers most of pubic area
V	Adult distribution; spread to medial thighs and lower abdomen
Genital development	
I	Prepubertal
II	Testicular enlargement (>4 mL volume); slight rugation of scrotum
III	Further testicular enlargement; penile lengthening begins
IV	Testicular enlargement continues; increased rugation of scrotum; increased penile breadth
V	Adult

47. What is the normal progression of sexual development and growth for girls during puberty?

About 85% of girls begin puberty with the initiation of breast enlargement, whereas 15% have axillary hair as the first sign. Menarche usually occurs about 18–24 months after the onset of breast development. For girls, the duration of puberty is about 4.5 years, which is longer than that of boys (Fig. 1-2).

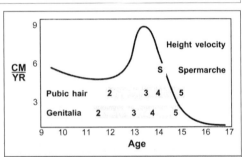

Figure 1-1. Summary of pubertal development in boys. (From Rosen DS: Physiologic growth and development during adolescence. Pediatr Rev 25:194–200, 2004.)

48. When do boys develop the ability to reproduce?

The average age of spermarche (as demonstrated by the presence of spermatozoa in the first morning urine) is 13.3 years. Unlike what occurs in girls (in whom menarche follows the peak height velocity), in boys spermarche occurs before the growth spurt.

49. When is delayed sexual development a concern?

The first easily recognizable sign of puberty in most females is a breast bud, which occurs at a mean age of 11 years. In boys, it is testicular enlargement, which on average begins at 11.5 years. Evaluation should be considered in girls with no breast development by 13 years or no menarche by 15 years and in boys with no testicular enlargement by age 14. By statistical definition, this is 3% of teenagers. If the norms for the onset of puberty are adjusted, the timing of concerns for delayed development may also change.

50. Why should the sense of smell be tested in a teenager with delayed puberty?

Kallmann's syndrome is characterized by a defect in GnRH with resultant gonadotropin deficiency and hypogonadism. Maldevelopment of the olfactory lobes occurs, with resultant anos-

TABLE 1-3.	TANNER STAGES FOR GIRLS
Stage	**Description**
Pubic hair	
I	None
II	Countable; straight; increased pigmentation and length; primarily on medial border of labia
III	Darker; begins to curl; increased quantity on mons pubis
IV	Increased quantity; coarser texture; labia and mons well covered
V	Adult distribution with feminine triangle and spread to medial thighs
Breast development	
I	Prepubertal
II	Breast bud present; increased areolar size
III	Further enlargement of breast; no secondary contour
IV	Areolar area forms secondary mound on breast contour
V	Mature; areolar area is part of breast contour; nipple projects

mia or hyposmia. Less commonly, cleft palate, congenital deafness, and color blindness can occur. These patients require hormonal therapy to achieve puberty and fertility.

51. **Which tests should you consider in a boy or girl with delayed puberty?**
If history or physical examination does not suggest an underlying cause (e.g., anorexia nervosa), tests should include **LH, FSH, testosterone** (male), and **bone age**.

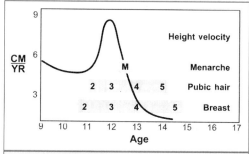

Figure 1-2. Summary of pubertal development in girls. (From Rosen DS: Physiologic growth and development during adolescence. Pediatr Rev 25:198, 2004.)

These tests help categorize the condition as hypergonadotropic (implying possible gonadal defects, androgen insensitivity, or enzyme defects) or hypogonadotropic (implying constitutional delay or primary hypothalamic-pituitary problems).

Further testing is predicated on the results of these initial tests. For example, a 14.5-year-old male with a bone age of 11.5 years and a total testosterone of 23 ng/dL (normal prepubertal level is <10 ng/dL) will probably begin to show outward evidence of puberty within the subsequent few months. Therefore, no further studies are warranted. On the other hand, if this boy has a bone age of 12.5 years, a testosterone level of <10 ng/dL, and no elevation of FH and LSH, specific testing of the hypothalamic-pituitary axis is indicated.

52. **What is the most common cause of primary gonadal failure in boys?**
Klinefelter syndrome. The frequency of this condition is 1 in every 500–1000 males. It is characterized in adolescence by gynecomastia and small, firm testes with seminiferous tubule

dysgenesis, and it is found in >80% of XXY males (i.e., males with 47 chromosomes). Levels of FSH and LH are elevated in these patients.

53. Can puberty be safely accelerated?
In some teenagers—more commonly boys—the constitutional delay in puberty has significant psychological effects. Studies have shown that, in **boys**, puberty can be accelerated without any compromise in expected adult height. In boys >14 years old with plasma testosterone levels of <10 ng/dL, 50–100 mg of intramuscular testosterone enanthate can be given monthly for 4–6 months. Treatment for **girls** who are constitutionally delayed is less well studied. Conjugated estrogen (0.3 mg [e.g., Premarin]) or ethinyl estradiol (5–10 μg) daily for 2–3 months has been used in girls >13 years old without breast buds.

KEY POINTS: SEXUAL DEVELOPMENT

1. If no signs of puberty by age 13 in girls and age 14 in boys, evaluate for an underlying pathologic medical cause.

2. Most cases of late puberty are constitutional (genetic) delay.

3. Nearly all boys begin puberty with testicular enlargement; 85% of girls begin puberty with breast enlargement.

4. Gynecomastia occurs in up to 50–75% of boys during Tanner genital stages II and III.

5. Mean time between the onset of breast development and menarche is slightly more than 2 years.

54. How do you evaluate a breast lump noted by a teenage girl on self-examination?
Although the incidence of cancerous lesions is extremely low in adolescents, it is not zero, and breast lumps do require careful evaluation. **Fibrocystic changes** (i.e., the proliferation of stromal and epithelial elements, ductal dilatation, cyst formation) are common in later adolescence and are characterized by variations in size and tenderness with menstrual periods. The most common tumor (up to 95%) is a *fibroadenoma*, which is a firm, discrete, rubbery, smooth mass that is usually found laterally. Other causes of masses include lipomas, hematomas, abscesses, and, rarely, adenocarcinoma (especially if a bloody nipple discharge is present).

The size, location, and other characteristics of a mass should be documented and reevaluated over the next one to three menstrual periods. A persistent or slowly growing mass should be evaluated with **fine-needle aspiration**. **Ultrasound** can be helpful for distinguishing cystic from solid masses. **Mammography** is a very poor tool for identifying distinct pathologic lesions in teenagers because the breast density of adolescents makes interpretation difficult.

Neinstein LS: Breast disease in adolescents and young women. Pediatr Clinic North Am 46:607–629, 1999.

SEXUALLY TRANSMITTED DISEASES

55. How does the prevalence of STDs in adolescents compare with that of adults?
Among sexually active people, adolescents have a **higher likelihood** than adults of being infected with an STD. About 25% of adolescents contract at least one STD by the time of high school graduation. Reasons for the increased susceptibility include the following:

- Cervical ectropion: *Neisseria gonorrhoeae* and *Chlamydia trachomatis* more readily infect columnar epithelium, and the adolescent ectocervix has more of this type of epithelium than does that of an adult.

- Cervical metaplasia in the transformation zone (for columnar to squamous epithelium) is more susceptible to human papillomavirus infection.
- There is less frequent use of barrier methods of contraception among this population.

56. **Is the presence of an ectropion noted on pelvic examination a concern?**
An **ectropion** is the outward rolling of a margin. A cervical ectropion is the extension of the erythematous columnar epithelium from the os onto the duller, pink cervix. It is a relatively common finding in adolescents. However, large ectropions extending to the vaginal wall or an abnormal cervical shape can be associated with diethylstilbestrol exposure in utero or chronic cervicitis.

57. **Which teenage girls should have pap smears done?**
Although carcinoma is rare in teenagers, cervical dysplasia is not. This is due in large part to the widespread acquisition of human papilloma virus (HPV), of which a number of subtypes are oncogenic. Most national organizations recommend that females who are sexually active and/or ≥18 years of age should have at least an annual Pap test. Because the false-negative rate of the test can be up to 30%, those teenagers at particularly high risk (e.g., multiple sexual partners, recurrent STDs) should be considered for more frequent testing. There is controversy in this area, however. Because the incidence of in situ carcinoma is very low in teenagers, debate centers around whether the specter of a pelvic examination may be a deterrent to teenagers initially seeking reproductive health care.

Kahn JA, Hillard PA: Human papillomavirus and cervical cytology in adolescents. Adolesc Med 15:301–321, 2004.

58. **What is the best way to screen for STDs?**
The gold standard for STDs, particularly in any case of possible sexual abuse, is **culture**. However, nonculture techniques involving nucleic acid amplification tests (e.g., polymerase chain reaction, ligase chain reaction, transcription-mediated amplification) are widely used and widely studied. They are emerging specifically as alternative first-line tests for diagnosing gonorrheal or chlamydial urethritis in males or cervicitis in females because of superior sensitivity and use in urine samples. The tests are not recommended for vaginal, rectal, or pharyngeal swabs. The CDC (and the courts) view the nonculture techniques as having a greater potential for false positivity, and the result of a single nonculture test is presumptive. Additional information from the CDC is available at:

http://www.cdc.gov/std/

59. **Are pelvic examinations with specula always required to obtain specimens in teenagers?**
A number of studies have demonstrated the following:
- Urine testing for chlamydia and gonorrhea using nucleic acid amplification techniques approaches the sensitivity and specificity of specimens obtained using a speculum.
- Vaginal specimens obtained without the use of a specula have a high screening validity for trichomonas, bacterial vaginosis, and yeast infections.
- Self-collection by teenagers of vaginal specimens yielded comparable polymerase chain reaction results as compared with physician-obtained cervical and vaginal specimens.
Future trends in screening for STDs in teenage girls may shift from endocervical sampling to urine-based and vaginal self-collection.

Shafer MB: Is the routine pelvic examination needed with the advent of urine-based screening for sexually transmitted diseases? Arch Pediatr Adolesc Med 153:119–125, 1999.

60. **Which STD is most closely linked to cervical cancer?**
HPV affects 20–40% of sexually active adolescent females. More than 80 HPV types have been identified, with variable presentations. These include anogenital condyloma acuminatum and cervical infection that may lead to cervical dysplasia. In the latter infection, the association of HPV with the potential for cervical carcinoma increases the urgency of screening for HPV in

sexually active teenagers. Visualization of anogenital warts can be enhanced by wetting the area with 3–5% acetic acid (vinegar), which whitens the lesions. HPV is also a cause of non-sexually transmitted disease, including deep plantar warts, palmar warts, and common warts.

61. Describe the appearance of condylomata acuminata.
Condyloma acuminata (anogenital warts) are soft, fleshy, wet, polypoid or pedunculated papules that appear in the genital and perianal area (Fig. 1-3). They may coalesce and take on a cauliflower-like appearance.

62. How do you treat condylomata and HPV infection?
A common approach for mucosal involvement is 25% podophyllin resin in benzoin applied carefully to the lesion and a 2–3 mm margin of surrounding skin and washed off completely after 3–6 hours. Reapplications can be done, but failure rates can be >50%. Other approaches, particularly on nonmucosal surfaces, include liquid nitrogen, 85% trichloroacetic acid, topical 5-fluorouracil, alpha-interferon, imiquimod cream 5%, and ablative therapy (e.g., laser surgical excision).

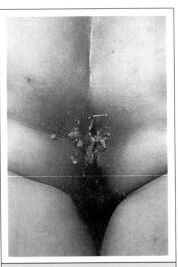

Figure 1-3. Perianal condylomata acuminata. (From Gates RH: Infectious Disease Secrets, 2nd ed. Philadelphia, Hanley & Belfus, 2003, p 221.)

63. What is the typical presentation of chlamydial genital infections in both female and male teenagers?
These are **asymptomatic infections**, which can persist for several months. In patients with symptoms, the disease should be suspected if vaginal discharge and bleeding are noted, especially after intercourse; this may be due to endocervical friability.

Peipert JF: Genital chlamydial infections. N Engl J Med 349:2424–2430, 2003.

64. A sexually active 17-year-old girl with adnexal and RUQ tenderness probably has what condition?
Fitz-Hugh-Curtis syndrome. This is an infectious perihepatitis that is caused by gonococci or, less commonly, by chlamydiae. It should be suspected in any patient with pelvic inflammatory disease (PID) who has RUQ tenderness. It may be mistaken for acute hepatitis or cholecystitis. The pathophysiology is felt to be the direct spread from a pelvic infection along the paracolic gutters to the liver, where inflammation develops and capsular adhesions form (the so-called "violin-string adhesions" seen on surgical exploration). If RUQ pain persists despite treatment for PID, ultrasonography should be done to rule out a perihepatic abscess.

65. A teenage girl develops migratory polyarthritis, fever, and scattered petechial lesions several days prior to menses. What condition should be suspected?
Gonococcal-arthritis-dermatitis syndrome (GADS). After a migratory polyarthritis or polyarthralgia, the arthritis settles in one or two large joints. The patient then develops painful tenosynovitis over the tendon sheaths in addition to a characteristic crop of embolic skin lesions over the trunk and extremities. Diagnosis is confirmed by culturing gonococci from blood, synovial fluid, and/or rectal or genitourinary sites.

66. **What is the typical appearance of *Neisseria gonorrhoeae* on Gram stain?**
Intracellular gram-negative diplococci (Fig. 1-4).

KEY POINTS: SEXUALLY TRANSMITTED DISEASES ✓

1. Regardless of the pathogen, most STDs in adolescents are *asymptomatic.*

2. Adolescents have a higher likelihood than adults of being infected with an STD.

3. Nucleic acid amplification tests for chlamydia and gonorrhea are particularly useful when screening for urethritis in males and cervicitis in females.

4. Vaginitis in adolescents has three main causes: (1) candidiasis, (2) trichomonas, and (3) bacterial vaginosis.

5. Despite higher rates of STDs being found among adolescents than any other age group, clinicians frequently do not inquire about sexual activity, risk factors, or means of reducing risks.

67. **What is the minimal criteria for the diagnosis of PID?**
Any one of the following must be present:
   - Uterine tenderness
   - Cervical motion tenderness
   - Adnexal tenderness

68. **What additional criteria support the diagnosis of PID?**
   - Oral temperature >38.3°C (101°F)
   - Abnormal cervical or vaginal discharge (with leukocytes > epithelial cells)
   - Elevated erythrocyte sedimentation rate (usually >15 mm/h)
   - Elevated C-reactive protein
   - Cervical infection with *Neisseria gonorrhoeae* or *Chlamydia trachomatis* (the former by culture, the latter by nonculture tests such as nucleic acid amplification)
   Because no single clinical aspect or laboratory test is definitive for PID, a constellation of findings is used to support the diagnosis.

   Centers for Disease Control and Prevention: Sexually transmitted diseases treatment guidelines, 2002. Mortal Morb Wkly Rep 55(RR-6):48, 2002.

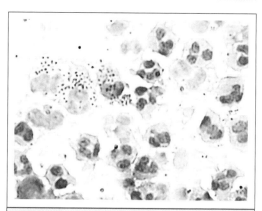

Figure 1-4. Gram stain of *Neisseria gonorrhoeae*. (From Gates RH: Infectious Disease Secrets, 2nd ed. Philadelphia, Hanley & Belfus, 2003, p 207.)

69. **How is the diagnosis of PID *definitively* made?**
   - **Endometrial biopsy** with histopathologic evidence of endometritis
   - **Transvaginal or abdominal ultrasonography** revealing tubo-ovarian abscess or fallopian tube abnormalities (e.g., thickened, fluid-filled fallopian tubes with or without free pelvic fluid)
   - **Laparoscopy** revealing abnormalities consistent with PID

   American Academy of Pediatrics: Pelvic inflammatory disease. In Pickering LK (ed): 2003 Red Book, 26th ed. Elk Grove Village, IL, American Academy of Pediatrics, 2003, p 469.

70. **What are the sequelae of PID?**
    Twenty-five percent of patients with a history of PID will have one or more major sequelae of the disease, including the following:
    - **Tubo-ovarian abscess:** Approximately 15–20% of all adolescents with PID
    - **Recurrent infection**
    - **Chronic abdominal pain:** May include exacerbated dysmenorrhea and dyspareunia related to pelvic adhesions in approximately 20% of patients with PID
    - **Ectopic pregnancy:** Risk is increased threefold to sevenfold
    - **Infertility:** Up to 11% after one episode of PID, 30% after two episodes, and 55% after three or more episodes

    Bortot AT, Risser WL, Cromwell, PF: Coping with pelvic inflammatory disease in the adolescent. Contemp Pediatr 21:33–48, 2004.

71. **Which adolescents with PID should be hospitalized for intravenous antibiotics?**
    Those with any of the following conditions:
    - Surgical emergency (e.g., appendicitis or ectopic pregnancy [or if such a diagnosis cannot be excluded])
    - Severe illness (e.g., pelvic or tubo-ovarian abscess, overt peritonitis)
    - Immunodeficiency (e.g., human immunodeficiency virus [HIV] infection with low CD4 lymphocyte count, immunosuppressive therapy)
    - Pregnancy
    - Expected unreliable compliance or follow-up or inability to tolerate outpatient regimen
    - Failure of outpatient therapy (e.g., compliance or tolerance problems or worsening symptoms at 48–72 hours)

    American Academy of Pediatrics: Pelvic inflammatory disease. In Pickering LK (ed): 2003 Red Book, 26th ed. Elk Grove Village, IL, American Academy of Pediatrics, 2003, p 470.

72. **When should laparoscopic exploration be considered in the setting of PID?**
    It should be considered in the following settings:
    - To evaluate medical treatment failures
    - To exclude surgical emergencies (if required)
    - In cases of rupture of a tubo-ovarian abscess
    - In patients with no response of a tubo-ovarian abscess to medical management within 48–72 hours

    Burstein GR, Murray PJ: Diagnosis and management of sexually transmitted diseases among adolescents. Pediatr Rev 24:119–127, 2003.

73. **When do the symptoms of endocervicitis occur in relation to menses?**
    Gonorrhea is much more likely to present during menstruation. Of patients with gonorrhea, 85% develop symptoms during the first 7 days of menses as compared with only 33% of patients with chlamydial infections.

74. **What is the most common cause of chronic pelvic pain in adolescents without a history of pelvic inflammatory disease?**
    Endometriosis. This condition results from the implantation of endometrial tissue at ectopic locations within the peritoneal cavity. The pain is both noncyclic (may occur with intercourse or defecation) and cyclic (often most severe just before menses), and it is poorly controlled by nonsteroidal anti-inflammatory medications or oral contraceptives. Intermenstrual bleeding is common. Although adult women classically have tender nodules that are noted in the posterior vaginal fornix and along the uterosacral ligaments, nodularity is rare in adolescents, and this

often masks clinical diagnosis. Definitive diagnosis is by laparoscopy and biopsy. Therapy can be medical (e.g., danazol) and/or surgical (e.g., excision, coagulation, laser vaporization).

Attaran M, Gidwani GP: Adolescent endometriosis. Obstet Gynecol Clin North Am 30:379–390, 2003.

KEY POINTS: PELVIC INFLAMMATORY DISEASE

1. The highest rate of PID occurs in adolescents.

2. No single clinical aspect or laboratory test is definitive for PID.

3. Key clinical finding: Adnexal, cervical motion or lower abdominal tenderness.

4. Cultures are often negative in PID because the disease is in the upper genital tract; however, specimens are obtained from the lower tract.

5. Ectopic pregnancy can mimic PID.

6. Hospitalization: Indicated for patients with PID with surgical emergencies, severe illness, immunodeficiency, pregnancy, unreliable compliance, or failure of outpatient therapy.

75. **How are the genital ulcer syndromes differentiated?**
    Genital ulcers may be seen in herpes simplex, syphilis, chancroid, lymphogranuloma venereum, and granuloma inguinale (donovanosis). Herpes and syphilis are the most common, and granuloma inguinale is very rare. Although there is overlap, clinical distinction is summarized in Table 1-4.

TABLE 1-4. DIFFERENTIATION OF GENITAL ULCER SYNDROMES

	Herpes simplex	Syphilis (primary, secondary)	Chancroid	Lymphogranuloma venereum
Agent	Herpes simplex virus	*Treponema pallidum*	*Haemophilus ducreyi*	*Chlamydia trachomatis*
Primary lesions	Vesicle	Papule	Papule-pustule	Papule-vesicle
Size (mm)	1–2	5–15	2–20	2–10
Number	Multiple, clusters (coalesce ±)	Single	Multiple (coalesce ±)	Single
Depth	Superficial	Superficial or deep	Deep	Superficial or deep
Base	Erythematous, nonpurulent	Sharp, indurated, nonpurulent	Ragged border, purulent, friable	Varies
Pain	Yes	No	Yes	No
Lymphadenopathy	Tender, bilateral	Nontender, bilateral	Tender, unilateral, may suppurate, unilocular fluctuance	Tender, unilateral, may suppurate, multilocular fluctuance

From Shafer MA: Sexually transmitted disease syndromes. In McAnarmey ER, Kreipe RE, Orr DP, Comerci GD (eds): Textbook of Adolescent Medicine. Philadelphia, W.B. Saunders, 1992, p 708.

76. **How do recurrent episodes of genital herpes simplex infections compare with the primary episode?**
    - Usually less severe, with faster resolution
    - Less likely to have prodromal symptoms (buttock, leg, or hip pain or tingling)
    - Less likely to have neurologic complications (e.g., aseptic meningitis)
    - More likely to have asymptomatic infections
    - Duration of viral shedding is shorter (4 versus 11 days)

    Kimberlin DW, Rouse DJ: Genital herpes. N Engl J Med 350:1970–1977, 2004.

77. **How are the three most common causes of postpubertal vaginitis clinically distinguished?**
    Candidal vaginitis: Vulvar itching and erythema, vaginal discharge (thick, white, curdlike) (*see* Fig. 1-5, *A*).
    Trichomonal vaginitis: Vulvar itching and erythema, vaginal discharge (gray, yellow-green, frothy; rarely malodorous) (*see* Fig. 1-5, *B*).
    Bacterial vaginosis: Minimal erythema, vaginal discharge (malodorous; thin white discharge clings to vaginal walls).

78. **How does the vaginal pH help indicate the cause of a vaginal discharge?**
    Ordinarily, the vaginal pH of a pubertal girl is <4.5 (as compared with 7.0 in prepubertal girls). If the pH is >4.5, infection with *Trichomonas* or bacterial vaginosis should be suspected.

79. **How does evaluation of the vaginal discharge help to identify the etiology?**
    See Table 1-5.

80. **What are "clue cells"?**
    Clue cells are vaginal squamous epithelial cells to which many bacteria are attached. This gives the cell a stippled appearance when viewed in a normal saline preparation. Clue cells are characteristic—but not diagnostic—of bacterial vaginosis (*see* Fig. 1-5, *C*).

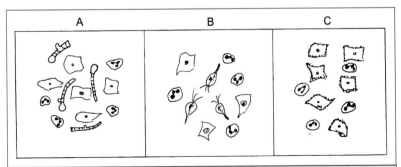

Figure 1-5. Cytologic findings in various forms of vaginitis. In all vaginal smears, one may see desquamated epithelial vaginal cells and inflammatory cells (neutrophils). *A, Candida albicans* vaginitis. The smear contains fungal hyphae. *B, Trichomonas vaginalis.* The smear contains ciliated protozoa. *C, Gardnerella vaginalis.* The smear contains "clue cells" (i.e., squamous cells with clumped nuclei, folded cytoplasm, and numerous bacteria attached to their surface). (From Damjanov I [ed]: Pathology Secrets. Philadelphia, Hanley & Belfus, 2002, p 364).

TABLE 1-5. EVALUATION OF VAGINAL DISCHARGE

	Candidal vaginitis	Trichomonal vaginitis	Bacterial vaginosis
pH	≤ 4.5	>4.5	>4.5
KOH prep	Mycelia pseudohyphae	Normal	Fishy odor (positive "whiff" test)
NaCl prep	Few WBCs	Many WBCs; motile trichomonads	Few WBCs

KOH = potassium hydroxide, NaCl = sodium chloride (salt), WBCs = white blood cells.

81. **What is the etiology of bacterial vaginosis?**

Formerly called nonspecific, *Gardnerella*, or *Haemophilus* vaginitis, bacterial vaginosis is the replacement of normal vaginal lactobacilli with a variety of bacteria, including *Gardnerella vaginalis*, genital mycoplasmas, and an overgrowth of anaerobic species. *G vaginalis* can be found in small numbers in up to 30% of nonsexually active adolescents, so vaginal cultures are of limited value.

82. **Is there an effective treatment for bacterial vaginosis?**

Optimal management remains unclear. Acceptable treatment options include oral metronidazole (Flagyl), 0.075% metronidazole gel, or 2% clindamycin cream. Treatment failure is about 15%. Relapse rates as high as 30% may occur within 3 months.

Nyirjesy P: Vaginitis in the adolescent patient. Pediatr Clin North Am 46:733–745, 1999.

83. **What is the most common STD in sexually active teenage males?**

Urethritis, both gonococcal and nongonococcal. Nongonococcal urethritis, particularly that due to *Chlamydia trachomatis*, is more common and is often asymptomatic. Other, less-common causes of nongonococcal urethritis include *Ureaplasma urealyticum, Trichomonas vaginalis*, herpes simplex, human papillomavirus, and yeast.

84. **How should asymptomatic, sexually active teenage males be screened for urethritis?**

Chlamydia trachomatis is the most common cause of *asymptomatic* urethritis. The most definitive screening method is to obtain urethral swabs for culture, although this method is invasive and not cost-effective. Nonculture methods (e.g., enzyme immunoassay, direct fluorescent antibody, nucleic acid amplification tests such as polymerase chain reaction) can also be done on the swabbed specimen. A less-invasive strategy is to test centrifuged, first-void urine for infection by culture or nonculture methods. A third strategy is to obtain 15 mL of unspun first-void urine and test it for leukocyte esterase (a dipstick test for the presence of white blood cells). If positive, more specific studies can be done for *C trachomatis* on spun urine or a urethral swab. This approach is about 70% sensitive. Precise guidelines for screening remain controversial. Generally, unless a precise STD exposure is known, studies for gonorrhea are not done, because this organism is more commonly associated with symptoms (dysuria or penile discharge).

U.S. Preventive Services Task Force. Screening for chlamydial infection. Available at: http://www.ahrq.gov/clinic/ajpmsuppl/chlarr.htm section1

SUBSTANCE ABUSE

85. **What are the stages of alcohol and drug abuse by teenagers?**
    Stage 1: Potential for abuse (decreased impulse control, peer pressure, ready availability)
    Stage 2: Experimentation (learning the euphoria; few consequences, little behavior change)
    Stage 3: Regular use (seeking the euphoria; increased frequency; use alone; buying or stealing drugs)
    Stage 4: Regular use (preoccupation with the "high"; daily use, loss of control, risk taking, estrangement from "sober" friends)
    Stage 5: Burnout (use of drugs to feel normal; multiple addictions, physical and mental deterioration, self-destructive behavior)

    Barangan CJ, Alderman EM: Management of substance abuse. Pediatr Rev 23:123–130, 2002.

86. **What are the categories of abused drugs?**
    - **Sedative-hypnotics:** Alcohol, barbiturates, benzodiazepines, gammahydroxybutyrate, rohypnol, other sedatives
    - **Stimulants:** Caffeine, cocaine, amphetamines, decongestants
    - **Tobacco**
    - **Cannabinoids:** Marijuana, hashish, Marinol
    - **Opioids:** Heroin, opium, pharmaceutical opioid pain killers, methadone, OxyContin
    - **Hallucinogens:** Lysergic acid diethylamide (LSD), phencyclidine, mescaline, psilocybin, hallucinogenic mushrooms, ecstasy
    - **Inhalants:** Aliphatic, halogenated, and aromatic hydrocarbons; nitrous oxide; ketones; esters
    - **Steroids**

    Liepman MR, Calles JL, Kizilbash L, et al: Genetic and nongenetic factors influencing substance abuse by adolescents. Adolesc Med 13:375–401, 2002.

87. **What is the CRAFFT screen?**
    This is a six-item screening test for adolescent substance abuse. Two or more "yes" answers indicate a >90% sensitivity and a >80% specificity for significant substance abuse. A number of screening instruments are available for interviewing adolescents, and the search for alcohol or drug use should be part of routine medical care.

    C — **C**ar: Have you driven a car (or ridden with a driver) under the influence of drugs or alcohol
    R — **R**elax: Do you use drugs or alcohol to relax, feel better, or fit in?
    A — **A**lone: Do you use drugs or alcohol while you are alone?
    F — **F**orget: Do you sometimes forget what you did while using drugs or alcohol?
    F — **F**amily/**F**riends: Do they ever tell you to cut down on drug or alcohol use?
    T — **T**rouble: Have you gotten into trouble when using drugs or alcohol?

    Mersy DJ: Recognition of alcohol and substance abuse. Am Fam Physician 67:1529–1536, 2003.
    National Institutes of Health. National Institute on Drug Abuse Web site. Available at: http://www.nida.nih.gov

88. **What are characteristic physical signs of illicit drug use?**

Physical Sign	Drug of Abuse
Increased heart rate	Amphetamine, cocaine, marijuana
Increased blood pressure	Amphetamine, cocaine, phencyclidine
Conjunctival redness	Marijuana
Pinpoint pupils	Heroin, morphine, other opiates
Sluggish pupillary response	Barbiturates
Irritation/ulceration of nasal mucosa	Intranasal cocaine, heroin, inhalants
Oral sores/burns, perioral pyodermas,	Inhalants
Cutaneous scars ("tracks")	Intravenous use
Gynecomastia, small testes	Marijuana

Subcutaneous fat necrosis	Intravenous and intradermal use
Tattoos in antecubital fossa	Intravenous use
Skin abscesses and cellulitis	Intravenous and intradermal use
Icterus	Intravenous use

Kaul P, Coupey SM: Clinical evaluation of substance abuse. Pediatr Rev 23:85–94, 2002.

89. **Are teens who drink excessively likely to become adults who drink excessively?**
In a study of 940 adolescents evaluated at ages 14–18 and again at age 24, the majority of those who demonstrated problematic alcohol use as teenagers also had the problem in early adulthood.

Rohde P, Lewinsohn PM, Kahler CW, et al: Natural course of alcohol use disorders from adolescence to young adulthood. J Am Acad Child Adolesc Psychiatr 40:83–90, 2001.

90. **Should an adolescent be screened for drug abuse without his or her consent?**
This is an area of contention. The official position of the American Academy of Pediatrics is that testing should not be done without consent in a competent older adolescent, even if a parent wishes otherwise. Others have argued that a teenager's right to privacy and confidentiality does not supersede potential risks of serious damage from drug abuse, particularly if there is strong clinical suspicion or parental concern. The legal ramifications are evolving and vary from state to state. In 1995, the U.S. Supreme Court ruled that random drug testing of high-school athletes was legal.

91. **A teenager who is being screened for drug abuse submits a suspicious urine specimen for testing. How can you tell if it is urine?**
   - pH should be between 4.6 and 8.0.
   - Temperature should range between 90.5°F and 98.6°F (32.5–37°C).
   - Urine submitted at body temperature will exceed 90.5°F (32.5°C) for 15–20 minutes. If the temperature is below this level during the first 4 minutes, the specimen should be considered suspect.
   - Urine creatinine concentration should exceed 0.2 mg/mL.
   - Urine specific gravity should be not <1.003.

92. **How long do illicit drugs remain detectable in urine specimens?**
There is variability depending on a patient's hydration status and method of intake, but, as a rule, metabolites can be detected after ingestion as shown in Table 1-6. Most urine screens are very sensitive and may detect drugs up to 99% of the time in concentrations established as analytic cutoff points. However, the screens can be much less specific, sometimes with false-positive rates of up to 35%. Therefore, second tests using the analytic methodology most specific for the suspected drug should be used.

AAP Task Force on Substance Abuse: Substance Abuse: A Guide for Health Professionals. Elk Grove Village, IL, American Academy of Pediatrics, 1988, p 55.

TABLE 1-6. DETECTION OF ILLICIT DRUG METABOLITIES	
Amphetamines	48 hours
Barbiturates (short acting)	24 hours
Benzodiazepines	3 days
Cocaine	2–3 days
Marijuana	3 days for light smoker; 21–27 days for heavy smoker
Morphine	48 hours
Phencyclidine	3 days for casual use; 8 days for heavy use

93. **What is the genetic predisposition of alcoholism?**
A male child of an alcoholic father is four times more likely to become an alcoholic than a child with a nonalcoholic father. If a *monozygotic twin* is an alcoholic, the likelihood of the other twin becoming an alcoholic is 55%; for *dizygotic twins*, the likelihood is 25%.

94. **Which type of substance abuse is more common in younger adolescents than older adolescents?**
Inhalants. In some surveys, up to 20% of eighth graders report recent use of inhalants (or "huffing") as compared with about 15% of twelfth graders. Household products are typically abused, including aliphatic hydrocarbons (e.g., gasoline, butane in cigarette lighters), aromatic hydrocarbons (e.g., benzene and toluene in glues and acrylic paints), alkyl halides (e.g., methylene chloride and trichloroethylene in paint thinners and spot removers) and ketones (e.g., acetone in nail polish remover). Inhalant abusers appear to have a greater risk of long-term substance abuse as compared with users of other psychoactive drugs. Inhalants have short durations of action and usually cannot be detected by toxic screen. However, they can cause cerebral atrophy and death (by asphyxiation or cardiac arrhythmia).

Anderson CE, Loomis GA: Recognition and prevention of inhalant abuse. Am Fam Physician 68:869–876, 2003.

95. **What are the toxicities of chronic marijuana use?**
Pulmonary: Decreased pulmonary function. As compared with cigarette smoke, marijuana smoke contains more carcinogens and respiratory irritants and produces higher carboxyhemoglobin levels and greater tar deposition. Long-term studies will determine if there is a link between chronic marijuana smoke exposure and lung cancer.
Endocrine: Associated with decreased sperm count and motility; may interfere with hypothalamic/pituitary function and increase the likelihood of anovulation; antagonizes insulin, which may affect diabetic management.
Behavioral: Short-term memory impairment, interference with learning, possible "amotivational syndrome."

96. **List the potential side effects of anabolic steroids.**

Endocrine	In males—testicular atrophy, oligospermia, gynecomastia
	In females—hirsutism, masculinization
Musculoskeletal	Premature epiphyseal closure
Dermatologic	Acne, alopecia, temporal hair recession
Hepatic	Impaired excretory function with cholestatic jaundice, elevated liver function test results, peliosis hepatitis (a form of hepatitis in which hepatic lobules have microscopic pools of blood), benign and malignant tumors
Cardiovascular	Hypertension, decreased high-density lipoprotein cholesterol, increased low-density lipoprotein cholesterol
Psychological	Aggressive behavior, mood swings, increased libido

Bagatell CJ, Bremner WJ: Androgens in men: Uses and abuses. N Engl J Med 334:707–714, 1996.

97. **Is androstenedione a safe, natural way for teenagers to increase muscle mass?**
No. "Andro," which is a precursor to testosterone, is normally produced in the adrenal glands and testes and converted in the peripheral tissues by 17-betahydroxysteroid dehydrogenase. It is a compound that is also found in plants and in highly publicized homerun hitters. However, studies show that it is more likely to result in increases in serum estradiol than testosterone or muscle mass. If teenage males know that breasts—rather than biceps—are more likely to emerge, they will likely steer clear of androstenedione.

Leder BZ, Longcope C, Catlin DH, et al: Oral androstenedione administration and serum testosterone concentrations in young men. JAMA 283:779–782, 2000.

98. What are the risks of smokeless tobacco?

As a result of the decreased gingival blood flow caused by nicotine, chronic ischemia and necrosis can occur. Chronic use results in **gingival recession** and **inflammation**, **periodontal disease**, and **oral leukoplakia** (a premalignant change). The risk of oral and pharyngeal cancer is increased. Although more commonly used by males, smokeless tobacco used by pregnant females may be associated with low-birthweight infants and premature birth. Smokeless tobacco, like cigarettes, is addictive.

99. When does cigarette smoking begin?

In the United States, about three quarters of daily adult smokers started smoking when they were between the ages of 13 and 17 years old. Worldwide, the average age is lower. Cigarette smoking remains the major preventable cause of premature death in the world. Clearly, the development of effective early intervention programs for adolescents is vital.

100. What are the 5 "As" of smoking cessation counseling?

- **A**sk about tobacco use
- **A**dvise to quit
- **A**ssess willingness to attempt quitting
- **A**ssist in attempt to quit (e.g., pharmacotherapy such as nicotine gum or patch)
- **A**rrange follow-up

Klein JD, Camenga DR: Tobacco prevention and cessation in pediatric patients. Pediatr Rev 25:17–26, 2004.

101. How effective are school-based youth smoking cessation programs?

In general, success rates are low (5–17%) when looking at cessation at 6–7 months after the intervention. This is true for a variety of programs: structured educational courses, nicotine replacement therapy, and computer-based education. Clearly, this is an area in which new approaches and strategies are needed.

Wiehe SE, Garrison MM, Christakis DA, et al: A systemic review of school-based smoking prevention trials with long-term follow-up. J Adol Health 36:162–169, 2005.

102. Are tattoos a tip-off to high-risk behaviors?

Yes. Permanent tattoos are obtained by 10–16% of adolescents between the ages of 12 and 18 years in the United States. They are strongly associated with high-risk behaviors, including substance abuse, early initiation of sexual intercourse, interpersonal violence, and school failure.

Roberts TA, Ryan SA: Tattooing and high-risk behavior in adolescents. Pediatrics 110:1058–1063, 2002.

TEENAGE MALE DISORDERS

103. How common is gynecomastia in teenage boys?

As many as 50–75% of boys between the ages of 12 and 14½ years have some breast development. In about 25%, it lasts for > l year and, in 7%, for >2 years. It occurs most commonly during Tanner genital stages II and III, and it usually consists of subareolar enlargement (breast bud). It may be unilateral or bilateral. The breast bud may be tender, which indicates the recent rapid growth of tissue. Obese boys often have breast enlargement due to the deposition of adipose tissue, and differentiation from gynecomastia (true breast budding) is sometimes difficult.

104. Why does gynecomastia occur so commonly?

Early during puberty, the production of estrogen (a stimulator of ductal proliferation) increases relatively faster than does that of testosterone (an inhibitor of breast development). This slight imbalance causes the breast enlargement. In obese teenagers, the enzyme aromatase (found in higher concentrations in adipose tissue) converts testosterone to estrogen.

105. What drugs are associated with gynecomastia?

The drugs that cause this effect can be easier to recall using the CHEST acronym:

C: Calcium-channel blockers: verapamil, nifedipine

H: Hormonal medications: anabolic steroids, oral contraceptives

E: Experimental/illicit drugs: marijuana, heroin, amphetamines, methadone

S: pSychoactive drugs: phenothiazines, tricyclic antidepressants, diazepam

T: Testosterone antagonists: spironolactone, ranitidine, cimetidine, ketoconazole

106. What other entities, besides drugs, are associated with gynecomastia?

The overwhelming majority of cases of gynecomastia in adolescent males occur as part of normal pubertal development. In addition to drugs, other causes include the following:

- **Recovery from chronic disease**
- **Inadequate androgen production:** Klinefelter syndrome, testicular failure, isolated LH deficiency (fertile eunuch)
- **Excess estrogen production:** Feminizing tumors (usually adrenal)
- **Pseudogynecomastia:** Carcinoma of the breast, neurofibromatosis, hemangiomas, lipomas, abscess, bruise
- **Other:** Pituitary tumor, testicular tumor, hypo- or hyperthyroidism, liver disease

  Braunstein GD: Gynecomastia. N Engl J Med 492:490–495, 1993.

107. Which boys with gynecomastia warrant further evaluation?

- Prepubertal boys
- Pubertal-age boys with little or no virilization and small testes
- Hepatomegaly or abdominal mass palpated
- Child with central nervous system complaints

Evaluations may include testing for hypothalamic or pituitary disease, feminizing tumors of the adrenal or testes, and genetic abnormalities (e.g., Klinefelter syndrome). Although breast cancer is nearly reportable if it occurs in boys and is extremely rare in men (0.2%), in patients with Klinefelter syndrome, the rate increases to 3–6%.

108. What treatment options are available for developmental gynecomastia?

Treatment usually depends on the amount of breast tissue present and the degree of psychological problems that this causes. There are three primary options.

- **Reassurance:** Explanation of the process and expected resolution usually suffices for most adolescents. They should be told that resolution can take up to 24 months.
- **Medications:** These may include antiestrogens (clomiphene citrate, tamoxifen), aromatase inhibitors (testolactone), nonaromatizable androgens (dihydrotestosterone), and weak androgens (danazol).
- **Surgery:** This should be done by a plastic surgeon who has experience in breast reduction.

109. What are the clinical manifestations of testicular torsion?

Testicular torsion in adolescents usually presents with acute-onset hemiscrotal pain that radiates to the groin and lower abdomen. Nausea and vomiting are common, but fever is rare. The testis is acutely tender and swollen, and it may be high riding. The cremasteric reflex is absent. Many patients report previous episodes of severe acute scrotal pain. Radionuclide imaging of the scrotum with Tc-99m pertechnetate and/or color Doppler ultrasound demonstrates low or absent blood flow and can be helpful in equivocal cases. However, testis salvage depends on the timely restoration of blood flow, and obtaining such studies should not delay a highly suspect case from surgical exploration. The spermatic cord sometimes can be untwisted manually; this will give temporary relief, but surgical exploration is still required for fixation to prevent recurrence. Both testes may be secured because the underlying suspension defect is often bilateral.

110. **How is testicular torsion clinically differentiated from other causes of the acute painful scrotum?**

Epididymitis: Usually slower in onset; pain initially localized to epididymis, but as inflammation spreads, whole testis may become painful; not usually associated with vomiting; pain does not usually radiate to the groin; usually associated with dysuria, pyuria, and discharge; often caused by *Neisseria gonorrhoeae* and *Chlamydia trachomatis;* history of STDs is suggestive; unusual in prepubertal boys and in nonsexually active teenagers

Orchitis: Usually slower in onset; often systemic symptoms (nausea, vomiting, fever, chills) as a result of diffuse viral infection; in patients with mumps, occurs about 4–6 days after parotitis; bilateral involvement more common

Torsion of appendix testis: Sudden onset of pain; localized tender nodule at upper pole (often with bluish discoloration); nausea and vomiting uncommon

Incarcerated hernia: Acute onset; pain not localized to hemiscrotum; usually palpable inguinal mass; testes not painful; symptoms and signs of bowel obstruction (vomiting, abdominal distension, guarding, rebound tenderness)

Kadish HA, Bolte RG: A retrospective review of pediatric patients with epididymitis, testicular torsion, and torsion of testicular appendages. Pediatrics 102:73–76, 1998.

111. **How does the Prehn sign help distinguish between epididymitis and testicular torsion?**

Classically, relief of pain with elevation of the testis (*negative Prehn sign*) is associated with epididymitis, whereas persistent pain (*positive Prehn sign*) is more indicative of testicular torsion. However, there is considerable overlap, and this relatively nonspecific sign should be interpreted in the context of other signs and symptoms.

112. **If complete testicular torsion has occurred, how long is it before irreversible changes develop?**

Irreversible changes develop in 4–6 hours. However, it is clinically impossible to distinguish partial from complete torsion, and thus duration of symptoms should not be used as a gauge for determining viability. Duration of symptoms does correlate with abnormal testicles on follow-up examination, which underscores the need for prompt diagnosis. Two thirds of patients with testicles salvaged between 12 and 24 hours after the onset of symptoms have palpable evidence of testicular atrophy during later evaluation as compared with only 10% when the diagnosis is made in <6 hours.

113. **What is the most frequent solid cancer in older adolescent males?**

Testicular cancer. The most common type is a seminoma, which, if detected when confined to the testicle (stage I), has a cure rate of up to 97% with orchiectomy and radiation. Although its overall effectiveness is debated, most authorities recommend that all adolescent males be taught testicular self-examination so that irregularities or changes in size can be noted early.

114. **What is the significance of a varicocele in a teenager?**

A *varicocele* is an enlargement of either the pampiniform or cremasteric venous plexus of the spermatic cord, which results in a boggy enlargement ("bag of worms") of the upper scrotum. These are rare before puberty. About 15% of boys between the ages of 10 and 15 years have a varicocele, and, in 2%, the varicoceles are very large. Most are asymptomatic. Longitudinal studies of adolescents show that large varicoceles may interfere with normal testicular growth and result in decreased spermatogenesis. Surgical correction can prevent the progressive damage.

Kass EJ: Adolescent varicocele. Pediatr Clin North Am 48:1559–1570, 2001.

115. **Which varicoceles warrant surgical intervention?**

- >20% volume difference between testes, implying a hypotrophic testes
- Large varicocele

- Bilateral varioceles (higher potential for infertility)
- Testicular pain
- Poor patient compliance with follow-up

Raj GV, Wiener JS: Varicoceles in adolescents: When to observe, when to intervene. Contemp Pediatr 21:39–56, 2004.

116. **On which side do varicoceles more commonly occur?**
The left side. The left spermatic vein drains into the left renal vein, and the right spermatic vein drains into the inferior vena cava. These hemodynamics favor higher left-sided pressures, which predispose patients to left-sided varicoceles. Unilateral left-sided varicoceles are the most common types, occurring in 90% of patients; the remainder are bilateral. A unilateral right-sided lesion is rare, and many experts consider its finding a reason to search for other causes of venous obstruction, such as a renal or retroperitoneal tumor, using ultrasound, computed tomography, or magnetic resonance imaging.

117. **An adolescent who boasts of his overpowering "hircismus" is likely in need of what?**
Both a dictionary and a shower. Hircismus is offensive axillary odor.

TEENAGE PREGNANCY

118. **How common is teenage pregnancy in the United States?**
About 1 in 10 young women under the age of 20 years become pregnant each year (about 1 million pregnancies). The likelihood that an adolescent will become pregnant before age 20 is about 1 in 4. Up to 90% of these pregnancies are unplanned. About 50% progress to delivery, 35% are terminated by abortion, and 15% end by miscarriage.

119. **What factors make it more likely that a teenager will become pregnant?**
- **Early initiation of sexual intercourse:** Risk factors for early initiation include low socioeconomic status, low future-achievement orientation, and academic difficulties.
- **Influence from peers and sisters:** If surrounded by sexually active friends and siblings, a teenager is more likely to be permissive with regard to sexual behavior and pregnancy itself. Many teens do not view pregnancy as a negative experience.
- **Family history of early parenting**
- **Lack of family support and structure**
- **Improper use or lack of use of contraceptives**
- **History of repeated negative pregnancy tests**
- **Race:** Blacks and Hispanics have higher rates of pregnancy than whites, although rates significantly vary by race according to socioeconomic status.

Emans SJ, Smith VAM, Laufer MR: Teenage pregnancy. In Emans SJ, Laufer MR, Goldstein DP (eds): Pediatric and Adolescent Gynecology, 4th ed. Philadelphia, Lippincott-Raven, 1998, pp 675–713.

120. **If a teenager has been pregnant once, how likely is she to become pregnant again during her teenage years?**
Repeat adolescent pregnancy is common. Up to 30% of these patients become pregnant again within 1 year, and 25–50% become pregnant again within 2 years. Factors associated with a likely second teen pregnancy include age <16 years at first conception, boyfriend >20 years, school dropout, below expected grade level at the time of first pregnancy, welfare dependency after the first pregnancy, complications during the first pregnancy, and departure from the hospital without birth control.

121. **What are the risks for infants of teenage mothers?**
Teenage mothers have a disproportionately increased risk of having babies who are low-birth-weight, premature, or small for gestational age. In addition, infant mortality is two to three times greater for the infants of teenage mothers. Studies conflict with regard to whether these risks are due to inherent biologic difficulties with pregnancy at a young age or to sociodemographic factors associated with teenage pregnancy (e.g., poverty, inadequate prenatal care).

> Fraser AM, Brockert JE, Ward RH: Association of young maternal age with adverse reproductive outcomes. N Engl J Med 332:1113–1117, 1995.

122. **How soon after conception will a urine pregnancy test be positive?**
Human chorionic gonadotropin (hCG) is a glycoprotein (with alpha and beta subunits) that is produced by trophoblastic tissue. Urine levels of 25 mIU/mL are detectable by the most sensitive methods (i.e., radioimmunoassay or enzyme immunoassay to the beta subunit) by about 7 days after fertilization. Although many home pregnancy tests can detect these low levels, some are less sensitive and detect levels of hCG that are around 1500 mIU/mL. This occurs, on average, about 3 weeks after fertilization (or 1 week after the missed menstrual period).

123. **In what setting should ectopic pregnancy be suspected?**
Amenorrhea with unilateral abdominal or pelvic **pain** and irregular **vaginal bleeding** is ectopic pregnancy until proven otherwise. Sequential hCG levels can help with differentiating an ectopic from an intrauterine pregnancy. Ordinarily, the doubling time of hCG levels is about 48 hours; in ectopic pregnancy, there is usually a significant lag. Other causes of lag include missed abortion and spontaneous abortion. Abdominal or transvaginal ultrasound is also useful for diagnosis. Laparoscopy may be necessary if the diagnosis remains unclear.

124. **How likely are teenagers to use contraception at the time of first intercourse?**
About one third of teenagers use no contraception at the time of first intercourse. The approximate time between onset of intercourse and seeking medical services for adolescent females is nearly 1 year. This in large part explains why 20% of all adolescent pregnancies occur during the first month after initiating sexual activity and why 50% occur within the first 6 months. If abstinence is not an option for a teenager, discussion of contraception should be initiated by the clinician early during adolescence to prevent unintended pregnancy.

> Rimsza ME: Counseling the adolescent about contraception. Pediatr Rev 24:162–170, 2003.

125. **Is a pelvic examination mandatory before starting a patient on oral contraceptive pills?**
No. Numerous professional organizations, including the American College of Obstetricians and Gynecologists, have advised that a pelvic examination is not required for safe use of oral contraception. A large percentage of teenagers will delay seeking contraceptive care if they believe a pelvic examination is required. Annual screening should subsequently be done for STDs and possible cervical dysplasia. The estimated risk of death from contraceptive use in a nonsmoking teenager (0.3/100,000) is substantially less than the risk of death during childbirth in the same age group (11.1/100,000).

> Rimsza ME: Counseling the adolescent about contraception. Pediatr Rev 24:162–170, 2003.

126. **What oral treatments are effective for emergency postcoital contraception (e.g., in a rape case)?**
Two hormonal methods for emergency contraception are approved by the FDA.
1. Preven (0.25 mg of levonorgestrel and 50 mcg of ethinyl estradiol): two tablets taken as soon as possible and repeated in 12 hours
2. Plan B (0.75 mg of levonorgestrel): a progestin-only method with 1 tablet taken as soon as possible and repeated in 12 hours

Emergency contraception pills likely work by inhibiting or delaying ovulation. Oral contraceptive pills are also used for emergency contraception. Emergency oral contraceptives are most effective when given within 72 hours of unprotected intercourse.

127. **When evaluating a teenager, what is the progression of cervicouterine changes that suggest pregnancy?**
- **4–6 weeks:** Softening of the lower uterine segment (*Hegar sign*) and softening of the cervix (*Goodell's sign*)
- **6 weeks:** Vagina and cervix assume a bluish hue (*Chadwick sign*)

Uterine size changes
- **Nongravid:** Lemon
- **8 weeks:** Tennis ball or orange
- **10 weeks:** Baseball
- **12 weeks:** Softball or grapefruit (unless uterus retroflexed)
- **>12 weeks:** Palpable above the symphysis
- **16 weeks:** Palpable between the symphysis and umbilicus
- **20 weeks:** Level of the umbilicus

TEENAGE SUICIDE

128. **How commonly do adolescents attempt suicide in the United States?**
About 2,000 teenagers die from suicide each year, but data about the frequency of attempts are hampered by underreporting. For each death by suicide, there are an estimated 50–200 attempts that fail, placing the number of attempts between 250,000–1,000,000. From 1950 to 1990, the suicide rate for adolescents in the 15- to 19-year-old group increased by 300% as compared with a 17% increase for the general population.

129. **Who are more likely to attempt suicide, males or females?**
Up to nine times as many females as males attempt suicide. However, males (particularly white males) are much more likely to succeed, due in large part to the choice of more lethal methods (especially firearms). Females more commonly try ingestions or wrist slashing.

130. **Which adolescents are at increased risk for suicide?**
Those with any of the following characteristics:
- History of previous attempts, especially those involving very lethal methods and those within the past 2 years (1–10% of failed suicides will be successful in future attempts)
- Signs of major depression (e.g., fatigue, sadness, loss of appetite, sleep irregularities)
- Substance abuse (up to 50% of victims between the ages of 18–24 years have blood alcohol levels ≥0.10%)
- Family history of psychiatric problems, including suicide and depression
- Personal history of "acting out" behavior (e.g., delinquency, truancy, sexual promiscuity)
- Living out of the home (in a correctional facility or group home)
- History of physical or sexual abuse

American Academy of Pediatrics. Committee on Adolescence: Suicide and suicide attempts in adolescents. Pediatrics 105:871–874, 2000.

131. **Which adolescents who have attempted suicide should be hospitalized?**
Although many programs admit all patients, even if they are medically stable, those adolescents with failed attempts who should strongly be considered for inpatient evaluation include the following:

- All with recurrent attempts
- Evidence of psychosis or persisting pervasive wish to die
- Method other than ingestion (e.g., jumping, use of firearm, attempted asphyxiation by hanging or carbon monoxide inhalation)
- Attempt at remote location (with less likelihood of discovery)
- Inadequate home, social, and supervisory situation

The American Academy of Child and Adolescent Psychiatry: Practice Parameter for the Assessment and Treatment of Children and Adolescents with Suicidal Behavior. J Am Acad Child Adolesc Psychiatry 40: 245–515, 2001.

CHAPTER 2

BEHAVIOR AND DEVELOPMENT

Mark F. Ditmar, MD

ATTENTION-DEFICIT/HYPERACTIVITY DISORDER

1. **What characterizes attention-deficit/hyperactivity disorder (ADHD)?**

   ADHD is a *chronic* neurodevelopmental/behavioral disorder that is diagnosed on the basis of the number, severity, and duration of three clusters of behavioral problems: *inattention, hyperactivity,* and *impulsivity.* It is the most commonly diagnosed behavior disorder in children. According to the *Diagnostic and Statistical Manual of Mental Disorders IV Text Revision* (DSM-IV-TR), symptoms of inattention, hyperactivity, and impulsivity must have lasted for >6 months and be inconsistent with the child's developmental level. These symptoms have to involve more than one setting and result in significant impairment at home, school, or in social settings. Some symptoms must have begun before the age of 7 years.

   Rappley MD: Attention-deficit/hyperactivity disorder. N Eng J Med 352:165–173, 2005.

2. **Is there a genetic predisposition to ADHD?**

   ADHD has a **high rate of heritability.** In studies of identical twins raised apart, if one twin has ADHD, the other has up to a 50% likelihood of being diagnosed with ADHD. In nonidentical twin studies, the concordance rate is as high as 33%. Studies of siblings of patients with ADHD indicate a 20–30% likelihood. About 25% of children with ADHD have at least one parent with symptoms and/or diagnosis of ADHD.

   Greenhill LL, Pliszka S, Dulcan MK, et al: American Academy of Child and Adolescent Psychiatry: Practice parameter for the use of stimulant medications in the treatment of children, adolescents, and adults. J Am Acad Child Adolesc Psychiatry 41(2 Suppl):26S–49S, 2002.

3. **What conditions can mimic ADHD?**

   Medical: Lead toxicity, iron deficiency, thyroid dysfunction, visual/hearing impairment, sleep disorders, mass lesions (e.g., hydrocephalus), seizures, complex migraines, fetal alcohol syndrome, fragile X syndrome, Williams syndrome, neurofibromatosis, tuberous sclerosis, medication side effects (e.g., cold preparations, steroids), and substance abuse.

   Developmental or learning disorders: Mental retardation (MR), autistic spectrum disorders (e.g., pervasive developmental disorder, Asperger syndrome), and specific learning disabilities. Central auditory processing difficulties have also been investigated, although it is still unclear as to whether such difficulties are a different disorder or if they represent the cognitive deficits seen with ADHD.

   Behavioral or emotional disorders: Affective disorders (e.g., dysthymia, bipolar disorder), anxiety disorders, stress reactions (e.g., posttraumatic stress disorder, adjustment disorder), other disruptive behavior disorders (e.g., oppositional defiant disorder), and personality disorders.

   Psychosocial factors: Family dysfunction, parenting dysfunction, and abuse.

4. **What are the comorbid disorders commonly seen with ADHD?**
   - Anxiety
   - Bipolar disorder

- Conduct disorder
- Depression
- Language problems
- Learning disorders
- MR
- Oppositional defiant disorder
- Sleep problems
- Tic disorders

5. **Is there a definitive diagnostic test for ADHD?**

No. Diagnosis requires evidence of characteristic symptomatology occurring in high frequency over an extended period of time. This information, which is ideally obtained from two settings or sources (e.g., school and home), can be garnered from observation, narrative histories, and the use of various standardized rating scales. A practitioner's ADHD toolkit, with scales for diagnosis, is available from the National Initiative for Children's Healthcare Quality at www.nichq.org/resources/toolkit.

Reiff MI, Stein MT: Attention-deficit hyperactivity disorder evaluation and diagnosis: A practical approach in office practice. Pediatr Clin North Am 50:1019–1048, 2003.

6. **How should ADHD be treated?**

A multimodal approach is recommended, which may include psychotropic medication, behavioral therapies, family education and counseling, and educational interventions.

American Academy of Pediatrics. Clinical practice guideline: Diagnosis and management of the child with attention-deficit/hyperactivity disorder. Pediatrics 105:1158–1170, 2000.

National Institutes of Health Consensus Development Conference Statement: Diagnosis and treatment of attention deficit hyperactivity disorder (ADHD). J Am Acad Child Adolesc Psychiatry 39:182–193, 2000.

7. **What are the best medications for treating ADHD?**

Stimulant medications (methylphenidate and dextroamphetamine). Randomized, controlled trials support their benefits, usually by demonstrating the improvement of core ADHD symptoms in 70–80% of children. Of the 20–30% of nonresponders to one medication, about half will respond to the other stimulant. Other medications used include tricyclic antidepressants, bupropion, and atomoxetine (a nonstimulant approved in 2003). There is controversy about the possible overuse of stimulants in children of all ages.

American Academy of Pediatrics. Subcommittee on Attention-Deficit/Hyperactivity Disorder and Committee on Quality Improvement: Clinical practice guideline: Treatment of the school-aged child with attention-deficit/hyperactivity disorder. Pediatrics 108:1033–1044, 2001.

Wender EH: Managing stimulant medication for attention-deficit/hyperactivity disorder. Pediatr Rev 23:234–236, 2002.

8. **Is a positive response to stimulant medication diagnostic of ADHD?**

A positive response is *not* diagnostic because (a) children without symptoms of ADHD given stimulants demonstrate positive responses in sustained and focused attention, and (b) observer bias (i.e., parent or teacher) can be considerable. Thus, many experts recommend a placebo-controlled trial when stimulant medication is used.

Nahlilk J: Issues in diagnosis of attention-deficit/hyperactivity disorder in adolescents. Clin Pediatr 43:1–10, 2004.

9. **How young is "too young" to diagnose ADHD and prescribe stimulant medications?**

The diagnosis is considered difficult to make in children <4–6 years old because the validity and reliability of the diagnosis of ADHD in these age groups have not been demonstrated. Methylphenidate carries a warning against its use in children <6 years old. Concerns exist regarding the unproven treatment of children at such a young age and the potential deleterious effect of psychotropic drugs on brain development. However, there has been a dramatic increase in the "off-label" use of stimulant medication in the 1990s for children 2–4 years old. The evaluation and most ideal treatment of these younger children remain a challenge.

Coyle JT: Psychotropic drug use in the very young child. JAMA 283:1059–1060, 2000.

Zito JM, Safer DJ, dosReis S, et al: Trends in the prescribing of psychotropic medications to preschoolers. JAMA 283:1025–1030, 2000.

10. **What are the risks of adolescents with ADHD?**

Increased high-risk behaviors, including higher rates of sexually transmitted diseases and pregnancies, and **increased school problems**, including higher rates of grade failure, dropping out, and expulsion. *Untreated* ADHD has also been found to be a significant risk factor for future substance abuse.

Robin AL: Attention-deficit/hyperactivity disorder in adolescents. Pediatr Ann 31:485–491, 2002.

Wilens TE, Faraone SV, Biederman J, Gunawardene S: Does stimulant therapy of attention-deficit/hyperactivity disorder beget later substance abuse? A meta-analytic review of the literature. Pediatrics 111:179–185, 2003.

KEY POINTS: THE "I"SSENTIALS OF ADHD

Inattention

Increased activity

Impulsiveness

Impairment in multiple settings

Inappropriate (for developmental stage)

Incessant (persists for >6 months)

11. **Is the Feingold diet of any value for the treatment of ADHD?**

Dr. Benjamin Feingold hypothesized in the early 1970s that hyperactivity in children was due to the ingestion of low-molecular-weight chemicals such as salicylates and artificial additives that are used for color and flavor. He recommended a diet devoid of these substances and claimed up to a 50% improvement in children on such a diet. Few controlled studies, however, have been able to demonstrate such an effect.

12. **Does sugar make children hyperactive?**

Although it would be gratifying if complex behavioral problems could be attributable solely or in large measure to dietary causes, this has not been shown to be the case. In a double-blind, controlled trial involving excessive dietary intakes of sucrose or aspartame, no adverse behavioral or cognitive changes were noted.

Wolraich ML, Wilson DB, White JW: The effect of sugar on behavior or cognition in children. A meta-analysis. JAMA 274:1617–1621, 1995.

13. **Do children with ADHD become teenagers and adults with ADHD?**

Ongoing observations of children initially diagnosed with ADHD note that **70-80%** will continue to have symptoms present during adolescence and up to **60%** will show symptoms as adults. These adolescents and adults also have continued problems with anxiety and depression as well as with tobacco and substance abuse. Motor vehicle infractions, employment difficulties, and intimate relationships have also been described as problematic for adults. Children and adolescents with symptoms of conduct disorder as well as ADHD are at the highest risk for severe problems as adults.

Wolraich ML, Wibbelsman CJ, Brown TE, et al: Attention-deficit/hyperactivity disorder among adolescents: A review of the diagnosis, treatment, and clinical implications. Pediatrics 115:1734–1746, 2005.

BEHAVIOR PROBLEMS

14. **What are the most common types of behavior problems in children?**
    - Problems of daily routine (e.g., food refusal, sleep abnormalities, toilet difficulties)
    - Aggressive-resistant behavior (e.g., temper tantrums, aggressiveness with peers)
    - Overdependent-withdrawing behavior (e.g., separation upset, fears, shyness)
    - Hyperactivity
    - Undesirable habits (e.g., thumb sucking, head banging, nail biting, playing with genitals)
    - School problems

    Chamberlin RW: Prevention of behavioral problems in young children. Pediatr Clin North Am 29:239–247, 1982.

15. **How much do babies normally cry each day?**
    In Brazelton's oft-quoted 1962 study of 80 infants, it was found that, at 2 weeks old, the average crying time was nearly 2 hours per day. This increased to nearly 3 hours per day at 6 weeks and then declined to about 1 hour per day at 12 weeks.

    Brazelton TB: Crying in infancy. Pediatrics 29:579–588, 1962.

16. **What is infantile colic?**
    Colic is excessive crying or fussiness, which occurs in 10–20% of infants. For study purposes, it is defined as paroxysms of crying in an otherwise healthy infant for >3 hours per day on >3 days per week. The typical picture is that of a baby (usually between the ages of 2 weeks and 3 months) who cries intensely for several hours at a time, usually during the late afternoon or evening. Often the infant appears to be in pain and has a slightly distended abdomen, with the legs drawn up; occasional temporary relief occurs if gas is passed.

    The symptoms nearly always resolve by the time the infant is 3 to 4 months old, but the problem can have repercussions, including early discontinuation of breastfeeding, multiple formula changes, heightened maternal anxiety and distress, diminished maternal-infant interaction, and increased risk for child abuse.

17. **What causes colic?**
    No precise cause has been identified, and the etiology is likely multifactorial. Theories have involved intolerance or allergy to cow milk or soy protein, immaturity of the gastrointestinal tract and/or the central nervous system, difficult infant temperament, and interaction problems between the infant and the caregiver (e.g., misinterpreted infant cues, transfer of parental anxiety).

18. **Are there any treatments that are useful for colic?**
    As is the case for most self-resolving conditions without a known cause, **counseling** is the most effective treatment. However, multiple interventions with minimal effectiveness are often tried, and these often involve the gastrointestinal tract: elimination of cow milk from the breastfeeding mother's diet, formula changes (to soy or to protein hydrolysates), or a trial of simethicone to decrease intestinal gas. Medications such as phenobarbital and diphenhydramine are used empirically in clinical practice for severe crying because they produce a sedating effect. They are not routinely recommended, especially for long-term use.

    Lucassen PL, Assendelft WJ, Gubbels JW, et al: Effectiveness of treatments for infantile colic: Systematic review. BMJ 316:1563–1569, 1998.

19. **How should children be punished?**

The goal of punishment should be to teach children that a specific behavior was wrong and to discourage the behavior in the future. To meet this goal, punishment should be consistent and relatively brief. It should be carried out in a calm manner as soon as possible after the infraction. Time-out from ongoing activity and removal of privileges are two punishment techniques that can be used. The use of corporal punishment is controversial. Although spanking and other physical forms of punishment are widely practiced, most developmental authorities argue against their use because they do not foster the internalization of rules of behavior and may legitimize violence.

Larsen MA, Tentis E: The art and science of disciplining children. Pediatr Clin North Am 50:817–840, 2003.

20. **How valid is the proverb "spare the rod and spoil the child" as a defense for corporal punishment?**

The actual biblical proverb (Proverbs 13:24) reads, "He who spares the rod hates his son, but he who loves him is careful to discipline him." Although the proverb has often been used as a justification for spanking, in actuality it does not refer to specific discipline strategies but rather to the need for love and discipline. In addition, the rod may refer to the shepherd's staff, which was used to guide—rather than hit—sheep.

Carey TA: Spare the rod and spoil the child: Is this a sensible justification for the use of punishment in child rearing? Child Abuse Negl 18:1005–1010, 1994.

21. **Is physical injury a concern in children with head banging?**

Head banging, which is a common problem that occurs in 5–15% of normal children, rarely results in physical injury. When injury does occur, it is usually in children with autism or other developmental disabilities. Normal children often show signs of bliss as they bang away, and the activity usually resolves by the time the child is 4 years old. (It may resume spontaneously during national board examinations.)

22. **What is the difference between a "blue" breath-holding spell and a "white" breath-holding spell?**

Both of these are syncopal attacks that occur commonly in children between the ages of 6 months and 4 years. A **"blue"** or **cyanotic spell** is more common. Vigorous crying provoked by physical or emotional upset leads to apnea at end of expiration. This is followed by cyanosis, opisthotonus, rigidity, and loss of tone. Brief convulsive jerking may occur. The episode lasts from 10–60 seconds. A short period of sleepiness may ensue. A **"white"** or **pallid spell** is more commonly precipitated by an unexpected event that frightens the child. On testing, children prone to these spells demonstrate increased responsiveness to vagal maneuvers. This parasympathetic hypersensitivity may cause cardiac slowing, diminished cardiac output, and diminished arterial pressure, which result in a pale appearance.

DiMario FJ Jr: Breathholding spells in childhood. Curr Probl Pediatr 29:281–289, 1999.

23. **When should a diagnosis of seizure disorder be considered rather than a breath-holding spell?**
    - Precipitating event is minor or nonexistent
    - History of no or minimal crying or breath holding
    - Episode lasts >1 minute
    - Period of post-episode sleepiness lasts >10 minutes
    - Convulsive component of episode is prominent and occurs before cyanosis
    - Occurs in child <6 months or >4 years old

24. **Does treatment with iron decrease the frequency of breath-holding spells?**

The relationship between anemia, iron deficiency, and breath-holding spells is unclear. In the 1960s, it was observed that children with breath-holding spells had lower hemoglobin levels than controls. Treatment with iron has decreased the frequency of breath-holding spells in some children. Interestingly, some of the children whose breath-holding spells respond to iron are not anemic, and the mechanism by which iron decreases breath-holding spells is not known.

Boon R: Does iron have a place in the management of breath-holding spells? Arch Dis Child 87:77–78, 2002.

25. **When does prolonged thumb-sucking warrant intervention?**
If frequent thumb-sucking persists in a child who is more than 4–5 years old or in whom permanent teeth have begun to erupt, treatment is usually indicated. Treatment commonly has two components: (1) application of a substance with an unpleasant taste at frequent intervals (such products are commercially available), and (2) behavior modification with positive reinforcement (small rewards) given when a child is observed not sucking his or her thumb. Occlusive dental appliances are generally not needed. Persistent thumb-sucking after the eruption of permanent teeth can lead to malocclusion.

26. **When should "toilet training" be started?**
When the child is physically and emotionally ready, training can be begun. The physical prerequisite of the neurologic maturation of bladder and bowel control usually occurs between 18 and 30 months of age. The child's emotional readiness is often influenced by his or her temperament, parental attitudes, and parent-child interactions. The "potty chair" should be introduced when the child is between 2 and 3 years old. Most children will achieve daytime bladder and bowel control by the age of 3½ years. A recent study indicates that intensive attempts at training before 27 months were not associated with earlier completion.

Blum NJ, Taubman B, Nemeth N: Relationship between age of toilet training and duration of training: A prospective study. Pediatrics 111(4 Pt 1):810–814, 2003.

27. **Are girls or boys toilet trained earlier?**
On average, **girls** are toilet trained earlier than boys. With regard to most other developmental milestones during the first years of life, however, there do not seem to be significant sex differences (i.e., in walking or running, sleep patterns, or verbal ability). Girls do show more rapid bone development.

28. **When is masturbation in a child considered pathologic?**
Masturbation (the rhythmic self-manipulation of the genital area) is considered a normal part of sexual development. However, if masturbation occurs to the exclusion of other activities, if it occurs in public places when the child is >6 years old, or if the child engages in activities that mimic adult sexual behavior, evaluation for sexual abuse, central nervous system abnormalities, or psychological pathology would be appropriate.

CRANIAL DISORDERS

29. **How many fontanels are present at birth?**
Although there are six fontanels present at birth (two anterior lateral, two posterior lateral, one anterior, and one posterior); only two (the anterior and posterior fontanels) are usually palpable on physical examination (Fig. 2-1).

30. **When does the anterior fontanel close?**
Usually when the infant is between 10 and 14 months old. However, it may not be palpable as early as 3 months, or it may remain open until 18 months.

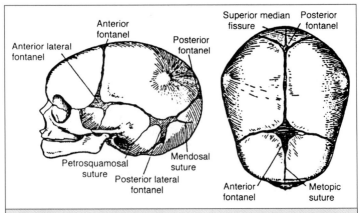

Figure 2-1. The cranium at birth, showing major sutures and fontanels. No attempt is made to show molding or overlapping of bones, which sometimes occurs at birth. (From Silverman FN, Kuhn JP [eds]: Caffey's Pediatric X-ray Diagnosis, 9th ed. St. Louis, Mosby, 1993, p 5.)

31. **Which conditions are most commonly associated with premature or delayed closure of the fontanel?**
    Premature closure: Microcephaly, high calcium/vitamin D ratio in pregnancy, craniosynostosis, hyperthyroidism, or variation of normal
    Delayed closure: Achondroplasia, Down syndrome, increased intracranial pressure, familial macrocephaly, rickets, or variation of normal

32. **When is an anterior fontanel too big?**
    The size of the fontanel can be calculated using the formula: (length + width)/2, where length equals anterior-posterior dimension and width equals transverse dimension. However, there is wide variability in the normal size range of the anterior fontanel. Mean fontanel size on day 1 of life is 2.1 cm, with an upper limit of normal of 3.6 cm in white infants and 4.7 cm in black infants. These upper limits may be helpful for identifying disorders in which a large fontanel may be a feature (e.g., hypothyroidism, hypophosphatasia, skeletal dysplasias, increased intracranial pressure). Of note is that the *posterior fontanel* is normally about the size of a fingertip or smaller in 97% of full-term newborns.

    Kiesler J, Ricer R: The anterior fontanel. Am Fam Physician 67:2547–2552, 2003.

33. **What are the types of primary craniosynostosis?**
    Craniosynostosis is the premature fusion of various cranial suture lines that results in the ridging of the sutures, asymmetric growth, and deformity of the skull. Suture lines (with resultant disorders listed in parentheses) include sagittal (scaphocephaly or dolichocephaly), coronal (brachycephaly), unilateral coronal or lambdoidal (plagiocephaly), and metopic (trigonocephaly). Multiple fused sutures can result in a high and pointed skull (oxycephaly or acrocephaly) (Fig. 2-2).

34. **What is the most common type of primary craniosynostosis?**
    Sagittal (60%); coronal synostosis accounts for 20% of cases.

35. **What causes craniosynostosis?**
    Most cases of isolated craniosynostosis have no known etiology. *Primary* craniosynostosis may be observed as part of craniofacial syndromes, including Apert, Crouzon, and Carpenter syndromes. *Secondary* causes can include abnormalities of calcium and phosphorus

metabolism (e.g., hypophosphatasia, rickets), hematologic disorders (e.g., thalassemia), mucopolysaccharidoses, and hyperthyroidism. Inadequate brain growth (e.g., microcephaly) can lead to craniosynostosis.

Kabbani H, Raghuveer TS: Craniosynostosis. Am Fam Physician 69:2863–2870, 2004.

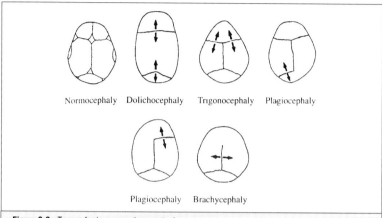

Figure 2-2. Types of primary craniosynostosis

36. **What is positional plagiocephaly?**

Since the implementation of the "back-to-sleep" program by the American Academy of Pediatrics in 1992 to reduce the risk of sudden infant death syndrome, about 1 in 60 infants has developed occipital flattening (posterior plagiocephaly) due to transient calvarial deformation from prolonged supine sleeping positions. Simple positional modifications (alternating left and right occipital sleep positions) usually suffice for correction, particularly if intervention is begun at an early age.

American Academy of Pediatrics. Committee on Practice and Ambulatory Medicine: Prevention and management of positional skull deformities in infants. Pediatrics 112.119–202, 2003.

37. **How is positional plagiocephaly differentiated from plagiocephaly caused by craniosynostosis?**

Synostotic plagiocephaly is much more rare, it is usually associated with ridging of the involved suture lines, and it causes a different pattern of frontal bossing and ear displacement when the infant's head is viewed from above (Fig. 2-3).

38. **What conditions are associated with skull softening?**
   - Cleidocranial dysostosis
   - Craniotabes
   - Lacunar skull (associated with spina bifida and major central nervous system anomalies)
   - Osteogenesis imperfecta
   - Multiple wormian bones (associated with hypothyroidism, hypophosphatasia, and chronic hydrocephalus)
   - Rickets

39. **What is the significance of craniotabes?**

In this condition, abnormally soft, thin skull bones buckle under pressure and recoil like a ping-pong ball. It is best elicited on the parietal or frontal bones and is often associated with rickets

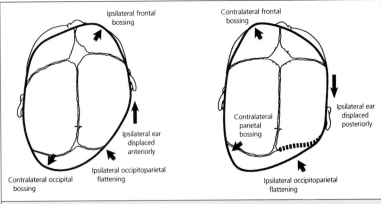

Figure 2-3. Factors distinguishing (*left*) positional plagiocephaly from (*right*) lambdoidal craniosynostosis. (From Kabbani H, Raghuveer TS: Craniosynostosis. Am Fam Physician 69:2866, 2004.)

in infancy. It may also be seen in hypervitaminosis A, syphilis, and hydrocephalus. Craniotabes may be a normal finding during the first 3 months of life.

40. **What evaluations should be done in a child with microcephaly?**
   The extent of evaluation depends on various factors: prenatal versus postnatal acquisition, presence of minor or major anomalies, developmental problems, and neurologic abnormalities. The diagnosis can be as straightforward as a simple familial variant (autosomal dominant) in a child with normal intelligence, or it can range to a variety of conditions associated with abnormal brain growth (e.g., intrauterine infections, heritable syndromes, chromosomal abnormalities). Evaluation may include the following:
   - Parental head-size measurements
   - Ophthalmologic evaluation (abnormal optic nerve or retinal findings may be in found in various syndromes)
   - Karyotype
   - Neuroimaging (cranial magnetic resonance imaging [MRI] or computed tomography scanning to evaluate for structural abnormalities or intracranial calcifications)
   - Metabolic screening
   - Cultures/serology if suspected intrauterine infection

41. **What are the three main general causes of macrocephaly?**
   - **Increased intracranial pressure:** Caused by dilated ventricles (e.g., progressive hydrocephalus of various causes), subdural fluid collections, intracranial tumors, or benign increased intracranial pressure (i.e., pseudotumor cerebri) from various causes
   - **Thickened skull:** Caused by cranioskeletal dysplasias (e.g., osteopetrosis) and various anemias
   - **Megalencephaly** (enlarged brain): May be familial or syndromic (e.g., Sotos syndrome) or caused by storage diseases, leukodystrophies, or neurocutaneous disorders (e.g., neurofibromatosis)

DENTAL DEVELOPMENT AND DISORDERS

42. When do primary and secondary teeth erupt?
Mandibular teeth usually erupt first. The central incisors appear by the age of 5–7 months, with approximately 1 new tooth per month thereafter until 23–30 months, at which time the second molars (and thus all 20 primary or deciduous teeth) are in place. Of the 32 secondary teeth, the central incisors erupt first between 5 and 7 years, and the third molars are in place by 17–22 years.

43. What is the significance of natal teeth?
Occasionally, teeth are present at birth (natal teeth) or erupt within 30 days after birth (neonatal teeth). When x-rays are taken, 95% of natal teeth are primary incisors, and 5% are supernumerary teeth or extra teeth. Very sharp teeth that can cause tongue lacerations and very loose teeth that can be aspirated should be removed. Females are affected more commonly than males, and the prevalence is 1:2,000–3,500. Most cases are familial and without consequence, but natal teeth can be associated with genetic syndromes, including the Ellis-van Creveld and Hallermann-Streiff syndromes.

44. How common is the congenital absence of teeth?
The congenital absence of primary teeth is very rare, but up to 25% of individuals may have an absence of one or more third molars, and up to 5% may have an absence of another secondary or permanent tooth (most commonly the maxillary lateral incisors and mandibular second premolar).

45. What are mesiodentes?
These are peg-shaped supernumerary teeth that occur in up to 5% of individuals, and they are most commonly situated in the maxillary midline. They should be considered for removal because they interfere with the eruption of permanent incisors.

46. Which teeth constitute the 32 permanent teeth?
The upper and lower central incisors, lateral incisors, cuspids, first bicuspids, second bicuspids, first molars, second molars, and third molars.

47. What is a ranula?
A large mucocele, usually bluish, painless, soft, and unilateral, that occurs under the tongue. Most of these self-resolve. If a patient has a large one, surgical marsupialization can be done. If the ranula is recurrent, excision may be needed.

48. Where are Epstein pearls located?
These white, superficial, mobile nodules are usually midline and often paired on the hard palate in many newborns. They are keratin containing cysts that are asymptomatic, do not increase in size, and usually exfoliate spontaneously within a few weeks.

49. How common is dental caries in children?
Very common. By 17 years old, only 15–20% of individuals are free from dental caries, and the average child has 8 decayed, missing, or filled tooth surfaces. Prevention of dental caries involves decreasing the frequency of tooth exposure to carbohydrates (frequency is more important than total amount), using fluoride, brushing the teeth, and using sealants.

American Academy of Pediatric Dentistry: www.aapd.org

50. What are milk-bottle caries?

Frequent contact of cariogenic liquids (e.g., milk, formula, breast milk, juice) with teeth, as occurs in infants who fall asleep with a bottle or who are breast fed frequently at night after the age of 1 year ("nursing caries"), has been associated with a significant increase in the development of caries (Fig. 2-4). The American Academy of Pediatrics recommends that infants not be put to sleep with a bottle (unless it is filled with water), that nocturnal ad lib breast feeding be limited as dental development progresses, and that cup feedings be introduced when the child is 1 year old.

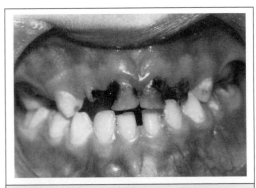

Figure 2-4. Classic nursing bottle decay involving the maxillary anterior teeth. Mandibular incisors are protected by the tongue during feeding and are usually caries-free. (From Gessner IH, Victorica BE: Pediatric Cardiology: A Problem-Oriented Approach. Philadelphia, W.B. Saunders, 1993, p 232.)

51. How does fluoride minimize the development of dental caries?
- Topical fluoride from toothbrushing is thought to increase the remineralization of enamel.
- Bacterial fermentation of sugar into acid plays a major role in the development of caries, and fluoride inhibits this process.
- As teeth are developing, fluoride incorporates into the hydroxyapatite crystal of enamel, thereby making it less soluble and less susceptible to erosion.

52. What is fluorosis?

Exposure to excessive levels of fluoride during tooth development, primarily in a patient <8 years old, can damage enamel, causing changes that range from mild (lacy white markings) to severe (pitting, mottling, striations).

53. How long should fluoride supplementation be continued?

Fluoride supplementation should continue until a child is 14–16 years old, when the third molar crowns are completely calcified.

Lewis CW, Milgrom P: Fluoride. Pediatr Rev 24:327–336, 2004.

KEY POINTS: DENTAL PROBLEMS

1. Prolonged pacifier use beyond the age of 18 months can result in oral and dental distortions.

2. Appropriate use of fluoride and dental sealants could prevent caries in most children.

3. Use of formula or breast feeding at bedtime after dental eruption leads to higher incidences of caries.

4. Excessive fluoride is associated initially with a white, speckled, or lacy appearance of the enamel.

54. **How effective are dental sealants for preventing cavities?**
Dental sealants may reduce the development of caries by up to 80% as compared with rates in untreated teeth. Although fluoride acts primarily by protecting smooth surfaces, dental sealants (commonly bisphenol A and glycidyl methacrylate) act by protecting the pits and fissures of the surface, especially in posterior teeth. Reapplication may be needed every 2 years. As a preventive dental procedure, it is relatively underused.

55. **How common is gingivitis in children?**
Gingivitis is extremely common, affecting nearly 50% of children. The disorder is usually painless and is manifested by the bluish-red discoloration of gums, which are swollen and bleed easily. The cause is bacteria in plaque deposits between teeth; the cure is improved dental hygiene and daily flossing.

56. **What is the largest health-related expense before adulthood for normally developing children?**
Dental braces. More than 50% of children have dental malocclusions that could be improved with treatment, but only 10–20% have severe malocclusions that require treatment. For others, the costs and benefits of braces need to be weighed individually. Besides the financial expense, the costs of braces include physical discomfort and some increases in the risk for tooth decay and periodontal disease.

57. **What causes halitosis is children?**
Halitosis (bad breath) is usually the result of oral factors, including microbial activity on the dorsal tongue and between the teeth. Conditions associated with postnasal drip, including chronic sinusitis, upper and lower respiratory tract infections, and various systemic diseases are also causes.

Amir E, Shimonov R, Rosenberg M: Halitosis in children. J Pediatr 134:338–343, 1999.

DEVELOPMENTAL ASSESSMENT

58. **Why do infants have primitive reflexes, and when should they disappear?**
Primitive reflexes are *automatisms* that are usually triggered by an external stimulus. Examples are rooting, which is triggered by touching the corner of the mouth, and the asymmetric tonic neck reflex (ATNR), which is triggered by rotating the head. Some reflexes (e.g., rooting, sucking, and grasp) have survival value. Others, such as the ATNR or the tonic labyrinthine reflex, have no obvious purpose. Placing and stepping reflexes usually disappear by 2 months. Moro and grasp reflexes and the ATNR usually disappear by 3 months.

59. **What three primitive reflexes, if persistent beyond 4–6 months, can interfere with the development of the ability to roll, sit, and use both hands together?**
Moro reflex: Sudden neck extension results in extension, abduction, and then adduction of the upper extremities with flexion of fingers, wrists, and elbows.
Asymmetric tonic neck reflex: In a calm supine infant, turning of the head laterally results in relative extension of the arm and leg on the side of the turn and flexion of both on the side away from the turn (the "fencer" position).
Tonic labyrinthine reflex: In an infant who is being held suspended in the prone position, flexion of the neck results in shoulder protraction and hip flexion, whereas neck extension causes shoulder retraction and hip extension.

Zafeiriou DI: Primitive reflexes and postural reactions in the neurodevelopmental examination. Pediatr Neurol 31:1–8, 2004.

60. **At what age do children develop handedness?**
Usually by **18–24 months**. Hand preference is usually fixed by the time a child is 5 years old. Handedness before 1 year may be indicative of a problem with the nonpreferred side (e.g., hemiparesis, brachial plexus injury).

61. **What percentage of children are left-handed?**
Various studies put the prevalence at **between 7% and 10%.** However, in former premature infants without cerebral palsy, the rate increases to 20–25%. Although antecedent brain injury has been hypothesized to account for this increase in prevalence of left-handedness, studies of unilateral intraventricular hemorrhage and handedness have not demonstrated a relationship. Of note is that animals such as mice, dogs, and cats show paw preferences, but, in these groups, 50% prefer the left paw and 50% prefer the right paw.

   Marlow N, Roberts BL, Cooke RW: Laterality and prematurity. Arch Dis Child 64:1713–1716, 1989.

62. **What are the major developmental landmarks for motor skills during the first 2 years of life?**
See Table 2-1.

TABLE 2-1. MAJOR DEVELOPMENTAL LANDMARKS FOR MOTOR SKILLS	
Developmental landmark	**Age range (in months)**
Major gross motor	
Steadiness of head when placed in supported position	1–4
Sits without support for >30 seconds	5–8
Cruises or walks holding on to things	7–13
Stands alone	9–16
Walks alone	9–17
Walks up stairs with help	12–23
Major fine motor	
Grasp	2–4
Reach	3–5
Transfers objects from hand to hand	5–7
Fine pincer grasp with index finger and thumb apposition	9–14
Spontaneous scribbling	12–24

63. **What are the most common causes of gross motor delay?**
Normal variation is the most common, followed by **MR**. **Cerebral palsy** is a distant third, and all other conditions combined (e.g., spinal muscular atrophy, myopathies) run a distant fourth. The most common pathologic cause of gross motor delay is MR, although most children with this condition have normal gross motor milestones.

64. **Do infant walkers promote physical strength or development of the lower extremities?**
No. On the contrary, published data confirm that infants in walkers actually manifest mild but statistically significant gross motor *delays*. Infants with walkers were found to sit, crawl, and walk later than those without walkers. Safety hazards can include head trauma, fractures, burns, finger entrapments, and dental injuries. Most of the serious injuries involve falls down stairs.

65. **Do twins develop at a rate that is comparable to infants of single birth?**
Twins exhibit **significant verbal and motor delay** during the first year of life. The difficulty lies not in the lack of potential but in the relative lack of individual stimulation. In general, children who are more closely spaced in a family have slower acquisition of verbal skills. Twins with significant language delay or with excessive use of "twin language" (language understood only by the twins themselves) may be candidates for interventional therapy.

66. **Do premature infants develop at the same rate as term infants?**
For the most part, premature infants do develop at the same rate as term infants. In ongoing developmental assessments, they eventually "catch up" to their chronologic peers not by accelerated development but rather through the arithmetic of time. As they age, their degree of prematurity (in months) becomes less of a percentage of their chronologic age. Early in life, the extent of prematurity is key and must be taken into account during assessments. Such "correction factors" are generally unnecessary after the age of 2–3 years, depending on the degree of prematurity.

67. **When can an infant smell?**
The sense of smell is present **at birth**. Newborn infants show preferential head turning toward gauze pads soaked with their mother's milk as opposed to the milk of another woman.

68. **What are the best measures of cognitive development?**
Ideally, cognitive development should be assessed in a fashion that is free of motor requirements. **Receptive language** is the best measure of cognitive function. Even an eye blink or a voluntary eye gaze can be used to assess cognition independently of motor disability. Adaptive skills such as tool use (e.g., spoon, crayon) are also useful, although they may be delayed because of purely motoric reasons. Gross motor milestones such as walking raise concerns about MR if they are delayed, but normal gross motor milestones cannot be used to infer normal cognitive development.

    National Institute of Child Health and Human Development: www.nich.nih.gov

69. **What do the stages of play tell us about a child's development?**
A well-taken history of a child's play is a valuable adjunct to more traditional milestones such as language and adaptive skills (Table 2-2).

70. **What can one learn about a child's developmental level with regard to the use of a crayon?**
A lot. At <9 months, the infant will use the crayon as a teething object. Between 10 and 14 months, the infant will make marks on a piece of paper, almost as a byproduct of holding the crayon and "banging" it against the paper. By 14–16 months, the infant will make marks spontaneously, and, by 18–20 months, he or she will make marks with vigorous scribbling. By 20–22 months, an infant will begin copying specific geometric patterns as presented by the examiner (Table 2-3). The ability to execute these figures requires visual-perceptual, fine motor, and cognitive abilities. Delay in the ability to complete these tasks suggests difficulty with one or more of these underlying streams of development.

71. **What is the value of the Goodenough-Harris drawing test?**
This "draw a person" test is a screening tool used to evaluate a child's cognition and intellect, visual perception, and visual-motor integration. The child is asked to draw a person, and a point is given for each body part drawn with pairs (e.g., legs) that is considered as one part. An average child that is 4 years and 9 months will draw a person with 3 parts; most children by the age of 5 years and 3 months will draw a person with 6 parts.

TABLE 2–2. PLAY ACTIVITY AND CHILD DEVELOPMENT

Age range (in months)	Play activity	Underlying skills
3	Midline hand play	Sensorimotor; self-discovery
4–5	Bats at objects	Ability to affect environment
6–7	Directed reaching; transfers	
7–9	Banging and mouthing objects	
12	Casting ("I throw it down, and you pick it up for me"); explores objects by visual inspection and handling rather than orally	Object permanence; social reciprocity; use of pointing, joint attention (eye gaze), and simple language to effect response in caregiver
16–18+	Stacking and dumping; exploring; lids; light switches; simple mechanical toys (jack-in-the-box; shape ball)	Means-ends behavior: experimenting with causality
24	Imitative play ("helping" with the dishes; doll play with a physical doll)	Language and socialization; development of "inner language"
36	Make-believe play (e.g., doll play with a pillow to represent the doll)	Distinguish between "real" and "not real"
48	Simple board games, rule-based playground games (e.g., "tag")	Concrete operations (Piaget)

www.parentcenter.com

TABLE 2–3. CRAYON USE AND DEVELOPMENT LEVEL

Age	Task
20–22 months	Alternates from scribble to stroke on imitation of examiner
27–30 months	Alternates from horizontal to vertical on imitation of examiner
36 months	Copies circle from illustration
3 years	Copies cross
4 years	Copies square
5 years	Copies triangle
6 years	Copies "Union Jack"

LANGUAGE DEVELOPMENT AND DISORDERS

72. **What are average times for the development of expressive, receptive, and visual language milestones?**
See Table 2-4.

TABLE 2-4.	DEVELOPMENT OF EXPRESSIVE, RECEPTIVE, AND VISUAL LANGUAGE		
Age in months	**Expressive**	**Receptive**	**Visual**
0–3	Coo	Alerts to voice	Recognizes parents; visual tracking
4–6	Monosyllabic babbling, laugh, "raspberry"	Turns to voice and sounds	Responds to facial expressions
7–9	Polysyllabic babbling; mama/dada, nonspecific	Recognizes own name; inhibits to command "No"	Imitates games (patty cake; peek-a-boo)
10–12	Mama/dada specific; first word other than mama/dada or names of other family members or pets	Follows at least one one-step command without a gestural cue (e.g., "Come here," "Give me")	Points to desired objects
16–18	Uses words to indicate wants	Follows many one-step commands; points to body parts on command	
22–24	Two-word phrases	Follows two-step commands	
30	Telegraphic speech	Follows prepositional commands	
36	Simple sentences		

73. **What are the warning signs of delayed language development?**
See Table 2-5.

74. **Do deaf infants babble?**
Yes. Babbling begins at about the same time in both deaf and hearing infants, but deaf infants stop babbling without the normal progression to meaningful communicative speech.
American Society for Deaf Children: www.deafchildren.org

75. **At what age does a child's speech become intelligible?**
Intelligibility increases by about 25% per year. A 1-year-old child has about 25% intelligibility, a 2-year-old has 50%, a 3-year-old has 75%, and a 4-year-old has 100%. Significantly delayed intelligibility should prompt a hearing and language evaluation.

76. **What are the most common causes of so-called "delayed speech"?**
The most common causes of speech or language delay include the following: developmental language disorders (i.e., normal cognition, impaired intelligibility, and delayed emergence of phrases, sentences, and grammatical markers), MR, hearing loss, and autistic spectrum disorder.
Feldman HM: Evaluation and management of language and speech disorders in preschool children. Pediatr Rev 26:131–142, 2005.

TABLE 2-5.	SIGNS OF LANGUAGE PROBLEMS NEEDING FURTHER EVALUATION
0–6 months	Child does not respond to sounds or turn toward a speaker who is out of sight.
	Child makes only crying sounds (no cooing or comfort sounds).
1 year	Child shows only inconsistent responses to sound.
	Child has stopped babbling or does not babble yet.
2 years	Child does not understand or pay attention when addressed.
	Child does not use any words.
	Vocabulary is minimal (<8–10 words) and is not growing.
	Speech primarily echoes what others say.
2½ years	Child is not combining words.
	Child has difficulty following commands or answering simple questions.
3 years	Child still echoes.
	Sentences are not used.
	Vocabulary is <100 words.
4 years	Child has difficulty formulating statements and questions.
	Child has deficient conversational skills and has difficulty learning concepts and/or sequences, such as numbers and the alphabet.
	Language usage is deviant and not appropriate for social interaction.
5 years	Child cannot retain and follow verbal directions.
	Child has difficulty learning sound-symbol relationships.
	Sentence structure is noticeably faulty, and word order in sentences is poor.
	Child cannot describe an event or outing.

Blum NJ, Baron M: Speech and language disorders. In Schwartz MW, Curry TA, Sargent J, et al (eds): Pediatric Primary Care: A Problem Oriented Approach. St. Louis, Mosby, 1997, pp 845–849.

77. **What causes flat tympanograms?**

    Tympanometry is an objective measurement of the compliance of the tympanic membrane and the middle ear compartment that involves varying the air pressure in the external ear canal from approximately –200 to +400 mmH$_2$O while measuring the reflected energy of a simultaneous acoustic tone. A normal tracing looks like an inverted "V," with the peak occurring at an air pressure of 0 mmH$_2$O; this indicates a functionally normal external canal, an intact tympanic membrane, and a lack of excess of middle ear fluid. Flat tympanograms occur with perforation of the tympanic membrane, occlusion of the tympanometry probe against the wall of the canal, obstruction of the canal by a foreign body or impaction by cerumen, or large middle ear effusion. Flat tympanograms due to middle ear effusion are usually associated with a 20–30 dB conductive hearing loss, although in occasional instances the loss may be as great as 50 dB.

78. **What methods are used to test hearing at different ages?**

    The gold standard remains pure tone testing under headphones (usually not achievable until the child is about 30 months old), but there are clinically valid methods that can be used at any age (*see* Table 2-6). Hearing testing should never be put off "until the child is older" if an indication for audiologic evaluation exists.

    American Academy of Audiology: www.audiology.org

TABLE 2-6.	METHODS TO TEST HEARING	
Age	**Method**	**Comment**
Any	Otoacoustic emissions	Useful for newborn screening; occasional false positives
Any	Brainstem auditory evoked response	Sensitive, specific; often requires sedation in younger children
0–6 months	Alerting to sound	Sound-field; assesses hearing in the better of the two ears if an asymmetry exists
6–18 months	Conditioned orienting	Sound-field; assesses hearing in the better of the two ears if an asymmetry exists
24+ months	Play audiometry	Picture pointing and so on; tests speech reception threshold; tests each ear separately
30+ months	Pure tones under headphones	

Cunningham M, Cox EO: Hearing assessment in infants and children: Recommendations beyond neonatal screening. Pediatrics 111:436–440, 2003.

79. **A toddler with a bifid uvula and hypernasal speech most likely has what condition?**
Velopharyngeal insufficiency with a possible submucosal cleft palate. The velum (soft palate) moves posteriorly during swallowing and speech, thereby separating the oropharynx from the nasopharynx. Velopharyngeal insufficiency exists when this separation is incomplete, which may occur after cleft palate repair or adenoidectomy (usually transient). In severe cases, nasopharyngeal regurgitation of food may occur. In milder cases, the only manifestation may be hypernasal speech as a result of the nasal emission of air during phonation. If a bifid uvula is present, one should palpate the palate carefully for the presence of a submucous cleft

KEY POINTS: LANGUAGE DEVELOPMENT

1. Very red flags: No meaningful words by 18 months or no meaningful phrases by 2 years.

2. Intelligibility should increase yearly by 25%, from 25% at 1 year of age up to 100% at 4 years of age.

3. Stuttering is common in younger children, but beyond the age of 5–6 years, it warrants speech evaluation.

4. Autism, MR, and cerebral palsy can present with speech delay.

5. Evaluation of hearing is mandatory in any setting of significant speech delay.

80. **When is stuttering abnormal?**
Stuttering is a common characteristic of the speech of preschool children. However, the vast majority of children do not persist with stuttering beyond 5 or 6 years of age. Preschoolers at increased risk for persistence of stuttering include those with a positive family history of stuttering and those with anxiety-provoking stress related to talking. A child older than 5 or

6 years who stutters should be referred to a speech-language pathologist for assessment and treatment.

81. **What advice should be given to parents of a child who stutters?**
   - Do not give the child directives about how to deal with his or her speech (e.g., "Slow down" or "Take a breath").
   - Provide a relaxed, easy speech model in your own manner of speaking to the child.
   - Reduce the need/expectations for the child to speak to strangers, adults, or authority figures or to compete with others (such as siblings) to be heard.
   - Listen attentively to the child with patience and without showing concern.
   - Seek professional guidance if speech is not noticeably more fluent in 2–3 months.

82. **Which infants with "tongue tie" should have surgical correction?**

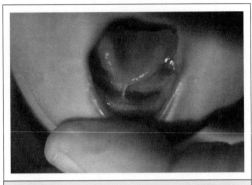

Figure 2-5. Newborn with ankyloglossia. (From Clark DA: Atlas of Neonatology. Philadelphia, W.B. Saunders, 2000, p 146.)

"Tongue tie," or **partial ankyloglossia**, is the restriction of mobility of the tongue due to a short or thickened lingual frenulum (Fig. 2-5). In theory, partial ankyloglossia can interfere with breast feeding and speech. The vast majority of infants (particularly those who can extend the tip of the tongue past the lips) accommodate and eventually develop normal lingual mobility. Indications for surgical correction are imprecise, but children with persistent speech problems after 2–4 years should be considered.

Ballard JL, Auer CE, Khoury JC: Ankyloglossia: Assessment, incidence, and effect of frenuloplasty on the breastfeeding dyad. Pediatrics 110:e63, 2002.
Lalakea ML, Messner AH: Ankyloglossia: does it matter? Pediatr Clin North Am 50:381–397, 2003.

83. **What are the autism spectrum disorders?**
Also called pervasive developmental disorders, these are five conditions (as listed in DSM-IV-TR) that are characterized by problems with social interaction, verbal and nonverbal communication, and repetitive behaviors with varying degrees of severity. They include the following (1) autistic disorder (autism); (2) Asperger syndrome; (3) Rett syndrome; (4) childhood disintegrative disorder (Heller syndrome); and (5) pervasive developmental disorder, not otherwise specified.

American Psychiatric Association. Diagnosis and Statistical Manual of Mental Disorders: DSM-IV-TR. Washington, DC: American Psychiatric Association, 2000.
Autism Society of America: www.autism-society.org

KEY POINTS: THREE ESSENTIAL FEATURES OF AUTISM

1. Impaired social interaction

2. Absent or abnormal speech and language development

3. Narrow range of interest and stereotyped or repetitive responses to objects

84. **What are the three essential features of autism?**
    - Impaired social interaction (extreme aloneness, failure to make eye contact)
    - Absent or abnormal speech and language development
    - Narrow range of interest and stereotyped or repetitive responses to objects

85. **Which behaviors of children should arouse suspicion of possible autism?**
    - Avoidance of eye contact during infancy
    - Relating to only part of a person's body (e.g., the lap) rather than to the whole person
    - Failure to acquire speech or speech acquisition in an unusual manner (e.g., echolalia [repeating another person's speech])
    - Repetition of television commercials and singing out of context and without communicative purpose
    - Spending long periods of time in repetitive activities and fascination with movement (e.g., spinning records, dripping water)
    - Interest in small visual details or patterns
    - Unusual abilities (e.g., early letter and number recognition)
    - Early reading with minimal comprehension
    - Absence of pointing to show or request something
    - Excessively lining up toys or other objects

    Coplan J: Counseling parents regarding prognosis in autistic spectrum disorder. Pediatrics 105:e65, 2000.

86. **What distinguishes Asperger syndrome from autism?**
    Asperger syndrome is commonly referred to as a "higher-functioning autism." Problems with social interactions and stereotypical behaviors exist, but patients with this condition have no clinically significant delay of language development. Unlike patients with autistic disorder—many of whom have MR and learn best by rote memorization—patients with Asperger syndrome usually do not have mental handicaps and can engage in more abstract thinking.

87. **What conditions are associated with autism?**
    - MR (about 25% with an intelligence quotient [IQ] of >70)
    - Seizures (up to 25%)
    - Fragile X syndrome (2–5%)
    - Tuberous sclerosis (1–4%)

88. **What laboratory evaluations should be considered in the evaluation of a child with suspected autism?**
    - **Metabolic screening:** Urine for organic acids, serum for lactate, amino acids, ammonia, and very-long-chain fatty acids (if developmental regression, MR, dysmorphic features, hypotonia, vomiting/dehydration, or feeding intolerance)
    - **Chromosomal analysis** (if dysmorphic features or MR)
    - **DNA fragile X analysis** (if MR)
    - **Electroencephalogram** (especially in patients with staring spells to rule-out absence seizures)
    - **Neuroimaging with MRI** (especially if abnormal head shape or circumference, focal neurologic abnormalities, or seizures)
    - **Lead level** (if history of pica)

    Roberts G, Palfrey JS, Bridgemohan C: A rational approach to the medical evaluation of a child with developmental delay. Contemp Pediatr 21:76–100, 2004.

MENTAL RETARDATION

89. **How is MR defined?**
    This condition is defined as significantly subaverage intellectual functioning (−2 standard deviations on a standardized measure) **plus** deficits in two or more of the following areas:

communication, self-care, home living, social skills, community use, self-direction, health, or safety. The American Association on Mental Retardation stipulates that this definition "refers to . . . limitations in *present functioning*" [emphasis added], thereby stripping the definition of MR of prognostic value. In fact, however, IQ and adaptive scores show sufficient stability over time (especially among individuals functioning in the mentally retarded range) that the diagnosis of MR does, in fact, carry prognostic value as well.

Batshaw ML: Mental retardation. Pediatr Clin North Am 40:507–522, 1993.

Gillberg C: Practitioner review: Physical investigations in mental retardation. J Child Psych Psychiatr 38:889–897, 1997.

90. **How is intelligence classified with IQ scores?**
Most IQ tests are constructed to yield a mean IQ of 100 and a standard deviation of 15 points (Table 2-7).

TABLE 2-7. CONSTRUCTION OF INTELLIGENCE QUOTIENT SCORES		
Intelligence quotient	**Standard deviation**	**Category**
>130	>+2	Very superior
116–130	+1 to +2	High average to superior
115–85	Mean ± 1	Average
84–70	−1 to −2	Low average to borderline MR
69–55	−2 to −3	Mild MR
54–40	−3 to −4	Moderate MR
39–25	−4 to −5	Severe MR
<25	<−5	Profound MR

91. **What features can indicate cognitive problems in infants and young children?**
In younger infants and toddlers, fine motor skill development and especially language development are the usual best correlates of cognitive achievement. As the child ages, the various milestones can be evaluated. Significant sequential delay should warrant referral for formal developmental testing to evaluate the possibility of MR (Table 2-8).

First LR, Palfrey JS: The infant or young child with developmental delay. N Engl J Med 330: 478–483, 1994.

TABLE 2-8. SIGNS OF SEQUENTIAL DELAY IN COGNITIVE ACHIEVEMENT	
2–3 months	Not alerting to mother with special interest
6–7 months	Not searching for dropped object
8–9 months	No interest in peek-a-boo
12 months	Does not search for hidden object
15–18 months	No interest in cause-and-effect games
2 years	Does not categorize similarities (e.g., animals versus vehicles)
3 years	Does not know own full name
4 years	Cannot pick shorter or longer of two lines
4½ years	Cannot count sequentially
5 years	Does not know colors or any letters
5½ years	Does not know own birthday or address

92. **What findings in a child with MR should prompt a cranial MRI?**
   - Cerebral palsy or motor asymmetry
   - Multiple somatic anomalies
   - Abnormal head size or shape
   - Neurocutaneous findings
   - Craniofacial malformation
   - Seizures
   - Loss or plateau of developmental skills
   - IQ <50

   Palmer FB, Capute AJ: Mental retardation. Pediatr Rev 15:473–479, 1994.

93. **Worldwide, what is the most common preventable cause of MR?**
   Iodine deficiency leads to maternal and fetal hypothyroxinemia during gestation, which causes brain developmental injury. Severe endemic iodine deficiency can cause cretinism (characterized by deaf-mutism, severe intellectual deficiency, and often hypothyroidism) and may occur in 2–10% of isolated world communities. Moderate iodine deficiency, which is even more common, leads to milder degrees of cognitive impairment.

   Cao XY, Jiang XM, Dou ZH, et al: Timing of vulnerability of the brain to iodine deficiency in endemic cretinism. N Engl J Med 331:1739–1744, 1994.

PSYCHIATRIC DISORDERS

94. **What is the prevalence of childhood psychiatric disorders?**
   Overall, 15–20% of children 4–20 years old in community samples are diagnosed with a specific psychiatric disorder. The most common disorders are as follows:
   - Attention deficit hyperactivity disorder (4–10%)
   - Separation anxiety (3–5%)
   - Oppositional disorder (5–10%)
   - Overanxious disorder (2–5%)
   - Conduct disorder (1–5%)
   - Depression (2–6%)

   National Institute of Mental Health: www.nimh.nih.gov

95. **If a parent has an affective disorder, what is the likelihood that an offspring will have similar problems?**
   Approximately 20–25% of these children will develop a major affective disorder, and as many as 40–45% will have a psychiatric problem.

96. **How does mania differ in children and adolescents?**
   Mania occurs in approximately 0.5–1% of adolescents and occurs less frequently in prepubertal children. **Younger children** may present with extreme irritability, emotional lability, and aggression. Dysphoria, hypomania, and agitation may be intermixed. Hyperactivity, distractibility, and pressured speech often occur in all age groups. Symptoms in **adolescents** more closely resemble those seen in adults. They include elated mood, flight of ideas, sleeplessness, bizarre behavior, delusions of grandeur, paranoia, and euphoria.

97. **What ritualistic behaviors are common in children with obsessive-compulsive disorder?**
   The most common rituals involve excessive cleaning, repeating gross motor rituals (e.g., going up and down stairs), and repetitive checking behaviors (e.g., checking that doors are locked or that homework is correct). Obsessions most commonly deal with fear of contamination. Symptoms tend to wax and wane in severity, and the specific obsessions or

compulsions change over time. Most children attempt to disguise their rituals. Anxiety and distress that interfere with school or family life can occur when children fail in their efforts to resist the thoughts or activities. Counseling and serotonin-reuptake-inhibiting medications (e.g., clomipramine, fluoxetine, sertraline, paroxetine, fluvoxamine, citalopram) can be beneficial.

Lewin AB, Storch EA, Adkins J, et al: Current directions in pediatric obsessive-compulsive disorder. Pediatr Ann 34:128–137, 2005.

98. **What distinguishes a conduct disorder from an oppositional defiant disorder?**
Both are disruptive behavior disorders of childhood and early adolescence. **Conduct disorder** is the more serious disorder in that it is diagnosed when the child's behaviors violate the rights of others (e.g., assault) or are in conflict with major societal norms (e.g., stealing, truancy, setting fires). Children with conduct disorder are at risk for developing the antisocial personality disorder seen in adults. **Oppositional defiant disorder** is characterized by recurrent negative and defiant behaviors toward authority figures.

99. **What are common symptoms of depression in children and adolescents?**
- Sadness
- School problems
- Tearfulness
- Somatic complaints
- Irritability
- Suicidal ideation
- Negative self-imagery
- Changes in appetite
- Lack of concentration
- Unintended weight changes
- Decreased interest in usual activities
- Sleep problems, including hypersomnia
- Fatigue
- Delusions

100. **How is depression in children diagnosed?**
The DSM-IV-TR criteria require the presence of five or more symptoms from the categories of sleep, interest, guilt, concentration, appetite, psychomotor, and suicide during the same 2-week period. A variety of ratings scales (e.g., the Hamilton Depression Rating Scale, the Childhood Depression Inventory, the Child Behavioral Checklist) are available to assist with evaluation.

101. **What are treatments for major depressive disorder in children and adolescents?**
Psychotherapy: Various types of therapy may be used, including cognitive-behavioral therapy, interpersonal therapy, and family therapy.
Psychopharmacology: Selective serotonin-reuptake inhibitors have been recommended by the American Academy of Child and Adolescent Psychiatry as the treatment of choice for children who warrant pharmacotherapy. There have been warnings by regulatory agencies in Britain and the United States that one of these drugs (paroxetine) may be associated with an increased risk of suicide.
Electroconvulsive therapy: This treatment is reserved for psychotic or life-threatening depression that is unresponsive to other treatments.

National Institute of Mental Health. Antidepressant medications for children and adolescents: Information for parents and caregivers. Available at http://www.nimh.nih.gov/healthinformation/antidepressant_child.cfm

Vitiello B, Swedo S: Antidepressant medications in children. N Engl J Med 350:1489–1491, 2004.

102. Are any laboratory tests indicated in the evaluation of possible depression in children?

Depending on the history and the physical examination, laboratory and radiographic studies may be indicated if an organic cause of symptoms is suspected. Thyroid function studies, a complete blood count to evaluate for anemia, pregnancy testing in postpubertal girls, and toxicology testing (if drug abuse is suspected) should be considered.

> Varley CK: Don't overlook depression in youth. Contemp Ped 19:70–76, 2002.

103. What are types of anxiety disorders in children?

Separation anxiety disorder: Developmentally inappropriate, unrealistic, persistent fears of separation from caregivers that interfere with daily activities

Panic disorder: Recurrent, discrete periods of intense fear or discomfort; rare in prepubertal children; may occur with or without *agoraphobia* (fear/distress in or about places that may limit egress, such as a restaurant)

Social anxiety disorder: Extreme anxiety about social interactions with peers and adults; may manifest as generalized or specific (e.g., public speaking)

PSYCHOSOCIAL FAMILY ISSUES

104. How likely is it that children in the United States will experience the separation or divorce of their parents?

More than 50% of first marriages end in divorce. In the United States, about 1.5 million children experience parental divorce each year. It is estimated that nearly 75% of black children and 40% of white children born to married parents will experience their parents' divorce before they are 18 years old. An addition to this stressor is that 50% of individuals who divorce will remarry within 5 years, thus creating another major family transition for a child.

105. How do children of different ages vary in their response to parental divorce?

Preschool age (2½–5 years): Most likely to show regression in developmental milestones (e.g., toilet training); irritability; sleep disturbances; preoccupation with fear of abandonment; demanding with remaining parent

Early school age (6–8 years): Most likely to demonstrate open grieving; preoccupied with fear of rejection and of being replaced; half may have a decrease in school performance

Later school age (9–12 years): More likely to demonstrate profound anger at one or both parents; more likely to distinguish one parent as the culprit causing the divorce; deterioration in school performance and peer relationships; sense of loneliness and powerlessness

Adolescence: Significant potential for acute depression and even suicidal ideation; acting-out behavior (substance abuse, truancy, sexual activity); self-doubts about own potential for marital success

> Hetherington EM: Divorce and the adjustment of children. Pediatr Rev 26:163–169,2005.
> Kelly JB: Children's adjustment in conflicted marriage and divorce: A decade review of research .I Am Acad Child Adolesc Psychiatry 39:963–973, 2000.

106. What factors are central to a good outcome after a divorce?

- Ability of parents to set aside or resolve conflicts without involving children
- Emotional and physical availability of custodial parent to the child
- Parenting skills of custodial parent
- Extent to which child does not feel rejected by noncustodial parent
- Child's temperament
- Presence of supportive family network
- Absence of continuing anger or depression in the child

> Cohen GJ: Helping children deal with divorce and separation. Pediatrics 110:1019–1023, 2002.
> Wallerstein JS: Separation, divorce, and remarriage. In Levine MD, Carey W, Crocker A (eds): Developmental-Behavioral Pediatrics, 3rd ed. Philadelphia, W.B. Saunders, 1999, pp 149–161.

107. **What is the "vulnerable child syndrome"?**

The *vulnerable child syndrome* is characterized by excessive parental concern about the health and development of their child. It usually occurs after a medical illness in which the parents are understandably upset or worried about the child's health (e.g., prematurity, congenital heart disease). However, this concern persists despite the child's recovery. Problems of the syndrome can include pathologic separation difficulties for parent and child, sleep problems, overprotectiveness, and overindulgence. Children are at risk for behavior, school, and peer-relationship problems.

108. **How does the cognitive understanding of death evolve?**

Toddler (<3 years): Death as separation, abandonment, or change

Preschool (3–6 years): Prelogical thought with magical and egocentric beliefs that the child may be responsible for the death; death as temporary and reversible

School-age (6–11 years): Concrete logical thinking; death as permanent and universal but due to a specific illness or injury rather than as a biologic process; death is something that occurs to others

Adolescence (≥12 years): Abstract logical thinking; more complete comprehension of death; death as a possibility for self

American Academy of Pediatrics. Committee on Psychosocial Aspects of Child and Family Health: The pediatrician and childhood bereavement. Pediatrics 105:445–447, 2000.

109. **Should adopted children be informed of their adoption?**

Yes. It should not occur as a one-time event, but rather increasing amounts of information can be given over time. Most preschool children will not understand the process or meaning of adoption, and for them disclosure should be guided by what the child wants to know. School-age children should be aware of their adoption and feel comfortable discussing it with their parents.

Borchers D; American Academy of Pediatrics Committee on Early Childhood, Adoption, and Dependent Care: Families and adoption: The pediatrician's role in supporting communication. Pediatrics 112:1437–1441, 2003.

110. **How common is domestic violence?**

Statistics indicate that 10–40% of families are afflicted by domestic violence. The potential impact on children in these families is enormous, including behavioral problems, developmental delay, and abuse. The American Academy of Pediatrics has recommended that all pediatricians incorporate screening for domestic violence as part of anticipatory guidance.

Parkinson GW, Adams RC, Emerling FG: Maternal domestic violence screening in an office-based pediatric practice. Pediatrics 108:e43–e51, 2001.

111. **Does participation in day care during infancy and the toddler years have negative effects on cognitive development?**

This question has been examined in a large multisite study funded by the National Institute of Child Health and Human Development. At 24 and 36 months of age, there has been no demonstrable relationship between the number of hours in day care and any of the measures of cognitive or language development. However, child care of higher quality was associated with better language and cognitive outcomes. The frequency of language stimulation in the child care setting seemed to be the most important variable.

112. **Who are "latchkey" children?**

The term refers to the millions of children <18 years old who are in unsupervised care after school because they are members of families in which one or two parents work. Because of the enormous variability of circumstances, the consequences may be positive (e.g., increased maturity, self-reliance) or negative (e.g., isolation, feelings of neglect). Increased after-school programs may minimize negative consequences.

113. **What are the effects of heavy television watching in children?**

At one point or another, television viewing has been blamed for many of the problems facing children today. Studies have documented the effects of heavy television viewing in the following areas: increased aggressive behavior, increase in general level of arousal, desensitization to violence, increased obesity, and decreased school performance. There does not seem to be a large effect of television viewing on cognition or attention.

SCHOOL PROBLEMS

114. **How is "learning disability" (LD) defined?**

The term dates back to 1963, when Dr. Samuel Kirk first used it to refer to children with normal intelligence who had difficulties with learning academic skills. Various definitions have since been proposed; a currently accepted one was proposed by the National Joint Committee on Learning Disabilities (NJCLD) in 1990. According to the NJCLD, the term "refers to a heterogenous group of disorders manifest by significant difficulties in the acquisition and the use of listening, speaking, reading, writing, reasoning, or mathematics abilities." The NJCLD notes that these disorders are lifelong and "intrinsic to the individual." Such difficulties are not due to visual, hearing, or motor handicaps; emotional problems; MR; or environmental, social, cultural, or economic issues.

National Joint Committee on Learning Disabilities. Learning disabilities: Issues on definition. ASHA Suppl 5:18–20, 1991.

115. **How are the LDs classified?**

Various classification systems have been proposed. DSM-IV-TR lists four types of LDs: reading, mathematics, writing, and "not otherwise specified." Often a distinction is made between verbal (language) and nonverbal (performance) abilities, but there can be considerable overlap in a child. Social-emotional disabilities are often considered part of the nonverbal grouping. Neuropsychologists investigate the role of specific brain processes (e.g., memory, attention, phonemic awareness) in creating difficulties for children with learning disabilities.

Capin DM: Developmental learning disorders: Clues to their diagnosis and management. Pediatr Rev 17:284–290, 1996.

116. **What distinguishes dyslexia, dyscalculia, and dysgraphia?**

Dyslexia is a reading LD. It is the most common LD, affecting 5–17% of school-aged children. Characterized by problems decoding single words, it is usually the result of deficits in phonological processing. Reading disabilities are heritable in many cases, although the mode of transmission appears variable; linkage studies have found loci on chromosomes 1 and 6.

Dyscalculia, or specific mathematics disability, affects 1–6% of children. Mathematics disabilities involve difficulties in computation, math concepts, and/or the application of those concepts to everyday situations.

Dysgraphia, or disorder of written expression, affects 2–8% of children. Difficulties with writing have several possible etiologies, including problems with fine motor control, linguistic abilities, visual-spatial skills, attention, memory, and sequencing.

Beitchman JH, Young AR: Learning disorders with a special emphasis on reading disorders: A review of the past 10 years. J Am Acad Child Adolesc Psychiatry 36:1020–1032, 1997.

Shaywitz SE, Shaywitz BA: Dyslexia. Pediatr Rev 24:147–152, 2003.

117. **In addition to learning disabilities, what factors may contribute to academic underachievement?**
- Hearing or visual problems
- MR
- Developmental language disorders
- ADHD

- Emotional/psychiatric disorders
- Disorganized home environment
- Lack of social support
- Sleep problems
- Chronic medical conditions
- Medications (e.g., anticonvulsants, antihistamines)

118. Is waiting to start school until a child is older a problem?

Although parents and schools often want to delay the start of school for children who have difficulty learning academic skills or who have problems with behavioral regulation, studies suggest that this is not usually an effective intervention. If delayed school entry results in a child being older than most classmates, this has been associated with later behavioral and school problems.

119. Is the term "school phobia" outdated?

Yes. There are multiple reasons why children refuse to go to school, and most of them are not related to phobias. Both separation anxiety disorder and generalized anxiety disorder are associated with school avoidance in children and should be considered. Depression, learning problems, and family stressors may also contribute to refusal to go to school. Understanding these underlying factors is important for developing an intervention that is likely to be successful.

Fremont WP: School refusal in children and adolescents. Am Fam Physician 68:1555–1564, 2003.

120. How much of a problem are bullies?

Bullying is defined as "intentional, unprovoked abuse of power by one or more children to inflict pain or cause distress to another child on repeated occasions." It is a universal problem in schools worldwide. The victims frequently experience a range of psychological, psychosomatic, and behavioral problems that include anxiety, insecurity, low self-esteem, sleeping difficulties, bedwetting, sadness, and frequent bouts of headache and abdominal pain.

Lyznicki JM, McCaffree MA, Robinowitz CB: Childhood bullying: Implications for physicians. Am Fam Physician 70:1723–1728, 2004.

Nansel TR, Overpeck M, Pilla RS, et al: Bullying behaviors among US youth: Prevalence and association with psychosocial adjustment. JAMA 285:2094–2100, 2001.

SLEEP PROBLEMS

121. What is the average daily sleep requirement by age?

- Birth: 16 hours
- 6 months: 14.5 hours
- 12 months: 13.5 hours
- 2 years: 13 hours
- 4 years: 11.5 hours
- 6 years: 9.5 hours
- 12 years: 8.5 hours
- 18 years: 8 hours

122. What are the effects of sleep deprivation on humans?

Decreased attention, decreased motivation, increased problems with emotional self-regulation, and problems with short-term memory and memory consolidation. In preschoolers, the amount of night and 24-hour sleep is clearly related to daytime behavior problems. Sleeping less at night is correlated with "acting out" behaviors: hyperactivity, oppositional or noncompliant behavior, and aggression (i.e., externalizing behavior problems). No relationship has been noted between sleep and internalizing behavior problems (e.g., anxiety) in younger children.

Lavigne JV, Arend R, Rosenbaum D, et al: Sleep and behavior problems among preschoolers. J Dev Behav Pediatr 20:164–169, 1999.

123. **Why is the supine sleeping position recommended for infants?**
In countries that have advocated the supine sleeping position as a preventive measure for sudden infant death syndrome (SIDS), there have been dramatic decreases in the incidence of the syndrome. Hypotheses on why the prone position is more dangerous for infants have included the potential for airway obstruction and the possibility of rebreathing carbon dioxide, particularly when soft bedding is used.

124. **When do infants begin to sleep through the night?**
By the time they are about 3 months old, approximately 70% of infants (slightly more for bottle-fed babies and slightly less for breast-fed babies) will not cry or awaken their parents between midnight and 6 AM. By 6 months, 90% of infants fit into this category, but between 6 and 9 months, the percentage of infants with night awakenings increases.

125. **What advice to parents may minimize the problem of night waking?**
   - After a parent-child bedtime routine, place the infant in the sleep setting while he or she is still awake (i.e., do not rock an infant to sleep).
   - The parent should not be present as the child falls asleep.
   - Gradually eliminate night feedings (infants by 6 months receive sufficient daytime nutrition to allow this).
   - Transitional objects (e.g., blanket, teddy bear) may minimize separation issues.
   - Create a consistent sleep schedule and a bedtime routine.
   - Avoid giving a child items in late afternoon or evening that contain caffeine (e.g., chocolate, soda).

   Meltzer LJ, Mindell JA: Nonpharmacologic treatments for pediatric sleeplessness. Pediatr Clin North Am 51:135–151, 2004.

126. **What are the pros and cons of co-sleeping among parents and children?**
Co-sleeping (or bed sharing) is a practice that has much variance worldwide. In the United States, it varies widely by race.
Pros: A more natural process; may promote breast feeding; may foster a greater sense of connection between child and family
Cons: May inhibit the development of self-soothing skills in infants; may be overstimulating (emotionally and sexually) to older children; risk factor for infant death from entrapment of infant in adult bed or suffocation from overlaying adult

   Riter S, Wills L: Sleep wars: Research and opinion. Pediatr Clin North Am 51:1–13, 2004.
   Willinger M, Ko CW, Hoffman HJ, et al; National Infant Sleep Position study: Trends in infant bed sharing in the United States, 1993-2000: The National Infant Sleep Position study. Arch Pediatr Adolesc Med 157:43–49, 2003.

127. **How common are sleep problems in elementary school-aged children?**
Approximately 40% of children between 7 and 12 years old experience sleep-onset delay, 10% experience night awakening, and 10% have significant daytime sleepiness. Some studies have shown that the extent of sleep is also inversely related to teacher reported psychiatric symptoms.

   Aronen ET, Paavonen EJ, Fjallberg M, et al: Sleep and psychiatric symptoms in school-age children. J Am Acad Child Adolesc Psychiatr 39:502–508, 2000.
   Owens JA: Sleep habits and sleep disturbances in elementary school-aged children. J Dev Behav Pediatr 21:27–36, 2000.

128. **What are parasomnias?**
Parasomnias are undesirable physical phenomena that occur during sleep. Examples include night terrors, nightmares, sleepwalking, sleeptalking, nocturnal enuresis, sleep bruxism, somniloquy, and body rocking. Between the ages of 3 and 13 years, nearly 80% of all children will have had at least one parasomnia.

   Laberge L, Tremblay RE, Vitaro F, Montplaisir J: Development of parasomnias from childhood to early adolescence. Pediatrics 106(1 Pt 1):67–74, 2000.

129. **At what age do sleepwalking and sleeptalking occur?**

    Sleepwalking occurs most commonly between the ages of 5 and 10 years. As many as 15% of children between the ages of 5 and 12 years may have somnambulated once, and as many as 10% of 3- to 10-year-old children may sleepwalk regularly. The sleepwalking child is clumsy, restless, and walking without purpose, and the episode is not remembered. Injury is common during this outing. **Sleeptalking** is monosyllabic and often incomprehensible. Both conditions usually end before the age of 15 years. Severe cases may benefit from diazepam or imipramine therapy.

130. **What is the difference between nightmares and night terrors?**

    Nightmares are frightening dreams that occur during rapid eye movement (REM) sleep (usually during the last half of the night) and that may be readily recalled on awakening. The child is aroused without difficulty and is usually easily consolable, but returning to sleep after a nightmare may be problematic.

    Night terrors are brief episodes that occur during non-REM stage IV sleep. They usually last 30 seconds to 5 minutes, during which a child sits up, screams, and appears aroused, often staring and sweating profusely. The child cannot be consoled, rapidly goes back to sleep, and does not recall the episode in the morning. The onset of night terrors in an older child or persistent multiple attacks may indicate more serious psychopathology.

131. **What recommendation should be given to a parent whose child is having night terrors?**

    An explanation of the phenomenon to the parent, with emphasis on the fact that the child is still asleep during the episode and should not be awakened, is all that is needed. If stress or sleep deprivation coincide with the night terrors, these factors should be addressed. If this is not successful, other approaches may be considered.

    - When night terrors occur at the same time each night, the parent may awaken the child 15 minutes before the anticipated event over a 7-day period and keep him or her awake for at least 5 minutes. This often disrupts the sleep cycle and results in resolution of the problem.
    - Rarely, for severe night terrors, a short course of diazepam will suppress REM sleep, reset the sleep cycles, and result in cessation of the problem.

VISUAL DEVELOPMENT/DISORDERS

132. **How well does a newborn see?**

    Because of the short diameter of the eye as well as retinal immaturity, a newborn's visual acuity is roughly 20/200 to 20/400. The human face is the most preferred object of fixation during early infancy. The light sense is one of the most primitive of all visual functions and is present by the 7th fetal month.

133. **Do babies make tears?**

    Alacrima, or the absence of tear secretion, is not uncommon during the newborn period, although some infants may produce reflexive tearing at birth. In most others, tearing is delayed and typically not seen until the infant is 2–4 months old. Persistent lack of tearing is seen in Riley-Day syndrome (familial dysautonomia). This is a rare genetic syndrome seen in the Ashkenazi Jewish population, affecting 1 in 10,000 newborns. Other symptoms include diaphoresis, skin blotching or marbling, hyporeflexia, and indifference to pain.

134. **At what age does an infant's eye color assume its permanent color?**

    A neonate's eyes will never be lighter than they are at birth. The pigmentation of the iris in all races increases over the first 6–12 months. The eye color is usually defined by 6 months and always by 1 year.

135. **A 2-week-old infant with intermittent eye discharge and clear conjunctiva has what likely diagnosis?**
Nasolacrimal duct obstruction, seen in roughly 5% of newborns, is typically due to an intermittent blockage at the lower end of the duct. Massaging the area and watchful waiting are generally all that is needed. Almost all cases (95%) resolve by 6 months, and a few resolve thereafter. Ophthalmologic referral during the first 6 months is usually unnecessary, unless there are multiple episodes of acute dacryocystitis or a large congenital mucocele. Most ophthalmologists advise referral between 6 and 13 months, because during this period simple probing of the duct is curative in 95% of patients. After 13 months, the cure rate by probing alone falls to 75%, and silicone intubation of the duct is often necessary.

Chiesi C, Guerra R, Longanesi L, et al: Congenital nasolacrimal duct obstruction: Therapeutic management J Pediatr Ophthalmol Strabismus 36:326–330, 1999.

136. **What is normal visual acuity for children?**
Birth–6 months: Gradually improves from 20/400 to 20/80
6 months–3 years: Improves from 20/80 to 20/50
2–5 years: Improves to 20/40 or better, with a <2-line difference between
                                      left and right eyes on visual charts
>5 years: 20/30 or better, with a <2-line difference between eyes on visual charts
        It should be noted that almost 20% of the pediatric population require eyeglasses for correction of refractive errors before adulthood.

137. **When do binocular fixation and depth perception develop in children?**
Binocularity of vision depends primarily on the adequate coordination of the extraocular muscles and is normally established by 3–6 months of age. At about 6–8 months, early evidence of depth perception is seen, but it is still poorly developed. Depth perception becomes very accurate at 6 or 7 years and continues to improve through the early teenage years.

Hartmann EE, Dobson V, Hainline L, et al: Preschool vision screening: Summary of a Task Force report. Behalf of the Maternal and Child Health Bureau and the National Eye Institute Task Force on Vision Screening in the Preschool Child. Pediatrics 106:1105–1115, 2000.

138. **How does refractive capacity vary with age?**
The newborn infant is typically slightly hyperopic (farsighted). The mild hyperopia actually increases slowly for about the first 8 years. It then decreases gradually until adolescence, when vision is emmetropic (no refractive error). After 20 years, there is a tendency for myopia (nearsightedness).

139. **How are the degrees of blindness classified?**
The World Health Organization defines blindness as follows:
Visual impairment: Snellen visual acuity of ≤20/60 (best eye corrected)
Social blindness: Snellen visual acuity of ≤20/200 or a visual field of ≤20°
Virtual blindness: Snellen visual acuity of <20/1200 or a visual field of ≤10°
Total blindness: No light perception

140. **What is strabismus?**
Strabismus is the misalignment of the eyes with either an in-turning (esotropia), out-turning (exotropia), or up-turning (hypertropia) of one eye.

141. **A 2-month-old baby is noted to have eyes that appear to turn outward rather than looking forward. Is this strabismus?**
Yes, but intervention is not needed unless the symptom persists beyond 3–4 months of age. Strabismus is defined as any deviation from perfect ocular alignment. However, the majority of infants will be found to have an **exodeviated** alignment (i.e., looking somewhat out) rather than

an **orthotropic** (i.e., straight) alignment. The majority of infants will become orthotropic by the time they are 4 months old.

Infants do not focus well because the macula and fovea are poorly developed at birth. Therefore, it is not uncommon for infants to occasionally have an inward crossing of the eyes or for their eyes to be turned slightly outward to 10° or 15°. Persistent in-turning of the eyes for more than a few seconds or outward deviation of >10–15° requires ophthalmologic referral.

142. **Name the most common types of childhood strabismus.**
- **Strabismus of visual deprivation** occurs when normal vision in one or both eyes is disrupted by any cause. The most serious varieties occur with tumors (e.g., retinoblastoma). In children with ocular tumors, strabismus may be the presenting sign.
- **Infantile** or **congenital esotropia** occurs within the first few months of life, usually as an isolated conditions. Corrective surgery is usually required.
- **Accommodative esotropia** commonly occurs between the ages of 2 and 4 years in very farsighted (hyperopic) children. These children use extra lens accommodation because of their visual problems, which leads to persistent convergence. Eyeglasses to correct the hyperopia usually correct the esotropia.
- **Childhood exotropia** appears between the ages of 2 and 5 years as intermittent misalignment that is often brought on by fatigue, visual inattention, or bright sunlight. There is a strong hereditary component. Surgery is often necessary after the correction of refractive errors and the elimination of any pathology that might have caused visual deprivation.

Trobe J: Physician's Guide to Eye Care, 2nd ed. San Francisco, Foundation of the American Academy of Ophthalmology, 2001.

143. **What separates pseudostrabismus from true strabismus?**
Often a cause of unnecessary ophthalmologic referrals, *pseudostrabismus* is the appearance of ocular misalignment (usually esotropia) that occurs in children with a broad and flat nasal bridge and prominent epicanthal folds. The iris appears to be shifted to the midline, with differing amounts of white sclera on each side (Fig. 2-6). This is a common condition that may occur in up to 30% of newborns. No treatment is required. It may be distinguished from true esotropia (or strabismus) by the observation of full extraocular movements, by symmetric reflections of a flashlight on the cornea from a distance of about 12 inches (although this test as a measure of strabismus is more accurate in infants ≥6 months old), and by normal visualization of red reflexes by direct ophthalmoscopy.

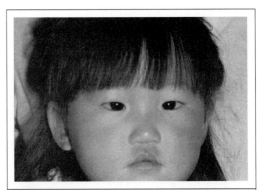

Figure 2-6. Pseudoesotropia. Note that the wide nasal bridge and prominent epicanthal folds create the illusion of an esotropia. The corneal light reflexes are centered in each eye; therefore, the eyes are straight. (From Gault JA: Ophthalmology Pearls. Philadelphia, Hanley & Belfus, 2003, p 45.)

Ticho BH: Strabismus. Pediatr Clin North Am 50:173–188, 2003.

144. **What is amblyopia?**
Amblyopia refers to decreased visual acuity in one eye that is not correctable by glasses and is a result of decreased visual stimulation of that eye. The visual cortex adheres to the concept of "use it or lose it." Amblyopia is the most common cause of vision loss in children <6 years old, and it occurs in 1–2% of this age group and 2–2.5% of the general population.

145. **What are the causes of amblyopia?**
- **Strabismus:** Input from one eye is suppressed to avoid double vision.
- **Anisometropic amblyopia:** Significant refraction differences cause the suppression of images from the weaker eye.
- **Deprivation:** Images received are unclear (e.g., from congenital cataracts or ptosis).
- **Occlusion amblyopia:** This is typically iatrogenic. Prolonged covering of the preferred eye as a treatment for amblyopia can cause changes in visual acuity in the preferred eye.

    Mittelman D: Amblyopia. Pediatr Clin North Am 50:189–196, 2003.

146. **How are cataracts diagnosed during the newborn period?**
By an abnormal red reflex. A black or white reflex, partial or complete, or asymmetry between the two eyes should prompt referral to an ophthalmologist.

147. **Why is early diagnosis and treatment critical for patients with congenital cataracts?**
Delay in treatment can lead to irreversible vision loss as a result of deprivation amblyopia. Cataracts undiagnosed for as little as 4–8 weeks after birth can result in permanent deficits. In general, the younger the child, the more urgent the need for evaluation if cataracts are suspected.

148. **What is ectopia lentis?**
Ectopia lentis refers to the displacement or dislocation of the lens. It may be due to trauma, but it has also been associated with systemic diseases such as Marfan syndrome, homocystinuria, and congenital syphilis.

149. **What diseases may present with a white pupil?**
Leukocoria, or white pupil, may be a result of any mass behind the pupillary space. This includes cataracts, retinoblastoma, and infants with retinopathy of prematurity that develop retinal detachment.

150. **How common are unequally sized pupils?**
Up to 20% of the normal population can have **physiologic anisocoria** (inequality of pupil size) of up to 2 mm. The percentage of difference remains the same in bright or dim lighting.

151. **Is heterochromia normal?**
Yes, if it is an isolated finding. Heterochromia, or different colored irises, can be a familial autosomal dominant trait. It is also seen in some syndromes (e.g., Waardenburg, Horner). However, changes in color can occur from trauma, hemorrhage, inflammation (uveitis, iridocyclitis), malignancy (retinoblastoma, neuroblastoma), glaucoma, or after intraocular surgery.

KEY POINTS: VISION

1. Red reflex testing should be done routinely for all infants.

2. Suspected cataracts require urgent evaluation, particularly in newborns and younger infants.

3. Uncorrected visual acuity errors in children <8 years old can cause irreversible, lifelong problems.

4. Amblyopia accompanies strabismus in 30–60% of cases.

5. Pseudoesotropia, a normal variant, mimics strabismus as a result of widened epicanthal folds. Unlike strabismus, corneal light reflections are equal.

152. **Which children are at high risk for visual abnormalities?**
- Prematurity (birth weight <1250 gm)
- Family history of congenital ocular abnormality (e.g., cataract, retinoblastoma), strabismus, or amblyopia
- Maternal intrauterine or cervicovaginal infection or substance abuse
- Systemic condition with vision-threatening ocular manifestations

   Trobe J: Physician's Guide to Eye Care, 2nd ed. San Francisco, Foundation of the American Academy of Ophthalmology, 2001.

153. **How is color blindness inherited?**
Color blindness typically involves the variable loss of the ability to distinguish colors, especially red, green, and blue. The defects can be partial (anomaly) or complete (anopia). Defects in appreciating red or green color are transmitted in an X-linked recessive manner and affect up to 1% and 6%, respectively, of the male population. Blue color blindness is an autosomal dominant phenomenon and occurs in 0.1% of the population.

ACKNOWLEDGMENT

The editors gratefully acknowledge contributions by Drs. Nathan J. Blum, Mark Clayton, and James Coplan that were retained from the first three editions of *Pediatric Secrets*.

CHAPTER 3

CARDIOLOGY

Thomas J. Starc, MD, MPH, Constance J. Hayes, MD, and Allan J. Hordof, MD

CLINICAL ISSUES

1. **Is mitral valve prolapse (MVP) always pathologic?**
   Some studies show that up to 13% of normal children have some degree of posterior leaflet prolapse on echocardiography. There likely is a spectrum of anatomic abnormalities, the most minor of which are a variation of normal. Those children with clinical features of mitral valve insufficiency constitute the pathologic category. Whenever auscultation reveals the classic findings of MVP, referral to a pediatric cardiologist is recommended. This allows for evaluation of the child for possible accompanying cardiac abnormalities (e.g., mitral insufficiency, secundum atrial septal defects) and confirmation of the diagnosis.

2. **What connective tissue diseases may be associated with MVP?**
   Marfan syndrome, Ehlers-Danlos syndrome, pseudoxanthoma elasticum, osteogenesis imperfecta, and Hurler syndrome.

3. **Do patients with MVP require prophylaxis against subacute bacterial endocarditis?**
   This is controversial. The incidence of endocarditis in patients with MVP *and* systolic murmur is 1 in 2,000 per year. Three factors—**male gender, advanced age,** and the presence of **systolic murmur**—seem to be associated with an increased risk of endocarditis in patients with MVP. Some experts argue that all patients should receive treatment, and others recommend selectively treating only patients with MVP *and* systolic murmur (mitral regurgitation) or thickened leaflets.

4. **Can a patient with heart disease simultaneously be polycythemic and iron deficient?**
   Yes. Patients with **cyanotic** heart disease may develop both clinical entities. Initially, as a response to cyanosis, the hematocrit rises. In patients with iron deficiency, the hematocrit may remain elevated, and the mean corpuscular volume will be lower than normal. Detailed studies of iron stores often reveal a concurrent deficiency. Those children with a history of poor nutrition and blood loss (e.g., previous surgery) are especially at risk for developing iron deficiency.

5. **What are the most common vascular rings and slings?**
   Vascular rings occur when the trachea and/or the esophagus are encircled by aberrant vascular structures. *Vascular slings* are compressions (typically anterior) that are caused by non-encircling aberrant vessels (*see* Table 3-1).

6. **What evaluations may be done if a vascular ring is suspected?**
   - **Chest x-ray:** For detection of possible right-sided aortic arch
   - **Barium esophagram:** Considered the gold standard for diagnosis; confirms external indentation of esophagus in up to 95% of cases (Fig. 3-1)

- **Magnetic resonance imaging:** Noninvasive and used in some centers as the primary diagnostic modality
- **Rigid bronchoscopy:** May confirm diagnosis by detecting pulsatile indentation of trachea
- **Arteriogram:** Precise delineation of vascular anatomy; rarely needed because of magnetic resonance imaging
- **Echocardiogram:** Not helpful for identifying the ring itself, but important when evaluating for possible congenital heart disease, which occurs in up to 25% of patients with vascular rings

TABLE 3-1. VASCULAR RINGS AND SLINGS

	Frequency	Symptoms	Treatment
"Complete" rings			
Double aortic arch	50%	Respiratory difficulty, worsened by feeding or exertion (onset <3 months)	Surgical division of a smaller arch (usually the left)
Right aortic arch with left ligamentum arteriosum	45%	Mild respiratory difficulty (onset later in infancy); swallowing dysfunction	Surgical division of ligamentum arteriosum
"Incomplete" rings			
Anomalous innominate artery	<5%	Stridor and/or cough in infancy	Conservative management or surgical suturing of artery to the sternum
Aberrant right subclavian artery	<5%	Occasional swallowing dysfunction	Usually no treatment necessary
Vascular sling or anomalous left pulmonary artery	Rare	Wheezing and cyanotic episodes during first weeks of life	Surgical division of anomalous left pulmonary artery (from right pulmonary artery) and anastomosis to the MPA

Adapted from Park MK: Cardiology for Practitioners, 4th ed. St. Louis, Mosby, 2002, p 242.

7. **Describe four categories of cardiomyopathy in children.**
   - **Dilated cardiomyopathy** is the most common. Etiology is usually unknown. Anatomically, the heart is normal, but both ventricles are dilated. Older children present symptoms of congestive heart failure (CHF). Infants show symptoms of poor weight gain, feeding difficulty, and respiratory distress. In all pediatric age groups, a more acute presenting symptom can be shock.
   - **Hypertrophic cardiomyopathy with left ventricular (LV) outflow obstruction** is also known as *idiopathic hypertrophic subaortic stenosis* and *asymmetric septal hypertrophy*. Of

patients with this condition, the majority have some degree of LV outflow tract obstruction as a result of abnormal hypertrophy of the subaortic region of the intraventricular septum. Most of these defects are inherited in an autosomal dominant fashion. This cardiomyopathy is associated with ventricular dysrhythmias and sudden death.

- **Hypertrophic cardiomyopathy without LV outflow obstruction** is also usually of unknown etiology. It may be associated with systemic metabolic disease, particularly storage disease. Cardiomegaly is a constant feature.

- **Restrictive cardiomyopathy** is associated with abnormal diastolic function of the ventricles. The ventricles may be of normal size, or they may be hypertrophied with normal systolic function. The atria are typically enlarged. The etiology is usually unknown but may be storage disease.

Maron BJ: Hypertrophic cardiomyopathy in childhood. Pediatr Clin North Am 51:1305–1346, 2004.

Shaddy RE: Cardiomyopathies in adolescents: Dilated, hypertrophic, and restrictive. Adolesc Med 12:35–45, 2001.

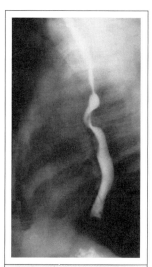

Figure 3-1. Barium swallow in a toddler with posterior compression of the esophagus and trachea from a vascular ring. (From Zitelli BJ, Davis HW: Atlas of Pediatric Physical Diagnosis, 4th ed. St. Louis, Mosby, 2002, p 540.)

8. **What are the cardiac causes of sudden cardiac death in young athletes?**

Sudden death occurs because of ventricular fibrillation in the setting of myocardial or coronary abnormalities or primary rhythm disorders. The main structural causes are hypertrophic cardiomyopathy (particularly with extreme LV hypertrophy), anomalies of the coronary artery, Marfan syndrome, and arrhythmogenic right ventricular (RV) dysplasia. Abnormal coronary arteries as a sequelae of Kawasaki syndrome may be a consideration. Prolonged QT syndrome and Wolff-Parkinson-White (WPW) syndrome have also been implicated. Children with congenital heart disease (e.g., aortic stenosis, Ebstein anomaly) are at higher risk for sudden death.

Despite the notoriety of sudden death (especially in professional or college athletes), it should be noted that this is relatively rare in younger athletes. Of the approximately 5 million high-school-age children who participate in athletics each year, only 25 (1 in 200,000) die of atraumatic causes during sports.

Spirito P, Bellone P, Harris KM, et al: Magnitude of left ventricular hypertrophy and risk of sudden death in hypertrophic cardiomyopathy. N Engl J Med 342:1778–1785, 2000.

Wren C, O'Sullivan JJ, Wright C: Sudden death in children and adolescents. Heart 83:410–413, 2000.

9. **What historical features can identify the patient who is at risk for sudden death?**
- Some common causes of sudden death may be associated with previous symptoms of exertional chest discomfort; dizziness or prolonged dyspnea with exercise; syncope; or palpitations.
- Family history of cardiovascular disease at an early age or sudden death may be associated with these patients. For example, although 40% of cases of hypertrophic cardiomyopathy are sporadic, 60% are inherited in an autosomal dominant fashion.
- History of seizures may be associated with prolonged QT syndrome.

Berger S, Dhala A, Friedberg DZ: Sudden cardiac death in infants, children, and adolescents. Pediatr Clin North Am 46:221–234, 1999.

Maron BJ: Sudden death in young athletes. N Engl J Med 349:1064–1075, 2003.

10. **How can the preparticipation sports physical identify patients at risk for sudden death?**
    - **Marfanoid features:** Tall and thin habitus, hyperextensible joints, pectus excavatum, click and murmur suggestive of MVP
    - **Pathologic murmurs:** Particularly a systolic murmur that increases with expiration and standing or decreases with squatting and is associated with an increased LV impulse (e.g., hypertrophic cardiomyopathy) or one that is associated with a suprasternal thrill (e.g., valvular aortic stenosis)
    - **Dysrhythmia:** Present

    Berger S, Dhala A, Friedberg DZ: Sudden cardiac death in infants, children, and adolescents. Pediatr Clin North Am 46:221–234, 1999.
    Maron BJ: Sudden death in young athletes. N Engl J Med 349:1064–1075, 2003.

11. **In which patients is syncope more likely to be of a cardiac nature?**
    - Sudden onset without any prodromal period of dizziness or imminent awareness
    - Syncope during exercise or exertion
    - Complete loss of awareness and muscle tone so that fall results in injury
    - History of palpitations or abnormal heartbeat before event
    - Very fast or very slow heart rate after event
    - Family history of sudden death

12. **What arrhythmias may be associated with syncope?**
    See Table 3-2.

TABLE 3-2. SYNCOPE		
Diagnosis	**History/Physical Exam**	**ECG Findings**
WPW	Family history of WPW, known hypertrophic cardiomyopathy, or Ebstein's anomaly	Short PR interval, presence of delta waves
Prolonged QT syndrome	Family history of prolonged QT, sudden death, and/or deafness	$QT_c = > 0.44$ sec
Atrioventricular block	Myocarditis, Lyme disease, acute rheumatic fever, maternal history of lupus	1°, 2°, or 3° heart block.
Arrhythmogenic right ventricular dysplasia	Syncope, palpitations, positive family history	PVCs, V tach, left bundle branch block
Ventricular tachycardia in a structurally normal heart	Majority of ventricular tachycardia occurs in abnormal hearts; requires extensive evaluation.	V tach

WPW = Wolff-Parkinson-White syndrome, PVCs = premature ventricular contractions, V tach = ventricular tachycardia, QT_c = corrected QT interval.
From Feinberg AN, Lane-Davies A: Syncope in the adolescent. Adolesc Med 13:553-567, 2002.

13. **What is the most common cause of syncope in children?**
In otherwise healthy children, **neurocardiogenic syncope** is most common. This entity goes by a number of terms, including *vasovagal syncope, neurally mediated syncope,* and *autonomic syncope.* Individuals who experience an orthostatic challenge may paradoxically respond with a decreased heart rate and increased peripheral vasodilation, which results in hypotensive syncope. Treatment for recurrent episodes may involve mineralocorticoids, salt and extra fluids, beta-blockers, and disopyramide.

Massin MM, Bourguignont A, Coremans C, et al: Syncope in pediatric patients presenting to an emergency department. J Pediatr 145:223–228, 2004.
Sapin SO: Autonomic syncope in pediatrics. Clin Pediatr 43:17–23, 2004.

KEY POINTS: SYNCOPE MORE LIKELY TO BE OF A CARDIAC NATURE

1. Occurring during exercise

2. Sudden onset without prodromal symptoms or awareness

3. Complete loss of tone or awareness leading to injury

4. Palpitations or abnormal heartbeat noted before event

5. Abnormal heart rate (fast or slow) after event

6. Family history of sudden death

14. **What are the most common clinical signs of coarctation of the aorta (Fig. 3-2) in older children?**
- Differential blood pressure: arms > legs (100%)
- Systolic murmur or bruit in the back (96%)
- Systolic hypertension in the upper extremities (96%)
- Diminished or absent femoral or lower-extremity pulses (92%)

Ing FF, Starc TJ, Griffiths SP, Gersony WM: Early diagnosis of coarctation of the aorta in children: A continuing dilemma. Pediatrics 98:378–382, 1996.

CONGENITAL HEART DISEASE

15. **What are the proven etiologies for congenital heart disease (CHD)?**
Only a small percentage of cases have identifiable causes:
- **Primary genetic factors** (e.g., chromosomal abnormalities, single gene abnormalities): 10%
- **Environmental factors** (e.g., chemicals; drugs such as isotretinoin or Accutane; viruses such as rubella; maternal disease): 3–5%
- **Genetic-environmental interactions** (i.e., multifactorial): 85%

16. **What prenatal maternal factors may be associated with cardiac disease in the neonate?**
See Table 3-3.

17. **In a cyanotic newborn, how can you distinguish pulmonary disease from cyanotic congenital heart disease?**
With the **hyperoxia test**. The infant is placed in 100% oxygen, and an arterial blood gas level is obtained. A $PaO_2 > 100$ mmHg is usually achieved in infants with primary lung disease, whereas a $PaO_2 < 100$ mmHg is characteristic of heart disease. Typically, children with cyanotic heart disease also have a low or normal pCO_2, whereas children with lung disease have an elevated pCO_2. Unfortunately, the hyperoxia test does not usually distinguish children with cyanotic heart disease from those with persistent pulmonary hypertension.

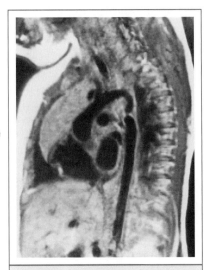

Figure 3-2. MRI of coarctation of the aorta. (From Clark DA: Atlas of Neonatology. Philadelphia, W.B. Saunders, 2000, p 119.)

18. **Which congenital heart lesions commonly appear with cyanosis during the newborn period?**
Independent pulmonary and systemic circulations (severe cyanosis)
- Transposition of great arteries with an intact ventricular septum

Inadequate pulmonary blood flow (severe cyanosis)
- Tricuspid valve atresia
- Pulmonary valve atresia with intact ventricular septum
- Tetralogy of Fallot
- Severe Ebstein anomaly of the tricuspid valve

TABLE 3-3. PRENATAL MATERNAL FACTORS ASSOCIATED WITH CARDIAC DISEASE IN NEONATES

Prenatal historic factor	Associated cardiac defect
Diabetes mellitus	Left ventricular outflow obstruction (asymmetric septal hypertrophy, aortic stenosis), D-transposition of great arteries, ventricular septal defect
Lupus erythematosus	Heart block, pericarditis, endomyocardial fibrosis
Rubella	Patent ductus arteriosus, pulmonic stenosis (peripheral)
Alcohol use	Pulmonic stenosis, ventricular septal defect
Aspirin use	Persistent pulmonary hypertension syndrome
Lithium	Ebstein anomaly
Diphenylhydantoin	Aortic stenosis, pulmonary stenosis
Coxsackie B infection	Myocarditis

From Gewitz MH: Cardiac disease in the newborn infant. In Polin RA, Yoder MC, Burg FD (eds): Workbook in Practical Neonatology, 3rd ed. Philadelphia, W.B. Saunders, 2001, p 269.

Admixture lesions (moderate cyanosis)
- Total anomalous pulmonary venous return
- Hypoplastic left heart syndrome
- Truncus arteriosus

> Victoria BE: Cyanotic newborns. In Gessner IH, Victoria BE (eds): Pediatric Cardiology: A Problem Oriented Approach. Philadelphia, W.B. Saunders, 1993, p 101.

19. **In the patient with suspected heart disease, what bony abnormalities seen on a chest x-ray increase the likelihood of CHD?**
    - **Hemivertebrae, rib anomalies:** Associated with tetralogy of Fallot, truncus arteriosus, and VACTERL syndrome (vertebral abnormalities, anal atresia, cardiac abnormalities, tracheoesophageal fistula and/or esophageal atresia, renal agenesis and dysplasia, and limb defects)
    - **11 ribs:** Seen in patients with Down syndrome
    - **Skeletal chest deformities** (scoliosis, pectus excavatum, narrow anterior-posterior [AP] diameter): Associated with Marfan syndrome and mitral valve prolapse
    - **Bilateral rib notching:** Coarctation of the aorta (usually seen in older children)

KEY POINTS: CARDIAC CAUSES OF CYANOSIS IN THE NEWBORN

1. Transposition of the great arteries
2. Tetralogy of Fallot
3. Truncus arteriosus
4. Pulmonary atresia
5. Total anomalous pulmonary venous return
6. Tricuspid atresia
7. Hypoplastic left heart

20. **How do pulmonary vascular markings on a chest x-ray help in the differential diagnosis of a cyanotic newborn with suspected cardiac disease?**
    The chest x-ray may help to differentiate the types of congenital heart defects. The increase or decrease in pulmonary vascular markings is indicative of pulmonary blood flow:
    Decreased pulmonary markings (diminished pulmonary blood flow)
    - Pulmonary atresia or severe stenosis
    - Tetralogy of Fallot
    - Tricuspid atresia
    - Ebstein anomaly

    Increased pulmonary markings (increased pulmonary blood flow)
    - Transposition of great arteries
    - Total anomalous pulmonary venous return
    - Truncus arteriosus

21. **What electrocardiogram (ECG) findings are considered characteristic for various congenital heart malformations?**
    - **Left axis deviation:** Atrial septal defect (primum), endocardial cushion defect, tricuspid atresia

- **WPW syndrome:** Ebstein anomaly, L-transposition of the great arteries (L-TGA)
- **Complete heart block:** L-TGA, polysplenia syndrome

22. **What chest x-ray findings (Fig. 3-3) are considered characteristic for various congenital heart diseases?**
    - **Boot-shaped heart:** Tetralogy of Fallot, tricuspid atresia
    - **Egg-shaped heart:** Transposition of great arteries
    - **Snowman silhouette:** Total anomalous pulmonary venous return (supracardiac)
    - **Rib notching:** Coarctation of the aorta (older children)

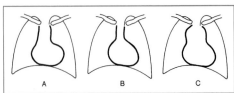

Figure 3-3. Abnormal cardiac silhouettes. *A,* Boot-shaped heart seen in cyanotic tetralogy of Fallot or tricuspid atresia. *B,* Egg-shaped heart seen in transposition of the great arteries. *C,* Snowman silhouette seen in total anomalous pulmonary artery venous return (supracardiac type). (From Park MK: Pediatric Cardiology for Practitioners, 4th ed. St. Louis, Mosby, 2002, p 54.)

23. **Which are the ductal-dependent cardiac lesions?**

    Ductal-dependent pulmonary blood flow
    - Critical pulmonic stenosis
    - Pulmonary atresia
    - Tricuspid atresia with pulmonary stenosis or pulmonary atresia

    Ductal-dependent systemic blood flow
    - Coarctation of the aorta
    - Hypoplastic left heart syndrome
    - Interrupted aortic arch

24. **Which types of CHD are associated with right aortic arch?**
    - Tetralogy of Fallot with pulmonary atresia (50%)
    - Truncus arteriosus (35%)
    - Classic tetralogy of Fallot (25%)
    - Double-outlet right ventricle (25%)
    - Single ventricle (12.5%)

    Crowley JJ, Oh KS, Newman B, et al: Telltale signs of congenital heart disease. Radiol Clin North Am 31:573–582, 1993.

25. **Which genetic syndromes are most commonly associated with CHD?**
    See Table 3-4.

26. **Which infants with CHD should be evaluated for other anomalies?**
    In the evaluation of the newborn with heart disease, several known associations between CHD and other anomalies should be considered, especially for the patient with more complex disease. Syndromes such as CHARGE (coloboma, heart disease, choanal atresia, retarded growth and development *or* central nervous system anomalies, genital hypoplasia, and ear anomalies and/or deafness) or VACTERL may first be identified by the presence of heart disease. An association between conotruncal defects (tetralogy of Fallot, truncus arteriosus, and interrupted aortic arch) and deletions on chromosome 22 is often seen. Some of these patients may have DiGeorge syndrome or velocardiofacial syndrome, but others may have only minimal palatal dysfunction. For this reason, patients with conotruncal cardiac defects should undergo screening for deletions on chromosome 22; if these are found, these patients should be referred to a geneticist for special testing and evaluation.

TABLE 3-4. GENETIC SYNDROMES ASSOCIATED WITH CONGENITAL HEART DISEASE

Syndrome	Percentage of patients with CHD	Predominant heart defect(s)
Down	50%	ECD, VSD, TOF
Turner	20%	COA
Noonan	65%	PS, ASD, ASH
Marfan	60%	MVP, AoAn, AR
Trisomy 18	90%	VSD, PDA
Trisomy 13	80%	VSD, PDA
DiGeorge	80%	IAA-B, TA
Williams	75%	SVAS, peripheral PS

CHD = congenital heart disease, ECD = endocardial cushion defect, VSD = ventricular septal defect, TOF = tetralogy of Fallot, COA = coarctation of the aorta, PS = pulmonic stenosis, ASD = atrial sepal defect, ASH = asymmetric septal hypertrophy, MVP = mitral valve prolapse, AoAn = aortic aneurysm, AR = aortic regurgitation, PDA = patent ductus arteriosus, IAA-B = interrupted aortic arch-type B, TA = truncus arteriosus, SVAS = supravalvular aortic stenosis.
From Frias JL: Genetic issues of congenital heart defects. In Gessner IH, Victoria BE (eds): Pediatric Cardiology: A Problem Oriented Approach. Philadelphia, W.B. Saunders, 1993, p 238.

27. **Describe the clinical manifestations of a large patent ductus arteriosus (PDA).**
    - Tachypnea and tachycardia
    - Wide pulse pressures
    - Bounding pulses
    - Labile oxygenation (premature infant)
    - Hyperdynamic precordium
    - Apnea (premature infant)
    - Systolic murmur (premature infant)
    - Continuous murmur (older child)

28. **How commonly do PDAs occur in premature infants?**
    They are evident in 40–60% of infants with a birth weight of 501–1,500 gm.

29. **When should indomethacin be administered to newborns with a PDA?**
    Indomethacin is effective for closing a PDA within the first 10 days of life. The drug is indicated for preterm infants with a hemodynamically significant PDA, which is defined as one in which there is deteriorating respiratory status (e.g., tachypnea, apnea, CO_2 retention, increased ventilatory support, failure to wean ventilatory support) or evidence of congestive heart failure.
    Wyllie J: Treatment of patent ductus arteriosus. Semin Neonatal 8:425–432, 2003.

30. **How often does a PDA reopen after indomethacin therapy?**
    Reopening after successful closure with indomethacin occurs in approximately 25% of infants (33% of infants <1,000 gm). The ductus is more likely to reopen when indomethacin therapy is initiated beyond the first week of life. In most cases, permanent constriction does not occur after a single dose; second and third doses are recommended at 12 and 36 hours after the initial dose.

31. **When should the ductus arteriosus be surgically ligated?**
    Surgical ligation is generally indicated in symptomatic infants who have failed two courses of medical management, including indomethacin. Although controversial, surgery is commonly

chosen for infants weighing ≤1,000 gm in whom there has been a single "failed-course" of indomethacin.

32. What are the contraindications for indomethacin therapy?

Indomethacin is contraindicated if the blood urea nitrogen level is >30 mg/dL, the creatinine level is >1.8 mg/dL, the platelet count is <60,000/mm^3, and if there is evidence of a bleeding diathesis.

33. How do an ostium primum and an ostium secundum defect differ?

Atrial septal defects are categorized in large part by their location. Defects may be isolated to the atrial septum itself, or they may extend into the ventricles (e.g., endocardial cushion defects). An **ostium secundum** is an isolated defect that involves a persistently enlarged opening at the fossa ovalis, which is approximately in the center of the septum. An **ostium primum** defect is located more inferiorly and is part of an atrioventricular(AV) canal defect, often in association with a regurgitant mitral valve.

34. How do the presenting symptoms of ventricular septal defect (VSD) and atrial septal defect (ASD) differ?

VSD: In an infant with a *large* VSD, signs indicative of congestive heart failure generally appear at 4–8 weeks of age, when the pulmonary vascular resistance drops and pulmonary blood flow increases. Congestive heart failure can occasionally be seen at 1–2 weeks of age in infants with large shunts in whom vascular resistance falls more quickly. The child with a *small* VSD may have a systolic murmur during the first few weeks of life. These infants do not develop congestive heart failure, and spontaneous closure often occurs.

ASD: Most children with an isolated ASD are not diagnosed until they are 3–5 years old. The majority are asymptomatic at the time of diagnosis. Rarely, infants with an ASD demonstrate signs of congestive heart failure during the first year of life. The congestive heart failure is due to a large left-to-right shunt and increased pulmonary blood flow, and it may be associated with failure to thrive or recurrent lower respiratory infections.

35. What are the four structural abnormalities of tetralogy of Fallot?

- Right ventricular outflow tract stenosis
- VSD
- Dextroposition of the aorta
- Right ventricular hypertrophy

36. What occurs during a "Tet spell"?

"Tet spells" are cyanotic and hypoxic episodes that occur in patients with tetralogy of Fallot. The pathophysiology is felt to be related to a change in the balance of systemic to pulmonary vascular resistance. Spells may be initiated by events that cause a decrease in systemic vascular resistance (e.g., fever, crying, hypotension) or by events that cause an increase in pulmonary outflow tract obstruction. Both types of events cause more right-to-left shunting and increased cyanosis. Hypoxia and cyanosis lead to metabolic acidosis and systemic vasodilatation, which cause a further increase in cyanosis. Anemia may be a predisposing factor. Although most episodes are self-limited, a prolonged Tet spell can lead to stroke or death; therefore, such a spell is an indication that surgery may be necessary.

37. After what age does a presumed peripheral pulmonic branch stenosis murmur deserve more detailed study?

The murmur of peripheral pulmonic branch stenosis—a low-intensity systolic ejection murmur heard frequently in newborns—is the result of the relative hypoplasia of the pulmonary arteries as well as the acute angle of the branching of pulmonary arteries in the early newborn period. This murmur usually persists until **3–6 months of age**.

38. What should parents be told about the risk of recurrence for common heart defects?

Recurrence risks for cardiovascular anomalies vary from 1–4% and are usually higher with the more common lesions (e.g., the recurrence risk for VSD is 3%, and the recurrence risk for Ebstein anomaly is 1%). The risk of CHD in pregnancies after the birth of one affected child is about 1–4%. With two affected first-degree relatives, the risk is tripled. With three affected children, the family may be considered at even higher risk.

Congenital Heart Information Network: www.tchin.org

CONGESTIVE HEART FAILURE

39. Identify the clinical signs and symptoms associated with CHF in children.

These may be grouped into three categories:

- **Signs/symptoms of impaired myocardial performance:** Cardiomegaly, tachycardia, gallop rhythm, cold extremities or mottling, growth failure, sweating with feeding, pallor
- **Signs/symptoms of pulmonary congestion:** Tachypnea, wheezing, rales, cyanosis, dyspnea, cough
- **Signs/symptoms of systemic venous congestion:** Hepatomegaly, neck vein distention, peripheral edema (seen in the older patient)

40. What acid-base changes are associated with CHF?

- **Mild CHF:** *Respiratory alkalosis* as a result of tachypnea (stimulation of J receptors secondary to increasing pulmonary edema)
- **Moderate or severe CHF:** *Respiratory acidosis* as a consequence of pulmonary edema and reduced compliance; *metabolic acidosis* as a result of decreased tissue perfusion

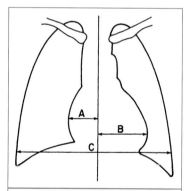

41. How is heart size assessed in older children?

Cardiothoracic (CT) ratio: This is derived by comparing the largest transverse diameter of the heart to the widest internal diameter of the chest: CT ratio = (A + B) / C, as shown in Fig. 3-4. A CT ratio >0.5 indicates cardiomegaly.

Figure 3-4. The cardiothoracic ratio is obtained by dividing the largest horizontal diameter of the heart (A + B) by the longest internal diameter of the chest (C). (From Park MK: Pediatric Cardiology for Practitioners, 4th ed. St. Louis, Mosby, 2002, p 51.)

42. In infancy, how does the likely cause of CHF vary by age?

See Table 3-5.

KEY POINTS: COMMON CARDIAC CAUSES OF CONGESTIVE HEART FAILURE IN A 6-WEEK-OLD INFANT

1. Ventricular septal defect

2. Atrioventricular canal

3. Patent ductus arteriosus

4. Coarctation of the aorta

TABLE 3-5. CAUSES OF CONGESTIVE HEART FAILURE

Age of Onset	Cause
At birth	HLHS
	Volume overload lesions:
	Severe tricuspid or pulmonary insufficiency
	Large systemic arteriovenous fistula
First week	TGA
	PDA in small premature infants
	HLHS
	TAPVR, particularly those with pulmonary venous obstruction
	Others:
	Systemic arteriovenous fistula
	Critical AS or PS
1–4 weeks	COA with associated anomalies
	Critical AS
	Large left-to-right shunt lesions (VSD, PDA) in premature infants
	All other lesions previously listed
4–6 weeks	Some left-to-right shunt lesions such as ECD
6 weeks–4 months	Large VSD
	Large PDA
	Others such as anomalous left coronary artery from the PA

AS = aortic stenosis, COA = coarctation of the aorta, ECD = endocardial cushion defect, HLHS = hypoplastic left heart syndrome, PA = pulmonary artery, PDA = patent ductus arteriosus, PS = pulmonary stenosis, TAPVR = total anomalous pulmonary venous return, TGA = transposition of the great arteries, VSD = ventricular septal defect.
From Park, Myung K: Pediatric Cardiology for Practitioners, 4th ed. St. Louis, Mosby, 2002, p 400.

43. **If a patient develops CHF and cardiomegaly during the newborn period but no murmur is heard, what is the differential diagnosis?**
    - Myocarditis
    - Cardiomyopathy as a result of asphyxia, hypoglycemia, or hypocalcemia
    - Glycogen storage disease (Pompe disease)
    - Cardiac dysrhythmia
        □ Paroxysmal supraventricular tachycardia
        □ Congenital heart block
    - Atrial flutter and/or fibrillation
    - Arteriovenous malformations (e.g., central nervous system, vein of Galen)
    - Sepsis

44. **If a patient develops CHF and cardiomegaly outside of the newborn period but no murmur is heard, what is the differential diagnosis?**
    Myocardial diseases
    - Endocardial fibroelastosis

- Myocarditis (viral or idiopathic)
- Glycogen storage disease (Pompe disease)

Coronary artery diseases resulting in myocardial insufficiency
- Anomalous origin of left coronary artery (LCA) from pulmonary artery
- Collagen disease (periarteritis nodosa)
- Kawasaki syndrome (acute vasculitis of infancy and early childhood)
- Calcification of the coronary arteries
- Medial necrosis of coronary arteries

CHD with severe heart failure
- Coarctation of the aorta in infants
- Ebstein anomaly

45. **When should afterload reduction be used in children?**
In settings of low cardiac output (CO) as a result of myocardial dysfunction with increased peripheral vascular resistance (cool extremities and poor capillary refill) and pulmonary congestion, afterload reduction can decrease overall cardiac work and myocardial O_2 consumption while increasing CO and oxygen delivery. It is often used to aid a failing heart during the immediate postoperative period and also may be of value in children with chronic ventricular dysfunction and those with mitral and/or aortic regurgitation or systemic-to-pulmonic shunts.

46. **What agents are used to treat afterload reduction in children?**
Agents that preferentially dilate arterioles (e.g., hydralazine), veins (e.g., nitrates), or both (e.g., sodium nitroprusside, captopril, other angiotensin-converting enzyme inhibitors) can be used. As a rule, arteriolar vasodilators tend to increase CO, and venous dilators tend to lessen pulmonary congestion. Afterload reduction may be of little use in shock states that occur as a result of causes other than myocardial failure. If the blood pressure remains unacceptably low (i.e., unstable shock), there is no role for afterload reduction. Volume replacement and inotropic support should first be used. Afterload reduction may also be of little benefit during the "warm phase," of septic shock when CO is actually increased and there is peripheral vasodilation.

ECG AND DYSRHYTHMIAS

47. **What are the characteristic features of the ECG of a premature infant?**
In the premature infant, there is less RV dominance. The R wave may be small in the right precordial leads, and there may be no significant S wave over the left precordium. The electrical axis is often in the normal quadrant (0–90°).

48. **How does the ECG of an infant differ from that of the older child?**
- **Birth:** At birth, the ECG reflects RV dominance. The QRS complex consists of a tall R wave in the right precordial leads (V_1–V_2) and an S wave in the left precordial leads (V_5–V_6). The axis is also rightward (90–150°).
- **Toddler age** (2–4 years): There is an axis shift from the right to the normal quadrant, and the R wave diminishes over the right precordial leads. The S wave disappears from the left precordium.
- **School age:** At this age the wave has a nearly adult tracing, with a small R and a dominant S in the right precordial leads and an axis in the normal quadrant.

49. **Describe the ECG abnormalities associated with potassium and calcium imbalances.**
See Fig. 3-5.

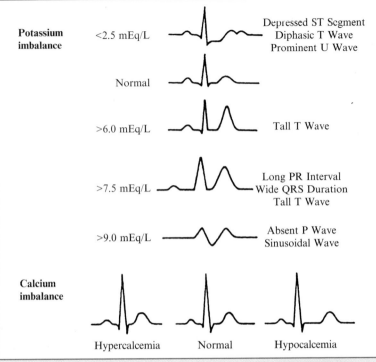

Figure 3-5. Electrocardiogram abnormalities associated with potassium and calcium imbalances. (From Park MK, Guntheroth WG: How to Read Pediatric ECGs, 3rd ed. St. Louis, Mosby, 1992, pp 106–107.)

50. **What is the corrected QT interval (QT$_c$)?**

The QT interval represents the time required for ventricular depolarization and repolarization. It begins at the onset of the QRS complex and continues through the end of the T wave. This interval varies with the heart rate. The QT$_c$ adjusts for heart rate differences. As a rule, a prolonged QT$_c$ interval is diagnosed when the QT$_c$ exceeds 0.44 seconds.

$$QTc = QT \text{ (in seconds)} / \sqrt{RR} \text{ (in seconds)}$$

Al-Khatib SM, LaPointe NM, Kramer JM, Califf RM: What clinicians should know about the QT interval. JAMA 289:2120–2127, 2003.

51. **What causes a prolonged QT interval?**

Congenital long QT syndrome
- Hereditary form
  □ Genetic defects in specific potassium and sodium channel genes
  □ Jervell-Lange-Nielsen syndrome (associated with deafness)
  □ Romano-Ward syndrome
- Sporadic type

Acquired long QT syndrome
- Drug-induced (especially antidysrhythmics, tricyclic antidepressants, phenothiazines)

KEY POINTS: ELECTROCARDIOGRAMS ✓

1. As compared with adults, newborns and infants normally have right-ventricular dominance.

2. Premature atrial beats in children are usually benign.

3. QT intervals must be corrected for heart rates.

4. A QT_C should not exceed 0.44 seconds, except in infants <6 months old, where up to 0.49 seconds may be normal.

- Metabolic/electrolyte abnormalities (hypocalcemia, hypokalemia, very-low-energy diets)
- Central nervous system and autonomic nervous system disorders (especially after head trauma or stroke)
- Cardiac disease (myocarditis, coronary artery disease)

52. What are the ECG findings in patients with complete heart block?
The atrial and ventricular activities are entirely independent. P waves are regular, and QRS complexes are also regular, with a rate slower than the P rate (Fig. 3-6).

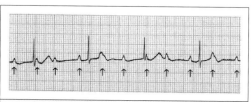

Figure 3-6. Complete heart block. Tracing demonstrates atrial activity (arrows) independent of slower ventricular rhythm. (From Zitelli BJ, Davis HW: Atlas of Pediatric Physical Diagnosis, 4th ed. St. Louis, Mosby, 2002, p 144.)

53. How abnormal are premature atrial contractions?
Premature atrial beats are usually benign, with the exception of patients with an electrical or anatomic substrate for supraventricular tachycardia (SVT) or atrial flutter.

54. How does SVT in children differ from physiologic sinus tachycardia?
SVT typically has the following features:
- Sudden onset and termination rather than a gradual change in rate
- Persistent ventricular rate of >180 bpm
- Fixed or almost fixed RR interval on ECG
- Abnormal P-wave shape or axis or absent P waves
- Little change in heart rate with activity, crying, or breath holding

55. When are isolated premature ventricular contractions (PVCs) usually benign in the otherwise healthy school-aged child?
- Structurally normal heart
- ECG intervals, especially QT_C, are normal
- No evidence of myocarditis, cardiomegaly, or ventricular tumor
- No history of drug use
- Electrolytes and glucose are normal
- They decrease with exercise

56. **Name the two most common mechanisms of SVT.**
    - WPW syndrome (due to an accessory bypass tract)
    - Atrioventricular nodal reentry

57. **What are the settings in which atrial arrhythmia (and SVT) may occur?**
    - Structurally normal heart: Accessory bypass tract or AV nodal reentry
    - Congenital heart disease (pre- or postoperatively): Ebstein anomaly, L-TGA with VSD and pulmonic stenosis; after Mustard, Senning, Fontan procedures
    - Hypertrophic cardiomyopathy
    - Dilated cardiomyopathy
    - Drug-induced: Sympathomimetics (e.g., cold medications, theophylline, beta agonists)
    - Infections: Myocarditis or fever
    - Hyperthyroidism

58. **What are some of the causes of a wide QRS?**
    - Premature ventricular contraction
    - Ventricular tachycardia
    - Premature atrial contraction with aberrancy
    - SVT with aberrancy
    - Bundle branch blocks
    - Preexcitation syndromes (WPW syndrome)
    - Electrolyte abnormalities
    - Myocarditis
    - Cardiomyopathy
    - Electronic ventricular pacemaker

59. **What vagal maneuvers are used to treat paroxysmal SVT in children?**
    Infants
    - Placement of an ice-soaked wet washcloth or rubber cloth filled with crushed ice over forehead and nose
    - Gagging with tongue blade

    Older children and adolescents
    - Above methods
    - Unilateral carotid massage
    - Valsalva maneuver (abdominal straining while holding breath)
    - Doing a headstand
      In general, the Valsalva maneuver and carotid massage are not as effective for children under the age of 4 years. Ocular pressure is not recommended because it has been associated with retinal injury. Vagal stimulation slows conduction in the AV node and prolongs refractoriness of the AV node, thereby interrupting the reentrant circuit.

60. **Other than vagal maneuvers, what treatments are used acutely for managing SVT?**
    If a patient's clinical condition has deteriorated rapidly, synchronized direct-current **cardioversion** is indicated. In patients who are stable and for whom vagal maneuvers have failed, **adenosine** has replaced digoxin and verapamil as the first drug of choice. An initial bolus of 100 μg/kg will exert an effect in 10–20 seconds by blocking conduction through the AV node. If this is ineffective, the dose can be increased in increments of 50–100 μg/kg every 1–2 minutes up to 300 μg/kg. The usual starting dose in adults is 6 mg and then 12 mg if the tachycardia persists.

    Etheridge SP, Judd VE: Supraventricular tachycardia in infancy: Evaluation, management and follow-up. Arch Pediatr Adolesc Med 153:267–271, 1999.

61. **Which children are candidates for transcatheter ablation techniques for SVT?**
Ablation therapy is used most commonly in children with dysrhythmias that are refractory to medical management and in those with life-threatening symptoms or possible lifelong medication requirements. Ablation is now commonly performed in children who are symptomatic from WPW or AV nodal reentrant tachycardia. Recommendations for transcatheter ablation are changing as increased experience with the safety and efficacy of the procedure are gathered. Recommendations vary with the age of the patient, the severity of the dysrhythmia, the type of lesion, the difficulty with medical control of the dysrhythmia, and the skill of the operator.

62. **How is WPW syndrome diagnosed on ECG?**
An accessory pathway bypasses the AV node, thereby resulting in early ventricular depolarization (pre-excitation). It is the most common cause of SVT in children. In infants and younger children with rapid heart rates, the delta wave may not be as evident. Additional clues that may be suggestive of WPW include the following:
- PR interval of <100 msec
- QRS duration of >80 msec
- No Q wave in left chest leads
- Left axis deviation

Perry JC, Giuffre RM, Garson A, Jr.: Clues to the electrocardiographic diagnosis of subtle Wolff-Parkinson-White syndrome in children. J Pediatr 117:871–875, 1990.

INFECTIOUS AND INFLAMMATORY DISORDERS

63. **How many blood cultures should be obtained to rule out subacute bacterial endocarditis?**
At least three separate blood cultures should be obtained. The use of multiple sites may decrease the likelihood of mistaking a contaminant for the true etiologic agent. In low-level bacteremia, additional specimen volume (≥3 mL) may increase the likelihood of positivity.

64. **Why might properly collected blood cultures be negative in the setting of clinically suspected bacterial endocarditis?**
- Prior antibiotic use
- The bacterial endocarditis may be right-sided
- Nonbacterial infection: Fungal (e.g., aspergillus, candida) or unusual organisms (e.g., rickettsia, chlamydia)
- Unusual bacterial infection: Slow-growing organisms or anaerobes
- Lesions may be mural or nonvalvular (i.e., less likely to be hematogenously seeded)
- Nonbacterial thrombotic endocarditis (sterile platelet-fibrin thrombus formations following endocardial injury)
- Incorrect diagnosis

Starke JR: Infectious endocarditis. In Feigin RD, Cherry JD, Demmler GJ, Kaplan S (ed): Textbook of Pediatric Infectious Diseases, 5th ed. Philadelphia, W.B. Saunders, 2004, p 362.

65. **Which cardiac lesions are at increased risk for bacterial endocarditis?**
- Cyanotic heart disease with or without a surgical shunt (e.g., tetralogy of Fallot with a Blalock-Taussig shunt)
- AV valve insufficiency (e.g., mitral insufficiency)
- Semilunar valve disease (e.g., aortic stenosis)
- Any lesion with an artificial valve
- Left-to-right shunts (e.g., VSD, patent ductus arteriosus)
- Coarctation of the aorta

66. **How reliable is the ECG for diagnosing bacterial endocarditis (BE)?**

Echocardiography can sometimes identify an intracardiac mass that is attached either to the wall of the myocardium or to part of the valve itself. Although the yield of echocardiography for diagnosing BE is low, the likelihood of a positive finding is increased under certain conditions (e.g., indwelling catheters, prematurity, immunosuppression, evidence of peripheral embolization). BE is still a clinical and laboratory diagnosis (physical examination and blood cultures, respectively) and *not* an "echocardiographic" diagnosis. A negative study does not rule out BE.

67. **How do Osler nodes and Janeway lesions differ?**

Both are noted in individuals with bacterial endocarditis. Pain is a key discriminator. **Osler nodes** are painful, tender nodules that are found primarily on the pads of the fingers and toes. **Janeway lesions** are painless, nontender, hemorrhagic nodular lesions seen on the palms and soles, especially on thenar and hypothenar eminences. Both lesions are rare in children with endocarditis.

Farrior JB, Silverman ME: A consideration of the differences between a Janeway's lesion and an Osler's node in infectious endocarditis. Chest 20:239–243, 1976.

68. **When should myocarditis be suspected?**

The presenting symptoms of myocarditis can be variable, ranging from subclinical to rapidly progressive CHF. It should be considered in any patient who experiences unexplained heart failure. Clinical signs include tachycardia out of proportion to fever, tachypnea, a quiet precordium, muffled heart tones, gallop rhythm without murmur, and hepatomegaly.

69. **What conditions are associated with the development of myocarditis?**

Infections
- Bacterial: Diphtheria
- Viral: Coxsackie B (most common), coxsackie A, human immunodeficiency virus, echoviruses, rubella
- Mycoplasmal
- Rickettsial: Typhus
- Fungal: Actinomycosis, coccidioidomycosis, histoplasmosis
- Protozoal: Trypanosomiasis (Chagas' disease), toxoplasmosis

Inflammatory
- Kawasaki disease
- Systemic lupus erythematosus
- Rheumatoid arthritis

Chemical/physical agents
- Radiation injury
- Drugs: Doxorubicin
- Toxins: Lead
- Animal bites: Scorpion, snake

70. **When should steroids be given to a child with myocarditis?**

The use of steroids in patients with myocarditis is controversial. Some authorities feel that the use of steroids may inhibit interferon synthesis and increase viral replication. If the inflammatory process is secondary to rheumatic fever, however, then steroids may be indicated.

71. **A child visiting from Mexico presents symptoms including unilateral eye swelling and new-onset acute CHF. What is a likely diagnosis?**
Acute myocarditis as a result of **Chagas' disease** (American trypanosomiasis) is likely. Seen in 25–50% of patients in endemic areas with early Chagas' disease, Romaña sign is unilateral, painless, violaceous, palpebral edema often accompanied by conjunctivitis. The swelling occurs near the bite site of the parasitic vector: the reduviid or Triatominae bug. Chagas' disease, a protozoan infection, is the most common cause of acute and chronic myocarditis in Mexico and in Central and South America.

72. **What are the common clinical signs and symptoms of pericarditis?**
   - **Symptoms:** Chest pain, fever, cough, palpitations, irritability, abdominal pain
   - **Signs:** Friction rub, pallor, pulsus paradoxus, muffled heart sounds, neck vein distention, hepatomegaly

73. **What is the position of comfort in the patient with pericarditis?**
The typical patient with pericarditis prefers to sit up and lean forward.

74. **What is Kawasaki disease?**
A multisystem disease characterized by a vasculitis of small and medium-sized blood vessels. If untreated, this can lead to coronary artery aneurysms and myocardial infarction.

75. **What are the principal diagnostic criteria for Kawasaki disease?**
The mnemonic **My HEART** may be helpful:
   M = **M**ucosal changes, especially oral and upper respiratory; dry and chapped lips; "strawberry tongue"
   H = **H**and and extremity changes, including reddened palms/soles and edema; desquamation from fingertips and toes is a late finding
   E = **E**ye changes, primarily a bilateral conjunctival infection without discharge
   A = **A**denopathy that is usually cervical, often unilateral, and ≥1.5 cm in diameter
   R = **R**ash that is usually a truncal exanthem without vesicles or crusts
   T = **T**emperature elevation, often to 104°F or above, lasting for >5 days

76. **How many diagnostic criteria are required for Kawasaki disease?**
The presence of fever and at least four of the other five features are needed for the classic diagnosis. However, a significant number of cases of *atypical* Kawasaki disease (20–60% of total) have been reported. These feature <5 of the criteria and occur particularly in children <1 year old; the symptoms are subsequently accompanied by the typical coronary artery changes. A high index of suspicion is important, because Kawasaki disease has replaced acute rheumatic fever as the leading cause of identifiable acquired heart disease in children in the United States.

Burns JC, Glode MP: Kawasak syndrome. Lancet 364:533–544, 2004
Council on Cardiovascular Disease in the Young, American Heart Association: Diagnostic guidelines for Kawasaki disease. Circulation 103:335–336, 2001.

77. **What is the typical age of children with Kawasaki disease?**
The majority of patients are **between 1 and 8 years old.** However, cases can occur in infants and teenagers. Both of these groups appear to be at increased risk of developing coronary artery sequelae. The diagnosis is often delayed, particularly in infants, because signs and symptoms of the illness may be atypical or subtle.

Genizi J, Miron D, Spiegel R, et al: Kawasaki disease in very young infants: High prevalence of atypical presentation and coronary arteritis. Clin Pediatr 42:263–267, 2003.

78. **What causes Kawasaki disease?**
Despite considerable progress in understanding the pathogenesis of this syndrome, the inciting agent remains undiscovered. Toxic agents (e.g., mercury, lead) and allergic and immunologic causes have been studied as potential causative factors. Numerous case reports and clinical series report that there are infectious agents associated with Kawasaki disease, including rickettsiae, *Klebsiella pneumoniae, Escherichia* sp., parainfluenza virus, Epstein-Barr virus, *Propionibacterium acnes*, retroviruses, and toxic shock syndrome toxin 1 staphylococci.

  Meissner HC, Leung DY: Kawasaki syndrome: Where are the answers? Pediatrics 112:672–676, 2003.

KEY POINTS: DIAGNOSTIC FEATURES OF KAWASAKI DISEASE

1. Erythema of oral cavity and dry, chapped lips

2. Conjunctivitis: Bilateral and without discharge

3. Edema/erythema and/or desquamation of hands and feet

4. Cervical lymphadenopathy

5. Polymorphous exanthem on trunk, flexor regions, and perineum

6. Fever, often up to 104°F, lasting ≥5 days

7. No other identifiable diagnostic entity to explain signs/symptoms

79. **Why should all children with Kawasaki disease receive intravenous immune globulin therapy?**
Intravenous immune globulin has been demonstrated to decrease the incidence of coronary artery abnormalities in children with Kawasaki disease. Additionally, fever and laboratory indices of inflammation resolve more quickly after treatment. The most common dosing is a single infusion over 12 hours of 2 gm/kg.
  Intravenous immuneglobulin improves outcome, with coronary artery dilation developing in <5% of patients and giant coronary aneurysms developing in <1% of patients. At present there is no reliable means of predicting which children with Kawasaki disease will develop coronary artery abnormalities. Therefore, all children with Kawasaki disease should receive parenteral gamma globulin.

  Fukunishi M, Kikkawa M, Hamana K, et al: Predictors of non-responsiveness to high-dose gamma-globulin therapy in patients with Kawasaki disease at onset. J Pediatr 137:172–176, 2000.
  Mori M, Imagawa T, Yasui K, et al: Predictors of coronary artery lesions after intravenous gamma-globulin treatment in Kawasaki disease. J Pediatr 137:177–180, 2000.

80. **Is aspirin therapy of benefit for children with Kawasaki disease?**
By itself, high-dose aspirin (80–100 mg/kg/day divided into doses taken every 6 hours) is effective for decreasing the degree of fever and discomfort in patients during the acute stages of illness. It is unclear if high-dose aspirin has an additive effect for decreasing the incidence of coronary artery abnormalities when used in conjunction with gamma globulin. Aspirin may be beneficial when administered in low doses after the resolution of fever due to its effects on platelet aggregation and prevention of the thrombotic complications seen in children with Kawasaki disease. Therefore, aspirin in low doses (3–5 mg/kg/day) is advised for about 6–8

weeks. If a follow-up echocardiogram at that time reveals no coronary abnormalities, therapy is usually discontinued. If abnormalities are present, therapy is continued indefinitely.

81. **If untreated, what percentage of children with Kawasaki disease will develop coronary artery ectasia or aneurysms?**
Between 15% and 25%.

82. **What factors are most strongly associated with the development of coronary artery disease in patients with Kawasaki disease?**
- Duration of fever of >16 days
- Recurrence of fever after an afebrile period of 48 hours
- Dysrhythmias (other than first-degree heart block)
- Cardiomegaly
- Male gender
- Age of <1 year

PHARMACOLOGY

83. **How valuable are digoxin levels?**
Digoxin levels are only useful as a guide to digoxin therapy. Digoxin levels may not be as helpful in infants and younger children because of the presence of endogenous digoxin-like immunoreactive substances, which cross-react with immunoassay antibodies to digoxin. Digoxin levels may be helpful, however, in older children and adolescents (especially in the presence of dysrhythmias).

84. **How long before oral digoxin begins to work?**
Oral digoxin reaches peak plasma levels 1–2 hours after administration, but a peak hemodynamic effect is not evident until 6 hours after administration (versus 2–3 hours for intravenous digoxin).

85. **A child with WPW syndrome and SVT is given digoxin, and the attending cardiologist is dismayed. Why?**
Digoxin can enhance conduction through a bypass tract while slowing down conduction through the AV node. Ventricular fibrillation has been reported in patients with WPW treated with digoxin. This effect is believed to be due to enhanced conduction down the bypass tract. For this reason, propranolol has replaced digoxin as the drug of choice for the treatment of children with SVT and WPW.

86. **What are the indications for prostaglandin E_1 (PGE_1) in the neonate?**
PGE_1 is indicated in cardiac lesions with inadequate pulmonary blood flow (e.g., pulmonary atresia with intact ventricular septum, tricuspid atresia with intact ventricular septum, critical pulmonary stenosis); inadequate systemic blood flow (e.g., critical coarctation of the aorta, interrupted aortic arch, hypoplastic left heart syndrome); or inadequate mixing (e.g., transposition of great vessels).

87. **What are the major side effects of PGE_1?**
Apnea, fever, cutaneous flushing, seizures, hypotension, and bradycardia/tachycardia.

88. **What are the side effects of indomethacin in the neonate?**
- Mild but usually transient decreased renal function
- Hyponatremia
- Hypoglycemia
- Platelet dysfunction producing a prolonged bleeding time

- Occult blood loss from the gastrointestinal tract
- Spontaneous perforation of the intestine

89. **How do alpha, beta, and dopaminergic receptors differ?**
    Alpha: In vascular smooth muscle, these cause vasoconstriction.
    Beta$_1$: In myocardial smooth muscle, these increase inotropic (contractile) force, chronotropic (cardiac rate) effect, and AV conduction (dromotropic).
    Beta$_2$: In vascular smooth muscle, these cause vasodilation.
    Dopaminergic: In renal and mesenteric vascular smooth muscle, these cause vasodilation.

90. **How do relative receptor effects differ by drug type?**
    See Table 3-6.

TABLE 3-6. RELATIVE RECEPTOR EFFECTS BY DRUG TYPE				
Drug	Alpha	Beta$_1$	Beta$_2$	Dopaminergic
Epinephrine	+++	+++	+++	0
Norepinephrine	+++	+++	+	0
Isoproterenol	0	+++	+++	0
Dopamine*	0 to +++ (dose-related)	++ to +++ (dose-related)	++	+++
Dobutamine	0 to +	+++	+	0

Effect of medication: 0 = none, + = small, ++ = moderate, +++ = large.
*For dopamine, at low doses (2–5 μg/kg/min), dopaminergic effects predominate. At high doses (5–20 μg/kg/min), increased alpha and beta effects are seen. At very high doses (>20 μg/kg/min), a markedly increased alpha effect with decreased renal and mesenteric blood flow occurs. For dobutamine, beta$_1$ inotropic effects are more pronounced than chronotropic effects are.

91. **How are emergency infusions for cardiovascular support prepared?**
    See Table 3-7.

TABLE 3-7. EMERGENCY INFUSIONS FOR CARDIOVASCULAR SUPPORT		
Catecholamine	Mixture	Dose
Isoproterenol, Epinephrine, Norepinephrine	0.6 mg × body wt (in kg), added to diluent to make 100 mL	1 mL/h delivers 0.1 μg/kg/min
Dopamine, Dobutamine	6 mg × body wt (in kg), added to diluent to make 100 mL	1 mL/h delivers 1 μg/kg/min

PHYSICAL EXAMINATION

92. **What causes the first heart sound?**
    The first heart sound is caused by the closure of the mitral and tricuspid valves.

93. **What causes the second heart sound?**
The second heart sound is caused by the closure of the aortic and pulmonary valves.

94. **In what settings can an abnormal second heart sound be auscultated?**
Widely split S_2
- Prolonged RV ejection time
- RV volume overload: Atrial septal defect, partial anomalous pulmonary venous return
- RV conduction delay: Right bundle branch block

Single S_2
- Presence of only one semilunar valve: Aortic or pulmonary atresia, truncus arteriosus
- P2 not audible: Tetralogy of Fallot, transposition of great arteries
- A2 delayed: Severe aortic stenosis
- May be normal in a newborn

Paradoxically split S_2 (A2 follows P2)
- Severe aortic stenosis
- Left bundle-branch block

Loud P2
- Pulmonary hypertension

95. **When can S_3 and S_4 be considered normal findings during a pediatric cardiac examination?**
An S_3 occurs early in diastole. It may be benign, but it can be abnormal in children with dilated ventricles and decreased compliance (e.g., in patients with CHF). An S_4 occurs late in diastole. It is usually abnormal in children.

96. **During physical examination, what patient maneuvers can increase the likelihood of detecting mitral valve prolapse (MVP) on auscultation?**
In patients with MVP, the leaflets of the mitral valve apparatus billow into the left atrium. Maneuvers that decrease LV size and volume (and thus increase the relative size of the leaflets) increase the likelihood of hearing the click or murmur. These include the straining phase of a Valsalva maneuver, inspiration, and change from a supine to a sitting position or from a squatting to a standing position. The left lateral decubitus position may also be facilitative.

97. **What is the difference between pulsus alternans and pulsus paradoxus?**
- **Pulsus alternans** is a pulse pattern in which there is alternating (beat-to-beat) variability of pulse strength due to decreased ventricular performance. This is sometimes seen in patients with severe CHF.
- **Pulsus paradoxus** indicates an exaggeration of the normal reduction of systolic blood pressure during inspiration. Associated conditions include cardiac tamponade (e.g., effusion, constrictive pericarditis), severe respiratory illness (e.g., asthma, pneumonia), and myocardial disease that affects wall compliance (e.g., endocardial fibroelastosis, amyloidosis).

98. **How is pulsus paradoxus measured?**
To measure a pulsus paradoxus, determine the systolic pressure by noting the first audible Korotkoff sound. Then retake the blood pressure by raising the manometer pressure to at least 25 mmHg higher than the systolic pressure, and allow it to fall very slowly. Stop as soon as the first sound is heard. Note that the sound disappears during inspiration.

Lower the pressure slowly, and note when all pulsed beats are heard. The difference between these two pressures is the pulsus paradoxus. Normally, in children, there is an 8–10 mmHg fluctuation in systolic pressure with different phases of respiration.

99. **Is palpation for femoral pulses a reliable screening tool for coarctation of the aorta in infants and older children?**
The detection of decreased lower extremity pulses seen in coarctation can be subtle and unreliable. In some **infants**, a patent ductus arteriosus may provide blood flow to the lower extremities, thus bypassing a severe coarctation. Upper and lower pulses may be equal as long as the ductus remains open. As the ductus closes, signs of coarctation of the aorta may appear with respiratory distress and cardiac failure. Decreased or absent pulses may then be noted. In **older children**, simultaneous palpation of upper and lower extremity pulses is important. If collaterals have developed, a delay in pulse rather than diminished volume may be noted. In a study of older patients (>1 year old) with documented coarctation, only 20% had absent lower extremity pulses, and distinguishing differences between upper extremity and lower extremity pulses was unreliable. Thus, some authors recommend that screening for coarctation of the aorta be done by measuring blood pressure in both arms and one leg.

Ing FF, Starc TJ, Griffiths SP, Gersony WM: Early diagnosis of coarctation of the aorta in children: A continuing dilemma. Pediatrics 98: 378–382, 1996.

100. **What is the differential diagnosis for a systolic murmur in each auscultatory area?**
See Fig. 3-7.

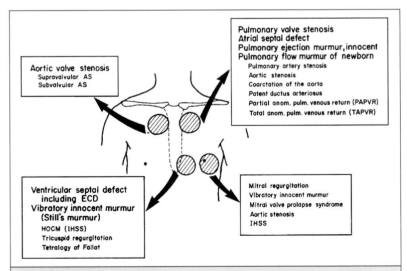

Figure 3-7. Systolic murmurs audible at various locations. Many may radiate to other areas. Less-common conditions are shown in smaller type. (From Park MK: Pediatric Cardiology for Practitioners, 4th ed. St. Louis, Mosby, 2002, p 32.)

101. What are the most common innocent murmurs?
See Table 3-8.

TABLE 3-8. MOST COMMON INNOCENT MURMURS		
Type (timing)	**Description of murmur**	**Common age group**
Classic vibratory murmur (Still murmur; systolic)	Maximal at MLSB or between LLSB and apex Grade 2–3/6 Low-frequency vibratory, "twanging string," or musical	3–6 years old; occasionally in infancy
Pulmonary ejection murmur (systolic)	Maximal at ULSB Early to midsystolic Grade 1–2/6 in intensity	8–14 years old
Pulmonary flow murmur of newborn (systolic)	Maximal at ULSB	Premature and full-term newborns; usually disappears by 3–6 months of age
	Transmits well to left and right chest, axillae, and back Grade 1–2/6 intensity	
Venous hum (continuous)	Maximal at right (or left) supra- and infra-clavicular areas Grade 1–2/6 intensity Inaudible in supine position Intensity changes with rotation of head and compression of jugular vein	3–6 years old
Carotid bruit (systolic)	Right supraclavicular area and over carotids Grade 2–3/6 intensity Occasional thrill over a carotid artery	Any age

MLSB = mid-left sternal border, LLSB = lower-left sternal border, ULSB = upper-left sternal border.

102. What features are suggestive of a pathologic murmur?
- Diastolic murmurs
- Late systolic murmurs

- Pansystolic murmurs
- Murmurs associated with a thrill
- Associated cardiac abnormalities (e.g., asymmetric pulses, clicks, abnormal splitting)
- Continuous murmurs

> McCrindle BW, Shaffer KM, Kan JS, et al: Cardinal clinical signs in the differentiation of heart murmurs in children. Arch Pediatr Adolesc Med 150:169–174, 1996.
> Rosenthal A: How to distinguish between innocent and pathologic murmurs in childhood. Pediatr Clin North Am 31:1229–1240, 1984.

103. **If a murmur is detected, what noncardiac factors suggest that the murmur is pathologic?**
   - Evidence of growth retardation (most commonly seen in murmurs with large left-to-right shunts)
   - Associated dysmorphic features (e.g., valvular disease in Hurler syndrome, Noonan syndrome)
   - Exertional cyanosis, pallor, or dyspnea, especially if associated with minor exertion such as climbing a few stairs (may be a sign of early CHF)
   - Short feeding times and volumes in infants (may be a sign of early CHF)
   - Syncopal or presyncopal episodes (may be seen in hypertrophic cardiomyopathy)
   - History of intravenous drug abuse (risk factor for endocarditis)
   - Maternal history of diabetes mellitus (associated with asymmetric septal hypertrophy, VSD, d-transposition), alcohol use (associated with pulmonic stenosis and VSD), or other medications
   - Family history of congenital heart disease

KEY POINTS: PATHOLOGIC MURMURS

1. Diastolic

2. Pansystolic

3. Late systolic

4. Continuous

5. Thrill present on examination

6. Additional cardiac abnormalities (e.g., clicks, abnormal splitting, asymmetric pulses)

SURGERY

104. **What are shunt operations?**
   Shunts between a systemic artery and the pulmonary artery are used to improve oxygen saturation in patients with cyanotic CHD and diminished pulmonary blood flow. Venoarterial shunts that connect a systemic vein and the pulmonary artery are also used for similar purposes.

105. **Name the major shunt operations (Fig. 3-8) for CHD.**
   - The **Blalock-Taussig** shunt consists of an anastomosis between a subclavian artery and the ipsilateral pulmonary artery. The subclavian artery can be divided and the distal end

anastomosed to the pulmonary artery *(classic BT shunt)*, or a prosthetic graft *(Gore-Tex)* can be interposed between the two arteries *(modified BT shunt)*.

- The **Waterston** shunt is an anastomosis between the ascending aorta and the right pulmonary artery. This procedure is rarely performed today.
- The **Potts** shunt is an anastomosis between the descending aorta and the left pulmonary artery. This procedure is rarely performed today.

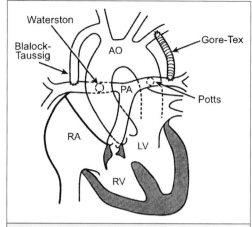

Figure 3-8. Major shunt operations. (From Park MK: Pediatric Cardiology for Practitioners, 4th ed. St. Louis, Mosby, 2002, p 194.)

106. **For which congenital heart disorder is the "switch operation" done?**
     Transposition of the great arteries. This procedure restores the aorta and the pulmonary artery to their correct anatomic positions, and it involves the reimplantation of the coronary arteries.

107. **What are the indications for surgical repair of VSD and ASD?**
     - **VSD:** Infants with a large VSD that is refractory to medical therapy (thereby causing failure to thrive and/or repeated lower respiratory tract infections) should be referred for surgery. Pulmonary hypertension is another indication for surgery. In older children with normal pulmonary artery pressure but with significantly increased pulmonary blood flow or left ventricular dilatation, surgical closure is sometimes advised.
     - **ASD:** Asymptomatic children should be scheduled for repair during the first 5 years of life. The rare infant with a symptomatic ASD should undergo surgery at the time of diagnosis.

108. **Is there any surgical therapy for hypoplastic left heart syndrome?**
     In patients with this condition, severe underdevelopment of the left ventricle, mitral valve, aortic valve, and ascending aortic arch occurs. Newborns develop signs of severe CHF and cyanosis. Two surgical options are available: **heart transplantation** and the **Norwood procedure**.

109. **What is the long-term prognosis for heart transplantation during infancy and childhood?**
     Survival statistics have improved dramatically over the last 10 years with the use of newer and safer immunosuppressive agents such as cyclosporine and FK506. However, children who receive transplanted hearts are at increased risk for cardiac rejection, infection, accelerated coronary artery disease, and lymphoproliferative syndromes. Recent estimated 5-year survival rates vary between 65% and 70%.

     Towbin JA: Cardiomyopathy and heart transplantation in children. Curr Opin Cardiol 17:274–279, 2002.

ACKNOWLEDGMENT

The editors gratefully acknowledge the contributions by Dr. Bernard J. Clark, III that were retained from the first three editions of *Pediatric Secrets*.

CHAPTER 4

DERMATOLOGY*

Maria C. Garzon, MD, and Kimberly D. Morel, MD

ACNE

1. **When is acne most likely to develop?**
   The development of micro comedones is typically the earliest sign of acne. Studies have shown that comedones occur in three fourths of premenarchal girls at an average age of 10 years and in about half of 10- to 11-year-old boys. They may herald (or predate) the onset of puberty.

2. **How do a "blackhead" and a "whitehead" differ histopathologically?**
   Both lesions are produced by obstruction and distention of the sebaceous follicle with sebum and cellular debris. When the follicular contents tent the overlying skin but are not exposed to the atmosphere, a **whitehead** occurs. If the contents project out of the follicular opening, oxidation of the exposed mass of debris produces a color change and a **blackhead**.

3. **What is the difference between neonatal acne and infantile acne?**
   Neonatal acne occurs in up to 20% of newborns and typically presents during the first 4 weeks after birth. Erythematous papulopustules develop on the face, especially the cheeks. It has been attributed to the transient elevation of androgenic hormones (both maternally derived and endogenous) that are present in a newborn infant. The lesions typically resolve within 1–3 months as androgen levels fall. *Neonatal cephalic pustulosis* is a term that has been proposed to replace neonatal acne. Since lesions have been shown to contain *Malassezia* species, neonatal "acne" may actually represent an inflammatory reaction to this yeast flora and not true acne at all.

KEY POINTS: MORPHOLOGIC DESCRIPTIONS OF PRIMARY CUTANEOUS LESIONS

1. **Macule:** A circumscribed, flat area, recognizable by color variation from surrounding skin, ≤1 cm

2. **Patch:** A large macule, >1 cm

3. **Papule:** A circumscribed elevation, <1 cm

4. **Plaque:** A large superficial papule, >1 cm

5. **Nodule:** A circumscribed solid elevation, ≤1 cm

6. **Vesicle** (small blister): A clear, fluid-filled elevation, ≤1 cm

7. **Bullae** (large blister): A fluid-filled elevation, >1 cm

8. **Pustule:** A circumscribed elevation of skin filled with pus

*The off-label use of medications will be discussed in this chapter.

Infantile acne affects a smaller number of infants on a delayed basis (3–6 months) and is characterized by greater degrees of inflammatory papules and pustules. Open and closed comedones and sometimes nodules are also present. This type is similar to acne vulgaris and may persist for years. The cause is unknown. Most patients with this condition have no evidence of precocious puberty or increased hormonal levels, although severe acne in this age group warrants evaluation for hyperandrogenism. Systemic therapy is sometimes required.

4. **Is an infant with acne more likely to be a teenager with acne?**
   The presence or severity of acne in an infant who is <3 months old is not felt to correlate with an increased likelihood of adolescent acne. However, delayed acne between 3 and 6 months of age (especially if persistent and severe) does have a higher correlation with the likelihood of more severe adolescent acne. Family history of severe acne also increases the likelihood of future problems.

   Herane MI, Ando I: Acne in infancy and acne genetics. Dermatology 206:24–28, 2003.

5. **What are the most severe forms of acne?**
   Acne fulminans is a rare but severe disorder that has also been called acute febrile ulcerative acne. It occurs in teenage boys as extensive, inflammatory, ulcerating lesions on the trunk and chest that are usually associated with fever, malaise, arthralgia, and leukocytosis. The etiology remains unclear, but immune complexes are thought to be involved. Treatment is systemic and includes the following: antibiotics, glucocorticoids, and retinoids.

   Acne conglobata is a severe form of acne that presents with comedones, papules, pustules, nodules, and abscesses. It is associated with significant scarring. It often arises in early adulthood, more typically in females. Systemic retinoid therapy is the treatment of choice.

   James WD: Acne. N Engl J Med 352:1463–1472, 2005.

6. **What is the therapeutic approach to acne?**
   Acne therapies, including comedolytics, antibacterial agents, and hormonal modulators, target various factors involved in the pathogenesis of acne. Topical agents including erythromycin, clindamycin, erythromycin–benzoyl peroxide, clindamycin–benzoyl peroxide, benzoyl peroxide, and azelaic acid reduce the population of *Propionibacterium acnes*. Systemic antibiotics (e.g., tetracycline and its derivatives) are most frequently used for moderate-to-severe papulopustular acne. The topical retinoid tretinoin (Retin-A, Avita) is comedolytic and prevents the formation of new keratin plugs. The systemic retinoid isotretinoin (Accutane) is used in cases of severe acne vulgaris. The exact mechanism of action of isotretinoin is not known but appears to be related to the inhibition of sebaceous gland activity. Other agents used in severe acne include intralesional corticosteroids. Hormonal modulation is most commonly accomplished with oral contraceptive pills, although antiandrogenic agents (e.g., spironolactone) have been used in teenage females with premenstrual flares, hirsutism, and male-pattern alopecia.

   Lee DJ, Van Dyke GS, Kim J: Update on pathogenesis and treatment of acne. Curr Opin Pediatr 15:405-10, 2003.
   Leyden JJ: A review of the use of combination therapies for the treatment of acne vulgaris. J Am Acad Dermatol 49:S200–S2010, 2003.

7. **When is the use of oral isotretinoin indicated in teenagers with acne?**
   Isotretinoin, which is 13-cis-retinoic acid (Accutane), is most appropriately used for nodulocystic acne, acne conglobata, or scarring acne that has been unresponsive to standard modes of treatment (e.g., oral/topical antibiotics, topical retinoids). Its most dangerous side effect is teratogenicity, and rigorous monitoring and definitive contraceptive counseling are mandatory.

   Haider A, Shaw JC: Treatment of acne vulgaris. JAMA 292:726–735, 2004.

8. **What serious side effects may be associated with systemic minocycline therapy for acne?**

Tetracyclines, including the derivative minocycline, are the most widely prescribed oral antibiotics for acne and have been used safely over long periods of time. They are contraindicated for patients <8 years old because of the potential for permanent dental staining. Rare reactions—particularly to minocycline—have included pneumonitis, autoimmune hepatitis, drug-induced lupus, serum-sickness-like reactions, and severe hypersensitivity reactions.

Eichenfield AH: Minocycline and autoimmunity. Curr Opin Pediatr 11:447–456, 1999.

Sturkenboom MC, Meier CR, Jick H, Stricker BH: Minocycline and lupuslike syndrome in acne patients. Arch Intern Med 159:493–497, 1999.

9. **What guidelines can help to maximize the compliance of teenagers with therapy for acne?**

- Reassure the teenager that acne is both common and treatable.
- Explain that acne cannot be scrubbed away.
- Do not overload teens with data. A few "take-home" messages are optimal.
- Allow teenagers to ask questions.
- Remember to treat the teenager's back and chest if they are involved, not just the face.
- Give the teenager choices whenever possible (e.g., Retin-A versus benzoyl peroxide).
- Be aware of the cost of the medications.
- Do not take noncompliance personally.

Strasburger VC: Acne: What every pediatrician should know about treatment. Pediatr Clin North Am 44: 1519–1520, 1997.

CLINICAL ISSUES

10. **What skin findings are suggestive of occult spinal dysraphism?**

Intraspinal anomalies without a detectable back mass may present with skin findings. Midline dermatologic findings in the lumbosacral area that are suggestive of occult spinal dysraphism include the following:

- Lipoma
- Hypertrichosis
- Pits: Dermal dimples or sinuses about the intergluteal cleft (particularly with lateral deviation of the cleft)
- Vascular lesions (hemangioma, port wine stain, telangiectases)
- Pigmentation variants (both hyperpigmentation, including lentigo and melanocytic nevus, and hypopigmentation)
- Aplasia cutis congenita
- Appendages (skin tags, tail)

Howard R: Congenital midline lesions: Pits and protuberances. Pediatr Ann 27.150–160, 1998.

11. **What conditions cause ring-like rashes on the skin?**

Not all rings are ringworm. Annular (ring-like) skin lesions can be seen in a wide variety of skin diseases in children. Common causes of these lesions include the following:

- Tinea corporis
- Dermatitis (atopic, nummular, or contact)
- Granuloma annulare (often composed of small papules without overlying scale)
- Erythema migrans
- Systemic lupus erythematosus

For online photo atlas, see www.dermatlas.med.jhmi.edu/derm

KEY POINTS: DIFFERENTIAL DIAGNOSES OF RING-LIKE SKIN RASHES

1. Tinea corporis

2. Dermatitis (atopic, nummular, or contact)

3. Granuloma annulare (often composed of small papules without overlying scale)

4. Erythema migrans

5. Systemic lupus erythematosus

12. **What is the natural history of molluscum contagiosum?**
Molluscum contagiosum is a common skin infection caused by a poxvirus. Lesions are small pinkish-tan, dome-shaped papules that often have a dimpled or umbilicated center. They are usually asymptomatic, but they may associated with an eczematous dermatitis and itch. Superinfection may complicate the course, require antibiotic therapy, and increase the likelihood of scarring after resolution. In healthy children, the course is self-limited but may last for 2 years. In some cases, persistent and widespread molluscum may require screening for congenital or acquired immunodeficiencies.

13. **What is the best way to eradicate molluscum contagiosum?**
If watchful waiting is not desired, therapeutic options are primarily destructive methods. Curettage (with core removal), cryotherapy, and peeling agents (salicylic and lactic acid preparations) can be used. An increasingly popular method is the use of cantharidin, a blistering agent, which is applied in the physician's office to individual lesions.

Ting PT, Dytoc MT: Therapy of external anogenital warts and molluscum contagiosum: A literature review. Derm Therapy 17:68–101, 2004.

14. **What are the common causes of acute urticaria in children?**
Acute urticaria may last for several weeks. If it persists beyond that period, it is typically characterized as *chronic urticaria*. In children, the most common causes of *acute urticaria* include the five "Is":
- Infection (viral and bacterial are the most frequent, but fungal pathogens may also cause urticaria)
- Infestation (parasites)
- Ingestion (medication and foods)
- Injections or infusions (immunizations, blood products, and antibiotics)
- Inhalation (allergens such as pollens and molds)

Weston W, Orchard D: Vascular reactions. In Schachner LA, Hansen RC (eds): Pediatric Dermatology, 3rd ed. St. Louis, Mosby, 2003 pp 801–831.

15. **Describe the characteristic clinical picture of erythema nodosum.**
A prodrome of fever, chills, malaise, and arthralgia may precede the typical skin findings. Crops of red to blue tender nodules appear over the anterior shins. Lesions may be seen on the knees, ankles, thighs, and, occasionally, the lower extensor forearms and face. They may evolve through a spectrum of colors that resemble a bruise. Often the changes are misdiagnosed as cellulitis or secondary to a traumatic event. This condition is associated with a variety of infectious (e.g., group A beta hemolytic streptococcus, tuberculosis) and noninfectious (e.g., ulcerative colitis, leukemia) causes.

16. **What, technically, are warts?**
Benign epidermal tumors caused by multiple types of human papillomaviruses.

KEY POINTS: MIDLINE LUMBOSACRAL LESIONS ASSOCIATED WITH OCCULT SPINAL DYSRAPHISM OR TETHERED CORD

1. Sacral pits (particularly with lateral deviation of the gluteal cleft)

2. Hairy patches

3. Appendages (skin tag or tail)

4. Sacral lipoma

5. Vascular lesions (hemangioma, port wine stain, telangiectasias)

6. Pigmentation variants (hyperpigmentation, including lentigo and melanocytic nevus, and hypopigmentation)

7. Aplasia cutis congenita

17. **How are plantar warts clinically distinguished from calluses?**
Plantar warts are painful warts on the soles of the feet. They are flat or slightly raised areas of firm hyperkeratosis with a collarette of normal skin (Fig. 4-1). Unlike calluses, with which they can be confused, plantar warts cause obliteration of the normal skin lines (dermatoglyphics).

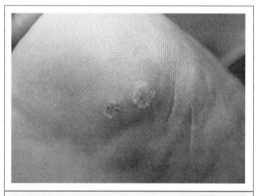

Figure 4-1. Plantar warts. Note disruption of skin lines. Characteristic black dots in the warts are thrombosed capillaries. (From Cohen BA: Pediatric Dermatology, 2nd ed. London, Mosby, 1999, p 115.)

18. **How can common warts be treated?**
The mode of therapy depends on the type and number of warts, the location on the body, and the age of the patient. No matter what treatment is used, warts can always recur; there are no absolute cures. The major goal is to remove warts without residual scarring. Of course, another option is no treatment at all because many warts self-resolve, but they may take years to do so. Therapies include liquid nitrogen (topical), topical tretinoin cream, cantharidin (if not facial), salicylic acid preparations, duct tape application, curettage, and electrodesiccation.

Other treatment modalities, including pulsed dye laser, topical imiquimod, and contact immunotherapy, have been used to treat recalcitrant warts in children. In some case reports, oral cimetidine has been effective, perhaps due to its immunomodulatory activity. Little data exists regarding the relative efficacy of many treatments of warts in children.

Siegfried EC: Warts on children: An approach to therapy. Pediatr Ann 25:79–90, 1996.

19. **What are the most common causes of lumps and bumps in the skin of children?**

    Although most parents fear malignancy, nodules, or tumors in the skin are very rarely malignant. A study of 775 excised and histologically diagnosed superficial lumps in children revealed the following.

    - **Epidermal inclusion cysts:** 59%
    - **Congenital malformations** (pilomatrixoma, lymphangioma, hemangioendothelioma, brachial cleft cyst): 17%
    - **Benign neoplasms** (neural tumors, lipoma, adnexal tumors): 7%
    - **Benign lesions of undetermined etiology** (xanthomas, xanthogranulomas, fibromatosis, fibroma): 6%
    - **Self-limited processes** (granuloma annulare, urticaria pigmentosa, persistent insect bite reaction): 6%
    - **Malignant tumors:** 1.4%
    - **Miscellaneous:** 4%

    Wyatt AJ, Hansen RC: Pediatric skin tumors. Pediatr Clin North Am 47:937–963, 2000.
    Knight PJ, Reiner CB: Superficial lumps in children: What, when, and why? Pediatrics 72:147–153, 1983.

20. **Why is a pyogenic granuloma neither pyogenic nor a granuloma?**

    A pyogenic granuloma, which is also called a lobular capillary hemangioma, is a common acquired lesion that develops typically at the site of obvious or trivial trauma on any part of the body. Local capillary proliferation occurs, often rapidly, and bleeding may develop (Fig. 4-2). Curettage and electrodesiccation of the base are curative. The lesion is neither an infectious pyoderma nor a granuloma on biopsy.

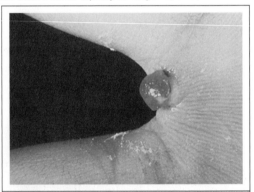

Figure 4-2. Pyogenic granuloma in the web space between fingers. (From Cohen BA: Pediatric Dermatology, 2nd ed. London, Mosby, 1999, p 127.)

21. **An 8-year-old has a hard, nontender, freely mobile nodule of the neck with a slightly bluish hue of the skin. What is the most likely diagnosis?**

    Pilomatrixoma. Also called *the benign calcifying epithelioma of Malherbe,* this is a benign tumor that often arises in children and adolescents on the face and neck. It is usually not confused with a malignant condition, but excision is often recommended for cosmetic reasons because these nodules may increase in size or become infected.

22. **What condition is classically diagnosed by the Darier sign?**

    Mastocytoma. This is a benign lesion composed of mast cells that arises at birth or during early infancy. It appears as a pink/tan plaque or nodule, often with a peau d'orange surface. **Darier sign** refers to the eliciting of erythema and an urticarial wheal by stroking or rubbing the lesion. The skin changes are caused by the release of histamine from the mechanically traumatized mast cells.

23. **What disorder can present as "freckles" associated with hives?**

    Urticaria pigmentosa (mastocytosis). Presenting at birth or during early infancy, multiple mastocytomas appear as brown macules, papules, or plaques (vesicle formation can also occur) and are often mistaken for freckles or melanocytic nevi. Lesions are usually only cutaneous but infrequently they may affect other organ systems (e.g., lungs, kidney, gastrointestinal tract, central nervous system). The Darier sign is a key feature of diagnosis.

24.   **What is impetigo?**
Impetigo is a superficial skin infection that is caused by *Staphylococcus aureus* or group A streptococcus. Historically, streptococcus was the most prevalent agent. However, over the last few decades, *S. aureus* appears to be the predominant organism, although mixed infections may also occur. Bullous impetigo is usually caused by *S. aureus*.

25.   **Is topical or systemic therapy better for impetigo?**
Treatment usually requires an antibiotic that is active against both streptococci and staphylococci. Topical antibiotics (mupirocin) can be used in localized disease. Systemic antibiotics are usually indicated for extensive involvement; outbreaks among household contacts, schools, or athletic teams; or if topical therapy has failed. Cephalosporins (e.g., cephalexin, cefadroxil), amoxicillin–clavulanate, and dicloxacillin are most effective. Erythromycin is unlikely to be useful because increasing numbers of staphylococci are resistant; local resistance patterns should determine its usage.

Sladden MJ, Johnston GA: Common skin infections in children. BMJ 329:95–99, 2004.

26.   **What dermatologic sign starts from a scratch?**
Dermographism occurs when the skin is stroked firmly with a pointed object. The result is a red line that is followed by an erythematous flare, which is eventually followed by a *wheal*. This "triple response of Lewis" usually occurs within 1–3 minutes. Dermographism (or skin writing) is an exaggerated triple response of Lewis and is seen in patients with urticaria. The tendency to be dermographic can appear at any age and may last for months to years. The cause is often unknown. White dermographism is seen in patients with an atopic diathesis, in whom the red line is replaced by a white line without a subsequent flare and wheal.

27.   **Do geographic tongues vary in the northern and southern hemispheres?**
Despite the Hubble telescope, more research awaits. *Geographic tongue* refers to the benign condition in which denudations of the filiform papillae on the lingual surface occur, giving the tongue the appearance of a relief map (Fig. 4-3). The patterns change over hours and days, and the histopathology resembles that of psoriasis. The patient is usually asymptomatic. No treatment is effective or necessary, because self-resolution is the rule. Etiology in either hemisphere is unknown.

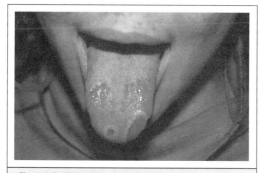

Figure 4-3. Geographic tongue. (From Sahn EE: Dermatology Pearls. Philadelphia, Hanley & Belfus, 1999, p 162.)

28.   **What diseases are associated with a strawberry tongue?**
Scarlet fever caused by group A beta hemolytic streptococcus and **Kawasaki disease** are the most common disorders associated with a strawberry tongue. The "strawberry-like" surface characteristics are caused by prominent lingual papillae. A white strawberry tongue is caused by fibrinous exudate overlying the tongue. Red strawberry tongues lack the fibrinous exudate.

ECZEMATOUS DISORDERS

29. **What is the difference between eczema and atopic dermatitis?**
The term *eczema* derives from the Greek word *exzein*, which means to erupt: *ex* (out) plus *zein* (to boil). To most physicians, eczema is synonymous with atopic dermatitis, a chronic skin disease manifested by intermittent skin eruption. **Eczema** is primarily a morphologic term used to describe an erythematous, scaling, inflammatory eruption with itching, edema, papules, vesicles, and crusts. There are other "eczematous eruptions" (nummular eczema, allergic contact dermatitis), but "garden variety" eczema is certainly the most common.
   Atopic dermatitis is a broader allergic tendency with multiple dermal manifestations that are mostly secondary to pruritus. Atopic dermatitis has been called an "itch that rashes, not a rash that itches." Its manifestations are dry skin, chronic and recurrent dermatitis, low threshold to pruritus, hyperlinear palms, eyelid pleats (Dennie-Morgan folds), pityriasis alba, and keratosis pilaris, among others.

30. **What is the usual distribution of rash in atopic dermatitis?**
Infant: Cheeks, trunk, and extensor surfaces of extremities, knees, and elbows
Child: Neck, feet, and antecubital and popliteal fossae
Older child: Neck, hands, feet, and antecubital and popliteal fossae

KEY POINTS: MAIN FEATURES OF ATOPIC DERMATITIS

1. Extensor surface involvement in infancy

2. Flexural surface involvement in older children

3. Lichenification with chronic scratching

4. Dennie-Morgan folds under eyes

5. Part of atopic triad: atopic dermatitis, asthma, and allergic rhinitis

31. **Describe the five key battle plans to treat atopic dermatitis.**
   1. **Reduce pruritus.** Topical corticosteroids and bland emollients help reduce pruritus. Oral antihistamines may also be used for their sedative effect at night and may reduce pruritus.
   2. **Hydrate the skin.** Emollients (petrolatum and fragrance-free ointments and creams) prevent the evaporation of moisture via occlusion and are best applied immediately after bathing, when the skin is maximally hydrated, to "lock in" moisture.
   3. **Reduce inflammation.** Topical steroids are invaluable as anti-inflammatory agents and can hasten the clearing of eruptions that are erythematous (inflamed). Medium-strength corticosteroids can be used on areas other than the face and occluded regions (diaper area); low-strength steroids (e.g., 1% hydrocortisone) may be used in these thin-skinned areas. Newer immunomodulators, such as topical tacrolimus and pimecrolimus, are approved for the intermittent treatment of moderate to severe atopic dermatitis in children 2 years old and older. However, their long-term side effects have not been fully evaluated.
   4. **Control infection.** Superinfection with *Staphylococcus aureus* is extremely common. First-generation cephalosporins such as cephalexin are the usual antibiotics of choice for infected atopic dermatitis.

5. **Avoid irritants.** Gentle fragrance-free soaps and shampoos should be used; wool and tight synthetic garments should be avoided; tight nonsynthetic garments may help minimize the "itchy" feeling; consider furniture, carpeting, pets, and dust mites as possible irritants and/or trigger factors.

> Hanifin JM, Cooper KD, Ho VC, et al: Guidelines of care for atopic dermatitis, developed in accordance with the American Academy of Dermatology (AAD)/American Academy of Dermatology Association "Administrative Regulations for Evidence-Based Clinical Practice Guidelines." J Am Acad Dermatol 50:391–404, 2004.

32. **Do soaps or clothes make any difference in atopic dermatitis?**
    - **Soaps:** Less drying, unfragranced, nondetergent soaps, such as Dove, are better than more drying soaps, such as Ivory. Other mild soaps include Cetaphil, Purpose, Aveeno, and Basis; the latter is a superfatted soap.
    - **Clothing:** Avoid woolen clothes: the fibers can irritate the skin and trigger the itch-scratch cycle. If woolens must be used, they should be lined. Soft fibers are the least irritating (e.g., cotton jerseys).

33. **What is the most common side effect of topical pimecrolimus and tacrolimus?**
    These topical immunomodulating creams are used for intermittent therapy. The most common side effect is burning or stinging, which can occur in up to 10% of patients, especially with initial use. This side effect tends to improve with continued use. Use on open skin sores should be avoided. The long-term side effects of chronic use are still under investigation. Patients should be instructed about the importance of sun protection while using topical immunosuppressive medications.

    > Eichenfield LF, Hanifin JM, Luger TA, et al: Consensus conference on pediatric atopic dermatitis. J Am Acad Dermatol 49:1088–1095, 2003.

34. **Why shouldn't fluorinated (halogenated) steroids be used on the face?**
    There are several reasons:
    - Facial skin is thinner and therefore percutaneous absorption is higher.
    - Telangiectasias or spider veins can occur.
    - Cutaneous atrophy can occur.
    - Perioral dermatitis or poststeroid rosacea can occur with rebound symptoms that are worse than the original rash.

35. **Is there a genetic basis for atopic dermatitis?**
    It is likely that both genetic and environmental factors play a role. Although specific genetic information is lacking, it has been strongly suggested that an individual's genotype determines whether he or she will develop atopic dermatitis. Many children with atopic dermatitis have a family history of atopy. If one parent has an atopic diathesis, 60% of offspring will be atopic; if two parents do, 80% of children are affected. Monozygotic twins are often concordant for atopic disease.

36. **Are there consistent immunologic alterations in children with atopic dermatitis?**
    Humoral changes include elevated immunoglobulin E levels and a higher-than-normal number of positive skin tests (type I cutaneous reactions) to common environmental allergens. Cell-mediated abnormalities have been found only during acute flares of the dermatitis; these include mild to moderate depression of cell-mediated immunity, a 30–50% decrease in lymphocyte-forming E-rosettes, decreased phagocytosis of yeast cells by neutrophils, and chemotactic defects of polymorphonuclear and mononuclear cells.

37. **What other skin conditions mimic atopic dermatitis?**
    - Seborrheic dermatitis
    - Scabies

- Contact dermatitis
- Langerhans cell histiocytosis
- Xerotic eczema (dry skin)
- Immunodeficiency disorders (e.g., Wiskott-Aldrich syndrome, hyperimmunoglobulin E syndrome, severe combined immunodeficiency)
- Nummular eczema
- Metabolic disorders (e.g., phenylketonuria, essential fatty acid deficiency, biotinidase deficiency)

38. **What is the "atopic march"?**
    Approximately half of infants with atopic dermatitis will develop asthma, and two thirds will develop allergic rhinitis. Thus, the one condition in infancy marches toward others. Currently under study are ways to interrupt this progression.

    Spergel JM, Paller AS: Atopic dermatitis and the atopic march. J Allergy Clin Immunol 112: S118–S127, 2003.

39. **What features help to differentiate seborrheic from atopic dermatitis during infancy?**
    See Table 4-1.

TABLE 4-1. SEBORRHEIC DERMATITIS VERSUS ATOPIC DERMATITIS		
	Seborrheic dermatitis	**Atopic dermatitis**
Color	Salmon	Pink or red (if inflamed)
Scale	Yellowish, greasy	White, not greasy
Age	Infants <6 months or adolescents	May begin at 2–12 months and continue through childhood
Itching	Not present	May be severe
Distribution	Face, postauricular scalp, axillae, and groin	Cheeks, trunk, and extensors of extremities
Associated features	None	Dennie pleats, allergic shiners, palmar creases
Lichenification	None	May be prominent
Response to topical steroids	Rapid	Slower

40. **How should parents cope with cradle cap?**
    Seborrheic dermatitis of the scalp—also known as "cradle cap"—during infancy presents as a yellow, greasing, scaling adherent rash on the scalp which may extend to the forehead, eyes, ears, eyebrows, nose, and the back of the head. It appears during the first few months of life and generally resolves in several weeks to a few months. Treatment includes the application of mineral oil followed by shampooing with a mild antidandruff shampoo that contains selenium (e.g., Selsun Blue). Parents should be cautioned to take extra care when washing the scalp because these shampoos may irritate the infant's eyes. A mild-potency topical steroid such as hydrocortisone (1–2.5%) may be needed for inflamed lesions. Families should be advised not to scrub or pick off the scale because the underlying skin is often tender and inflamed.

41. **What condition causes bumps on the cheeks, upper arms, and thighs?**
    Keratosis pilaris. Associated both with atopic dermatitis and ichthyosis vulgaris, this condition runs in families and is asymptomatic. It is characterized by spiny follicular papules, giving

involved areas a "chicken skin" or "gooseflesh" feel. Usual treatment is with bland emollients or emollients that contain a mild peeling agent, such as alphahydroxy acid preparation.

42. **What are the causes of irritant contact diaper rash?**
A variety of local factors are involved. Diapers contribute to the chafing of the skin and the prevention of moisture evaporation, thus increasing epidermal hydration and permeability to irritants. Proteolytic enzymes in urine and stool and ammonia in urine irritate chafed skin. Seasoned pediatricians will advise that alcohol-based diaper wipes also feed the flames of diaper rash.

43. **What features of diaper rash suggest more sinister diseases?**
    - Marked tenderness, rapid onset (staphylococcal scaled skin syndrome)
    - Deep ulcerations, vesicles (herpes simplex)
    - Beefy red, erosive, extensive lesions (particularly intertriginous) that are poorly responsive to topical steroids and antifungals (Langerhans cell histiocytosis, acrodermatitis enteropathica, immunodeficiency states)
    - Extensive and severe lesions with pungent odor (abuse or neglect with infrequent changing)
    Boiko S: Making rash decisions in the diaper area. Pediatr Ann 29:50–56, 2000.

44. **Are cloth diapers "better" than disposables?**
There is no clear answer here, although there are parties who swear by one or the other. Studies, however, have shown both a decreased incidence of diaper rash with disposable diapers and a documented decrease in skin moisture and incidence of rash with superabsorbent diapers as a result of decreased leakage and less alkaline pH. The adjective "better" implies a value judgment, and other factors such as cost, environmental impact, and convenience must be considered. More than 97% of the diapers used in the United States are of the disposable variety.

45. **Are topical steroid/antifungal preparations useful for treating children with diaper dermatitis?**
Most diaper dermatitis is usually diagnosed as either irritant contact dermatitis or candidal dermatitis. Irritant diaper dermatitis responds well to very-low-potency topical corticosteroids (as a result of their anti-inflammatory properties) and a topical barrier such as zinc oxide ointment. Candidiasis of the diaper area responds well to topical antifungal preparations; rarely, an oral anticandidal medication is also necessary. In both types of diaper dermatitis, frequent diaper changes, exposure to air, and avoidance of excessive moisture are helpful. Combination preparations containing both antifungal and corticosteroid medications are not recommended to treat diaper dermatitis because the strength of the steroid component in these products is usually too high for use in the diaper area.
   Kazaks EL, Lane AT: Diaper dermatitis. Pediatr Clin North Am 47:909–920, 2000.

46. **Which dietary deficiencies may be associated with an eczematous dermatitis?**
Zinc, biotin, essential fatty acids, and protein (kwashiorkor).

47. **What are the two main types of contact dermatitis?**
Irritant and allergic. Irritant contact dermatitis arises when agents such as harsh soaps, bleaches, or acids have direct toxic effects when they come into contact with the skin. Allergic contact dermatitis is a T-cell mediated inflammatory immune reaction that requires sensitization to a specific antigen.

48. **What type of agents can cause allergic contact dermatitis in children?**
Allergic contact dermatitis can occur in all age groups, but it is often under recognized in pediatric patients. Sensitizers include plant resins (poison ivy, sumac, or oak), nickel in jewelry,

metal snaps and belts, topical neomycin ointment, preservatives (formaldehyde releasers), and materials used in shoes, including adhesives, rubber accelerators, and leather tanning agents.

49. **When does the rash in poison ivy appear relative to exposure?**
    Poison ivy, or rhus dermatitis, is a typical delayed hypersensitivity reaction. The time between exposure and cutaneous lesions is usually **2–4 days.** However, the eruption may appear as late as a week or more after contact in individuals who have not been previously sensitized (this explains why lesions continue to erupt after the initial "outbreak" of rash).

50. **Are the vesicles in poison ivy contagious?**
    No. The contents of blisters do not contain the allergen. Washing the skin removes all surface oleoresin and prevents further contamination.

51. **What is the "id" reaction?**
    Your superego will be stroked if you identify the "id" reaction in a confusing dermatologic case. This reaction is the generalization of a local inflammatory dermatitis (e.g., contact dermatitis, tinea capitis following treatment) to sites that have not been directly involved with the offending agent. The exact mechanism remains unclear, but it may be immune-complex mediated.

52. **How does the vehicle used in a dermatologic preparation affect therapy?**
    In general, **acute lesions** (moist, oozing) are best treated with aqueous, drying preparations. **Chronic, dry lesions** fare better when a lubricating, moisturizing vehicle is used. As a rule, any vehicle that enhances hydration of the skin enhances the percutaneous absorption of topical medications (most of which are water-soluble). Thus, in preparations of equal concentration, the potency relationship is ointment > cream > gel > lotion (Box 4-1).

BOX 4-1. VEHICLES USED IN DERMATOLOGIC PREPARATIONS

Drying vehicles
Lotion: A suspension of powder in water. Therapeutic powder remains after aqueous phase evaporates. Useful in hairy areas, particularly the scalp.
Gel: Transparent emulsion that liquifies when applied to skin. Most useful for acne preparations and tar preparations for psoriasis.
Pastes: Combination of powder (usually cornstarch) and ointment; stiffer than ointment.

Moisturizing vehicles
Creams: Mixture of oil in a water emulsion. More useful than ointments when environmental humidity is high and in naturally occluded areas. Less greasy than ointment.
Ointments: Mixture of water in an oil emulsion. Also has an inert petroleum base. Longer lubricating effect than cream.

FUNGAL INFECTIONS

53. **What are useful methods for diagnosing tinea infections?**
    Although the microscopic examination of **potassium hydroxide (KOH) preparations** is employed in the search for hyphae, the use of **dermatophyte test medium** is reliable, simple, inexpensive, and more definitive. Samples from hair, skin, or nails are obtained by scraping with a scalpel, cotton-tipped applicator, or toothbrush (the latter especially for tinea capitis), and these are inoculated directly onto the test medium. After approximately 1–2 weeks, a color

change from yellow to red in the agar surrounding the dermatophyte colony indicates positivity. If the most definitive diagnosis is needed, culture on Sabouraud medium is the test of choice.

54. **Why is it necessary to culture for tinea capitis?**
Tinea capitis can be caused by a variety of dermatophyte fungal organisms, and, over the last decade, resistance to commonly used treatments (griseofulvin) has been noted. Children with tinea capitis are requiring longer courses of treatment and higher doses of medication to eradicate the fungal infection. Moreover, other conditions (e.g., alopecia areata, psoriasis of the scalp) may be confused with tinea capitis. Therefore, just like for other pediatric infections, it is important to document the type of infection so that proper treatment may be administered.

KEY POINTS: MAIN FEATURES OF TINEA CAPITIS ✔

1. Scaly alopecia

2. Black-dot hairs often observed

3. Associated with posterior cervical adenopathy

4. Potassium hydroxide test often positive

5. Diagnosis confirmed by positive fungal culture

6. Most common cause: *Trichophyton tonsurans*

55. **How can a culture be obtained if fungal culture medium is not available in the office?**
The simplest method is to take a cotton swab culturette and moisten it with water. Then, take the swab and rub it over the affected areas and all four quadrants of the scalp. The cotton swab can be used to directly inoculate the fungal culture media if you have it in the office or transported back to the laboratory for inoculation.

Friedlander SF, Pickering B, Cunningham BB, et al: Use of the cotton swab method in diagnosing tinea capitis. Pediatrics 104:276–279, 1999.

56. **What are the clinical presentations of tinea capitis?**
Tinea capitis occurs more commonly in African-American children in the United States. It can present with scalp scaling, "black dot" tinea, inflammation, or a kerion (a boggy, tender mass) (Fig. 4-4). Scalp scaling can occur without hair loss and should not be attributed to seborrheic dermatitis after infancy and before puberty. The "black dot" presentation occurs when

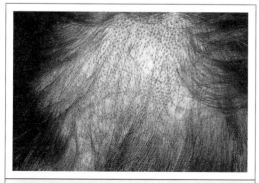

Figure 4-4. Black dot tinea. (From Schachner LA, Hansen RC [eds]: Pediatric Dermatology, 3rd ed. Edinburgh, Mosby, 2003, p 1096.)

the infected hair shaft breaks at the surface of the scalp, leaving a bald patch with black dots (or lighter dots, depending on hair color). Some patients will have inflammatory papules, pustules, erythema, and scaling or with a kerion. Regional adenopathy is very common with inflammatory tinea.

Hubbard TW: Predictive value of symptoms in diagnosing childhood tinea capitis. Arch Pediatr Adolesc Med 153:1150–1153, 1999.

57. Is a Wood lamp helpful for screening for tinea capitis?

In 1930, yes. In the new millennium, no. The reason is the changing epidemiology of tinea. Previously, more cases were caused by *Microsporum canis*, which is an ectothrix fungus (i.e., one that stays on the outside of the hair shaft) that fluoresces yellow-green with a Wood lamp. Now more cases are caused by *Trichophyton tonsurans*, which is an endothrix fungus (i.e., one that invades the inner part of the hair shaft) and does not fluoresce. In certain scenarios, a Wood lamp can be helpful, but as a screening tool, it is not.

58. Why is topical therapy alone insufficient for tinea capitis?

The dermatophytes (i.e., fungi) that cause tinea can thrive deep in the hair shaft, beyond the reach of topical therapy alone. Recommended therapy is a combination of oral griseofulvin (microsize or ultramicrosize preparation), which is given after milk, ice cream, or a fatty meal to facilitate absorption, and biweekly shampooing with 1% or 2.5% selenium sulfide or ketoconazole shampoo to decrease the spread of spores. Of note is that relative resistance by tinea to griseofulvin is being increasingly observed, and higher, longer dosing may be needed to achieve clinical cure. Although newer systemic antifungals are available and have been used in selected cases, they are currently not approved for the treatment of tinea capitis in children.

Pomeranz AJ, Sabnis SS: Tinea capitis: Epidemiology, diagnosis and management strategies. Pediatr Drugs 4:779–783, 2002.

59. How should children who are receiving griseofulvin for tinea capitis be monitored?

The incidence of hepatitis or bone-marrow suppression from griseofulvin in children is rare. Children who are undergoing an acute course of treatment (6–8 weeks) do not need obligatory blood counts or liver function tests. However, a history of hepatitis or its risk factors would warrant a pretreatment evaluation of liver function and intermittent monitoring. For those rare cases in which griseofulvin is going to be used for >2 months, one should consider obtaining complete blood counts and liver function tests on an every-other-month basis.

60. Is a kerion a bacterial or fungal entity?

A kerion is a fluctuant and tender mass that occurs in some cases of tinea capitis. Occipital or posterior cervical lymph nodes are often enlarged. A kerion is felt to be primarily an excessive inflammatory response to tinea, and thus initial treatment consists of antifungal agents, principally griseofulvin and selenium sulfide shampoo. However, bacterial cultures of kerions will demonstrate *Staphylococcus aureus* or a mixture of gram-negative bacteria in two thirds of cases. Because most kerions resolve without antibiotics, the role of these bacteria in the pathogenesis is unclear. Short courses of oral steroids should be considered in those lesions that are exquisitely painful.

Honig PJ, Caputo GL, Leyden JJ, et al: Microbiology of kerions. J Pediatr 123:422–424, 1993.

61. What puts the "versicolor" in tinea versicolor?

A very common superficial disorder of the skin, tinea versicolor (also known as pityriasis versicolor) is caused by the yeast *Malassezia furfur* (formerly known as *Pityrosporum orbiculare*). It appears as multiple macules and patches with fine scales over the upper trunk, arms, and occasionally the face and other areas (Fig. 4-5). Lesions are "versatile" in color (i.e., light tan, reddish, or white) and "versatile" by season (i.e., lighter in summer and darker in winter as compared with surrounding skin). The yeast interferes with melanin production, possibly by the disruption of tyrosinase activity, at the involved sites. Diagnosis can be confirmed with a KOH preparation of a scraping from the involved skin, which has characteristic fungal hyphae and a grapelike spore pattern referred to as a "spaghetti and meatball" appearance. Wood's light will also display yellow-brown fluorescence.

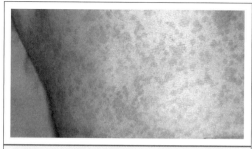

Figure 4-5. Tinea versicolor on the chest. (From Gawkrodger DJ: Dermatology: An Illustrated Colour Text, 3rd ed. London, Churchill Livingstone, 2002, p 38.)

62. **How is tinea versicolor treated?**
    - **Selenium sulfide 2.5% lotion:** The shampoo or lotion is applied over the affected area overnight nightly during the first week, with decreasing frequency over the ensuing weeks.
    - **Ketoconazole 2% shampoo:** The shampoo is applied to wet skin and lathered. Patients are instructed to let the shampoo remain in place without washing for 3–5 minutes. Treatment is repeated for 1–3 days in a row. Monthly prophylactic treatments are suggested to prevent recurrence.
    - **Oral ketoconazole, fluconazole, and itraconazole:** These treatments, which are sometimes effective after a single one-time dose, may be considered for use in older children and adolescents. However, side effects, including liver toxicity, may occur.

63. **After the sneaker is removed, how do you distinguish between "shoe dermatitis" and "athlete's foot"?**
    - **Allergic contact dermatitis** (shoe dermatitis): This condition often involves the dorsa of the toes and the distal third of the foot. The rash is red, scaly, and vesicular. KOH preparations of scrapings for fungus are negative.
    - **Tinea pedis** (athlete's foot): Presentations can include redness and scaling, primarily on the instep or the entire weight-bearing surface, or erythema and maceration between the toes, especially the third and fourth web spaces. A less-common presentation is one in which vesicular lesions develop, called *bullous tinea pedis*. In tinea pedis, the nails may be yellowed and thickened. *KOH preparations* are *positive* for hyphae. Tinea pedis is much less common in prepubertal children.

HAIR AND NAIL ABNORMALITIES

64. **How fast does hair grow?**
    About 1 cm per month.

65. **On what parts of the skin is hair not normally found?**
    Palms, soles, genitalia, and medial/lateral aspects of toes and fingers.

66. **What causes sparse or absent hair in children?**
    - **Congenital localized:** Nevus sebaceous, aplasia cutis, incontinentia pigmenti, focal dermal hypoplasia, intrauterine trauma (e.g., scalp electrodes), infection (e.g., herpes, gonococcal)

- **Congenital diffuse:** Loose anagen syndrome, Menkes syndrome, trichoschisis, genetic syndromes (e.g., ectodermal dysplasia, lamellar ichthyosis, Netherton syndrome)
- **Acquired localized:** Tinea capitis, alopecia areata, traumatic scarring (e.g., trichotillomania), androgenic alopecia, Langerhans cell histiocytosis, lupus erythematosus
- **Acquired diffuse:** Telogen effluvium, anagen effluvium, acrodermatitis enteropathica, endocrinopathies (e.g., hypothyroidism)

Datloff J, Esterly NB: A system for sorting out pediatric alopecia. Contemp Pediatr 3:53–56, 1986.

67. **How can alopecia areata be differentiated from tinea capitis?**

In **tinea capitis,** the fungal organism invades the hair shaft but is also present in the epidermis (the top layer of the skin). There are usually changes of scaling and inflammatory lesions that are intermingled with black dots representing broken hairs. In **alopecia areata,** the scalp is smooth, although there may be a pink discoloration. Some hairs within the patch may have a tapered appearance, with the wider end distally and a thinner end at the base of the scalp (i.e., the "exclamation point hair") (Fig. 4-6). There is no lymphadenopathy in patients with alopecia areata, but this is not uncommon in patients with tinea capitis.

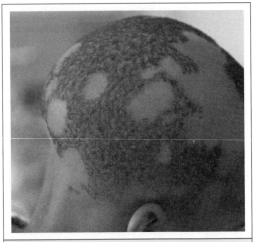

Figure 4-6. Well-demarcated, hairless patches of alopecia areata.

68. **What are poor prognostic indicators for recovery of hair in patients with alopecia areata?**
    - Atopy
    - Presence of other immune-mediated disease (e.g., thyroid disease, vitiligo)
    - Family history of alopecia areata (about 25% of patients)
    - Young age at onset
    - Nail dystrophy
    - Extensive hair loss

Madani S, Shapiro J: Alopecia areata update. J Am Acad Dermatol 42:549–566, 2000.

69. **What are treatments for alopecia areata?**

Treatment is based on the extent of disease: patchy, totalis (loss of all scalp hair), or universalis (loss of all body hair). Although the cause is unknown, alopecia areata is generally considered to be a T-cell-mediated autoimmune disorder. Treatments include the following: intralesional and topical corticosteroids, systemic corticosteroids (rarely used chronically due to side effects), topical minoxidil with anthralin (as an irritant, anthralin is designed to cause a mild dermatitis and alter localized immune function), topical sensitizers, topical immunosuppressors (e.g., cyclosporine), and photochemotherapy with psoralens.

Harrison S, Sinclair R: Optimal management of hair loss (alopecia) in children. Am J Clin Dermatol 4:757–770, 2003.

National Alopecia Areata Foundation: www.naaf.org

70. **Are most hairs growing or resting?**

Most infants and children have about 90% of scalp hair in the growing (anagen) and about 10% in the resting (telogen) state. On average, a single scalp hair will grow for about 3 years, rest for 3 months, and then, upon falling out, be replaced by a new growing hair.

71. **What is the likely diagnosis in a child who develops diffuse hair loss 3 months after major surgery?**

Telogen effluvium. This is the most common cause of diffuse acquired hair loss in children. In a healthy individual, most hairs are present in a growing (anagen) phase. After a physical or emotional stress such as a significant fever, illness, pregnancy, birth, surgery, or large weight loss, a large number of scalp hairs can convert to the resting (telogen) phase. About 2–5 months after the stressful event, the hair begins to shed, at times coming out in large clumps. The condition is temporary and usually does not produce a loss of more than 50% of the hair. When the hair roots are examined, there is a characteristic lighter-colored root bulb, which characterizes a telogen hair. The hair loss can continue for 6–8 weeks, at which time new, short, regrowing hairs should be visible.

Anagen effluvium, which the loss of growing hairs, is most commonly seen during radiation and chemotherapy treatments for cancer.

72. **What puzzling cause of asymmetric hair loss in a child will sometimes cause an intern to pull his or her hair out?**

Trichotillomania is hair loss as a result of self-manipulation, such as rubbing, twirling, or pulling. Hair loss is asymmetric. The most common physical finding is unequal hair lengths in the same region without evidence of epidermal changes of the scalp. Parents often do not observe the causative behavior, and convincing them of the likely diagnosis may take some effort. Behavior modification, along with the application of petroleum or oil to the hair to make pulling more difficult, is the treatment of choice. Rarely a child will swallow the hair and develop vomiting because of the formation of a gastric trichobezoar (hairball).

73. **What is the "flag sign"?**

The term *flag sign* refers to alternating bands of decreased pigment or structural changes of the hair shaft. It most commonly occurs after nutritional deficiency.

Wade MS, Sinclair RD: Disorders of hair in infants and children other than alopecia. Clin Dermatol 20:16–28, 2002.

74. **What causes green hair?**

Besides hair dye in a rebellious teenager, children with blond or light-colored hair can develop green hair after long-term exposure to chlorinated swimming pools. It is the result of the incorporation of copper ions into the hair matrix. Over-the-counter chelating shampoos are available for prevention and treatment.

75. **How should ingrown toenails be managed?**

Soaks, open-toed sandals, properly fitting shoes, topical or systemic antibiotics, incision and drainage, or surgical removal of the lateral portion of the nail may all be used. Control is best obtained by letting the nail grow beyond the free end of the toe. Proper instruction on nail care, including straight rather than arc trimming, is mandatory.

76. **Which pathogens are responsible for paronychia?**

Acute paronychia (inflammation of the nailfold, usually with abscess formation) is most commonly caused by *Staphylococcus aureus*. The proximal or lateral nailfolds become intensely erythematous and tender. If a collection of pus develops at this site, it should be incised and drained. The treatment of acute paronychia includes the oral administration of antistaphylococcal antibiotics.

Chronic paronychia is most often caused by *Candida albicans* and often involves a history of chronic water exposure (e.g., dishwashing, thumb sucking). Although rarely inflamed, there is edema of the nailfolds and separation of the folds from the nail plate. The nails may become ridged and develop a yellow-green discoloration. A bacterial culture may reveal a variety of gram-positive and gram-negative organisms. Therapy includes topical antifungal agents and avoidance of water. There is no place for griseofulvin in the treatment of chronic paronychia.

77. **A healthy 7-year-old child who develops progressive yellowing and increasing friability of all nails over a period of 12 months likely has what condition?**
    Twenty nail dystrophy (trachyonychia). The progressive development of rough nails with longitudinal grooves, pitting, chipping, ridges, and discoloration occurring in isolation in school-aged children has been given this name, although not all nails need be involved. The etiology remains unclear, and a majority of cases resolve spontaneously without scarring. The nail changes, however, may herald other conditions, such as alopecia areata, lichen planus, and psoriasis.

INFESTATIONS

78. **How do lice differ?**
    - *Pediculosis capitis* (head lice): *Pediculus capitis*, the smallest and most common of the three human lice, is an obligate human parasite. Spread occurs directly by contact with an infected individual or indirectly through the use of shared combs, brushes, or hats. For unknown reasons, infestation is nearly 35 times more likely among whites than blacks.
    - *Pediculosis corporis* (body lice): *Pediculus humanus*, the largest (2–4 mm) of the three types, is usually associated with poor hygiene. It does not live on the body but instead in the seams of clothing. It can be a vector for other diseases, such as epidemic typhus, trench fever, and relapsing fever.
    - *Pediculosis pubis* (pubic lice): *Phthirus pubis* is also known as the crab louse because it is a broad insect with legs that look like claws. It is sometimes mistaken for a brown freckle. Acquisition is primarily through sexual contact.

79. **What are the clinical findings of head lice infestation?**
    Scalp pruritus is most common, but many children are **asymptomatic**. A search for lice should be made in any school-aged child presenting with scalp itching. Nits (lice eggs) are found in greatest density on the parietal and occipital areas.

80. **How is the diagnosis of head lice made?**
    On physical examination, an actual louse (wingless, grayish insects about 3–4 mm) may be difficult to find, although one should easily be able to find nits. The nits are attached to the hair close to the surface of the scalp and are oval and flesh colored (Fig. 4-7). Those that have not hatched are *not* easily removed from the hair shaft (as compared with hair casts, dander, and external debris). Overdiagnosis is common. Microscopic evaluation of a few hairs can confirm the diagnosis. When the louse emerges, the empty egg case, or nit, appears white in color (*see* Fig. 4-7).

    Pollack RJ, Kiszewski AE, Spielman A: Overdiagnosis and consequent mismanagement of head louse infestations in North America. Pediatr Infect Dis J 19:689–693, 2000.

81. **What types of treatment are available for head lice?**
    - **Permethrin:** 1% and 5% (Nix, Elimite)
    - **Pyrethrins** (RID, A-200, R&C)

- **Malathion:** 0.5% (Ovide)
- **Lindane:** 1% (Kwell)
- **Asphyxiants:** Petroleum jelly (Vaseline), mayonnaise, olive oil
- **HairClean 1–2–3:** A combination product of ylang ylang, anise, coconut oil, isopropyl alcohol, and rubbing alcohol
- **Trimethoprim–sulfamethoxazole:** After it is taken orally by the patient, the antibiotic is ingested by the lice during a blood feeding, and it may kill symbiotic bacteria required for nutrition and reproduction.
- **Nit picking** (*see* question 82)

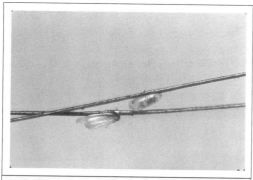

Figure 4-7. Viable head louse egg (*right*) and hatched empty nit (*left*) attached to a child's hair. (From Schachner LA, Hansen RC [eds]: Pediatric Dermatology, 3rd ed. Edinburgh, Mosby, 2003, p 1143.)

Jones KN, English JC 3rd: Review of common therapeutic options in the United States for the treatment of pediculosis capitis. Clin Infect Dis 36:1355–1361, 2003.

82. **Should parents nit pick?**

Once an infestation of lice has been properly treated, the nits are not viable or contagious. Despite this, many schools will not allow children with nits to attend, although this nit-free policy has not been shown to be of benefit for controlling outbreaks. Increasing resistance to therapy may make removal more important to avoid diagnostic confusion. Manual removal (nit picking) is the most effective method, although it is time consuming and tedious. Fine-toothed combs, especially the LiceMeister comb (available through the National Pediculosis Association [www.headlice.org]), aid in the removal.

83. **How is a skin scraping for scabies or "scabies prep" done?**

Because the highest percentage of mites are usually concentrated on the hands and feet, the web spaces between digits are the best places to look for the characteristic linear burrows. Moisten the skin with alcohol or mineral oil, scrape across the area of the burrow with a small, rounded scalpel blade (e.g., No. 15), and place the scrapings on a glass slide with a drop of KOH (or additional mineral oil, if used) and a cover slip. Burrows, if unseen, can be more precisely localized by rubbing a washable felt-tip marker across the web space and removing the ink with alcohol. If burrows are present, ink will penetrate through the stratum corneum and outline the site. Under the microscope, mites, eggs, and/or scybala (mite feces) may be seen.

84. **What treatment eliminates the scabies' babies?**

The treatment of choice for treating scabies is permethrin 5% cream (Elimite, Acticin). It may be used in children as young as 2 months old. It is more effective than Lindane (the previously accepted treatment for scabies), and it has a much lower risk of neurotoxicity.

The cream is applied from the neck to the toes at night with removal after 8–14 hours by bathing or showering. Retreatment in 1 week may be considered. Physicians must make patients aware of the fact that lesions and pruritus may linger for 1–2 weeks after effective therapy. One must be supportive during this time to prevent unnecessary retreatment by parents. Antihistamines and low-potency topical steroids may help control symptoms. It must be stressed that all family members and close contacts should be treated simultaneously.

Flinders DC, DeSchweinitz P: Pediculosis and scabies. Am Fam Physician 69:341–350, 2004.

85. **What was the first human disease with a cause that was precisely identified?**

Scabies. The etiologic agent, *Sarcoptes scabiei*, was first identified in 1687. The itch for knowledge, it seems, initially was stronger than the thirst for knowledge (*see* Fig. 4-8).

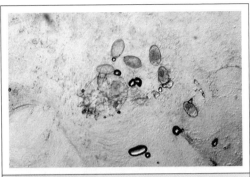

Figure 4-8. Scabies mite and eggs. (From Gates RH [ed]: Infectious Disease Secrets, 2nd ed. Philadelphia, Hanley & Belfus, 2003, p 356.)

86. **After a weekend class trip during which he stayed overnight at a hotel, a teenager develops two linear clusters of itchy red bumps on his legs. What is the most likely cause of his rash?**

Bed bug bites, usually caused by *Cimex lectularius,* often present as pink papules occurring in groups of two or three instead of single bites. This has led some to describe the bites as "breakfast, lunch, and dinner bites." They may inhabit furniture and bedding in homes, dormitories, or hotels. The itching will resolve with time, but superinfection with bacterial organisms may occur.

NEONATAL CONDITIONS

87. **What are the most common birthmarks?**
    - **Salmon patches** (vascular stains or nevi): These are faint, pink-red, macular patches composed of distended dermal capillaries and found on the glabella, eyelids, and the nape of the neck. Seen in 70% of white infants and 60% of black infants. Usually fade, but may persist indefinitely, becoming more prominent during crying.
    - **Mongolian spots** (dermal melanosis): These blue-black macules are found on the lumbosacral area and occasionally on shoulders and backs. Seen in 80–90% of oriental, black, and Native American babies but ≤10% of white infants. Most Mongolian spots fade by age 2 and disappear by age 10.

88. **How concerning are pustular lesions in the newborn period?**
    When presented with pustules in the newborn, it is very important to rule out infectious etiologies, because some may be life-threatening. The purulent material should be evaluated with a Gram stain, KOH, Tzanck preparation, and bacterial and viral cultures. A Wright stain will reveal the presence of neutrophils or eosinophils.

89. **What is the differential diagnosis of vesicles or pustules in the newborn?**

Noninfectious	Infectious
Miliaria	Candidiasis
Erythema toxicum	Staphylococcal folliculitis
Transient neonatal pustular melanosis	Herpes simplex
Infantile acropustulosis	Congenital syphilis
Incontinentia pigmenti	Varicella
Langerhans cell histiocytosis	Bacterial sepsis

Roberts LJ: Dermatologic diseases. In McMillan JA, DeAngelis CD, Feigin RD, et al (eds): Oski's Pediatrics, Principles and Practice, 3rd ed. Philadelphia, Lippincott Williams & Wilkins, 1999, p 376.

90. **Should a newborn with a sharp red line down the center of the body prompt a call to the neonatal intensive care unit?**

Not unless the caller wants to be red faced. This is likely the **"harlequin color"** change, a relatively common entity seen in up to 10% of newborns, particularly premature infants. It consists of a reddening of one side of the body with a sharp line of demarcation along the midline. The change occurs only when the child is lying on one side. The superior half is light, whereas the dependent half is dark and subfused. The cause is thought to be an imbalance in the autonomic regulation of peripheral blood vessels. If the infant is flipped, the color pattern reverses. If the infant is placed prone or supine, the color change disappears.

91. **What is the medical significance of cutis marmorata?**

Cutis marmorata is the bluish mottling of the skin often seen in infants and young children who have been exposed to low temperatures or chilling. The reticulated marbling effect is the result of dilated capillaries and venules causing darkened areas on the skin; this disappears with warming. Cutis marmorata is of no medical significance, and no treatment is indicated. However, persistent cutis marmorata is associated with trisomy 21, trisomy 18, and Cornelia de Lange syndromes. There is also a congenital vascular anomaly called *cutis marmorata telangiectatic congenita* that has persistent purple reticulate mottling of the skin.

92. **A healthy infant with scattered reddish nodules on the back skin most likely has what condition?**

Subcutaneous fat necrosis consists of sharply circumscribed, indurated nodular lesions usually seen in healthy, term newborns and infants during the first few days to weeks of life. The stony hard areas of panniculitis are generally movable and slightly elevated, and the overlying skin is a reddish, violaceous color. Although the cause is unknown, it is thought that obstetric trauma and pressure on bony prominences may contribute to the problem. The usual sites (cheeks, back, buttocks, arms, and thighs) are consistent with this. Histologically, the lesions display extensive inflammation in the subcutaneous tissue with large fat lobules. Most lesions are self-limiting and require no therapy. However, occasionally they may extensively calcify and spontaneously drain with subsequent scarring. Remember that significant hypercalcemia may be present in a small number of patients. Therefore, a serum calcium level should be ordered whenever the disorder is suspected; it should be rechecked periodically until the condition resolves and for several months thereafter.

93. **What should the family of a newborn with a yellow, hairless patch with a cobblestone texture be advised to do?**

The lesion is likely a **nevus sebaceous**. This hamartomatous neoplasm usually presents as a yellow-pink hairless plaque on the scalp or face at the time of birth and is composed primarily of malformed sebaceous glands. Under the influence of androgens at puberty, the glands may hypertrophy and lead to the development of other neoplasms (e.g., basal cell carcinoma). The risk of neoplastic (usually benign) development is 10–15%. Some experts advise excision during the preteen, prepubertal years. Careful monitoring of the lesion for new growths or nonhealing ulcerations at all ages is advised, especially during adolescence.

94. **Aplasia cutis congenita of the scalp may be associated with which chromosomal abnormality?**

Aplasia cutis congenita (congenital absence of the skin) presents on the scalp as solitary or multiple well-demarcated ulcerations or atrophic scars. Of variable depth, the lesions may be limited to epidermis and upper dermis or occasionally extend into the skull and dura. Although most children with this lesion are normal without multiple anomalies, other associations include epidermolysis bullosa, placental infarcts, teratogens, sebaceous nevi, and limb anomalies. Aplasia cutis is a feature of **trisomy 13 syndrome**.

95. **Describe the appearance and distribution of transient neonatal pustular melanosis.**

Consisting of small vesicopustular lesions 3–4 mm in size, transient pustular melanosis occurs in almost 5% of black and <1% of white newborns. It may be present at birth or appear shortly after birth. The lesions most often cluster on the neck, chin, palms, and soles, although they may occur on the face and trunk. The pustules rupture easily and progress to brown, pigmented macules with a fine collarette of scale. Microscopic examination of the contents of the pustules reveals neutrophils with no organisms. There are no associated systemic manifestations, and the eruption is self-limited, although the hyperpigmentation may last for months.

96. **Is erythema toxicum neonatorum really toxic?**

Not in the least. *Erythema toxicum* is a common eruption composed of erythematous macules, papules, and pustules that occur in newborns, usually during the first few days of life. The lesions may start as irregular, blotchy, red macules, varying in size from millimeters to several centimeters. They often develop into 1–3-mm, yellow-white papules and pustules on an erythematous base, giving a "flea-bitten" appearance. They occur all over the body except on the palms and soles, which are spared because the lesions occur in pilosebaceous follicles, which are absent on the palmar and plantar surfaces. The rash is less common in premature infants, with incidence proportional to gestational age and peaking at 41–42 weeks. Although it may be seen at birth, it is most common during the first 3–4 days of life and is occasionally noted as late as 10 days of life. Erythema toxicum usually lasts 5–7 days and heals without pigmentation. Other than the rash, the newborn appears healthy.

97. **How is the diagnosis of erythema toxicum confirmed?**

Erythema toxicum is often confused with a variety of other skin disorders, including impetigo neonatorum, herpes simplex, transient neonatal pustular melanosis, milia, and miliaria. The diagnosis can be confirmed by staining the contents of a pustule with Wright or Giemsa stain. Clusters of eosinophils confirm the presence of erythema toxicum.

98. **How are the most common neonatal papular lesions distinguished?**

See Table 4-2.

TABLE 4-2.	COMMON NEONATAL PAPULAR LESIONS		
	Neonatal cephalic pustulosis	Milia	Erythema toxicum
Distribution	Face	Face and other areas	Face, trunk, and extremities
Appearance	Papule or pustule	Yellow or white papule	Yellow or white papule
Erythematous	Yes	No	Yes
Contents on smear PMNs	Keratin + sebaceous material	Eosinophils	
Incidence	Occasional	40–50% of term infants	30–50% of term infants
Course	Last several months	Disappear in 3–4 weeks	Disappear in 2 weeks

PMNs = polymorphonuclear cells.

99. **For academic purposes (and ICD-9-CM coding), is it possible to be more scientific about the diagnosis of "prickly heat"?**

The scientific name for this condition is **miliaria rubra**. It is due to sweat retention, and its clinical morphology is determined by the level at which sweat is trapped. Sweat trapped at a superficial level produces clear vesicles without surrounding erythema (sudamina or crystallina); miliaria rubra (prickly heat, erythematous papules, vesicles, papulovesicles) is produced by sweat trapped at a deeper level; pustular lesions (miliaria pustulosa) and even abscesses (miliaria profunda) are produced with sweat retention at the deepest of levels (infants rarely develop these types). With the advent of air conditioning, miliaria rarely occurs in newborn nurseries.

PAPULOSQUAMOUS DISORDERS

100. **What diseases are associated with the Koebner reaction?**

Koebnerization is a response to local injury whereby skin lesions are found at the sites of trauma (e.g.. linear lesions at the sites of scratching). This is seen in patients with psoriasis (Fig. 4-9) as well as those with other conditions, including lichen planus and flat warts.

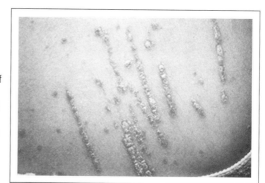

Figure 4-9. Koebner phenomenon in psoriasis with linear plaques at sites of excoriations. (From Cohen BA: Pediatric Dermatology, 2nd ed. St. Louis, Mosby, 1999, p 63.)

101. **A skin scale that easily bleeds on removal is characteristic of what condition?**

The appearance of punctate bleeding points after removal of a scale is the **Auspitz sign**. It is seen primarily in psoriasis and is related to the rupture of capillaries high in the papillary dermis, near the surface of the skin.

102. **What is the typical pattern of lesions in childhood psoriasis?**

Psoriasis presents as well-circumscribed, erythematous plaques with overlying white scale in children and adults. These occur on the scalp, elbows, knees (Fig. 4-10), sacrum, and genitalia. Psoriasis may also present with guttate (drop-like) lesions over the trunk and extremities. These children may have group A beta hemolytic streptococcus infection as an underlying precipitating factor.

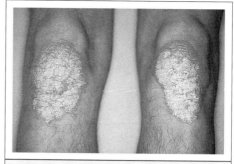

Figure 4-10. Plaques of psoriasis on the knees. (From Gawkrodger DJ: Dermatology: An Illustrated Colour Text, 3rd ed. London, Churchill Livingstone, 2002, p 27.)

103. **What percentage of children with psoriasis have nail involvement?**

Nail changes, most commonly pitting, may be the only manifestation of psoriasis. The reported incidence of nail pitting in children with psoriasis is as high as 40%. Other nail changes include onycholysis (separation of the nail plate from nailbed at the distal margin) and thickening of the nail plate, often with white-yellow discoloration. Subungual debris may occur.

104. What are treatment modalities for psoriasis?

Various therapies have been used to treat psoriasis. The choice of treatment will depend on the extent of involvement, previous treatments, and the age of the patient. Topical treatments include topical corticosteroids, calcipotriene (a vitamin D analog), retinoids, and tar. Other treatment modalities include phototherapy and, rarely, systemic retinoids and methotrexate.

Schön MP, Boehncke W-H: Psoriasis. N Engl J Med 352:1899–1912, 2005.

105. What are the eight Ps of lichen planus?

- **Papules:** Usually 2–6 mm in diameter; often seen in a linear pattern as a result of the Koebner reaction
- **Plaques:** Commonly generated from a confluence of papules with exaggerated surface markings of the overlying skin (Wickham striae)
- **Planar:** Individual lesions, usually flat-topped
- **Purple:** Distinctly violaceous
- **Pruritus:** Often intensely itchy
- **Polygonal:** Borders of papules are often angulated
- **Penis:** Common site of involvement in children
- **Persistent:** Chronic, with remissions and exacerbations for up to 18 months

106. How is pityriasis rosea distinguished from secondary syphilis?

Often with difficulty; both are primarily papulosquamous rashes. **Pityriasis rosea** classically consists of oval lesions that organize in parallel fashion on the trunk (the "Christmas tree" distribution) and are preceded in 40–80% of cases by a large annular erythematous lesion (herald patch). **Secondary syphilis** lesions occur 3–6 weeks after the chancre, and, as compared with pityriasis rosea, they have more involvement of the palms, soles, and mucous membranes and have accompanying lymphadenopathy. However, because atypical presentations are common, testing for syphilis should be performed in any sexually active individual who is diagnosed with pityriasis rosea.

107. What is the treatment for pityriasis rosea?

Pityriasis rosea is a self-limited condition that usually resolves in 6–12 weeks. Therefore, treatment is often not required, unless there is significant pruritus or cosmetic disfigurement. A wide range of treatments are reported. Topical corticosteroids help reduce pruritus, but they do not alter the course of the disease. Sunlight or ultraviolet B phototherapy results in clinical improvement in some individuals. In a recent clinical study, oral erythromycin was shown to be beneficial.

Sharma PK, Yadav TP, Gautam RK, et al: Erythromycin in pityriasis rosea: A double-blind, placebo-controlled clinical trial. J Am Acad Dermatol 42:241–244, 2000.

PHOTODERMATOLOGY

108. Why is limiting excessive sun exposure in children important?

Most people experience a significant percentage of their lifetime sun exposure early in life. Years of unprotected sun exposure will lead to freckling, wrinkling, and skin cancer formation, including melanoma. In an era of rising rates of melanoma (projected to be 1 in 75) and squamous and basal cell carcinomas, the use of sun-protection strategies (e.g., sunscreens) during the pediatric years could lower the risk to an individual. Broad-spectrum sunscreens may attenuate the number of nevi in white children, especially if they have freckles.

Gallagher RP, Rivers JK, Lee TK, et al: Broad-spectrum sunscreen use and the development of new nevi in white children: A randomized clinical trial. JAMA 283:2955–2960, 2000.

109. **What are good strategies for protection against sun exposure?**
- Avoid the sun, if possible, during peak hours (10 AM–3 PM) or seek shade.
- Apply sunscreen at least 30 minutes before sun exposure.
- Use a broad-spectrum sunscreen with a sun-protection factor (SPF) of 15–30.
- Apply liberal amounts of sunscreen (2 mg/body cm or about 30 mL for an adult or 15 mL for a 7-year-old child).
- Reapply sunscreen every 2 hours, even if it claims to be "waterproof."
- Wear lip protection that has sunscreen in it.
- Wear protective clothing, hats, and sunglasses.

110. **What types of sunscreens are available?**
Physical sunscreens are composed of zinc oxide or titanium dioxide and function by scattering ultraviolet light. Although they are opaque, newer micronized preparations are easier to apply and more acceptable to patients. **Chemical sunscreens** absorb either ultraviolet A (UVA) or ultraviolet B (UVB) light. Most commercially available sunscreens are combinations of various agents. For sunscreens to function well, they must be applied on all exposed surfaces in adequate quantities and reapplied throughout the day.

111. **How is the SPF of a sunscreen determined?**
SPF is the level of effectiveness of a sunscreen's ability to protect against UVB light; it is not a measurement of UVA light protection. The SPF rating is a ratio of the dose of ultraviolet light needed to produce minimal redness on sun-protected skin to the dose of ultraviolet light needed to produce minimal redness on unprotected skin.

112. **Should sunscreens be avoided in infants?**
This is controversial. There are concerns that the skin of infants <6 months old has different absorptive characteristics and that biologic systems that metabolize and excrete drugs may not be fully developed. However, there is no evidence that the limited use of sunscreen in infants is problematic. Physical protection (e.g., clothing, hats, shade, sunglasses) is most ideal, but if an infant's skin is not adequately protected, it may be reasonable to apply sunscreen to small areas, such as the face and the back of the hands. Physical sunscreens containing zinc oxide are preferred over chemical sunscreens for use on infant skin.

> Committee on Environmental Health: Ultraviolet light: A hazard to children. Pediatrics 104:328–333, 1999.

113. **Which "lime" disease is not transmitted by ticks?**
Limes contain psoralens that react with ultraviolet light and that can produce erythema, vesicles, and/or hyperpigmentation on areas of the skin that have come in contact with lime juice. This is known as **phytophotodermatitis** and is seen with other psoralen-containing plants, such as celery and figs. Additionally, berloque dermatitis (*berloque* is French for "pendant," which some lesions can resemble) is an irregularly patterned hyperpigmentation of the neck due to photosensitization by furocoumarins (i.e., psoralens) in perfumes. It is caused by fragrances that contain bergamot oil, an extract from the peel of a type of orange that is grown in southern France and Italy. Bergamot oil contains 5-methoxypsoralen, which enhances the erythematous and pigmentary response of UVA light.

114. **Which conditions are associated with marked sun sensitivity?**
- **Inherited disorders:** Porphyrias, xeroderma pigmentosum, Bloom syndrome, Rothmund-Thomson syndrome, Hartnup disorder
- **Exogenous agents:** Drugs (e.g., tetracyclines, thiazides), photoallergic contact dermatitis (associated with perfumes and para-aminobenzoic acid esters)

- **Systemic disease:** Lupus erythematosus, dermatomyositis
- **Idiopathic disorders:** Polymorphous light eruption, solar urticaria, actinic prurigo, hydroa vacciniforme

Garzon MC, DeLeo VA: Photosensitivity in the pediatric patient. Curr Opin Pediatr 9:377–387, 1997.

115. What is the appearance of polymorphous light eruption?

The most common pediatric photodermatosis, polymorphous light eruption is characterized by itchy red papules, plaques, or papulovesicles that appear several hours to days after ultraviolet light exposure. It can be diagnosed by phototesting (i.e., the induction of lesions by intentional ultraviolet light exposure) and by skin biopsy. It is usually suggested by the classic history and the exclusion of other photosensitivity disease.

Morison WL: Photosensitivity. N Engl J Med 350:1111–1117, 2004.

116. Is a child with sun sensitivity protected by sitting behind a window?

Yes and no, depending on the reason for the sensitivity. Ultraviolet light is divided into three wavelength groups: ultraviolet C (UVC), 200–290 nm; UVB, 290–320 nm; and UVA, 320–400 nm. UVC light is cytotoxic and can cause retinal injury, but fortunately it is almost completely absorbed by the ozone layer. UVB light causes sunburn, dermatologic flares (e.g., in patients with lupus erythematosus), and, with chronic exposure, skin cancer. UVA light (which is also emitted from the fluorescent lamps used in most schools) is responsible for psoralen and drug phototoxicity and porphyria flares, and it can cause skin cancer with chronic exposure. Windows block UVB light, but not UVA. Thus, children with UVA-sensitive disorders would not be protected by sitting behind a window.

PIGMENTATION DISORDERS

117. What disorders of childhood are associated with areas of hypopigmentation?

Hypopigmentation is caused by a decrease—not a total absence—of pigmentation or melanin. Conditions that feature hypopigmented lesions include tuberous sclerosis, tinea versicolor, pityriasis alba, nevus depigmentosus, hypomelanosis of Ito, leprosy, and postinflammatory hypopigmentation.

118. Is treatment helpful for children with postinflammatory hypopigmentation?

In children with **pityriasis alba** (postinflammatory hypopigmentation associated with atopic dermatitis), very-low-potency topical steroids, emolliation, and sun protection measures can make skin color more uniform. Treatment does not seem to help in other cases of postinflammatory hypopigmentation, such as those that occur after infection, abrasions, or burns, but sun protection is advisable (*see* Fig. 4-11).

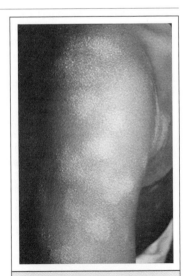

Figure 4-11. Pityriasis alba. Poorly demarcated areas of hypopigmentation in patient with atopic dermatitis. (From Cohen BA: Pediatric Dermatology, 2nd ed. London, Mosby, 1999, p 75.)

119. What treatments are available for vitiligo?

Vitiligo is a disorder of depigmentation (total absence of pigmentation with sharp demarcations; Fig. 4-12). The etiology is unknown but may be autoimmune in nature. There are rare associations with other autoimmune conditions, including thyroiditis and juvenile-onset diabetes. Treatment is often unsatisfactory. Potent topical steroids have been used for localized areas. Topical tacrolimus ointment has been used with some success to treat facial vitiligo in children. Ultraviolet light therapy has been employed for some children with severe, extensive disease. Dyes (including self-tanning agents) and coverage cosmetics are often helpful for camouflaging skin lesions.

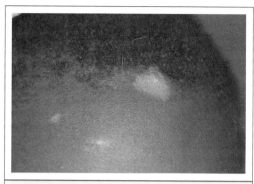

Figure 4-12. Vitiligo. Note well-demarcated areas of total depigmentation.

National Vitiligo Foundation: www.nvfi.org

120. What conditions are associated with congenital depigmentation of the skin?

Congenital depigmentation, or **albinism**, constitutes a number of genetically inherited syndromes that are characterized by disorders of melanin synthesis and that may affect the skin, hair, and eyes. **Generalized (oculocutaneous) albinism** is often complicated by ocular abnormalities, including visual impairment, photophobia, and nystagmus. Piebaldism is a distinct form of congenital depigmentation that affects segments of skin. Patients with this condition often have a forelock of white hair, which is caused by a genetic mutation that differs from generalized albinism. Localized congenital depigmentation associated with a white forelock, heterochromia irides, and congenital deafness characterizes Waardenburg syndrome.

121. What is the likely diagnosis if a patient taking trimethoprim–sulfamethoxazole develops an erythematous, sharply marginated, round lesion that leaves an area of hyperpigmentation upon resolution?

Fixed drug eruption. These 2–10 cm plaques, which may be solitary or multiple, are red to violaceous inflammatory reactions that occur after medication ingestion (commonly antibiotics), especially after trimethoprim–sulfamethoxazole and tetracycline. They are commonly mistaken for urticaria or erythema multiforme. The resultant hyperpigmentation helps to make the distinction.

Morelli JG, Tay YK, Rogers M, et al: Fixed drug eruptions in children. J Pediatr 134:365–367, 1999.

122. Why are Spitz nevi and malignant melanoma often confused?

The Spitz nevus can appear suddenly and grow rapidly. Histologically, it has many features that can be mistaken for malignancy. It actually was previously referred to as benign juvenile melanoma. "Benign" is the key word for this red to brown, dome-shaped papule, which usually appears on the face or extremity. Clinicopathologic correlation is the key to making this diagnosis. It is essential that an experienced pathologist interpret the biopsy when a Spitz nevus is suspected. Melanoma in childhood has been misdiagnosed as Spitz nevi, and Spitz nevi have been misdiagnosed as melanoma.

Murphy ME, Boyer JD, Stashower ME, Zitelli JA: The surgical management of Spitz nevi. Dermatol Surg 28:1065–1069, 2002.

123. What are the clinical features of familial dysplastic nevus syndrome?

The syndrome, which is also known as the *familial atypical mole syndrome,* is found in families who have acquired nevi that develop into melanoma. These nevi are 5–15 mm in diameter and are round to oval in shape. Furthermore, they have irregular and indistinct margins, exhibit variation in color within the same lesion, and have both macular and elevated components. They tend to occur in sun-protected areas.

124. In children with pigmented nevi, what factors increase the risk of melanoma?

Melanoma is rare during childhood. If there is a family history of melanoma or atypical moles, a history of severe sunburns before the age of 18 years, or the child has a giant congenital nevus, the risk is greater. Estimated risks vary for different-sized congenital nevi. The projected lifetime risk for a melanoma developing within a congenital nevus is controversial. For small congenital nevi, the risk is low. For giant congenital nevi, the risk is estimated to be 6–8%. Acquired nevi very rarely develop melanomas.

Eichenfield LF, Gibbs NF: Hyperpigmentation disorders. In Eichefield LF, Frieden IJ, Esterly NB (eds): Textbook of Neonatal Dermatology. Philadelphia, W.B. Saunders, 2001 pp 370–394.

125. What is the differential diagnosis of yellow-brown or orange nodules in children?

- Nevus sebaceous
- Benign cephalic histiocytosis
- Juvenile xanthogranuloma
- Langerhans cell histiocytosis
- Solitary mastocytoma
- Spitz nevus
- Urticaria pigmentosa
- Connective-tissue nevus

VASCULAR BIRTHMARKS

126. How are vascular birthmarks classified?

The updated biologic classification of vascular birthmarks is the most widely accepted classification of vascular birthmarks. It was first proposed in 1982 and was adapted recently to reflect new knowledge. Two broad categories of vascular birthmarks are described: vascular tumors and vascular malformations. There are many types of vascular tumors, but infantile hemangiomas are the most common. Vascular malformations are categorized on the basis of their flow characteristics and type of anomalous channels:

Vascular tumors (selected)	Vascular malformations
Infantile hemangioma	Capillary malformation (port wine stains, salmon patch)
Congenital hemangioma	Venous malformations
Kaposiform hemangioendothelioma	Lymphatic malformation (microcystic, macrocystic)
Tufted angioma	Arteriovenous malformations
Pyogenic granuloma	Mixed malformations

Enjolras O, Milliken J: Vascular tumors and vascular malformations, new issues. Adv Dermatol 13:375–423, 1998.

Mulliken JB, Glowacki J: Hemangiomas and vascular malformations in infants and children. Plast Reconstr Surg 69:412–420, 1982.

127. Describe the life history of hemangiomas.

Hemangiomas or, more specifically, infantile hemangiomas, are common benign vascular tumors. They are rarely fully developed at birth, but precursor lesions (an area of pallor, telangiectasia, or "bruise") may be detected on close inspection within the first few days of life. They may have superficial and/or deep components. Hemangiomas undergo a growth phase until the child reaches the age of 6–12 months, at which time the tumors start to involute. This process of involution occurs over several years at a rate of approximately 10% resolution each year. There still may be residual skin changes (e.g., skin redundancy, pallor, atrophy, telangiectasia) after the hemangioma has resolved. Plastic surgical intervention may be considered in selected cases. Because 90–95% of these tumors resolve spontaneously, it is important to avoid the temptation of early plastic surgery, cryotherapy, radiation therapy, or sclerosing agents, which can hasten resolution but lead to a higher likelihood of scarring.

Bruckner AL, Frieden IJ: Hemangiomas of infancy. J Am Acad Dermatol 48:477–493, 2003.

128. **What are the major goals of the management of hemangiomas?**
The decisions regarding which hemangiomas require treatment and the best therapeutic modalities may not always be easy ones. The major goals of management are as follows:
- Prevent or reverse life- or function-threatening complications.
- Treat ulcerated hemangiomas.
- Prevent permanent disfigurement caused by a rapidly enlarging lesion.
- Minimize psychosocial stress for the family and the patient.
- Avoid overly aggressive procedures that may result in scarring in lesions that have a good likelihood of involuting without significant residual lesions.

Frieden IJ: Which hemangiomas to treat—and how? Arch Dermatol 133:1593–1595, 1997.

129. **Which hemangiomas are especially worrisome?**
- **Multiple cutaneous hemangiomas:** May be associated with visceral hemangiomas (e.g., liver)
- **Large hemangiomas:** May cause significant disfigurement of underlying structures and may be associated with congestive heart failure
- **"Beard" hemangiomas:** May be a marker for underlying laryngeal or subglottic hemangioma that may impair respiratory function
- **Midline spinal hemangiomas:** May be a marker for underlying spinal cord abnormality
- **Head and neck hemangiomas:** Usually larger lesions, may be associated with other congenital anomalies, including central nervous system, cardiac, ocular, and sternal defects (e.g., **P**osterior fossa malformation, **H**emangioma, **A**rterial abnormalities, **C**oarctation, **E**ye abnormalities, **S**ternal defects [PHACES] syndrome).
- **Vulnerable anatomic locations:** Impair vital functions, cause disfigurement (e.g. periocular, neck, lip, nasal tip)
- **Ulcerated hemangiomas:** Increased risk of superinfection, cause pain and lead to scarring

Metry DW, Hebert AA: Benign cutaneous vascular tumors of infancy: When to worry, what to do. Arch Dermatol 136:905–914, 2000.

130. **When are systemic corticosteroids indicated for the treatment of infantile hemangiomas?**
Although the approach to palpable hemangiomas generally involves observation over time, indications for systemic corticosteroids (prednisone 2–3 mg/kg/day tapered over months) include the following:
- Lesions that interfere with normal physiologic functioning (i.e., breathing, hearing, eating, vision), especially periocular hemangiomas (to prevent amblyopia)
- Recurrent bleeding, ulceration, or infection
- A rapidly growing lesion that distorts facial features
- High-output congestive heart failure

Bruckner AL, Frieden IJ: Hemangiomas of infancy. J Am Acad Dermatol 48:477–493, 2003.

131. **If intralesional or systemic steroids have failed as options for hemangiomas requiring treatment, what else may be of benefit?**
- **Chemotherapeutic agents (vincristine):** These are usually used for life-threatening hemangiomas for which other modalities have failed.

- **Embolization**
- **Surgery**
- **Interferon alpha:** Used subcutaneously, it may act by blocking endothelial cell motility and inhibiting angiogenesis. However, neurotoxicity is a common and severe side-effect that has resulted in limiting the use of this drug.
- **Pulsed dye laser:** This may be used with other modalities but is usually of little benefit in situations in which intralesional or systemic corticosteroids were previously indicated. Limited penetration restricts use to superficial lesions. It can be useful for painful ulcerated hemangiomas that fail to respond to other treatment modalities. Controversy exists regarding its potential to cause scarring.

132. **Why is an infant with a vascular tumor and new-onset thrombocytopenia so worrisome?**

This can indicate the development of the **Kasabach-Merritt syndrome** (or phenomenon), a life-threatening condition of rapidly enlarging vascular tumors and progressive coagulopathy. Platelets are sequestered within the lesion(s), forming thrombi and consuming coagulation factors. Ecchymoses may develop initially around the vascular tumor, but a disseminated coagulopathy with microangiopathic hemolytic anemia can result. Aggressive therapy (systemic steroids, vincristine, interferon alpha, and surgery) is frequently needed. Kasabach-Merritt syndrome is not caused by common hemangiomas of infancy but rather by two rare vascular tumors (Kaposiform hemangioendothelioma and tufted angioma).

133. **How do superficial hemangiomas differ from port wine stains?**

Superficial hemangiomas are superficial, palpable, vascular tumors that usually involute with time. In the past, they were called "strawberry" hemangiomas. **Port wine stains,** which are sometimes called *nevus flammeus,* are flat vascular malformations composed of capillary and postcapillary venule-size vessels that do not involute. Some superficial hemangiomas may mimic port wine stains during the first few weeks of life; observation of their growth pattern is helpful for establishing the correct diagnosis (Box 4-2).

BOX 4-2. SUPERFICIAL HEMANGIOMAS VERSUS PORT WINE STAINS

Superficial hemangiomas	Port wine stains
Palpable	Flat, macular
Common (4–10% of children <1 year old)	Less common (0.1–0.3%)
Often not apparent at birth (more visible at 2–12 weeks)	Present at birth
Bright red	Pale pink to blue-red (darkens with age)
Well-defined borders	Borders variable
Pathology: Proliferating angioblastic endothelial cells with variable blood-filled capillaries	Pathology: Dermal capillary dilation
90–95% involute spontaneously by age 9	No involution: may worsen with darkening and hypertrophy
Rapid growth phase	Proportionate growth (as child grows)
Suggested therapy: Watchful waiting; active treatment for some lesions	Suggested therapy: Flash lamp pulsed-dye laser in children

134. **When are port wine stains associated with other anomalies?**
    Sturge-Weber syndrome refers to the association of a facial port wine stain (typically affecting the skin innervated by the first branch of the trigeminal nerve [Fig. 4-13]), an ocular vascular anomaly linked with glaucoma, and a leptomeningeal vascular anomaly associated with seizures and developmental delay.

    Klippel-Trenaunay syndrome refers to the association of a limb port wine stain (usually lower extremity) with ipsilateral soft tissue and bony overgrowth and venous varicosities.

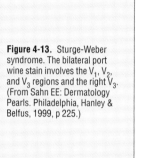

Figure 4-13. Sturge-Weber syndrome. The bilateral port wine stain involves the V_1, V_2, and V_3 regions and the right V_3. (From Sahn EE: Dermatology Pearls. Philadelphia, Hanley & Belfus, 1999, p 225.)

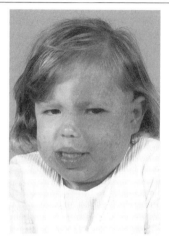

VESICOBULLOUS DISORDERS

135. **What is the Nikolsky sign?**
    This sign demonstrates **epidermal fragility**. Gentle lateral pressure placed on apparently intact skin causes an erosion, especially near preformed vesicles. This sign is positive in several autoimmune, infectious, and inherited blistering conditions, such as bullous pemphigoid, staphylococcal scalded skin syndrome (SSSS), and epidermolysis bullosa.

136. **What are causes of skin blistering in childhood?**
    - **Infectious:** Bacterial (bullous impetigo, SSSS), viral (herpes simplex virus, varicella)
    - **Contact dermatitis:** Poison ivy, phytophotodermatitis
    - **Inherited disorders:** Epidermolysis bullosa, bullous congenital ichthyosiform erythroderma
    - **Autoimmune disorders:** Linear immunoglobulin A disease, bullous pemphigoid, pemphigus vulgaris
    - **Other:** Erythema multiforme, toxic epidermal necrolysis, thermal injury (burns)

137. **How is SSSS differentiated from toxic epidermal necrolysis (TEN)?**
    Both are diffuse bullous diseases. **SSSS** commonly arises in young children <5 years old and develops after a localized staphylococcal infection with diffuse cutaneous disease caused by an exfoliative toxin. The level of blistering includes the superficial levels of the epidermis. **TEN** is believed to be a hypersensitivity reaction (often to a drug) and occurs in all age groups. The level of blistering is deep, and the entire epidermis is necrotic (Table 4-3).

TABLE 4-3. DIFFERENTIATION BETWEEN STAPHYLOCOCCAL SCALDED SKIN SYNDROME AND TOXIC EPIDERMAL NECROLYSIS

	Staphylococcal scalded skin syndrome	Toxic epidermal necrolysis
Etiology	Infectious; group II staphylococci	Immunologic; usually drug related
Morbidity/mortality	Low	High
Mucous membrane involvement	Rare	Frequent
Nikolsky sign	Present	Absent
Target lesions	Absent	Often present
Level of blister	Upper epidermis (below stratum corneum)	Subepidermal
Histopathology	No epidermal necrosis or dermal inflammation	Full-thickness epidermal necrosis; prominent perivascular dermal inflammation

Adapted from Roberts LJ: Dermatologic diseases. In McMillan JA, DeAngelis CD, Feigin RD, et al (eds): Oski's Pediatrics, Principles and Practice, 3rd ed. Philadelphia, Lippincott Williams & Wilkins, 1999, p 379.

138. **Why are neonates susceptible to SSSS?**
The answer lies in the fact that newborns share their susceptibility to SSSS with patients in renal failure. It is the reduced clearance of the exfoliative toxin by the newborn's immature kidneys that contributes to their increased susceptibility to SSSS.

139. **Where can the *Staphylococcus aureus* be found in patients with SSSS?**
Staphylococcus aureus commonly colonizes the nasopharynx and the umbilicus. The source of infection may also be present in the urinary tract, a wound, conjunctiva, or blood.

140. **What is epidermolysis bullosa (EB)?**
EB is a heterogeneous group of inherited disorders characterized by blister formation, either spontaneously or at sites of trauma. There are three general categories of EB: simplex, junctional, and dystrophic. The extent of blistering and the degree of scarring roughly correlates with the level of blister formation in the epidermis or dermis.
Dystrophic Epidermolysis Bullosa Research Association of America: www.debra.org

141. **Is steroid therapy beneficial for the treatment of Stevens-Johnson syndrome (SJS) or TEN?**
This is a continuing area of controversy; studies are inconclusive. Treatment may be considered early during the course of SJS if multiple mucosal surfaces are involved, but skin denudation is limited. The potential for steroids to increase medical complications (e.g., hemorrhage, infection) must be taken into account. If initiated, clinical response (or lack thereof) should be carefully followed, and steroids should be discontinued if the condition is worsening. Because the majority of cases of SJS will spontaneously resolve, other therapies are vital: skin care, nutritional support, ophthalmologic care, and the

treatment of secondary bacterial infections. Steroids have been reported to be associated with an increased mortality rate among patients with TEN.

Leaute-Labreze C, Lamireau T, Chawki D, et al: Diagnosis, classification, and management of erythema multiforme and Steven-Johnson syndrome. Arch Dis Child 83:347–352, 2000.

142. **What therapy should be considered for patients with rapidly progressive SJS or TEN?**
Intravenous immune globulin should be considered. Caution should be used, especially in patients with poor renal function, hypercoagulable states, and IgA deficiency.

143. **What infectious agent is most commonly associated with recurrent erythema multiforme?**
Herpes simplex virus.

144. **What common infectious agent should be considered in a child with SJS?**
Mycoplasma pneumoniae.

ACKNOWLEDGMENT

The editors gratefully acknowledge contributions by Drs. Robert Hayman and Leonard Kristal that were retained from the first three editions of *Pediatric Secrets.*

CHAPTER 5

EMERGENCY MEDICINE

Joan Bregstein, MD, Cindy Ganis Roskind, MD, and Steve Miller, MD

This chapter is dedicated to Steve Miller, MD, whose life ended tragically on October 19, 2004. Steve was our honored and respected division chief, a cherished colleague, and an irreplaceable friend. His memory will live on in the lives he touched, the students he taught, and the words he wrote.

BIOTERRORISM

1. **Why are children more vulnerable to biologic agents than adults?**
   - **Anatomic and physiologic differences:** Thinner dermis, increased surface-area-to-volume ratio, smaller relative blood volume, higher minute ventilation
   - **Developmental considerations:** Inability to flee dangerous situations, possible increased risk of posttraumatic stress disorder
   - **Some vaccines not licensed for children:** Anthrax (18–65 years), plague (18–61 years)
   - **Vaccines more dangerous in children:** Smallpox, yellow fever
   - **Antibiotics less familiar to pediatricians:** Tetracyclines, fluoroquinolones

     Cieslak TJ, Henretig FM: Bioterrorism. Pediatr Ann 32:145–165, 2003.
     Centers for Disease Control and Prevention: www.bt.cdc.gov

2. **What are the three routes of transmission of anthrax?**
   - **Inhalation:** Most feared; can lead to multiorgan hemorrhagic necrosis
   - **Cutaneous:** Inoculated through wound, causing a black, painless ulcer
   - **Ingestion:** May cause gastrointestinal or upper-respiratory symptoms

   A spore-forming, gram-positive rod, *Bacillus anthracis* can survive for extended periods before entering the body, when it will germinate and proliferate (Fig. 5-1).

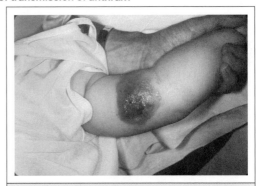

   Figure 5-1. Cutaneous anthrax in a child. (From Schachner LA, Hansen RC (eds): Pediatric Dermatology, 3rd ed. Edinburgh, Mosby, 2003, p 1033.)

3. **How are the lesions of smallpox distinguished from varicella (chickenpox)?**
   - Smallpox lesions predominate on the face and extremities (centrifugal), whereas varicella lesions are typically heaviest on the trunk (centripetal).

- The rash of smallpox progresses in similar stages (macules, papules, vesicles, crusting), whereas varicella is seen with multiple crops in differing stages.
- Smallpox rash develops more slowly than varicella rash.

4. **How can the presenting symptoms of bubonic plague be differentiated from that of plague resulting from bioterrorism?**
Bubonic plague—of "black death" fame—resulted from the bite of fleas, which led to large tender regional adenopathy (the "bubo") with subsequent hematogenous dissemination, multiorgan involvement, and septicemia. In bioterrorism, the organism *Yersinia pestis* would be aerosolized, and inhalation would result in presentations more typical of pneumonic plague, with fever, chills, tachypnea, cough, and bloody sputum; lymphadenitis would likely be a later finding.

Dennis DT, Chow CC: Plague. Pediatr Infect Dis J 23:69–71, 2004.

5. **Why should families living near nuclear power plants keep potassium iodide (KI) in their medicine cabinets?**
The American Academy of Pediatrics recommends that families living within 10 miles of a nuclear power plant (or 50 miles in densely populated areas, where evacuations may be more difficult) have KI on hand in the event of a nuclear radiation catastrophe. KI will inhibit the uptake of radioactive iodine (^{131}I) into the thyroid gland. Children are more susceptible than adults to the subsequent development of thyroid cancer if exposed. If KI is administered within 1 hour, 90% of ^{131}I is blocked, but after 12 hours there is little effect.

Committee on Environmental Health, American Academy of Pediatrics: Radiation disasters and children. Pediatrics 111:1455–1466, 2003.

CHILD ABUSE AND SEXUAL ABUSE

6. **How significant a problem is child abuse in the United States?**
Latest figures show that almost **1 million** children a year are confirmed by child protective service agencies as being victims of child maltreatment. The majority (60%) are victims of neglect; 23% are victims of physical abuse; 9% are of sexual abuse; and 9% are of emotional or other forms of maltreatment. Boys may be victimized as often as girls, but they may not be as likely to disclose the abuse.

American Academy of Pediatrics: Guidelines for the evaluation of sexual abuse of children: Subject review. Pediatrics 103:186–191, 1999.

7. **What is the most common cause of severe closed head trauma in infants <1 year old?**
Shaken impact or **shaken baby syndrome.** This injury is more likely to occur from severe shaking *and* impact; thus, the dual terminology. Violent shaking of an infant with sudden impact can result in subdural hematomas, subarachnoid hemorrhages, and cerebral infarcts. The diagnosis is suggested by the lack of a corroborating mechanism of injury in the face of a symptomatic child, or, rarely, a confession by the perpetrator. In many cases, physical examination reveals retinal hemorrhages (Fig. 5-2). Other signs of trauma are usually lacking. Diagnosis is confirmed by computed tomography (CT) scanning or magnetic resonance imaging (MRI). If a lumbar puncture is performed, the fluid may be bloody or xanthochromic. The prognosis is grim for an infant who is in coma from this abuse: 50% die, and nearly half of the survivors have significant neurologic sequelae.

American Academy of Pediatrics: Shaken baby syndrome: Rotational cranial injuries and technical report. Pediatrics 108:206–210, 2001.

8. **Why is the diagnosis of shaken baby/impact syndrome often overlooked?**

When an infant is unconscious with respiratory distress, apnea, and/or seizures, the diagnosis of shaken baby syndrome should be considered. However, depending on the degree of shaking and the degree of resulting damage, the symptoms can be mild and nonspecific and may mimic symptoms of a viral illness, feeding disorder/dysfunction, or even colic.
Victims may have a history of poor feeding, vomiting, lethargy, and/or irritability that may have gone on for days or weeks.

American Academy of Pediatrics: Shaken baby syndrome: Rotational cranial injuries and technical report. Pediatrics 108:206–210, 2001.

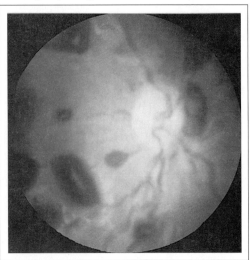

Figure 5-2. Retinal hemorrhages of victim of shaken baby/impact syndrome. (From Zitelli BJ, Davis HW: Atlas of Pediatric Physical Diagnosis, 4th ed. St. Louis, Mosby, 2002, p 181.)

9. **What diagnostic tests may be contributory if shaken baby/impact syndrome is suspected?**
   - **Head CT:** Good for demonstrating subarachnoid and large extra-axial hemorrhages and mass effect; may be falsely negative, especially early in the presentation
   - **MRI:** Good for diagnosing subdural hemorrhages and intraparenchymal lesions; may miss subarachnoid blood and fractures
   - **Spinal tap:** May yield bloody cerebrospinal fluid
   - **Chest x-ray:** May be normal or may reveal acute or healed rib fractures, which are suggestive of abuse
   - **Complete blood count:** May be normal or may show mild to moderate anemia
   - **Prothrombin time/partial thromboplastin time:** May show mild to moderate abnormalities or reveal frank disseminated intravascular coagulation
   - **Amylase:** May show an increase, signifying possible pancreatic damage
   - **Liver function tests:** Abnormalities may signify occult liver injury

   American Academy of Pediatrics: Shaken baby syndrome: Rotational cranial injuries and technical report. Pediatrics 108:206–210, 2001.

KEY POINTS: RETINAL HEMORRHAGES

1. May be the only sign in an infant of a nonaccidental shaking injury

2. Should always be assessed in an infant whose presenting symptoms include excessive irritability, lethargy, sepsis-like appearance, seizures, or coma

3. Should always be confirmed by an ophthalmologist

4. If found, should be followed by a skeletal series and cranial neuroimaging (computed tomography scanning and/or magnetic resonance imaging)

10. **What are important historic indicators of possible child abuse?**
    - Multiple previous hospital visits for injuries
    - History of untreated injuries
    - Cause of trauma not known or inappropriate for age or activity
    - Delay in seeking medical attention
    - History incompatible with injury
    - Parents unconcerned about injury or more concerned about unrelated minor problem (e.g., cold, headache)
    - History of abused siblings
    - Changing or inconsistent stories to explain injury

    Kottmeier P: The battered child. Pediatr Ann 16:343–351, 1987.
    Sirotnak AP, Grigsby T, Krugman RD: Physical abuse of children. Pediatr Rev 25:264–276, 2004.

11. **What important physical examination findings are indicators of possible child abuse?**
    - Burns, especially cigarette or immersion burns on the buttocks or perineum or burns in a stocking/glove distribution
    - Genital trauma or sexually transmitted infection in a prepubertal child
    - Signs of excessive corporal punishment (welts, belt or cord marks, bites)
    - Frenulum lacerations in young infants (associated with forced feeding)
    - Multiple bruises in various stages of resolution
    - Neurologic injury associated with retinal or scleral hemorrhages
    - Fractures suggestive of abuse (e.g., skull fractures in infants, metaphyseal fractures, posterior rib fractures, femur fractures in infants, scapular fractures)

    Kottmeier P: The battered child. Pediatr Ann 16:343–351, 1987.
    Sirotnak AP, Grigsby T, Krugman RD: Physical abuse of children. Pediatr Rev 25:264–276, 2004.

12. **When should child abuse be considered in the event of an unexplained death of a child?**
    Always. Sudden infant death syndrome (SIDS) should be a diagnosis of exclusion in any unexplained death. Deaths as a result of SIDS usually occur during the first year of life, most commonly (90%) in children less than 7 months old. All children who die suddenly of unclear causes should have a complete physical examination that looks for signs of external trauma (e.g., bruises, injury to the genitalia) and an ophthalmologic examination that looks for retinal hemorrhages.

13. **What are the causes of sudden and unexpected deaths in infancy?**
    SIDS accounts for about 85–90% of cases. Because the incidence of SIDS has been falling since more infants began sleeping in the supine position, the percentage of non-SIDS deaths has increased. In a 10-year study of 669 infants in Quebec, other causes included infection (7%), cardiovascular disease (2.7%), child abuse or neglect (2.6%), and metabolic diseases or genetic disorders (2.1%). The percentage of non-SIDS cases was significantly higher in ages that were atypical for SIDS: <1 month and >6 months of age.

    American Academy of Pediatrics, Committee on Child Abuse and Neglect: Distinguishing sudden infant death syndrome from child abuse fatalities. Pediatrics 94:124–126, 1994.
    Cote A, Russo P, Michaud J, et al: Sudden unexpected death in infants: What are the causes? J Pediatr 135:437–443, 1999.

14. **Which conditions with ecchymoses can be mistaken for child abuse?**
    - **Mongolian spots (dermal melanosis):** These are commonly mistaken for bruises, especially when they occur elsewhere than the classic lumbosacral area; unlike bruises, they do not fade with time.
    - **Coagulation disorders:** In 20% of cases of hemophilia, there is no family history of disease; bruising may be noted in unusual places in response to minor trauma.

- **Folk medicine:** Southeast Asian practices of spoon rubbing (*quat sha*) or coin rubbing (*cao gio*) can produce ecchymoses; the practice of cupping (the inversion of a heated cup on the back) produces circular ecchymoses.
- **Moxibustion:** This is the Southeast Asian practice of burning an herbal substance on the child's abdomen to cure disease.
- **Dyes:** Clothing dyes, especially from jeans, sometimes mimic bruising; they are easily removed with topical alcohol.

15. **How do the color changes of an ecchymosis progress?**

The visual aging of bruises is an inexact science with significant variability. Bruises on the face or genitalia heal more quickly than bruises on other parts of the body, because there is increased blood supply to these regions. In general, the better the blood supply and the more superficial the wound, the faster it will heal. It takes roughly 5–7 days for a bruise to become greenish yellow. The following table should only be used as a guideline.

0–1 days: Red/blue
1–5 days: Blue/purple
5–7 days: Green/yellow
8–10 days: Yellow/brown
1.5–4 weeks: Resolution

Schwartz AJ, Ricci LR: How accurately can bruises be aged in abused children? Literature review and synthesis. Pediatrics 97:254–257, 1996.

16. **How are fractures dated radiographically in children?**

After a fracture, the following will be seen:
- **1–7 days:** Soft-tissue swelling; fat and fascial planes blurred; sharp fracture line
- **7–14 days:** Periosteal new bone formation as soft callus forms; blurring of fracture line; occurs earlier for infants, later for older children
- **14–21 days:** More clearly defined (i.e., hard) callus forming as periosteal bone converts to lamellar bone
- **21–42 days:** Peak of hard callus formation
- **≥60 days:** Remodeling of bone begins with reshaping of the deformity (up to 1–2 years)

If the timing of an injury does not correlate with the dating of a fracture or if fractures at multiple stages of healing are present, child abuse should be suspected.

17. **What fractures are suggestive of child abuse?**

Spinal fractures, posterior and anterior rib fractures, skull fractures, metaphyseal chip fractures, and vertebral, femoral, pelvic, or scapular fractures. These are fractures that commonly result from twisting (spiral fractures), throwing, and beating. Metaphyseal chip fractures are the result of the forceful jerking of an extremity. Anterior and posterior rib fractures occur with severe side-to-side compression of the thorax; they are almost never caused by cardiopulmonary resuscitation (CPR). The description and forcefulness of injury should be consistent with the fracture. One should be especially suspicious if such fractures occur in a child who is not yet walking.

Oral R, Blum KL, Johnson C: Fractures in young children: are physicians in the emergency department and orthopedic clinics adequately screening for possible abuse? Pediatr Emerg Care 19:148–153, 2003.

Sirotnak AP, Grigsby T, Krugman RD: Physical abuse of children. Pediatr Rev 25:264–277, 2004.

18. **What constitutes the skeletal survey?**

Skeletal injuries, particularly multiple healed lesions, are strong indicators of a pattern of abuse, particularly in the absence of sufficient clinical evidence to justify such a diagnosis. The *skeletal survey* is a multiple-imaging series that provides multiple views of the following:

- **Appendicular skeleton:** Humeri, forearms, hands, femurs, lower legs, and feet
- **Axial skeleton:** Thorax, pelvis, (including mid and lower lumbar spine), lumbar spine, cervical spine, and skull

  "Body grams" (studies that encompass the entire child in one or two exposures) are not felt to be of sufficient sensitivity to be useful. If abuse is highly suspected and the initial study is normal, a follow-up series 2 weeks later will increase the diagnostic yield.

  American Academy of Pediatrics: Diagnostic imaging of child abuse. Pediatrics 105:1345–1348, 2000.

19. **Up to what age should a skeletal series be ordered?**
    If physical abuse is suspected, the American Academy of Pediatrics recommends that children up to the age of 2 years have a skeletal series.

20. **When are burn injuries suspicious for child abuse?**
    Burn injuries account for about 5% of cases of physical abuse. As with other injuries, the description of the incident causing the burn should be consistent with the child's development and the extent and degree of the burn observed. The following types are suspicious for abuse:
    - **Immersion burns:** Sharply demarcated lines on the hands and feet ("stocking-glove" distribution), buttocks, and perineum, with a uniform depth of burn; the immersion of a child in a hot bath is a classic example
    - **Geographic burns:** Burns, usually of second or third degree, in a distinct pattern, such as circular cigarette burns or steam iron burns
    - **Splash burns:** Pattern with droplet marks projecting away from the most involved area; splash marks on the back of the body usually require another person and may or may not be accidental

21. **How do you recognize Munchausen's syndrome by proxy?**
    In this form of child abuse, adults inflict illness on a child or falsify symptoms to obtain medical care for a child. Features include the following:
    - Recurrent episodes of a confusing medical picture
    - Multiple diagnostic evaluations at medical centers ("doctor shopping")
    - Unsupportive marital relationship, often with maternal isolation
    - Compliant, cooperative, and overinvolved mother
    - Higher level of parental medical knowledge
    - Parental history of extensive medical treatment or illness
    - Conditions resolve with surveillance of child in the hospital
    - Findings correlate with the presence of the parent

    Ludwig S: Child abuse. In Fleisher GR, Ludwig S (eds): Textbook of Pediatric Emergency Medicine, 4th ed. Baltimore, Lippincott Williams & Wilkins, 2000, p 1679.

    Schreier H: Munchausen by proxy defined. Pediatrics 110:985–988, 2002.

22. **How often is sexual abuse committed by an individual known previously by the child or adolescent?**
    Between 75% and 80% of the time. Relatives are the perpetrators in 50% of cases.

23. **In cases of suspected sexual abuse of a child, is it necessary to conduct a full sexual abuse examination immediately, or can the patient be referred to a child advocacy center and child abuse specialist at the earliest possible time?**
    If you believe the alleged sexual abuse has occurred within the past 96 hours or if there is ongoing bleeding or evidence of acute injury, it is important to complete the medical examination immediately. Accepted protocols for evaluating child sexual assault victims should be followed to properly secure biologic evidence such as semen, blood, and epithelial cells. If the history suggests an event occurring more than 72 hours earlier and there is no acute

injury, an emergency examination may not be necessary. The examination can be scheduled at the earliest possible time at a center that specializes in the evaluation of child and sexual abuse.

24. **After the documentation of history and a careful physical examination, what evidence should be collected in cases of suspected sexual abuse or assault of a postpubertal female?**

    With a suspected history of sexual contact, loss of consciousness, or poor history, the following should be obtained:
    1. **Pregnancy testing** if postmenarchal
    2. **Evidence of sexual contact,** including 2–3 swabbed specimens from each area of assault for the following substances:
       - Sperm (motile/nonmotile)
       - Acid phosphatase (secreted by the prostate; component of seminal plasma)
       - P_{30} (prostate glycoprotein present in seminal fluid)
       - Blood group antigens
    3. **Evidence to document perpetrator**
       - Foreign material on clothing
       - Suspected nonpatient hairs
       - DNA testing (controversial)

    Johnson CF: Child sexual abuse. Lancet 364:462–470, 2004.

25. **Should evidence of sexually transmitted diseases (STDs) be collected in cases of postpubertal sexual abuse or assault?**

    This is controversial. There are some who feel that these patients should be prophylactically treated with antibiotics but that cultures, which could falsely influence a jury if the case ultimately goes to court, are not necessary. There are others who feel that all patients who get treated should have cultures performed to prove the presence of an infection. If cultures are obtained, the following should be included:
    - Gonococcal cultures of the pharynx, vagina or cervix, and rectum
    - Chlamydial cultures of the pharynx, vagina or urethra, and rectum
    - Rapid plasmin reagin or Venereal Disease Research Laboratory test for syphilis; if positive, confirm with specific antibody testing

26. **What options should be offered to a postpubertal female after a sexual assault involving vaginal penetration?**

    After a negative pregnancy test, the following issues should be discussed:
    - **Gonococcal prophylaxis:** Especially if abuse occurs less than 48 hours before evaluation (as a result of organism incubating and potential for false-negative cultures).
    - **Human immunodeficiency virus (HIV) testing/prophylaxis:** Consensus guidelines do not exist regarding HIV testing and postexposure prophylaxis and must be individualized, depending on a variety of factors (e.g., extent of sexual contact, status of perpetrator, parental wishes). Prophylaxis is not indicated if >72 hours have passed since the exposure.
    - **Pregnancy prophylaxis:** Oral contraceptives (e.g, Ovral, 2 tablets × 2 given 12 hours apart) may be given within 72 hours of the sexual contact.

27. **How long does forensic evidence of sexual abuse persist after contact?**

    The lack of cervical mucus in prepubertal girls decreases the survival of motile sperm, and the utility of body swabbing in prepubertal girls is very low after 24 hours. Data are very limited with regard to the pharyngeal persistence of nonmotile sperm and the pharyngeal and rectal persistence of acid phosphatase. Both acid phosphatase and P_{30} can persist indefinitely on clothing if it is kept dry and not washed. See Table 5-1.

TABLE 5-1. TYPES OF FORENSIC EVIDENCE

Site	Motile sperm	Nonmotile sperm	Acid phosphatase	P_{30}
Pharynx	0.5–6 hours	6 hours (?)	6 hours (?)	Unknown
Rectum	0.5–8 hours	24 hours	24 hours (?)	Unknown
Vagina	0.5–8 hours	7–48 hours	12–48 hours	12–48 hours
Clothing	<0.5 hour	Up to 12 months	Up to 3 years	Up to 12 years

? = limited data.
From Reece RM: Child Abuse: Medical Diagnosis and Management. Philadelphia, Lea & Febiger, 1994, p 234.

28. **What is the best predictor of *Neisseria gonorrhoeae* infection in children <12 years old who are examined for sexual abuse?**
Vaginal or urethral discharge. Without evidence of discharge, the likelihood of a culture result being positive is near zero.

   Sicoli RA, Losek, JD, Hudlett JM, et al: Indications for *Neisseria gonorrhoeae* cultures in children with suspected sexual abuse. Arch Pediatr Adolesc Med 149:86–89, 1995.

29. **If a patient who is not sexually active is diagnosed with an infection caused by an STD-associated organism, how likely is sexual abuse the reason for acquisition?**
See Table 5-2.

TABLE 5-2. LIKELIHOOD OF SEXUAL ABUSE ACCORDING TO ORGANISM

Organism	Likelihood of sexual abuse
Neisseria gonorrhoeae	Diagnostic
Treponema pallidum (syphilis)	Diagnostic
Chlamydia trachomatis	Diagnostic
Human immunodeficiency virus	Diagnostic
Trichomonas vaginalis	Highly suspicious
Condylomata acuminata	Suspicious
Herpes (genital location)	Suspicious
Bacterial vaginosis	Inconclusive

Adapted from American Academy of Pediatrics: Sexually transmitted diseases. In Pickering LK (ed): 2003 Red Book, 26th ed. Elk Grove Village, IL, American Academy of Pediatrics, 2003, p 162.

30. **Is the size of the hymenal opening an important finding in the diagnosis of sexual abuse?**
The hymenal opening is measured with a child in the supine, frog-leg position, and various studies have attempted to determine a size that most likely correlates with sexual abuse. The ranges have been from 4–10 mm, but variations in technique, positioning, and relative relaxation of the patient have limited the value of absolute numbers. In addition, there is considerable overlap in diameter between sexually abused and nonabused girls. Thus, the size of the

hymenal opening has been deemphasized as a diagnostic or confirmatory test, particularly as an isolated finding. More important as part of the examination is inspection for scarring and tears of the hymen and surrounding tissues. Recent studies have reexamined the concept of hymenal size as a screening tool for abuse.

Pugno PA: Genital findings in prepubertal girls evaluated for sexual abuse: A different perspective on hymenal measurements. Arch Fam Med 8:403–406, 1999.

Heger A, Emans SJ: Introital diameter as the criteria for sexual abuse. Pediatrics 85:222–223, 1990.

KEY POINTS: SEXUAL ABUSE

1. Most common physical finding: Normal examination

2. Perpetrator known to victim in 75–80% of cases

3. Diagnostic of abuse: Gonorrhea, syphilis, chlamydia, human immunodeficiency virus

4. Indications for immediate medical examination: Alleged assault within 96 hours, ongoing bleeding, or evidence of acute injury

5. Use of accepted/standardized protocols important during evaluative process

31. What is the most common finding of the physical examination of a child who has been sexually abused?

A **normal physical examination** is the most common physical finding. It is crucial to know that a normal examination does not rule out sexual abuse.

32. If physical abuse is suspected, are physicians mandated to photograph physical findings?

No. A good drawing of the physical findings is sufficient. However, if photographs are taken, a card with the patient's name, date of birth, and the photographer's signatures must be included in the photo so that the patient can be clearly identified. In addition, the body part that is being photographed must be clearly identifiable. If abuse is suspected, it is not necessary to obtain parental consent to take photographs.

ENVIRONMENTAL INJURY

33. How do fresh and salt water drownings differ?

Fresh water injures the lung primarily by disrupting surfactant, thereby leading to alveolar collapse. Damage to the alveolar membranes leads to the transudation of fluid into the air spaces and pulmonary edema. **Salt water** pulls fluid into the air spaces directly by creating a strong osmotic gradient, and the accumulated water washes away surfactant, thereby leading to alveolar collapse. By either mechanism, patients develop ventilation-perfusion mismatch and hypoxemia, which may require aggressive mechanical support. Ultimately, management for either fresh- or salt-water drowning is the same.

Harries M: Near drowning. BMJ 327:1336–1338, 2003.

Ibsen LM, Koch T: Submersion and asphyxial injury. Crit Care Med 30: S402–S408, 2002.

34. What cardiovascular changes occur as body temperature falls?

- **31–32°C:** Elevated heart rate, cardiac output, and blood pressure; peripheral vasoconstriction and increased central vascular volume; normal electrocardiogram (ECG)

- **28–31°C:** Diminished heart rate, cardiac output, and blood pressure; ECG irregu-larities include premature ventricular contractions (PVCs), supraventricular dysrhythmias, atrial fibrillation, and T-wave inversion
- **<28°C:** Severe myocardial irritability; ventricular fibrillation, usually refractory to electrical defibrillation; often absent pulse or blood pressure; J waves on ECG

35. **What happens if you externally warm a severely hypothermic patient too rapidly?**
    - **Core temperature "afterdrop":** The body temperature drops because external rewarming causes peripheral vasodilation and the return of cold venous blood to the core.
    - **Hypotension:** Peripheral vasodilation increases total vascular space, thereby causing a drop in blood pressure.
    - **Acidosis:** Lactic acid returns from the periphery, thereby resulting in rewarming acidosis.
    - **Dysrhythmias:** Rewarming alters acid-base and electrolyte status in the setting of an irritable myocardium.

36. **What are acceptable rewarming methods for the hypothermic child?**
    For patients with mild hypothermia (32–35°C), passive rewarming by removing cold clothing and placing the patient in a warm, dry environment with blankets is generally sufficient. Active external rewarming involves the use of heating blankets, hot water bottles, and overhead warmers and is used for patients with acute hypothermia in the 32–35°C range as well. Active external rewarming should not be used for chronic hypothermia (>24 hours). More aggressive core rewarming techniques should be considered for patients with temperatures <32°C. These techniques include gastric or colonic irrigation with warm fluids, peritoneal dialysis, pleural lavage, and extracorporeal blood rewarming with partial bypass. Intravenous and other fluids should be heated to 43°C. Patients should be given warmed, humidified oxygen by face mask or endotracheal tube.

37. **What systems malfunction in patients with heatstroke?**
    Heatstroke is a medical emergency of multisystem dysfunction that includes a very high fever (usually >41.5°C). The systems that are affected include the following:
    - **Central nervous system:** Confusion, seizures, and loss of consciousness
    - **Cardiovascular:** Hypotension as a result of volume depletion, peripheral vasodilation, and myocardial dysfunction
    - **Renal:** Acute tubular necrosis and renal failure, with marked electrolyte abnormalities
    - **Hepatocellular:** Injury and dysfunction
    - **Heme:** Abnormal hemostasis, often with signs of disseminated intravascular coagulation
    - **Muscle:** Rhabdomyolysis

38. **How quickly can temperature rise inside a closed automobile as a result of sunlight?**
    In one study in New Orleans, with an outside air temperature at 93°F, temperature reached 125°F in 20 minutes and 140°F in 40 minutes. Leaving the window slightly open ("cracking the window") did not affect the rapid temperature elevation. The dangers of leaving a child unattended in a vehicle for even a few minutes become readily apparent.

    Gibbs LI, Lawrence DW, Kohn MA: Heat exposure in an enclosed automobile. J La State Med Soc 147:545–546, 1995.

39. **What is the "critical thermal maximum"?**
    42°C. This is the body temperature at which cell death begins as physiologic processes unravel. Enzymes denature, lipid membranes liquefy, mitochondria misfire, and protein production fails.

40.   **What two questions are key when considering the placement of an endotracheal tube in a patient who has been in a house fire?**

- **How extensive are the signs of heat exposure in the upper airway?** Physical examination may reveal carbonaceous sputum, singed nasal hairs, facial burns, or pulmonary abnormalities. These make the development of swelling of the upper airway more likely and thus prompt consideration of viewing the vocal cords directly to look for signs of impending upper airway obstruction. If significant swelling, erythema, or blistering is seen, intubation should be performed electively to protect the airway from progressive obstruction.
- **Are there signs or symptoms of impending airway obstruction as a result of mucosal injury and edema?** Yes. These include hoarseness, stridor, increasing respiratory distress, and difficulty handling secretions. If present (along with the physical exam [PE] signs as noted above), intubation should be undertaken. Intubation with an endotracheal tube should be done immediately for patients experiencing respiratory failure.

41.   **Which laboratory studies are needed for patients with suspected carbon monoxide poisoning?**

1. **Blood carboxyhemoglobin (HbCO) level**
   - 0–1%: Normal (smokers may have up to 5–10%)
   - 10–30%: Headache, exercise-induced dyspnea, confusion
   - 30–50%: Severe headache, nausea, vomiting, increased heart rate and respirations, visual disturbances, memory loss, ataxia
   - 50–70%: Convulsions, coma, severe cardiorespiratory compromise
   - > 70%: Usually fatal
2. **Hemoglobin level:** To evaluate correctable anemia
3. **Arterial pH:** To detect acidosis
4. **Urinalysis for myoglobin:** With carbon monoxide poisoning patients are susceptible to tissue and muscle breakdown with possible acute renal failure resulting from the renal deposition of myoglobin

42.   **What are the key aspects of treatment of carbon monoxide poisoning in children?**

- **Very close monitoring**
- **100% oxygen** until the HbCO level falls to 5%. The half life of HbCO is 4 hours if the patient is breathing room air (at sea level), 1 hour if the patient is breathing 100% oxygen (at sea level), and <1 hour if the patient is in a hyperbaric oxygen chamber with 100% oxygen.
- **Consider treating for cyanide poisoning,** especially when metabolic acidosis persists after adequate treatment with oxygen.
- Refer for use of **hyperbaric oxygen** if any of the following are true: (1) the patient has a history of coma, seizure, or abnormal mental status at the scene or in the emergency department; (2) there is persistent metabolic acidosis; (3) the patient is a neonate; (4) the patient is a pregnant woman; or (5) the HbCO level is >25%, even if the patient is neurologically intact.

43.   **Why is carbon monoxide such a deadly toxin?**

- It is odorless and invisible and can overwhelm a patient without warning.
- It is a product of partial combustion of nearly all fossil fuels, so it is ubiquitous in daily living (i.e., ranging from running cars to heating homes to barbecuing with charcoal).
- Early intoxication with this toxin is misdiagnosed as flu-type illness because of common symptoms such as headache, dizziness, and malaise.
- It develops a nearly irreversible bond with hemoglobin (with an affinity 200–300 times that of oxygen) that shifts the oxyhemoglobin dissociation curve to the left and changes its shape from sigmoidal to hyperbolic (with greatly diminished O_2 tissue release).
- It also develops a strong bond with other heme-containing proteins, particularly in the mitochondria, thereby leading to metabolic acidosis and cellular dysfunction (especially in cardiac and central nervous system tissues).

44. What are the different degrees of burn injuries?
See Table 5-3.

TABLE 5-3.	CLASSIFICATION OF BURN WOUNDS*		
Degree	**Depth**	**Clinical appearance**	**Cause**
First	Epidermis	Dry, erythematous	Sunburn, scald
Second	Superficial dermis	Blisters, moist, erythematous	Scald, immersion, contact
	Deep dermis	White eschar	Grease, flash fire
Third	Subcutaneous	Avascular—white/ dark, dry, waxy (yellow)	Prolonged immersion, flame, contact, grease, oil
Fourth	Muscle	Charred, skin surface cracked	Flame

*Alternatively, burns can be described as either superficial (first degree), partial (second degree), or full thickness (third and fourth degree).
Adapted from Coren CV: Burn injuries in children. Pediatr Ann 16:328–339, 1987.

45. How does the "rule of nines" apply in children?
The "rule of nines" is a device used to estimate the extent of burns in adults. For example, in adults, the entire arm is 9% of the total body surface area (TBSA), the front of the leg is another 9% of the TBSA, and so on. The resulting estimate of the extent of burns is particularly helpful for calculating fluid requirements. Correction for age is necessary with this formula because of differing body proportions. Therefore, for children, use the surface of a patient's palm, which represents about 1% of TBSA, as the tool for estimating the percentage of the TBSA affected by the burn (Fig. 5-3).

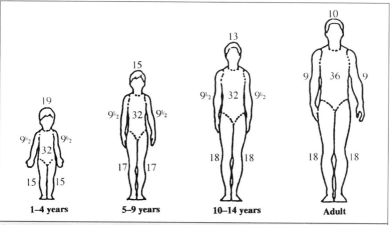

Figure 5-3. Rule of nines as applied to children. (From Carajel HF: Burn injuries. In Behrman RE (ed): Nelson Textbook of Pediatrics, 14th ed. Philadelphia, W.B. Saunders, 1992, p 235.)

46. Which burn injuries are indications for hospitalization?
- Second-degree burns covering >10% of the TBSA
- Third-degree burns covering >2% of the TBSA
- Significant burns involving the hands, feet, face, joints, or perineum
- Burns resulting from suspected child abuse
- Electrical burns
- Circumferential burns (which may predispose the patient to vascular compromise)
- Explosion, inhalation, or chemical burns (in which other organ trauma may be involved)
- Significant burns in children <2 years old

Rodgers GL: Reducing the toll of childhood burns. Contemp Pediatr 17:152–173, 2000.

KEY POINTS: ENVIRONMENTAL INJURIES

1. Anaphylaxis in children: Food (e.g., peanuts, tree nuts, seafood) is twice as common as bee stings as a cause.

2. Carbon monoxide poisoning is often misdiagnosed because the presenting symptoms can be flu-like.

3. Impending upper airway obstruction in house fires is more likely if there is the presence of carbonaceous sputum, singed nasal or facial hairs, or respiratory abnormalities (e.g., hoarseness, stridor).

4. Hospitalization is indicated for significant burns involving the hands, feet, joints, or perineum or if there are circumferential burns.

47. Why are alkali burns worse than acid burns in the eye?
Alkali burns are caused by lye (e.g., Drano, Liquid Plummer), lime, or ammonia, in addition to other agents; they are characterized by *liquefaction necrosis*. They are worse than acid burns because the damage is ongoing. When spilled in the eye, **acid** is quickly buffered by tissue and limited in penetration by precipitated proteins; *coagulation necrosis* results, which is usually limited to the area of contact. Alkali, however, has a more rapid and deeper advancement, thereby causing progressive damage at the cellular level by combining with membrane lipids. This underscores the importance of extensive irrigation of the burned eye, particularly in cases of alkali burns.

48. How do the injuries produced by lightning and high-voltage wires differ?
- **Lightning:** Consists of direct current of extremely high voltage (200,000–2,000,000,000 volts) delivered over milliseconds. Lightning exposure causes massive electrical counter-shock with asystole, respiratory arrest, and minimal tissue damage.
- **High-voltage wires:** Deliver alternating current of lower voltage (rarely exceeding 70,000 volts) over a longer period of time. High-voltage exposure causes ventricular fibrillation and deep-tissue injury. The resultant muscle necrosis can lead to substantial myoglobin release and renal failure.

49. In electrical injury, is alternating or direct current more hazardous?
At low voltages (e.g., those found in household electrical devices), alternating current is more dangerous than direct. Exposure to alternating current can provoke tetanic muscle contrac-tions so that the victim who has grasped an electrical source is unable to let go, thereby pro-longing the exposure and producing greater tissue injury. Direct current or high-voltage alternating current typically causes a single forceful muscular contraction that will push or throw the victim away from the source.

50. **If a toddler suffers a full-thickness burn to the corner of the mouth after biting on an electrical cord, what complications are possible?**
Severe burns of the oral commissure can become markedly edematous within the first several hours. An eschar develops at the site, which can detach and cause significant bleeding from the labial artery 1–3 weeks later. Scarring can be extensive, and plastic surgeons should be consulted early during the management of this kind of injury.

51. **What agents are the most common causes of anaphylaxis seen in U.S. emergency rooms?**
Food. Peanuts, tree nuts (e.g., almonds, hazelnuts) and seafood head the list and are twice as common as bee stings as a trigger. Severe reactions occur 1–2 hours after exposure. Anaphylaxis may occur without a skin reaction, so a high index of suspicion is needed in a child with unexplained sudden bronchospasm, laryngospasm, severe gastrointestinal symptoms, or poor responsiveness. In some adolescents, certain foods (e.g., wheat, celery, shellfish), if ingested within 4 hours of exercise, can lead to food-dependent, exercise-induced anaphylaxis. Risk factors for fatal anaphylactic reactions include a history of asthma, delayed diagnosis, and delayed administration of epinephrine.

> Sampson HA: Anaphylaxis and emergency treatment. Pediatrics 111:1601–1608, 2003.

LACERATIONS

52. **What advice should be given over the telephone regarding the transportation of an avulsed digit?**
Wrap the severed piece in a dry gauze (sterile, if possible). Place the wrapped piece in a small, sealed plastic bag to minimize its contact with water. Place this bag in a container filled with ice. It is incorrect to place the avulsed piece in any liquid, because this causes tissue swelling. Direct contact with ice is to be avoided to prevent tissue necrosis.

53. **Which lacerations should be referred to a surgeon or an emergency room physician who is familiar with wound repair?**
- Large, complex lacerations
- Stellate or flap lacerations
- Lacerations with questions of tissue viability
- Lacerations involving lip margins (vermilion border)
- Deep lacerations with nerve or tendon damage
- Knife and gunshot wounds

54. **How many days should sutures remain in place?**
Blood supply dictates healing: the more blood, the better and the faster the healing. In general, as the site of laceration proceeds, from head to toe, the length of time of suture placement increases: eyelids—3 days; face—5 days; trunk and upper extremities—7 days; and lower extremities—10 days.

55. **When should a nerve injury be suspected in a finger laceration?**
- **Abnormal testing of sensation** (diminished pain or two-point discrimination)
- **Abnormal autonomic function** (absence of sweat or lack of skin wrinkling after soaking in water)
- **Diminished range of motion of finger** (may also indicate joint, bone, or tendon disruption)
- **Pulsating blood emerging from the wound** (on the flexor aspect, the nerve is superficial to the digital artery, and arterial flow implies nerve damage)

56. **What should be done if nerve damage is suspected?**

For injuries to major nerves (e.g., the brachial plexus), immediate consultation is necessary. If the digital nerve is injured, immediate repair is not essential, and this is not a true emergency. Delayed nerve repair is very satisfactory, particularly in younger children. If an operating suite and personnel are not poised to proceed, skin closure can be done and the operation deferred (after surgical consultation). Care must be taken to avoid the use of a hemostat or clamp to stop arterial bleeding because this may cause further damage to the nerve. Simple pressure—often for extended periods—generally suffices.

57. **Which lacerations should not be sutured?**

Lacerations at high risk for infection should be considered for healing by secondary intention or delayed primary closure. As a general rule, these include cosmetically unimportant puncture wounds, human bites, lacerations involving mucosal surfaces (e.g., mouth, vagina), and wounds with a high probability of contamination (e.g., acquired in a garbage bin). Many authorities in the past recommended that wounds untreated for more than 6–12 hours on the arms and legs and for 12–24 hours to the face not be sutured. However, the type of wound and risk for infection are more important than any absolute time criterion. For example, a noncontaminated laceration of the face should be considered for suturing even 24 hours after the injury. A good rule of thumb is as follows: If you can irrigate and clean a wound to the point at which it looks "fresh," then you are safe to close it primarily. Otherwise, you should let it heal by secondary intention.

58. **Which are at greater risk for infection, dog bites or cat bites?**

Generally, infection rates are higher in **cat bites** because of the greater likelihood of a puncture wound rather than a laceration injury. Additionally, *Pasteurella multocida*, which is the most common pathogen responsible for infection, is present in higher concentrations in cat bites. Wounds caused by cat and dog bites usually contain multiple other organisms, including *Staphylococcus aureus, Moraxella, Streptococcus, Neisseria* species, and anaerobes.

Talon DA, Citron DM, Abrahamian FM, et al: Bacteriologic analysis of infected dog and cat bites. N Engl J Med 340(2):85–92, 1999.

59. **Should antibiotic prophylaxis be given for dog, cat, and human bites?**

This is a controversial topic. Studies indicate that antibiotic prophylaxis is not indicated for "low-risk" dog bites but that they should be considered for "high-risk" injuries such as cat and human bites, hand and foot wounds, puncture wounds, and wounds treated initially after 12 hours. More important is that all such wounds should first be irrigated under pressure, cleaned, and débrided as necessary.

Fleisher GR: The management of bite wounds. N Engl J Med 340:138–140, 1999.

Cummings P: Antibiotics to prevent infection in patients with dog bite wounds: A meta-analysis of randomized trials. Ann Emerg Med 23:535–540, 1994.

60. **What are the recommendations for tetanus prophylaxis in a child with a laceration?**

See Table 5-4.

61. **Which animal causes the most cases of rabies in the United States?**

In the United States, bats cause more cases of human rabies than any other form of wildlife. From 1980–1999, 21 (58%) of the 36 human cases of rabies resulting in death in the United States were associated with bats. In most other countries, dogs are the most significant sources of the virus. On average, from 1980–1997, only two cases per year of human rabies nationwide have been attributable to domestic dogs.

Center for Disease Control and Prevention: Human Rabies Prevention—United States, 1999. Recommendations of the Advisory Committee on Immunization Practices (ACIP). MMWR 48(RR-1):1–21, 1999.

TABLE 5-4.	RECOMMENDATIONS FOR TETANUS PROPHYLAXIS IN CHILDREN WITH A LACERATION		
No. of vaccinations	Previous booster	Most recent type of wound	Recommendation for children = 7 years old*
Unclear or <3	—	Clean, minor	Adult-type tetanus vaccine
		Tetanus-prone	Adult-type tetanus vaccine plus tetanus immunoglobulin
≥3	>10 years	Clean, minor	Adult-type tetanus vaccine
		Tetanus-prone	Adult-type tetanus vaccine
≥3	5–10 years	Clean, minor	None
		Tetanus-prone	Adult-type tetanus vaccine
≥3	<5 years	Clean, minor	None
		Tetanus-prone	None

*In children <7 years old, other tetanus-containing vaccines (DTAP, DT) should be given rather than the adult-type tetanus vaccine (TD), depending on the immunization status of the child and his or her previous reactions. *Clean, minor wounds* are generally defined as wounds that are <6 hours old; not infected or contaminated with feces, soil, or saliva; superficial enough to permit irrigation and débridement; and surrounded by viable tissues. In addition, most are linear. *Tetanus-prone wounds* include all other wounds but especially those caused by puncture, crush injury, burns, or frostbite.

62. **If at a local petting zoo a playful 20-month-old child is bitten by a duck, scratched by a rabbit (breaking skin), spit on by a camel, and licked on the face by a horse, should rabies prophylaxis be given?**
    In general, no prophylaxis is needed for any of these animal wounds unless the animal is actively rabid. The local health department should be contacted if there is any question. Immediate rabies vaccination and rabies immune globulin are recommended for bites or scratches from bats, skunks, raccoons, foxes, and most other carnivores if these injuries break the skin. Bites from dogs and cats generally do not necessitate prophylaxis if the animal is healthy and can be observed closely for a 10-day period. No case in the United States has been attributed to a dog or cat that has remained healthy for the confinement period of 10 days.
      American Academy of Pediatrics: Rabies. In Pickering LK (ed): 2003 Red Book, 26th ed. Elk Grove Village, IL, American Academy of Pediatrics, 2003, pp 514–521.

63. **When is the use of lidocaine with epinephrine contraindicated as a local anesthetic?**
    When there is a question of tissue viability and in any instance in which vasoconstriction might produce ischemic injury to an end organ without an alternative blood supply (e.g., tip of the nose, margin of the ear, tip of the finger or toe).

64. **Is there a maximum dose of lidocaine that is safe when the drug is used for local anesthesia?**
    Yes! No more than 4 mg/kg of lidocaine *without* epinephrine and 7 mg/kg of lidocaine *with* epinephrine should be used when infiltrating for local anesthesia. This is generally an issue only when suturing large wounds or when using a higher concentration of lidocaine (2% instead of 1%), in which case you would be delivering 20 mg/mL instead of 10 mg/mL.

65. **What are methods for decreasing the pain of local lidocaine infiltration?**
    - Infiltration into the subcutaneous layer
    - Infiltration at a slow rate
    - Buffering the anesthetic (e.g., with bicarbonate)
    - Warming the anesthetic to body temperature
    - Using a small-gauge needle (e.g., 30 gauge)
    - Distracting the patient/using hypnosis or biofeedback

    Noeller T, Cydulka RK: Laceration repair techniques. Emerg Med Reports 17:207–217, 1996.

66. **What are some of the ingredients in the alphabet soup of topical anesthetics?**
    - **LET** (**l**idocaine, **e**pinephrine, and **t**etracaine)
    - **TAC** (**t**etracaine, **a**drenaline, and **c**ocaine)
    - **LMX** (4% liposomal **l**idocaine)
    - **V-TAC** (**v**iscous TAC)
    - **PLP** (**p**rilocaine, **l**idocaine, and **p**henylephrine)
    - **EMLA** (**e**utectic **m**ixture of **l**ocal **a**nesthetics)

    TAC was among the first of these to be developed, but its higher costs and safety concerns (as a result of the cocaine component) have resulted in others—primarily LET—replacing it as first-line therapy.

    Stewart GM, Simpson P, Rosenberg NM: Use of topical lidocaine in pediatric laceration repair: A review of topical anesthetics. Ped Emerg Care 14:419–423, 1998.

67. **In what situations is EMLA cream useful?**
    EMLA, as noted above, is made up of an eutectic mixture of local anesthetics, which are lidocaine and prilocaine. EMLA is very useful for anesthetizing the skin before venipuncture, intravenous placement, injection, lumbar puncture, and circumcision. The cream is placed on the site and covered with an occlusive dressing for 1–2 hours. Obviously, its most practical use is for anticipated procedures.

68. **What are the advantages and disadvantages of using tissue glues or adhesives to close wounds and lacerations?**
    Advantages
    - Needleless, painless procedure
    - Does not require follow-up office or emergency department visit because adhesive falls off on its own
    - Generally a much quicker procedure than suturing
    - Less anxiety-producing for the patient and the patient's parents

    Disadvantages
    - Can be used only for a select type of wound
    - Cannot be used with bite or puncture wounds
    - Cannot be used with deep (more than 5 mm) or jagged wounds
    - Cannot be used with wounds on ears, hands, feet, or mucocutaneous areas
    - Minimally more expensive than sutures

69. **How is conscious sedation best managed in children?**
    There is **no single best method** for the conscious sedation of pediatric patients for diagnostic, radiologic, or minor surgical procedures. Surveys indicate that a wide variety of approaches are used in emergency rooms and radiology suites, including opioids (morphine, meperidine, fentanyl, butorphanol), benzodiazepines (diazepam, midazolam), barbiturates (pentobarbital, thiopental), and nonbarbiturate anesthetic/analgesic agents (ketamine). Although conscious

sedation, by definition, is a state of medically controlled depressed consciousness with a patent airway, maintained protective reflexes, and appropriate responses to stimulation on verbal command, the potential for rapidly developing problems should be anticipated. These can include hypoventilation, apnea, airway obstruction, and cardiorespiratory collapse. Consequently, pharmacologic agents used for conscious sedation should be administered under supervised conditions and in the presence of competent personnel who are capable of resuscitation, ongoing monitoring (especially pulse oximetry), and sufficient equipment for resuscitation (e.g, positive-pressure oxygen delivery system, suction apparatus). As a rule, few office settings are appropriate for conscious sedation.

Linzer JF: Conscious sedation: What you should know before and after. Clin Pediatr Emerg Med 1:306–310, 2000.

RESUSCITATION

70. **What are the signs and symptoms of respiratory distress in children?**
   - Tachypnea
   - Hyperpnea
   - Nasal flaring
   - Grunting
   - Head bobbing
   - Cyanosis
   - Stridor
   - Wheezing

71. **Can CPR cause rib fractures in infants?**
   Very unlikely. In one study of 91 infants who underwent autopsy and postmortem x-rays after CPR, none had rib fractures. Child abuse must always remain at the top of a list when rib fractures are identified.

   Spevak MR, Kleinman PK, Belanger PL, et al: Cardiopulmonary resuscitation and rib fractures in infants. A postmortem radiologic-pathologic study. JAMA 272:617–618, 1994.

72. **Are fixed and dilated pupils a contraindication to resuscitation for a patient in cardiac arrest?**
   No. Pupillary dilatation begins 15 seconds after cardiac arrest and is complete after approximately 1 minute and 45 seconds. It may only be a sign of transient hypoxia. The only absolute contraindications to resuscitation are rigor mortis, corneal clouding, dependent lividity, and decapitation.

73. **Why is the airway of an infant or child more prone to obstruction than that of an adult?**
   - An infant has a smaller margin of safety because of his or her smaller airway diameter. Because airflow is inversely proportional to the airway radius raised to the fourth power (the oft-cited Poiseuille law), small changes in the diameter of the trachea can result in very large drops in airflow.
   - The tracheal cartilage of an infant is softer and can result in collapse upon hyperextension. This is particularly important if CPR is performed with vigorous extension of the neck; air exchange may then be obstructed.
   - In an infant, the lumen of the oropharynx is relatively smaller than that of an adult as a result of the larger size of the tongue and the smaller size of the mandible.
   - Lower airways are smaller and less developed in children. The typical peanut and an infant's mainstem bronchus always seem to fit like a hand in a glove.

74. How can size and depth of endotracheal tubes (ETTs) be estimated?

1. For choosing a tube size, a good rule of thumb is as follows:

$$\frac{16 + age \ (in \ years)}{4} = internal \ diameter \ (mm)$$

For example, with this formula, a 2-year-old child would require a 4.5-mm tube. Because this is an approximation, the next smaller- and larger-sized tubes should be available. To convert internal diameter size to French catheter size, multiply by 4 (e.g., a 5-mm tube is a 20 Fr).

2. Another good guide is the rule of the "pinky"; the infant or child's pinky approximates the internal diameter of the correctly sized tube.

3. After the insertion of the ETT, appropriate depth (measured by markings at the gum line) can be approximated using the following formula for children >1 year old:

$$\frac{Age \ in \ years}{2} + 12 \ cm$$

75. At what ages should cuffed versus uncuffed ETTs be used?

In adolescents and adults, cuffed ETTs are used and inflated just enough to obliterate any audible air leak. However, in children <8 years old, an uncuffed ETT is advised because the cricoid cartilage is the narrowest part of the airway and serves as a functional cuff. Therefore, an uncuffed ETT should allow for minimal air leak at the cricoid ring. Absence of an air leak indicates that there may be excessive pressure at the cricoid cartilage.

76. What is the Sellick maneuver?

The Sellick maneuver is the application of pressure on the cricoid ring to prevent aspiration. Cricoid pressure should be initiated during preparation for intubation from the time sedation is administered or bag-mask ventilation is initiated until the airway is demonstrated to be secured.

77. What are the potential reasons for acute deterioration in an intubated patient?

These can be remembered using the DOPE acronym:

D = **D**isplacement of the endotracheal tube
O = **O**bstruction of the tube
P = **P**neumothorax
E = **E**quipment failure

American Heart Association: PALS Provider Manual. Dallas, American Heart Association, 2002, p 182.

78. What emergency drugs can be given via an endotracheal tube?

E-LAINE: **E**ndotracheally—**l**idocaine, **a**tropine, **i**soproterenol, **n**aloxone, and **e**pinephrine

79. What is the role of high-dose epinephrine in pediatric resuscitations?

Animal studies, anecdotal reports, and small clinical trials have shown that the use of epinephrine in higher doses (100–200 times the normal dose) may facilitate the return of spontaneous circulation better than the standard lower dose. However, evidence gained from larger prospective adult studies and a recent randomized clinical trial in children have demonstrated no benefit and possible adverse effects. The American Heart Association currently recommends that, after the standard first dose of epinephrine (0.01 mg/kg of a 1:10,000 solution), subsequent higher doses (0.1–0.2 mg/kg of a 1:1,000 solution) may be considered an acceptable alternative to standard doses.

Perondi MB, Reis AG, Paiva EF, et al: A comparison of high-dose and standard-dose epinephrine in children with cardiac arrest. N Engl J Med 350:1722–1730, 2004.

80. How effective is intratracheal epinephrine?

Epinephrine is poorly absorbed from the lung; if available, intraosseous or intravenous administration is preferable. If epinephrine is to be given via an endotracheal tube in an acute setting, it should be mixed with 1–3 mL of normal saline and instilled with a catheter or feeding tube beyond the end of the endotracheal tube to facilitate dispersal. The ideal endotracheal dose is unclear, but because of the poor absorption, higher initial doses (0.1–0.2 mg/kg of a 1:1,000 solution) should be used.

81. **When is atropine indicated during a resuscitation?**

Atropine may be administered to the child with symptomatic bradycardia after other resuscita-tive measures (i.e., oxygenation and ventilation) have been initiated. It is useful for breaking the vagally mediated bradycardia that is associated with laryngoscopy, and it may have some benefit during the initial treatment of atrioventricular block. The deleterious effects of a slow heart rate are more likely to occur in a younger child, whose cardiac output is more dependent on rate changes than volume or contractility changes. Atropine is no longer routinely recom-mended for the treatment of asystole in children.

82. **What risks are associated with administering an inappropriately low dose of atropine?**

If the dose of atropine is too small, paradoxically worsening bradycardia may result. This is as a result of atropine's central stimulating effect on the medullary vagal nerve at lower doses, which slows atrioventricular conduction and heart rate. Standard dosing of atropine in a set-ting of bradycardia is 0.02 mg/kg intravenously. However, at least 0.1 mg should be used, even in the youngest patient.

83. **When is the use of calcium indicated during a resuscitation?**

Routine use of calcium is no longer recommended during a resuscitation. There is evidence that calcium may increase postischemic injury in the intracranial reperfusion phase that fol-lows resuscitation. However, calcium use may be justified in three settings of resuscitation: (1) an overdose of a calcium-channel blocker; (2) hyperkalemia resulting in cardiac dysrhyth-mia; and (3) infants and children with low serum calcium.

84. **What are the indications for the placement of an intraosseous line?**

Because of the difficulty and delays with establishing intravenous access in pediatric resuscita-tions, intraosseous infusions have become the very early second line of therapy in emergency settings. Failure to achieve intravenous access in three attempts or 90 seconds (whichever is shorter) is an indication for intraosseous access. An intraosseous line is a rapid means of vas-cular access and uses the marrow cavity of bone, which drains into the central venous system. All medications and fluids that can be given intravenously can be given by the intraosseous route, at the same rate and dosages, with comparable distribution. The technique involves placing a needle, a bone marrow needle, or an intraosseous needle into the proximal tibia approximately 1–3 cm below and medial to the tibial tuberosity. Distal tibial and proximal femoral sites are less commonly used.

85. **What signs indicate that an intraosseous needle has been correctly placed?**

1. A soft pop should be felt as you break through the cortex.
2. The needle should be very stable.
3. There should be free flow of intravenous fluids without infiltration of the subcutaneous tissues.
4. Bone marrow aspiration—although it does confirm placement—may not always be possi-ble, even when needle placement is correct. Therefore, if you cannot aspirate marrow, you should rely on signs 1–3 for determination of placement.

86. **Is capillary refill still a useful clinical sign?**

Capillary refill is the return to normal color of the pulp of the finger or fingernail after it has been compressed. In healthy children, a normal value is approximately 2 seconds. In theory, a normal refill time is a measure of adequate peripheral perfusion and thus normal cardiac output and peripheral vascular resistance. It has been used as a measure of perfusion in the settings of trauma and possible dehydration. However, it must be used in conjunction with other clinical features, because studies of its usefulness as a sole indicator of dehydration have shown it to have a low sensitivity and specificity. In one study of children with 5–10% dehydration, only 50% had prolonged capillary refill. In addition, lower ambient temperature has a significant effect on delaying capillary refill. Capillary refill should be measured in the upper extremity.

Baraff LJ: Capillary refill: Is it a useful clinical sign? Pediatrics 92:723–724, 1993.

87. **Name the potentially reversible causes of clinical deterioration during a resuscitation.**
    - **4 Hs:** Hypoxemia, hypovolemia, hypothermia, and hyperkalemia/hypokalemia
    - **4 Ts:** Tamponade, tension pneumothorax, toxins, and thromboembolism

    American Heart Association: PALS Provider Manual. Dallas, American Heart Association, 2002, p 182.

88. **What rule of thumb defines hypotension in children (e.g., systolic blood pressure <5th percentile for age)?**

Age	Systolic blood pressure (mmHg)
<1 month	≤60
1 month to 1 year	≤70
1 to 10 years	≤70 + (2× age in years)
>10 years	≤90

    American Heart Association: PALS Provider Manual. Dallas, American Heart Association, 2002, p 426.

89. **How is shock defined in children?**
    It is defined as "a clinical condition in which tissue perfusion is inadequate to meet metabolic demands." Evaluation includes both **direct** cardiovascular assessment (heart rate, quality of proximal and distal pulses, and blood pressure, including pulse pressure) and **indirect** cardiovascular assessment to evaluate end-organ perfusion (central nervous system: alertness, responsiveness; skin: capillary refill, color, temperature; kidneys: urine output).

    American Heart Association: PALS Provider Manual. Dallas, American Heart Association, 2002, p 174.

90. **What are the signs and symptoms of shock?**
    - Tachycardia
    - Poor peripheral pulses
    - Slow capillary refill
    - Cool extremities
    - Hypotension
    - Altered mental status
    - Low urine output

91. **What types of shock can occur in children?**
    - **Hypovolemic:** Most common, often in the setting of gastroenteritis; peripheral vasoconstriction; narrow pulse pressure
    - **Distributive (septic):** Wide pulse pressure; hypo- or hyperthermia
    - **Cardiogenic:** Systemic or pulmonary edema or both; increased work of breathing; grunting; narrow pulse pressure
    - **Anaphylactic:** Laryngeal edema, urticaria, vomiting
    - **Obstructive:** Obstruction of blood flow as a result of tension pneumothorax, cardiac tamponade, pulmonary embolus; tachycardia, poor perfusion, narrowed pulse pressure

    American Heart Association: PALS Provider Manual. Dallas, American Heart Association, 2002, p 426.

92. **After a motor vehicle accident, an 8-year-old boy has right-sided pain, a heart rate of 150 bpm, a blood pressure of 110/70 mmHg, and a capillary refill time of 3.5 seconds. How should his initial fluid therapy be managed?**
It is important to recognize that this child is in **shock**, despite having a normal blood pressure for age. For children in shock, changes in blood pressure are often late and precipitous. Findings of tachycardia, prolonged capillary refill, and diminished pulses are indicative of hypovolemia in this patient, thereby requiring aggressive fluid resuscitation. Isotonic crystalloid (saline or lactated Ringer's solution) should be given in boluses of 20 mL/kg as quickly as possible. If, after 40 mL/kg of crystalloid, hemodynamic measures have not improved or have worsened, blood products should be given in 10 mL/kg boluses. Typed and cross-matched blood would be the ideal choice, but it is usually not ready in time to be used. Type-specific packed red blood cells should be available within 15 minutes and are the next option. O-negative packed red blood cells should be reserved for those in profound shock or with exsanguinating hemorrhage.

Pediatric Critical Care Medicine: www.pedsCCM.org

KEY POINTS: SIGNS AND SYMPTOMS OF SHOCK

1. Tachycardia

2. Poor peripheral pulses

3. Slow capillary refill

4. Cool extremities

5. Hypotension

6. Altered mental status

93. **What is the initial management algorithm for septic shock?**
Septic shock is accompanied by fever or hypothermia, metabolic acidosis, signs of vasodilation (e.g., a widened pulse pressure, hypotension), and, sometimes, altered mental status. Early recognition of sepsis and initiation of therapy are important to outcome.
- Control and/or maintain airway.
- Recognize poor perfusion/shock.
- Push 20 cc/kg up to 60 cc/kg of isotonic crystalloid solution.
- If there is still evidence of shock/poor perfusion, begin intravenous dopamine and titrate to perfusion status and normal blood pressure.

Hotchkiss RS, Karl IE: The pathophysiology and treatment of sepsis. N Engl J Med 348:138–150, 2003.

94. **What are the four classes of medications that can be used to support cardiac output?**
- **Inotropes:** Increase cardiac contractility and often heart rate (norepinephrine)
- **Vasopressors:** Increase vascular resistance and blood pressure (higher-dose dopamine and dobutamine)
- **Vasodilators:** Decrease vascular resistance and cardiac afterload and promote peripheral perfusion (sodium nitroprusside)
- **Inodilators:** Increase cardiac contractility and reduce afterload (milrinone)

95.   What are the signs and symptoms of a tension pneumothorax?

A tension pneumothorax appears with hypotension, respiratory distress, diminished breath sounds on the affected side, and tracheal deviation. Treatment begins with emergent needle decompression in the second intercostal space at the midclavicular line and is followed by a chest tube.

96.   What is the effect of body temperature on arterial blood gases?

CO_2 and O_2 are more soluble and exert less partial pressure at lower temperatures. Therefore, blood sampled from a hypothermic patient and warmed to the standard 37°C in the blood gas analyzer will have a higher partial pressure than exists in the patient. Similarly, blood sampled from the hyperthermic patient and cooled to 37°C will have a lower partial pressure than exists in the patient. For each 1°C difference from 37°C, the PaO_2 changes by about 7%, and the $PaCO_2$ changes by about 4.5%. Although much debate exists surrounding whether to use the "corrected" (patient body temperature) or "uncorrected" (37°C of blood gas analyzer) value, the difference in most clinical scenarios is not significant. In cases of extreme temperature differences (e.g., hypothermia in cold-water near-drowning patients), the difference may be considerable.

KEY POINTS: SHOCK IN PEDIATRIC TRAUMA

1. Often masked in pediatric patients because the inherent reserve in a child allows for the maintenance of vital signs in the normal range, even in the presence of severe hemodynamic compromise

2. Suspected in patients with tachycardia, a decrease in pulse pressure >20 mmHg, skin mottling, cool extremities, delayed capillary refill (>2 seconds), and altered mental status

3. Presence of hypotension in a child represents a state of uncompensated shock and indicates severe blood loss of >45% of circulating blood volume

4. Not explainable by head trauma alone, except in the case of an infant with open fontanels and unfused cranial sutures who may have a significant hemorrhage into the subgaleal or epidural space

5. May be associated with long bone (particularly femur) and pelvic fractures

6. Should quickly prompt an evaluation of the child's abdomen for the source of blood loss

97.   How do pediatric and adult defibrillation differ?

The following are characteristic of pediatric defibrillation.

- **Smaller dosing:** 2 W-sec/kg and then doubled as needed
- **Smaller paddles:** Standard pediatric paddles are 4.5 cm in diameter as compared with 8 cm for adults
- **Rarer use:** Ventricular fibrillation is uncommon in children

Samson RA, Berg RA, Bingham R; Pediatric Advanced Life Support Task Force, International Liaison Committee on Resuscitation for the American Heart Association; European Resuscitation Council: Use of automated external defibrillators for children: An update—an advisory statement from the Pediatric Advanced Life Support Task Force, International Liaison Committee on Resuscitation. Pediatrics 112(1 Pt 1): 163–168, 2003.

98. **What is the difference between livor mortis and rigor mortis?**
    - **Livor mortis:** Dependent lividity is the gravitational pooling of blood that results in a line of mauve staining in the dependent half of a recently deceased body. It usually is noticeable 30 minutes after death and is very marked at 6 hours.
    - **Rigor mortis:** This is the muscular stiffening and shortening that result from ongoing cellular activity and depletion of ATP after death, with increasing lactate and phosphate and salt precipitation. Neck and facial changes begin at 6 hours, shoulder and upper extremities changes begin at 9 hours, and trunk and lower extremity changes begin at 12 hours.
      Livor mortis and rigor mortis are absolute indications to not initiate a resuscitation. They should be looked for during the initial rapid assessment; in the confusion of the moment, they may be easily overlooked.

99. **When should a failing resuscitation be stopped?**
    Studies have suggested that, when **more than two rounds of medication** (i.e., epinephrine and bicarbonate) have been given and/or **more than 20 minutes** have elapsed since the initiation of resuscitation without clinical cardiovascular or neurologic improvement, the likelihood of death or survival with neurologic devastation greatly increases. Unwitnessed out-of-hospital arrests are nearly always associated with a poor outcome. In settings of hypothermia, asystolic patients should be rewarmed to 36°C before resuscitation is discontinued.

    Schindler M, Bohn D, Cox PN, et al: Outcome of out-of-hospital cardiac or respiratory arrest in children. N Engl J Med 335:1473–1479, 1996.

100. **What factors are predictive of good or bad outcomes for pediatric emergency department resuscitation?**
     See Table 5-5.

TABLE 5-5. PREDICTIVE FACTORS IN PEDIATRIC RESUSCIATION	
Predictors of good outcome after pediatric cardiac arrest	**Predictors of bad outcome after pediatric cardiac arrest**
Witnessed arrest	Unwitnessed arrest
Bystander CPR	No bystander CPR
EMS arrival time <10 minutes	Resuscitation efforts >30 minutes before ROSC
Resuscitation effort <20 minutes	>2 doses of epinephrine before ROSC
<2 doses epinephrine before ROSC	Rhythm of PEA or asystole
Rhythm of VF or VT	Cause of arrest: Sepsis, trauma, or SIDS
Prehospital ROSC	Cause of arrest: Submersion

CPR = cardiopulmonary resuscitation, EMS = emergency medical services, ROSC = return of spontaneous circulation, PEA = pulseless electrical activity, VF = ventricular fibrillation, VT = ventricular tachycardia, SIDS = sudden infant death syndrome.

101. **Why is resuscitation less successful in children than in adults?**
     Adults more commonly experience collapse and arrest from primary cardiac disease and associated dysrhythmias: ventricular tachycardia and fibrillation. These are more readily reversible and carry a better prognosis. **Children**, however, have cardiac arrest as a secondary phenomenon as a result of other processes (e.g., respiratory obstruction, apnea) that are often associ-

ated with infection, hypoxia, acidosis, or hypovolemia. Primary cardiac arrest is rare. The most common dysrhythmia associated with pediatric cardiac arrest is asystole. It is less frequently reversible, and by the time a child has cardiac arrest, severe neurologic damage is almost always present.

TOXICOLOGY

102. **What are the most common poisonings among children <6 years old?**

Nonpharmaceuticals	Pharmaceuticals
Cosmetics and personal care products	Analgesics
Cleaning substances	Cough and cold preparations
Plants, including mushrooms and tobacco	Topical agents
Batteries, toys, and other foreign bodies	Vitamins
Insecticides, pesticides, and rodenticides	Antimicrobials
Art, craft, and office supplies	Gastrointestinal preparations
Hydrocarbons	Antihistamines
	Hormone and hormone antagonists

Watson WA, Litovitz TL, Klein-Schwartz W, et al: 2003 annual report of the American Association of Poison Control Centers Toxic Exposure Surveillance System. Am J Emerg Med 22:335–404, 2004.
American Association of Poison Control Centers: www.aapcc.org.

103. **What common household products are generally nontoxic when ingested?**
   - Abrasives
   - Adhesives
   - Bleach (<5% sodium hypochlorite)
   - Deodorants
   - Cosmetics
   - Most ink, markers, and crayons

104. **What drugs are most likely to cause death in children <6 years old?**
   - Iron
   - Antidepressants
   - Cardiovascular medications
   - Antiepileptic medications

   Osterhoudt KC: The toxic toddler: Drugs that can kill toddlers in small doses. Contemp Pediatr 17:73–87, 2000.

105. **Name the toxicology "time bombs."**
   The time bombs are those medications that lack symptoms early after ingestion but have a profoundly toxic course later. They are as follows:
   - Acetaminophen
   - Iron
   - Alcohols (e.g., methanol, ethylene glycol)
   - Lithium
   - Time-release medications
   - Antiepileptic medications (e.g., Dilantin, carbamazepine)

106. **What empiric drug therapies are indicated for the poisoned child who has altered mental status?**
   All poisoned patients with depressed mental status should receive oxygen via a nonre-breather face mask. Blood glucose should be rapidly evaluated, or empiric treatment for

hypoglycemia with intravenous glucose 0.5 gm/kg should be initiated. Finally, naloxone may be given as a diagnostic and therapeutic measure in the event of suspected or known opioid ingestion.

107. What is the role of ipecac in the treatment of acute poisonings and overdoses?

Syrup of ipecac is a nonprescription emetic agent that was used in the past to remove toxic substances from the stomach. However, in 2003, the American Academy of Pediatrics advised that ipecac should not be administered routinely in the management of poisoned patients because there is no evidence from clinical studies that it improves the outcome of poisoned patients. In addition, its routine administration may delay the administration or reduce the effectiveness of activated charcoal, oral antidotes, and whole-bowel irrigation.

American Academy of Pediatrics Committee on Injury, Violence, and Poison Prevention: Poison treatment in the home. Pediatrics 112:1182–1185, 2003.

108. How does single-dose activated charcoal work? When should it be considered?

Single-dose activated charcoal is prepared as a liquid slurry and given orally to a poisoned patient. As it enters the stomach, it adsorbs toxins, thereby preventing absorption into the circulation. It is most efficacious when given within 1 hour of the time of poison ingestion. The dose in children is 1 gm/kg, and in adolescents and adults it is 50–100 gm. Charcoal is contraindicated in patients whose airway reflexes are compromised. In addition, it should not be given via a nasogastric tube unless the airway is protected with an endotracheal tube.

American Academy of Clinical Toxicology, European Association of Poisons Centres and Clinical Toxicologists: Position statement: Single-dose activated charcoal. J Toxicol Clin Toxicol 35:721–741, 1997.

109. Should activated charcoal be given to a sleepy 2-year-old child who consumed half a bottle of a liquid antihistamine 2 hours before the evaluation?

This would not be a good idea because of a potentially compromised airway (i.e., in a sleepy child) and the delay in administration. The effectiveness of activated charcoal decreases with time. In this setting, its use should only be considered if the following were true: (1) the patient had ingested, up to 1 hour previously, a potentially toxic amount of a poison known to be adsorbable to charcoal; and (2) airway protection was assured because the charcoal can cause vomiting and aspiration.

American Academy of Clinical Toxicology, European Association of Poisons Centres and Clinical Toxicologists: Position statement: Single-dose activated charcoal. J Toxicol Clin Toxicol 35:721–741, 1997.

110. In what settings is activated charcoal not advised?

- Unprotected airway
- Clinical appearance of ileus, hematemesis, or severe vomiting
- Drugs for which immediate oral antidotes are available (e.g., late recognition of pure acetaminophen ingestion)
- Hydrocarbons because of possible increased risk of aspiration
- Compounds for which it is ineffective: Acids, alcohols, alkalis, cyanide, iron, heavy metals, and lithium

American Academy of Clinical Toxicology, European Association of Poisons Centres and Clinical Toxicologists: Position statement: Single-dose activated charcoal. J Toxicol Clin Toxicol 35:721–741,1997.

KEY POINTS: ACETAMINOPHEN OVERDOSE

1. Significant ingestions may have no initial symptoms.

2. Assess for co-ingestions.

3. Administer charcoal if ingestion was within 4 hours of treatment.

4. Assess plasma acetaminophen level, and apply nomogram.

5. Administer the antidote N-acetylcysteine if ingestion was within 8 hours of treatment.

---

111. **Should all children with ingestions be given a cathartic?**
   No. Cathartics may help to decrease absorption and lessen the constipation caused by charcoal. Magnesium sulfate (250 mg/kg), magnesium citrate (4–8 mL/kg up to 300 mL), or sorbitol (70%, 1.5 gm/kg) are the usual choices. The contraindications are similar to those for activated charcoal. Care must be taken when cathartics are given to smaller children because large volume loss may result. The repeated administration of magnesium-containing cathartics can cause hypermagnesemia, which is manifested by hypotonia, altered mental status, and, in severe cases, respiratory failure. However, magnesium citrate is associated with less emesis than sorbitol.

   Perry H, Shannon M: Emergency department gastrointestinal decontamination. Pediatr Ann 25:19–26, 1996.

112. **In what setting would multiple-dose activated charcoal be advised?**
   Multiple-dose activated charcoal therapy involves the repeated administration (more than two doses of 0.5 to 1.0 gm/kg every 4 to 6 hours) of oral activated charcoal to enhance the elimination of drugs that are already absorbed into the body. The rationale behind its use is that drugs with a prolonged elimination half-life are more likely to have their elimination enhanced the longer an adsorptive agent remains in the gastrointestinal tract. Potential complications include bowel obstruction, constipation, regurgitation, and subsequent aspiration. Its use should be considered if a patient has ingested a life-threatening amount of carbamazepine, dapsone, phenobarbital, quinine, benzodiazepines, phenytoin, tricyclic antidepressants, or theophylline. Use in patients with salicylate poisoning is controversial.

   American Academy of Clinical Toxicology, European Association of Poisons Centres and Clinical Toxicologists: Position statement and practice guidelines on the use of multi-dose activated charcoal in the treatment of acute poisoning. Clin Toxicol 37:731–751, 1999.

113. **When is gastric lavage indicated?**
   Gastric lavage involves the passage of a large orogastric tube (e.g., 24-Fr orogastric for a toddler, 36-Fr orogastric for a teenager) and the sequential administration and aspiration of small volumes of normal saline (50–100 mL in smaller children, 150–200 mL in teenagers), with the intent of removing toxic substances that are present in the stomach. Efficacy remains unproven, and complications are possible (e.g., laryngospasm, esophageal injury, aspiration pneumonia). Its use is reserved for patients whose airways are protected and who have ingested a potentially life-threatening quantity of a poisonous substance within 1 hour of evaluation.

   American Academy of Clinical Toxicology, European Association of Poisons Centres and Clinical Toxicologists: Position statement: Gastric lavage. J Toxicol Clin Toxicol 35:711–719, 1997.

114. **What are the indications for whole-bowel irrigation in patients with acute ingestions?**

This is a method of gastrointestinal decontamination using a large volume of polyethylene-glycol–balanced electrolyte solution such as Colyte or GoLYTELY. These solutions are not known to cause electrolyte imbalance because neither one is significantly absorbed, and they do not exert an osmotic effect. Whole-bowel irrigation is indicated for toxic ingestions of sustained release or enteric-coated medications. It may also be helpful in cases of ingestions of iron, lead, or packets of illicit drugs. The usual recommended dosing is 500 mL/hour in toddlers and 2 L/hour in adolescents and adults (by mouth in cooperative patients or by nasogastric tube in uncooperative patients). The most important contraindication to whole-bowel irrigation is airway compromise.

American Academy of Clinical Toxicology, European Association of Poisons Centres and Clinical Toxicologists: Position statement: Whole bowel irrigation. J Toxicol Clin Toxicol 35:753–762, 1997.

KEY POINTS: TOXICOLOGY

1. Ipecac is no longer routinely recommended for poisoning.

2. Activated charcoal is most efficacious if given within 1 hour of ingestion.

3. Multiple-dose activated charcoal attempts should be used to remove agents previously absorbed.

4. Gastric lavage has unproven efficacy for most ingestions.

5. Whole-bowel irrigation is indicated for sustained-release or enteric-coated substances.

115. **How is the manipulation of urinary pH used when treating patients with poisonings?**

Acidification or alkalinization of the urine to enhance the excretion of weak acids and bases has been a traditional way to enhance the elimination of toxicologic agents. In recent years, its use has been limited because of the potential complications from fluid overload (e.g., pulmonary and cerebral edema), the risk of acidemia, and the use of other therapeutic advancements (e.g., hemodialysis). However, alkaline diuresis is still considered valuable for the management of acute overdoses of salicylates, barbiturates, and tricyclic antidepressants.

116. **Naloxone (Narcan) is considered an antidote for which kinds of ingestions?**

Naloxone is an antidote for opioid drugs. It reverses the central nervous system and respiratory depression of morphine and heroin, and it clears the depressed sensorium in overdoses that result from many of the synthetic opioids, including propoxyphene, codeine, dextromethorphan, pentazocine, and meperidine. It is a known antidote for clonidine, and its efficacy for reversing the signs and symptoms of tetrahydrozoline (over-the-counter eyedrop solutions and nasal decongestants) ingestion in children has been described. The pediatric dose is 0.01–0.1 mg/kg. However, many authorities now recommend the following regimen for all suspected opioid or opioid-like acute poisonings:

- Coma without respiratory depression: 1.0 mg
- Coma with respiratory depression: 2.0 mg

These doses may be repeated every 2–10 minutes up to a total dose of 8–10 mg. If intravenous access is not available, the drug can be given intramuscularly, sublingually, or endotracheally.

Holmes JF, Berman DA: Use of naloxone to reverse symptomatic tetrahydrozoline overdose in a child. Pediatr Emerg Care 15:193–194, 1999.

117. **Which ingestions are radiopaque on abdominal x-ray?**
The mnemonic **CHIPS** indicates possible suspects:
   C = **C**hloral hydrate
   H = **H**eavy metals (e.g., arsenic, iron, lead)
   I = **I**odides
   P = **P**henothiazines, psychotropics (e.g., cyclic antidepressants)
   S = **S**low-release capsules, enteric-coated tablets
The likelihood of radiopacity depends on numerous factors, including the weight of the patient, the size of the ingestion, and the composition of the pill matrix.

   Tenenbein M: General management principles for poisoning. In Barkin RM, Caputo GL, Jaffe DM, Knapp JE, Schafermeyer RW, Seidel J (eds): Pediatric Emergency Medicine Concepts and Clinical Practice, 2nd ed. St. Louis, Mosby, 1997, pp 527–534.

118. **What is a toxidrome?**
A toxidrome is a clinical constellation of signs and symptoms that is very suggestive of a particular poisoning or of a category of intoxication. For example, patients with salicylate overdose commonly have a fever, hyperpnea, tachypnea, abnormal mental status (ranging from lethargy to coma), tinnitus, vomiting, and, sometimes, oil of wintergreen odor from methylsalicylate.

   Shannon M: Ingestion of toxic substances by children. N Engl J Med 342:186–191, 2000.

119. **What is the toxidrome for anticholinergics such as antihistamines?**
   - Delirium, visual hallucinations
   - Tachycardia
   - Hypertension
   - Hyperpyrexia
   - Dilated, sluggish pupils
   - Dry skin
   - Facial flushing
   - Urinary retention
   - Hypoactive bowel sounds

   The mnemonic for anticholinergic ingestions is as follows: "Mad as a hatter, red as a beet, dry as a bone, blind as a bat, and hot as Hades."

120. **What breath odors may be associated with specific ingestions?**

Characteristic odor	Responsible toxin/drug
Wintergreen	Methylsalicylate
Bitter almond	Cyanide
Carrots	Cicutoxin (of water hemlock)
Fruity	Ethanol, acetone (nail polish remover), isopropyl alcohol, chloroform
Fishy	Zinc or aluminum phosphide
Garlic	Organophosphate insecticide, arsenic, thallium
Glue	Toluene
Minty	Mouthwash, rubbing alcohol
Mothballs	Naphthalene, p-dichlorobenzene, camphor
Peanut	Vacor rat poison (odor is from a flavoring agent)
Rotten egg	Hydrogen sulfide, N-acetylcysteine, disulfiram
Rope (burned)	Marijuana, opium
Shoe polish	Nitrobenzene

   Woolf AD: Poisoning in children and adolescents. Pediatr Rev 14:411–422, 1993.

121. **What are the limitations of the routine toxicology screen?**
Most toxicology screens are intended to detect the drugs that are encountered in substance abuse. Even in larger pediatric hospitals, comprehensive toxicology screens generally include

only a fraction of the drugs that are available to children. Most blood screens analyze for acetaminophen, salicylates, and alcohols. Urine is often screened for substances of abuse and other common psychoactive drugs, including antidepressants, antipsychotics, benzodiazepines, sedative-hypnotics, and anticonvulsants. Other potential toxins that can cause mental status changes (e.g., carbon monoxide, chloral hydrate, cyanide, organophosphates) or circulatory depression (e.g., beta-blockers, calcium-channel blockers, clonidine, digitalis) may not be included, but these may be assayed via individual blood tests. In clinical studies, toxicology screens are most valuable in quantitative settings (i.e., for assessing drug levels). Additionally, treatment of the acutely poisoned patient must begin long before the results of many toxicology screens are available.

Belson MG, Simon HK, Sullivan K, Geller RJ: The utility of toxicologic analysis in children with suspected ingestions. Pediatr Emerg Care 15:383–387, 1999.

122. How do the types of alcohol ingestions vary?

All alcohols can cause central nervous system disturbances that range from mild mentation and motor abnormalities to respiratory depression and coma. Each alcohol individually is associated with specific metabolic complications:

- **Ethanol** (e.g., beverages, colognes, perfumes, aftershave lotion, mouthwash, topical antiseptic, rubbing alcohol): In infants and toddlers, this can cause the classic triad of coma, hypothermia, and hypoglycemia; in adolescents, it can cause intoxication and mild neurologic findings. At levels of >500 mg/dL, it can be lethal.
- **Methanol** (e.g., antifreeze, windshield washer fluid): This agent can cause severe refractory metabolic acidosis and permanent retinal damage leading to blindness.
- **Isopropyl alcohol** (e.g., jewelry cleaners, rubbing alcohol, windshield deicers, cements, paint removers): These can cause gastritis, abdominal pain, vomiting, hematemesis, central nervous system depression, moderate hyperglycemia, hypotension, and acetonemia, without acidosis.
- **Ethylene glycol** (e.g., antifreeze, brake fluid): This causes severe metabolic acidosis. In addition, it is metabolized to oxalic acid, which can cause renal damage by the precipitation of calcium oxalate crystals in the renal parenchyma and can lead to hypocalcemia.

123. Which alcohol is considered the most lethal?

Methanol. Deaths can occur as a result of doses of as little as 4 mL of pure methanol. Unique to methanol is that it becomes more toxic as it is metabolized. Methanol is broken down by alcohol dehydrogenase to formaldehyde and formic acid; it is the formic acid that causes the refractory metabolic acidosis and ocular symptoms.

124. Why may fomepizole replace ethanol as the primary antidote for methanol and ethylene glycol ingestions in children?

Both methanol and ethylene glycol require the enzyme alcohol dehydrogenase to create their toxic metabolites. Ethanol, given either intravenously or orally (the latter is more commonly used), competitively inhibits the formation of these metabolites by serving as a substrate for the enzyme. However, it is inebriating, it may cause hypoglycemia, and its kinetics are widely variable. Fomepizole is a safer and more effective blocker of alcohol dehydrogenase. Although the drug itself is significantly higher in cost, it may lower other costs as a result of shorter and less-intensive hospital stays.

Casavant MJ: Fomepizole in the treatment of poisoning. Pediatrics 107:170, 2001.

125. How is the osmolar gap helpful for diagnosing ingestions?

The osmolar gap is the difference between the measured osmolarity (obtained from freezing point depression) and the calculated osmolarity (calculated = 2 [serum Na] + blood urea nitrogen/2.8 + glucose/18). Normal osmolarity is about 290 mOsm/L. A significant osmolar gap suggests an alcohol poisoning, which typically produces exogenous osmoles.

126. **What is "MUDPILES"?**

    MUDPILES is an acronym for metabolic acidosis with a high anion gap; this is associated with a variety of ingestions:

    M = **M**ethanol, **m**etformin
    U = **U**remia
    D = **D**iabetic ketoacidosis
    P = **P**araldehyde
    I = **I**soniazid, **i**ron, **i**nborn errors of metabolism
    L = **L**actic acidosis (seen with shock, carbon monoxide, and cyanide)
    E = **E**thanol, **e**thylene glycol
    S = **S**alicylates

127. **How can pupillary findings assist in the diagnosis of toxic ingestions?**

Miosis (pinpoint pupils)	Narcotics, organophosphates, phencyclidine, clonidine, phenothiazines, barbiturates (occasionally), ethanol (occasionally)
Mydriasis (dilated pupils)	Anticholinergics (atropine, antihistamines, cyclic antidepressants), sympathomimetics (amphetamines, caffeine, cocaine, lysergic acid diethylamide, nicotine)
Nystagmus	Barbiturates, ketamine, phencyclidine, phenytoin

128. **If a child has ingested a product that contains acetaminophen, when should the first acetaminophen level be obtained?**

    A plasma level obtained **4 hours** after ingestion is a good indicator of the potential for hepatic toxicity. Nomograms are available for determining risk. As a rule, doses <150 mg/kg are unlikely to be harmful.

129. **When should a "NAC attack" begin?**

    N-acetylcysteine ("NAC") is a specific antidote for acetaminophen hepatotoxicity. It works by serving as a glutathione-substitute for detoxifying the hepatotoxic metabolites. It should be used for any acetaminophen overdose with a toxic serum acetaminophen level within the first 24 hours after ingestion. It is especially effective if used during the first 8 hours after ingestion. If acetaminophen levels are not available on a rapid basis or the time since ingestion is not clear, it is preferable to initiate N-acetylcysteine, orally or intravenously, while awaiting consultation with a toxicologist or with a poison control center.

    Kociancic T, Reed MD: Acetaminophen intoxication and length of treatment: How long is long enough? Pharmacotherapy 23:1052–1059, 2003.

130. **What arterial blood gas is classic for salicylate poisoning?**

    Metabolic acidosis and **respiratory alkalosis**. Salicylates directly stimulate the medullary respiratory drive center, thereby causing tachypnea with diminished PCO_2 (respiratory alkalosis); bringing about lactic acidosis and ketoacidosis by inhibiting Krebs cycle enzymes; uncoupling oxidation phosphorylation; and inhibiting amino acid metabolism (metabolic acidosis).

131. **What are hidden salicylates?**

    These are salicylates that are found in over-the-counter products, such as Pepto-Bismol (bismuth salicylate). Salicylate absorption can be substantial, and, in the setting of influenza or chickenpox, Pepto-Bismol use has been discouraged because of the potential for complications such as the development of Reye's syndrome.

    Szap MD: Hidden salicylates. Am J Dis Child 143:142, 1989.

132. **What are the classic ECG findings associated with tricyclic antidepressants?**
Tricyclic antidepressants interfere with myocardial conduction and can precipitate ventricular tachycardias or complete heart block. A QRS interval >0.1 second is predictive of poor outcome in these patients. The presence of a large R wave in lead accelerated ventricular rhythm (AVR) is also associated with tricyclics. If these findings are noted, treatment with sodium bicarbonate should be initiated. Sodium bicarbonate helps prevent the sodium-channel blockade that is caused by these medications.

133. **What features suggest the possibility of lead toxicity in a child?**
Most children with elevated lead levels are asymptomatic. Plumbism (i.e., lead intoxication) should be suspected if a child has the following symptoms:
- Pica, including a history of accidental ingestions or foreign body insertion in the nose or ear
- Vague or increasing abdominal complaints, such as anorexia, recurrent abdominal pain, constipation, and vomiting
- Vague behavioral effects, such as hyperactivity, irritability, malaise, or lethargy
- Progressive ataxia or afebrile seizure
- A history of unexplained or iron-deficiency anemia
- Basophilic stippling of peripheral red blood cells

  Piomelli S: Childhood lead poisoning. Pediatr Clin North Am 49:1285–1304, 2002.

134. **Should all children be screened for elevated lead levels?**
Because of substantial regional and local variations in the prevalence of elevated lead levels, the recommendation to screen all children is controversial. Some states have adopted universal screening because increased lead levels—even at low concentrations (<10 µg/dL)—have been associated with slowed mental growth and behavior disorders. In general, it is advisable to screen high-risk children, including those with the following characteristics:
- Living in or visiting homes with peeling paint that were built before 1960 or that are undergoing renovation
- Having a sibling or playmate with an elevated lead level
- Living with an adult whose job or hobby involves lead
- Living near an industry that is likely to release lead (e.g., smelting plant, battery-recycling plant)

  Canfield RL, Henderson CR, Jr., Cory-Slechta DA, et al: Intellectual impairment in children with blood lead concentrations below 10 µg per deciliter. N Engl J Med 348:1517–1526, 2003.

135. **If elevated lead is discovered on a routine screen, what are the most likely sources of exposure?**
- **Lead-based paint:** Found in homes built before the 1960s (ban on residential use since 1977)
- **Home renovation:** Releases lead-containing dust into the environment
- **Soil:** Contamination from nearby industries like smelting, soldering, battery-recycling, sandblasting, and demolition
- **Drinking water:** Older, lead-containing pipes

  Infrequent sources of exposure are cooking in ceramic or pewter cookware, lead-containing folk remedies, moonshine liquor made with lead vats or tubes, or parental occupation or hobbies (stained-glass making, lead glazes for painting). In adolescents, inhaling leaded gasoline fumes can result in lead toxicity.

  Campbell C, Osterhoudt KC: Prevention of childhood lead poisoning. Curr Opin Pediatr 12:428–437, 2000.

136. **At what lead levels is chelation indicated?**
<25 µg/dL   Chelation is not indicated.
25–45 µg/dL   Chelation is not routinely indicated because no evidence exists that chelation prevents or reverses neurotoxicity. Some patients may benefit from (oral)

chelation (e.g., succimer), especially if elevated levels persist despite aggressive environmental intervention and abatement.

45–70 µg/dL   Chelation is indicated with either succimer or $CaNa_2EDTA$ (if no clinical symptoms suggestive of encephalopathy are present [e.g., headache, persistent vomiting]). If symptoms of encephalopathy are seen, chelation with dimercaprol and $CaNa_2EDTA$ are indicated. Before chelation, an abdominal radiograph scan should be taken to evaluate for the possible removable of enteral lead.

>70 µg/dL   Inpatient chelation therapy with dimercaprol and $CaNa_2EDTA$ is indicated.

Committee on Drugs: Treatment guidelines for lead exposure in children. Pediatrics 96:155–160, 1995.

137. Which clinical and laboratory features correlate with an acutely elevated serum iron level?

Serum iron levels obtained 4–6 hours after ingestion correlate with the severity of toxicity. Iron levels >300 µg/dl are associated with mild toxicity that consists of local gastrointestinal symptoms (e.g., nausea, vomiting, diarrhea). A serum iron level of 500 µg/dL is associated with serious systemic toxicity, and a level of 1000 µg/dL is associated with death. Other laboratory tests that correlate with an elevated iron level include leukocytosis (>15,000/mm^3) and hyperglycemia (>150 mg/dL). Sometimes radiopaque tablets may be demonstrated on abdominal x-ray.

138. If a toddler is suspected of swallowing too many multivitamins, how long should he/she remain under physician observation?

The toxic compound in multivitamin overdose is iron. There are a large variety of children's chewable multivitamins that contain different amounts of elemental iron (0–18 mg per tablet). The toxic dose of iron ingestion is ≥20 mg/kg of elemental iron, and the lethal dose of iron has been reported to be in the range of 60–180 mg/kg of elemental iron. In a small child, a toxic dose is about 300 mg of elemental iron, which is the equivalent of 20 tablets of multivitamins containing 15 mg of elemental iron per tablet. Frequently, the amount of ingestion is not known. Because iron can initially cause nausea, vomiting, and abdominal pain, a child with suspected iron poisoning of an unknown amount should be observed. A child who has no complaints and has a normal physical examination after 4–6 hours of observation can be safely allowed to go home.

139. What are the four clinical stages of iron toxicity, and what are their correlating pathophysiologies?

Although the presence, duration, and severity of these phases will vary considerably, the four phases (with time after ingestion given in parentheses) are as follows:

Stage 1 (0.5–6 hours): During this stage, iron exhibits a direct corrosive effect on the small bowel. Symptoms include nausea, vomiting, abdominal pain, and/or gastrointestinal hemorrhage.

Stage 2 (6–24 hours): Iron silently accumulates in the mitochondria during this period, which is relatively free of symptoms.

Stage 3 (4–40 hours): This phase is characterized by systemic toxicity with shock, metabolic acidosis, depressed cardiac function, and hepatic necrosis.

Stage 4 (2–8 weeks): During this phase, pyloric stenosis and obstruction can develop as a result of earlier local bowel irritation.

140. What is the preferred method of gastrointestinal decontamination in patients with iron overdose?

Whole-bowel irrigation is effective and is the method of choice for patients with symptoms of iron toxicity. Syrup of ipecac is no longer recommended, and activated charcoal will not adsorb iron. Many adult-strength iron-containing pills are very large and are often too large for orogastric lavage.

141. **How do the signs and symptoms of acute iron ingestion differ from those of other heavy metal poisonings?**

     Iron salt ingestion causes early gastrointestinal symptoms and, in severe cases, hemorrhagic gastritis, shock, and coma. After 24–48 hours, evidence of hepatic damage ensues.

     Lead poisoning may cause mild gastrointestinal symptoms; however, encephalopathy with cerebral vasculitis, increased intracranial pressure and coma, seizures, and severe neurologic damage are the most feared complications.

     Acute **mercury salt** poisoning causes both a hemorrhagic gastroenteritis and renal damage. The liver is generally not injured.

     Arsenic poisoning affects multiple organs, with marked skin and hair changes, neurologic effects (encephalopathy, peripheral neuropathy, tremor, coma, convulsions), fatty infiltration of the liver, renal tubular and glomerular damage, and cardiac involvement with conduction delays and dysrhythmias.

142. **What is the value of a deferoxamine challenge?**

     Deferoxamine challenge may occasionally be useful as an additional screening test for mild to moderate iron poisoning if "stat" iron levels are not available. In the asymptomatic or mildly symptomatic patient, a dose of 15 mg/kg (up to 1 gm maximum) may be given intramuscularly. A positive test (orange or "vin rose" tint to the urine) signifies the excretion of feroxamine (deferoxamine–iron chelate). All patients with a positive challenge test should be admitted for continuing chelation therapy. A negative challenge test in a patient with significant symptoms does not rule out iron toxicity and should not be deemed reliable.

143. **Which is worse: drinking dishwashing detergent or drinking toilet bowl cleaner?**

     You are better off with the toilet bowl cleaner, although both acid (toilet bowl cleaner) and alkali (dishwashing detergent) ingestions may cause severe esophageal burns. **Alkalis** cause injury by liquefaction necrosis (dissolving proteins and lipids), thereby allowing for deeper penetration of the caustic substance and greater local tissue injury. With **acids**, coagulation necrosis of the tissue occurs. This results in the formation of an eschar that limits the penetration of the toxin into deeper tissues. As compared with acids, alkalis are more typically in solid and paste form; this increases tissue contact time and potential for tissue injury.

144. **Are steroids helpful for patients with caustic ingestions?**

     Steroids are controversial for the treatment of caustic ingestions. They are purported to reduce scar formation and strictures, but they may interfere with wound healing and predispose the patient to perforation. Most authorities currently recommend steroids for all significant second-degree burns; alternatively, these authorities also advocate their omission for significant full-thickness burns (where their use might be hazardous as well as ineffectual) and for first-degree burns (which are expected to heal without scarring, regardless of treatment).

145. **Which hydrocarbons pose the greatest risk for chemical pneumonitis?**

     The household hydrocarbons with low viscosities pose the greatest aspiration hazard. These include furniture polishes, gasoline, kerosene, turpentine, other paint thinners, and lighter fuels.

146. **Which patients with hydrocarbon ingestions should be admitted?**

     All patients with significant clinical findings and patients with mild clinical findings and positive chest x-rays should be admitted. Children with a history of exposure are safe to discharge after 4–6 hours of observation if they have no symptoms; were treated as a result of accidental ingestion; have very transient coughing or gagging; have a normal physical examination; and will have reliable follow-up examinations.

147. **A patient receiving an antiemetic drug (e.g., promethazine) who develops involuntary, prolonged twisting and writhing movements of the neck, trunk, and arms likely has what condition?**
Acute dystonia. This dystonic reaction is classically seen as an adverse effect of antidopaminergic agents such as neuroleptics, antiemetics, and metoclopramide. In children, phenothiazines are the most common culprit. Treatment includes the administration of diphenhydramine (Benadryl) orally, intramuscularly, or intravenously at 1 mg/kg/dose. Benztropine (Cogentin) is also used in adolescents.

148. **What do SLUDGE and DUMBELS have in common?**
Both of these are acronyms that are used to assist with remembering the problems involved with organophosphate poisoning (i.e., lipid-soluble insecticides used in agriculture and terrorism, "nerve gas"). Organophosphates inhibit cholinesterase and cause all of the signs and symptoms of acetylcholine excess.
Muscarinic effects: Increased oral and tracheal secretions, miosis, salivation, lacrimation, urination, vomiting, cramping, defecation, and bradycardia; may progress to frank pulmonary edema
Central nervous system effects: Agitation, delirium, seizures, and/or coma
Nicotinic effects: Sweating, muscle fasciculation, and, ultimately, paralysis
SLUDGE: Salivation, **l**acrimation, **u**rination, **d**efecation, **g**astrointestinal cramps, **e**mesis
DUMBELS: Defecation, **u**rination, **m**iosis, **b**ronchorrhea/**b**radycardia, **e**mesis, **l**acrimation, **s**alivation

149. **What metal intoxication can mimic Kawasaki disease?**
Mercury. *Acrodynia* refers to one form of mercury salt intoxication that results in a constellation of signs and symptoms that is very similar to that currently recognized as Kawasaki syndrome. The classic presenting symptoms of acrodynia were described in children who were exposed to calomel (a substance used in teething powders), which was essentially mercurous chloride. The symptom complex included swelling and redness of the hands and feet, skin rashes, diaphoresis, tachycardia, hypertension, photophobia, and an intense irritability with anorexia and insomnia. Infants were often very limp, laying in a frog-like position, with impressive weakness of the hip and shoulder girdle muscles. Similar symptoms have been described in children exposed to other forms of mercury, including broken fluorescent light bulbs or diapers rinsed in mercuric chloride.

150. **Why is cyanide so toxic?**
Cyanide ions bind to the heme-containing cytochrome a_3 enzyme in the electron transport chain of mitochondria, which is the final common pathway in oxidative metabolism. Thus, with a significant exposure, virtually every cell in the body becomes starved of oxygen at the mitochondrial level and is unable to function. As with carbon monoxide poisoning, symptoms tend to be most prominent among the metabolically active organ systems. In particular, the central nervous system is rapidly affected; this causes headache and dizziness and may progress to prostration, convulsions, coma, and death. Less-severe ingestions may be noted initially by the burning of the tongue and mucous membranes, with tachypnea and dyspnea resulting from the cyanide stimulation of chemoreceptors.

151. **In what settings should cyanide poisoning be suspected?**
- **Suicidal ingestion,** often involving chemists who have access to cyanide salts as reagents
- **Fires** causing the combustion of materials such as wool, silk, synthetic rubber, polyurethane, and nitrocellulose, which results in the release of cyanide
- Patients who are on **nitroprusside continuous infusion**, an antihypertensive agent that contains 5 cyanide moieties per molecule

152. **What kinds of plants account for the greatest percentage of deaths from plant poisonings?**
Mushrooms account for ≥50% of these deaths. The most dreaded are the *Amanita* species, which initially cause intestinal symptoms as a result one toxin (phallotoxin) and then hepatic and renal failure as a result of a separate toxin (amatoxin). Other mushroom classes can cause a variety of early-onset (<6 hours) symptoms, including muscarinic effects (e.g., sweating, salivation, colic), anticholinergic effects (e.g., drowsiness, mania, hallucinations), gastroenteritis, and Antabuse-type effects (if taken with alcohol).

153. **After an enjoyable take-out meal of moo goo gai pan, an 8-year-old child has facial burning and headache. What is the likely diagnosis?**
Chinese restaurant syndrome. Several hours after the ingestion of Chinese food, a patient may complain of burning and numbness of the face and neck, headache, and, occasionally, severe chest pain. Symptoms can persist for up to 1–2 days. The pathophysiology remains unclear, but monosodium glutamate, a food additive, may be involved, with the glutamate acting as a neurotransmitter. Other studies suggest that the fermentation of typical ingredients in Chinese cooking (e.g., soy sauce, black beans, shrimp paste) may release histamines that account for the symptoms.

154. **Is mistletoe toxic?**
Mistletoe, the popular Christmas plant, is an evergreen with small white berries. Ingestion of small amounts of the berries, leaves, or stems may result in gastrointestinal symptoms, including pain, nausea, vomiting, and diarrhea. Rarely, large ingestions have resulted in seizures, hypertension, and even cardiac arrest. In some countries, extracts of mistletoe have been used for illegal abortifacients or brewed in teas that are particularly toxic. In the United States, the typical call to a poison center concerns a child who eats one or two mistletoe berries, which, in general, is unlikely to produce significant signs or symptoms.

155. **Should ingested disc batteries be removed?**
Although the concern is that a disc battery may produce corrosive intestinal injury, most traverse the gastrointestinal tract without incident. An initial x-ray for localization is indicated. If the disc battery is in the distal esophagus, removal is required. Otherwise, if the battery is in the stomach or beyond and the patient remains asymptomatic, watchful waiting is appropriate. If the battery is not seen in the stool by 5–7 days, a repeat x-ray should be obtained.

156. **What is the most common causes of aspirated foreign bodies resulting in respiratory symptoms and requiring bronchoscopic removal in children?**
Peanuts are easily the most common, causing nearly 40% of cases in some studies. Other causes include other nuts, other organic (food) materials, seeds (sunflower and watermelon), twigs, plastics, popcorn, pins, and screws. Because the clinical picture of aspiration can mimic viral upper respiratory infection, the diagnosis is often delayed.

> Black RE, Johnson DG, Matlak ME, et al: Bronchoscopic removal of aspirated foreign bodies in children. J Pediatr Surg 29:682–684, 1994.

157. **What is the best way to remove a foreign body from the esophagus?**
Three methods are used, and often local custom prevails regarding selection:
- **Esophagoscopy,** the most commonly used method, is done under general anesthesia.
- A **Foley catheter** can be inserted beyond the foreign body, inflated, and then pulled back to remove the object. This extraction method is used by various centers, particularly for coins if the ingestion is <24 hours old and no respiratory distress is present. Complications, such as airway obstruction by a displaced coin and esophageal perforation, are possible.
- In **bougienage**, the object is forced into the stomach.

TRAUMA

158. **In a child with head trauma, is a skull x-ray a good screening study?**
No. Use of skull films for the management of head trauma in children has been controversial. Skull films will reveal only bony abnormalities and not intracranial injuries. Although the presence of a skull fracture increases the relative risk for intracranial injury by almost fourfold, the absence of a skull fracture on plain x-ray does not rule out an intracranial injury. A normal skull film may be falsely reassuring. Plain x-rays are not considered to be sufficiently sensitive or specific to be clinically useful in most settings. Skull films may be considered in well-appearing children <3 months old with a history of nontrivial head trauma without hematoma present or in children between 3 months and 1 year old who have a moderate to severe skull hematoma. Presence of a fracture would warrant CT evaluation. Also, many practitioners consider films for temporal injuries given the proximity of the middle meningeal artery and the possibility of increased epidural bleeding that occurs with fracture at that site, even with a relatively minor injury. Parietal hematomas and large scalp hematomas—but *not* frontal hematomas—may also increase the risk of intracranial injury and therefore may warrant a CT scan.

Greenes DS, Schutzman SA: Clinical significance of scalp abnormalities in asymptomatic head-injured infants. Pediatr Emerg Care 17:88–92, 2001.

Isaacman DJ, Poirier MP, Loiselle JM, et al: Closed head injury in children. Pediatr Emerg Care 18:48–52, 2002.

159. **When should a CT scan be considered after head trauma?**
A model has yet to be perfected with regard to clinical indicators of traumatic brain injury in children. However, some indices to consider are as follows:
- Glasgow Coma Scale score <15
- Focal neurologic abnormality
- Seizure (early, focal, or prolonged)
- Skull fracture (especially depressed or basilar skull fracture)
- Full fontanel
- Loss of consciousness (especially if more than brief)
- Deteriorating or persistent altered level of consciousness, irritability, or behavior
- Unremitting vomiting (especially if >4–6 hours) or progressive headache
- Signs of penetrating skull trauma or bony abnormality
- Age <3 months with nontrivial trauma
- Age <2 years with significant scalp hematoma
- Amnesia
- Persistent headache

Schutzman SA: Head injury. In Fleisher GR, Ludwig S (eds): Textbook of Pediatric Emergency Medicine, 4th ed. Baltimore, Lippincott Williams &Wilkins, 2000, p 272.

Schutzman SA, Barnes P, Duhaime AC, et al: Evaluation and management of children younger than two years old with apparently minor head trauma: Proposed guidelines. Pediatrics 107:983–993, 2001.

160. **If a patient with head trauma has persistent hypotension and bradycardia despite resuscitative efforts, what should be considered?**
Neurogenic shock. Trauma to the cervical or high thoracic spinal cord can often injure or ablate the descending sympathetic pathways, which results in the loss of vasomotor tone and sympathetic control of the heart. The child may be in severe hypovolemic shock but will not be able to mount a tachycardic response. Treatment consists of cardiorespiratory support, atropine, fluid resuscitation, and sympathomimetics (particularly epinephrine). Although these patients are hypovolemic and need fluids, aggressive fluid resuscitation may lead to fluid overload and pulmonary edema as a result of the loss of vasomotor tone and the subsequent pooling of fluids.

161. **When intracranial pressure is acutely elevated, how long is it before papilledema develops?**
Generally, 24–48 hours.

162. **What are the components of the Glasgow Coma Scale?**
Developed in 1974 by the neurosurgical department at the University of Glasgow, the scale was an attempt to standardize the assessment of the depth and duration of impaired consciousness and coma, particularly in the setting of trauma. The scale is based on eye opening, verbal responses, and motor responses, with a total score that ranges from 3–15 (Table 5-6).

TABLE 5-6.   GLASGOW COMA SCALE

Best verbal response*
5 Oriented, appropriate conversation
4 Confused conservation
3 Inappropriate words
2 Incomprehensible sounds
1 No response

Best motor response to command or to pain (e.g., rubbing knuckles on sternum)
6 Obeys a verbal command
5 Localizes
4 Withdraws
3 Abnormal flexion (decorticate posturing)
2 Abnormal extension (decerebrate posturing)
1 No response

Eye opening
4 Spontaneous
3 In response to verbal command
2 In response to pain
1 No response

*Children <2 years old should receive full verbal scores for crying after stimulation.

---

163. **How do the signs of different types of central nervous system herniation differ?**
- **Tentorial herniation** (unilateral herniation of the temporal lobe from the middle to the posterior fossa through rigid tentorium): Ipsilateral third nerve findings (pupillary dilation, ptosis, loss of medial gaze) and contralateral hemiparesis and decerebrate posturing
- **Cerebellar tonsils through foramen magnum:** Abnormalities of tone, bradycardia, hypertension, and progressive respiratory distress (Cushing's triad)
- **Subfalcine herniation** (herniation of one cerebral hemisphere beneath the falx cerebri to the opposite side): Leg weakness and bladder abnormalities
   Be aware that these clinical findings tend to overlap, and an altered state of consciousness is often the initial symptom.

164. **How, when, and where are car seats to be used?**
All 50 states require that children riding in cars be restrained in an approved safety seat based on weight, height, and age as follows:
- Birth to 1 year of age and up to 20–22 lb: Rear-facing infant seat
- >1 year old and 20–40 lb: Forward-facing toddler seat
- 40–80 lb or <4'9": Belt-positioning booster seat
- >8 years or >4'9": Shoulder strap with belt
- All children ≤12 years old should ride in the back seat

   American Academy of Pediatricians: "Car safety seats: A guide for families, 2004." Available at: www.aap.org/family/carseatguide.htm
   Dowd MD: Motor vehicle injury prevention: current recommendations for child passenger safety. Pediatr Emerg Care 20:778–782, 2004.

165. **What are the dangers of air bags to children?**
Children *<13 years old* and *<5 feet tall* should not be seated in the front seat of cars with air bags. Air bag deployment has been associated with such life-threatening injuries as cervical spine injuries and closed head trauma. Other, less-serious injuries include facial, neck, and chest abrasions; facial and upper-extremity burns; and blunt and chemical ocular trauma.

   McCaffrey M, German A, Lalonde F, Letts M: Air bags and children: A potentially lethal combination. J Pediatr Orthop 19:60–64, 1999

166. **What are the major signs of a blow-out fracture?**
Traumatic force to the eye can result in a blow-out fracture affecting either the orbital floor or the medial wall. The fracture may result from either a sudden increase in intraorbital pressure or from a direct concussive force to the bony walls. Symptoms and signs can include the following:
- Pain on upward gaze
- Diplopia on upward gaze
- Enophthalmos (i.e., posterior displacement of the globe of the eye)
- Loss of sensation over the upper lip and gums on the injured side
- Inability to look upward on the affected side as a result of entrapment of the inferior rectus muscle
- Crepitus over the inferior orbital ridge

167. **Which eyelid injuries should be referred to a specialist for repair?**
- Wounds involving the medial canthus that may have involved the medial canaliculus
- Injury to the lacrimal sac or nasal lacrimal duct, which can potentially lead to obstruction if not repaired correctly
- Deep horizontal lacerations of the upper lid that may involve the levator muscle and result in ptosis
- Lacerations of the lid margin, which may lead to notching if not repaired properly

   American College of Surgeons Committee on Trauma: Advanced Trauma Life Support for Doctors, 6th ed. Chicago, American College of Surgeons, 1997, p 414.

168. **When evaluating a patient with an eye injury, when should you suspect a ruptured globe, and how should you handle it?**
The sudden onset of marked visual impairment in the face of eye trauma should raise your suspicion for a ruptured globe. The eye will be sunken as a result of decreased intraocular pressure, and the anterior chamber may be flattened or shallow. You may see a tear-shaped pupil, which is the result of the contents of the iris coming forward and plugging the laceration or puncture. A ruptured globe is a true emergency, and an ophthalmologist should be called immediately. The approach, which is summed up by the acronym **SANTAS**, should be as follows:

S = **S**terile dressing and **s**hield should be placed over the eye to protect from further damage.

A = **A**ntiemetics should be given to protect against increased pressure.

N = **N**PO (nothing by mouth) to prepare for surgery.

T = **T**etanus shot should be given.

A = **A**nalgesics, either parenteral or oral (avoid topical), should be administered.

S = **S**edation, if not contraindicated by other injuries, should be given.

American College of Surgeons Committee on Trauma: Advanced Trauma Life Support for Doctors, 6th ed. Chicago, American College of Surgeons, 1997, p 416.

Rahman WM, O'Connor TJ: Facial trauma. In Barkin RM (ed): Pediatric Emergency Medicine, Concepts and Clinical Practice. St. Louis, Mosby, 1997, pp 252–283.

169. **How does the location of cervical spine fractures vary between younger children and older children/adults?**
Younger children tend to have fractures of the *upper* cervical spine, whereas **older children and adults** have fractures more often involving the *lower* cervical spine, for the following reasons:
- Changing fulcrum of the spine: In an infant, the fulcrum of the cervical spine is at approximately C2–C3; in a child who is 5–6 years old, the fulcrum is at C3–C4; from 8 to adulthood, it is at C5–C6. These changes are in large part to the result of the relatively large head size of a child as compared with that of an adult.
- Younger children have relatively weak neck muscles.
- Younger children have poorer protective reflexes.

Woodward GA: Neck trauma. In Fleisher GR, Ludwig S (eds): Textbook of Pediatric Emergency Medicine, 4th ed. Baltimore, Williams &Wilkins, 2000, p 1318.

170. **Which patients may have SCIWORA?**
Up to two thirds of children with spinal cord injuries have **SCIWORA** (**s**pinal **c**ord **i**njury **w**ith**o**ut **r**adiographic **a**bnormality). Most of these patients are <8 years old and have signs and symptoms that are consistent with spinal cord injury, but x-ray and CT studies reveal no bony abnormalities. It is postulated that the highly malleable pediatric spine allows the cord to sustain injury from flexion/extension forces without causing bony disruption. The more recent use of MRI among these children may help to clarify the cause(s). The initial neurologic complaints of these children should be taken seriously. Even with normal x-rays, a patient with an altered sensorium or with neurologic abnormalities that are consistent with cervical cord injury (e.g., motor or sensory changes, bowel/bladder problems, vital sign instability) requires continued neck immobilization and more extensive evaluation.

171. **Are single lateral cervical spine radiographs sufficient to "clear" a patient after neck injury?**
No. In some studies, the sensitivity of a single view for fractures is only 80%. American College of Radiology guidelines recommend at least three views: (1) anteroposterior (including the C7-T1 junction, C1-C7); (2) lateral; and (3) open mouth (odontoid). The last view is often difficult to obtain in younger children. CT scanning and MRI imaging are reserved for more extensive evaluation for spinal cord injury when the initial three views are negative in symptomatic patients. The use of oblique films is controversial.

Keats TE, Dalinka MK, Alazraki N, et al: Cervical spine trauma. American College of Radiology. ACR Appropriateness Criteria. Radiology 215 Suppl:S243–S246, 2000.

172. **A 16-year-old boy has a stab wound to the mid abdomen. His vital signs are as follows: heart rate, 152 bpm; blood pressure, 80/50 mmHg; respiratory rate, 28 breaths per minute. What screening x-rays or diagnostic tests should be ordered?**
None! This child has a penetrating abdominal wound, is in shock from internal bleeding, and needs to go to the operating room immediately. The proper approach to this patient is to stabilize his airway, provide oxygen and fluids, and transport as quickly as possible to the operating room.

173. **If the abdominal CT scan is negative in a patient with blunt abdominal trauma, can you be certain that there is no intra-abdominal injury?**

No. CT scans may miss some gastrointestinal, diaphragmatic, and pancreatic injuries. If the CT shows free fluid in the abdominal cavity but no obvious organ injury, there may be injury to the gastrointestinal tract or the mesentery, and early surgical intervention is mandated.

American College of Surgeons Committee on Trauma: Advanced Trauma Life Support for Doctors, 6th ed. Chicago, American College of Surgeons, 1997, p 166.

174. **Why is left shoulder pain after abdominal trauma a worrisome sign?**

This may represent blood accumulating under the diaphragm, resulting in pain referred to the left shoulder (Kehr's sign). The sign can be elicited by left upper quadrant palpation or by placing the patient in the Trendelenburg's position. The finding is worrisome because it suggests possible solid organ abdominal injury—most commonly the spleen—and requires surgical consultation and radiographic studies (usually CT or ultrasound) to grade the extent of injury.

Powell M, Courcoulas A, Gardner M, et al: Management of blunt splenic trauma: significant differences between adults and children. Surgery 122:654–660, 1997.

175. **A 5-year-old child has ecchymosis of the lower abdomen after a motor vehicle crash. What should you immediately suspect?**

This child's injuries should immediately key you in to the possibility of a **lap-belt injury**. In children who are either too young (<8 years old) or too small (<4'9''), the lap-belt of a car rests abnormally high on the child's body and, instead of crossing the lap at the hips, crosses the lap at the lower abdomen. The most common injuries to suspect are lumbar spine injuries, particularly a flexion disruption (Chance) fractures and bowel or bladder perforations or disruptions.

Sivit CJ, Taylor GA, Newman KD, et al: Safety-belt injuries in children with lap-belt ecchymosis: CT findings in 61 patients. Am J Radiol 157:111–114, 1991.

176. **When are drops for pupillary dilation contraindicated?**

These drops should not be used in patients who require sequential neurologic examinations (e.g., after severe head trauma), in whom increasing intracranial pressure with herniation is possible. They are also contraindicated in the setting of acute-angle glaucoma. The risk of inducing glaucoma is very low in children, but if symptoms of glaucoma (e.g., moderate eye pain, decreased vision, cloudy cornea, asymmetric pupil size, poor pupillary reaction) are present, dilation should be deferred. All of these drops can have side effects, and these can be minimized by pressure over the medial canthus to avoid systemic absorption.

177. **When should an avulsed tooth be reimplanted?**

Avulsion is the complete displacement of the tooth from its socket. Primary teeth (i.e., baby teeth) should not be reimplanted because nerve root damage or dental ankylosis may result. Secondary teeth should be repaired within 30 minutes (<10 minutes may be most optimal) to maximize the chance of tooth viability. Thus, early insertion after gently rinsing the tooth is preferable (even if this does not result in a perfect fit, reimplantation may prevent the root from drying). It is important to disturb the root as minimally as possible. If not reimplantable (e.g., in the case of an uncooperative patient), a dislodged tooth should be gently rinsed, transported in milk or saliva or under a parent's tongue, and reimplanted temporarily until definitive dental care can be obtained.

Weiger R, Heuchert T: Management of an avulsed primary incisor. Endod Dental Traumatol 15:138–143, 1999.

178. **What are the three most important considerations when evaluating nasal trauma?**

- **Bleeding:** If persistent, bleeding should be controlled with pressure, topical vasoconstrictors, topical thrombin, cauterization, and anterior or posterior nasal packing.

- **Septal hematoma:** If the nasal septum is bulging into the nasal cavity, there is likely a hematoma that must be drained. If drainage is not performed, abscess formation or pressure necrosis can result and lead to a saddle-nose deformity.
- **Watery rhinorrhea:** This may be a sign of cribriform plate, suborbital ethmoid, sphenoid sinus, or frontal sinus fracture with cerebrospinal fluid leak. Radioisotope scans or CT scans with metrizamide dye can confirm the fracture; hospitalization is warranted if this is positive. More extensive facial trauma requires evaluation for many items, especially midface fractures and eye damage. Determining if the nose is fractured is a lower priority item because fracture reduction is done only if there is distortion of the nose. Furthermore, such distortion cannot be properly assessed acutely because of swelling.

179. **How long before a broken nose in a child must be reduced?**
If a nasal bone fracture causes asymmetry (which is noted as the swelling from acute trauma subsides), the fracture should be reduced within 4–5 days; a longer delay may result in malunion.

180. **How does one distinguish nasal mucosal drainage from cerebrospinal fluid leakage?**
This often becomes an issue when children have nasal rhinorrhea after trauma. The simplest test is to check the glucose concentration. The glucose level of cerebrospinal fluid is normally 40–80 mg/dL, whereas glucose concentration of nasal mucus is normally near 0 mg/dL.

181. **In a 7-year-old boy with an x-ray-proven pelvic fracture, what urologic procedure is needed, and what procedure is relatively contraindicated?**
The urethra, as it passes through the prostate, is very close to the pubic bone and is thus susceptible to injury from a pelvic fracture. Urethral damage should be suspected in all patients with pelvic fractures, even those without hematuria. The recommended diagnostic procedure is a **retrograde urethrogram**. A boggy, high-riding prostate found on rectal examination and/or blood seen at the urethral meatus are clinical signs of possible urethral disruption; these two findings are contraindications for passing a **Foley catheter**. A partial urethral disruption could potentially be made into a complete one with the passing of the catheter.

182. **How is zipper entrapment remedied?**
This situation most commonly occurs in boys with intact foreskins. After using a local anesthetic (1% lidocaine without epinephrine), release is accomplished by simple manipulation of the zipper, cutting the median bar of the zipper with a wire cutter, or dividing the zipper transversely.

Strait RT: A novel method for removal of penile zipper entrapment. Pediatr Emerg Care 15:412–413, 1999.

ACKNOWLEDGMENT

The editors gratefully acknowledge contributions by Drs. Meri Sonnett, Fred Henretig, and Jane M. Lavelle that were retained from the first three editions of *Pediatric Secrets*.

CHAPTER 6

ENDOCRINOLOGY

Sharon E. Oberfield, MD, and Daniel E. Hale, MD

ADRENAL DISORDERS

1. **What are the symptoms of adrenal insufficiency?**
   Newborns: Nonspecific findings of vomiting, irritability, and poor weight gain; may progress to cardiovascular shock
   Children: Lethargy, easy fatigability, poor weight gain, and vague abdominal complaints; hyperpigmentation (primary insufficiency); symptoms of hypoglycemia (secondary insufficiency); may also have intercurrent illness with vascular collapse

2. **What distinguishes primary and secondary adrenal insufficiency?**
   Primary: Abnormality of the adrenal gland itself
   Secondary: Hypothalamic or pituitary dysfunction

3. **What is the differential diagnosis of primary adrenal insufficiency?**
   - **Inherited enzymatic defects:** Congenital adrenal hyperplasia (multiple enzymatic defects)
   - **Autoimmune disease:** Isolated, autoimmune polyendocrine syndromes (APES) I and II, Schmidt syndrome
   - **Infectious disease:** Tuberculosis, meningococcemia, disseminated fungal infections
   - **Trauma:** Bilateral adrenal hemorrhage

4. **What are the most common causes of secondary adrenal insufficiency?**
   Secondary causes can include failure of the hypothalamic and/or pituitary gland as a result of tumor, central nervous system trauma, irradiation, infection, or surgery. The most common cause, however, is **prolonged glucocorticoid use** for the treatment of nonadrenal disease.

5. **Can clinical clues suggest that adrenal insufficiency is a primary rather than secondary problem?**
   - **Primary adrenal insufficiency:** Adrenocorticotropic hormone (ACTH) levels rise as a result of disruption of the hormonal feedback loop. Hyperpigmentation can result from these elevated levels. Primary deficiencies commonly lead to hyponatremia *and* hyperkalemia.
   - **Secondary adrenal insufficiency:** ACTH levels are low, and no hyperpigmentation occurs. Furthermore, in secondary insufficiency, the zona glomerulosa of the adrenal gland (responsible for aldosterone secretion) remains intact. Therefore, hyperkalemia and/or volume depletion are distinctly uncommon, but hyponatremia may occur as a result of decreased capacity to excrete a water load.

6. **What is the most common form of congenital adrenal hyperplasia (CAH)?**
   CAH refers to a group of autosomal recessive disorders that result from various enzymatic defects in the biosynthesis of cortisol. Depending on the enzyme involved, the blockade can result in excesses or deficiencies in the other steroid pathways (i.e., mineralocorticoids and androgens). **21-Hydroxylase deficiency** accounts for >90% of cases; the complete (salt-losing) and partial (simple virilizing) forms occur in about 1 in 12,000 births and have an equal

sex distribution. A late-onset or attenuated form (mild deficiency) manifests in adolescent females with hirsutism and menstrual irregularities.

Speiser PW, White PC: Congenital adrenal hyperplasia. N Engl J Med 349:776–788, 2003.

7. **In newborns with CAH, why are girls likely to be diagnosed earlier than boys?**
The most obvious clinical feature of CAH in the newborn period is **ambiguous genitalia** as a result of excess androgen. In boys, androgen excess does not cause any clearly abnormal appearance of the external genitalia. In girls, however, ambiguous genitalia are common. CAH should always be considered in the differential diagnosis of ambiguous genitalia, particularly in genetic females.

8. **How do the major steroid preparations vary in potency?**
See Table 6-1.

TABLE 6-1. RELATIVE POTENCIES OF GLUCOCORTICOIDS

Name	Relative gluco- corticoid potency	Relative dosing (mg)	Relative mineralo- corticoid potency
Cortisone	1	100	+
Hydrocortisone	1.25	80	++
Prednisone	5	20	+
Prednisolone	5	20	+
Methylprednisolone	6	16	0
9a-Fluorocortisol	20	5	+++++
Dexamethasone	50	1	0

Adapted from Donohoue PA: The adrenal cortex. In McMillan JA, DeAngelis CD, Feigin RD, Warshaw JB (eds): Oski's Pediatrics, Principles and Practice, 3rd ed. Philadelphia, J.B. Lippincott, 1999, p 1814.

9. **How do physiologic, stress, and pharmacologic doses of hydrocortisone differ?**
   - **Physiologic:** Careful studies have shown that adrenal glucocorticoid production in the normal individual is about 7–8 mg/m^2/24 h. Because 50–60% of oral hydrocortisone is absorbed, the recommended oral physiologic replacement is about 12–15 mg/m^2/24 h.
   - **Stress:** On the basis of studies performed before the development of high-quality radioim-munoassays, a consensus developed that production of glucocorticoid increased about threefold when individuals were physiologically stressed. Hence, when the term *stress dose* is used, it generally means 50 mg/m^2/24 h of hydrocortisone.
   - **Pharmacologic:** Glucocorticoids are extensively used in pharmacologic doses for the treatment of various inflammatory processes and in surgery or trauma to reduce or prevent swelling and inflammation. The doses are dependent on the underlying process and are often >50 mg/m^2/24 h of hydrocortisone.

10. **When does adrenal-pituitary axis suppression occur in prolonged glucocorticoid treatment?**
As a general rule, the longer the duration of treatment and the higher the dose, the greater the risk of adrenal suppression. If pharmacologic doses of glucocorticoids are used for <10 days, there is a relatively small risk of permanent adrenal insufficiency, whereas daily use for >30 days carries a high risk of transient or permanent adrenal suppression.

CALCIUM METABOLISM AND DISORDERS

11. **Is it the Chvostek or Trousseau sign that gets the tap?**

    Chvostek. Both are clinical manifestations of hypocalcemia or hypomagnesemia that occur because of neuromuscular irritability.

    - **Chvostek sign:** Tapping on the facial nerve in front of the ear results in movement of the upper lip.
    - **Trousseau sign:** Inflating a blood pressure cuff at pressures greater than systolic for 2 minutes results in carpopedal spasm.

12. **What are the causes of hypercalcemia?**

    Remember the "High **5-Is** rule": **H** (**h**yperparathyroidism) plus the five **Is** (**i**diopathic, **i**nfantile, **i**nfection, **i**nfiltrations, and **i**ngestions) and **S** (**s**keletal disorders).

    Hyperparathyroidism
    Familial
    Isolated
    Syndromic
    Idiopathic
    Williams syndrome
    Infantile
    Subcutaneous fat necrosis
    Secondary to maternal hypoparathyroidism
    Infections
    Tuberculosis
    Infiltrations
    Malignancy
    Sarcoidosis
    Ingestions
    Milk-alkali syndrome
    Thiazide diuretics
    Vitamin A intoxication
    Vitamin D intoxication
    Skeletal disorders
    Hypophosphatasia
    Immobilization
    Skeletal dysplasias

13. **An 8-year-old in a spica cast after hip surgery develops vomiting and a serum calcium of 15.3 mg/dL. What should be the level of concern?**

    A serum calcium concentration of >15 mg/dL or the presence of significant symptoms (i.e., vomiting, hypertension) constitutes a *medical emergency* and requires immediate intervention to lower the calcium level. The initial mainstay of treatment is isotonic saline at 2–4 times maintenance rates and furosemide at 1 mg/kg intravenously every 6 hours. Furosemide is a potent diuretic and calciuric agent. Meticulous monitoring of input and output and of serum and urinary electrolytes (including serum magnesium) is vital. Electrocardiogram monitoring is mandatory because hypercalcemia can be associated with conduction disturbances including premature ventricular contractions, ventricular tachycardia, prolonged PR interval, prolonged QRS duration, and atrioventricular block. Additional treatment with glucocorticoids and antihypercalcemic agents may also be needed.

14. **What is hypoparathyroidism?**

    Parathyroid hormone is a calcium regulatory hormone that increases serum calcium by increasing the resorption of Ca^{2+} from bone and by increasing gastrointestinal and urinary absorption of calcium via the increasing synthesis of calcitriol. Hypoparathyroidism can result from anomalies of the gland itself, destruction by surgery or autoimmune processes, synthetic abnormalities, or decreased distal cellular responsiveness to the hormone. The result can be acute and chronic hypocalcemia.

15. **In what clinical circumstances should hypoparathyroidism be suspected?**
    - Manifestations of hypocalcemia (e.g., carpopedal spasm, bronchospasm, tetany, seizures)
    - Lenticular cataracts (these can also occur with other causes of long-standing hypocalcemia)
    - Changing behaviors, ranging from depression to psychosis
    - Mucocutaneous candidiasis (seen in familial form)
    - Dry and scaly skin, psoriasis, and patchy alopecia
    - Brittle hair and fingernails
    - Enamel hypoplasia (if present during dental development)

16. **What are the main causes of hypocalcemia in children?**
    - **Nutritional:** Inadequate intake of vitamin D and/or calcium may cause this condition.
    - **Renal insufficiency:** This may be the result of the following: (1) increased serum phosphorus from a decreased glomerular filtration rate with depressed serum calcium and secondary hyperparathyroidism, or (2) decreased activity of renal α-hydroxylase, which is involved in converting the less-active 25-hydroxyvitamin D into the more active 1,25-$(OH)_2$ D.
    - **Nephrotic syndrome:** With lowered serum albumin, total calcium levels are reduced. Additionally, intestinal absorption of calcium is decreased, urinary losses of cholecalciferol-binding globulin are increased, and urinary losses of calcium are increased with prednisone therapy.
    - **Hypoparathyroidism:** In infants, this may result from primary aplasia, hypoplasia, or DiGeorge syndrome. In older children, autoimmune polyglandular disease or mitochondrial myopathy syndromes may cause it.
    - **Pseudohypoparathyroidism:** This is a peripheral resistance syndrome with elevated parathyroid hormone and normal renal function that can cause the condition.
    - **Disorders of calcium sensor genes**

    Umpaichitra V, Bastian W, Castells S: Hypocalcemia in children: Pathogenesis and management. Clin Pediatr 40:305–312, 2001.

17. **In what syndrome of hypocalcemia is a short fourth metacarpal seen?**
    Albright hereditary osteodystrophy, a type of pseudohypoparathyroidism, is characterized by short stature, obesity, developmental delay, and brachydactyly (the shortening of hand bones).

CLINICAL SYNDROMES

18. **How does the syndrome of inappropriate secretion of antidiuretic hormone (SIADH) develop?**
    Antidiuretic hormone (ADH) is released from the posterior pituitary gland and serves as a regulator of extracellular fluid volume. The secretion of ADH is regulated by changes in osmolality sensed by the hypothalamus and alterations in blood volume detected by carotid and left atrial stretch receptors. Intracranial pathology can increase the secretion of ADH directly by local central nervous system effects, and intrathoracic pathology can increase secretion by stimulating volume receptors. Medications can directly promote ADH release and enhance its renal effects. SIADH is usually asymptomatic until symptoms of water intoxication and hyponatremia develop. Nausea, vomiting, irritability, personality changes, progressive obtundation, and seizures can result.

19. **What are the five criteria for the diagnosis of SIADH?**
    1. Hyponatremia with reduced serum osmolality
    2. Urine osmolality elevated as compared with serum osmolality (a urine osmolality <100 mOsm/dL usually excludes the diagnosis)
    3. Urinary sodium concentration excessive for the extent of hyponatremia (usually >20 mEq/L)
    4. Normal renal, adrenal, and thyroid function
    5. Absence of volume depletion

20. **What clinical features suggest diabetes insipidus?**
    Because diabetes insipidus is caused by an insufficiency of ADH or the inability to respond to ADH, the signs and symptoms tend to be directly related to excessive fluid loss. The clinical spectrum may vary depending on the child's age. The infant may present symptoms of failure to thrive as a result of chronic dehydration, or there may be a history of repeated episodes of hospitalizations for dehydration. There may also be a history of intermittent low-grade fever.

    Often caretakers report a large-volume intake or an inability to keep a dry diaper on the infant. In the young child, diabetes insipidus may appear to be difficulty with toilet training. In the older child, the reappearance of enuresis, increasing frequency of urination, nocturia, or dramatic increases in fluid intake may herald the diagnosis. Frequent urination with large urinary volumes should lead to the suspicion of diabetes insipidus, and the absence of glucosuria is sufficient to rule out diabetes mellitus.

21. **How is the diagnosis of diabetes insipidus (DI) made?**
    Deprivation of water intake for a limited time and judicious monitoring of physical and biochemical parameters may be required. The diagnosis of DI rests on the demonstration of the following: (1) an inappropriately dilute urine in the face of a rising or elevated serum osmolality; (2) urine output that remains high despite the lack of oral input; and (3) changes in physical parameters that are consistent with dehydration (weight loss, tachycardia, loss of skin turgor, dry mucous membranes). A child who, with water deprivation, appropriately concentrates urine (>800 mOsm/L) and whose serum osmolality remains constant (<290 mOsm/L) is unlikely to have DI.

    If a child meets the criteria for the diagnosis of DI, the water-deprivation test is usually ended with the administration of some form of ADH, such as desmopressin and the provision of fluids. If the urine subsequently becomes appropriately concentrated, this confirms the diagnosis of ADH deficiency (central DI). Failure to concentrate suggests renal resistance to ADH (nephrogenic DI).

    Cheetham T, Baylis PH: Diabetes insipidus. Paeditr Drugs 4:785–796, 2002.

DIABETIC KETOACIDOSIS

22. **What is diabetic ketoacidosis (DKA)?**
    This is a state of severe metabolic derangement that results from both insulin deficiency and increased amounts of counter-regulatory hormones (catecholamines, glucagon, cortisol, and growth hormone). Its main features are hyperglycemia (glucose usually >300 mg/dL), ketonemia (serum ketones >3 mmol/L with ketonuria), and acidosis (venous pH <7.30 and serum HCO_3 <15 mEq/L).

23. **What percent of newly diagnosed diabetics present symptoms of DKA?**
    30%. The percentage is higher in younger children (<5 years old).

24. **What are the mainstays of therapy for DKA?**
    - Adequate initial **supportive care** (airway maintenance, supplemental oxygen as needed)
    - **Volume resuscitation,** especially if shock is present (with care taken to avoid the too-rapid correction of hyperosmolarity)

- **Insulin** administration
- **Frequent monitoring** of vital signs, electrolytes, glucose, and acid-base status

25. **How has the approach to fluid replacement in patients with DKA changed over the past decade?**

In an effort to prevent cerebral edema, recommendations for the initial fluid resuscitation in patients with DKA have undergone revision. Unless a patient is in shock, initial boluses of isotonic solution should ideally not exceed 10–20 mL/kg over 1–2 hours, and fluid replacement with a solution with a tonicity ≥45% over at least 48 hours is recommended.

Dunger DB, Sperling MA, Acerini CL, et al: European Society for Paediatric Endocrinology/Lawson Wilkins Pediatric Endocrine Society consensus statement on diabetic ketoacidosis in children and adolescents. Pediatrics 113:e133–e140, 2004.

26. **Why is a falling serum sodium concentration during the treatment of DKA of concern?**

Most patients with DKA have a significant sodium deficit of 8–10 mEq/kg, which needs to be replaced. Following initial fluid boluses, fluids containing 0.5 normal saline or greater may be required. As a general rule, the serum Na is low at the outset and rises throughout the course of treatment. An initial Na of >145 mEq/L suggests severe dehydration or hyperosmolarity. An initial Na that is normal or low and begins to fall with treatment merits prompt attention because it indicates either inappropriate fluid management or the onset of inappropriate diuretic hormone secretion (SIADH) and can signal impending cerebral edema.

27. **What is the typical potassium status in children with DKA?**

In almost all children in DKA, there is a **substantial potassium deficit** of 6–10 mEq/kg, although the initial serum K value is usually normal or high. If the initial K level is <3.5 mEq/L, 60 mEq/L should be added to the infusion, and close electrocardiogram monitoring should be instituted. If the initial K level is 3.5–5.5 mEq/L, 40 mEq/L of potassium is used. When the initial K level is >5.5 mEq/L, only 20 mEq/L is recommended. If the initial K level is >6 mEq/L, obtain an electrocardiogram and add K^+ only when the level falls to ≤5.5 mEq/L and the patient has voided.

28. **Why do potassium levels fall during the management of DKA?**

- Dilutional effects of rehydration
- Correction of acidosis (less K^+ exchanged out of cell for H^+ as pH rises)
- Insulin administration (increases cellular uptake of K^+)
- Ongoing urinary losses

Most patients are potassium depleted, although the serum K^+ is usually normal or elevated. A low K^+ is particularly worrisome, because it suggests severe potassium depletion.

29. **Should bicarbonate be used for the treatment of children with DKA?**

See Table 6-2.

30. **What are three clear indications for the use of bicarbonate?**

The establishment of an adequate intravascular volume and the provision of sufficient quantities of insulin are *far* more important in the treatment of DKA than bicarbonate. The decision to initiate bicarbonate therapy should be based on an arterial blood gas level and *not* a venous blood gas level. The three clear indications for bicarbonate therapy are as follows.

1. Symptomatic hyperkalemia
2. Cardiac instability
3. Inadequate ventilatory compensation

Each of these conditions requires admission to an intensive care unit, where appropriate monitoring can be undertaken and ventilatory assistance provided, if necessary.

TABLE 6-2.	PROS AND CONS OF BICARBONATE TREATMENT IN CHILDREN WITH DIABETIC KETOACIDOSIS
PRO	**CON**
Improved pH enhances myocardial contractility and response to catecholamines	Cardiac function problems are rare in children
Ventilatory response to acidosis blunted when pH is <7.0	Ventilatory response well maintained in children
No adverse effect of bicarbonate on oxygenation has been demonstrated clinically	May alter oxygen-binding of hemoglobin, potentially decreasing tissue oxygenation
Questionable relevance of central nervous system acidosis	Paradoxical central nervous system acidosis documented in humans
May be useful in the rare patient with hyperkalemia	Hypokalemia may result from uptake of K^+ as acidosis is corrected; low serum K is six times more common after bicarbonate treatment
	May be associated with increased hyperosmolarity and cerebral edema

31. **When should glucose be added to the infusate in patients with DKA?**
    When the glucose level approaches 300 mg/dL. It is usually wise to order the appropriate glucose-containing fluid in advance because it is not desirable to have a child become hypoglycemic. Many centers now use the "two-bag" method: they order two identical bags of intravenous fluid, one containing glucose and one without glucose. As the blood sugar approaches 200 mg/dL, glucose is added to the infusate (via a Y tube). With the two-bag system, it is possible to alter the concentration of glucose anywhere between 0% and 10%, with a goal of maintaining the blood sugar in the 100–200 mg/dL range, thereby avoiding hypoglycemia.

KEY POINTS: DIABETIC KETOACIDOSIS

1. Triad of metabolic derangement: Hyperglycemia, ketonemia, and acidosis.

2. Initial presentation in about one third of patients.

3. Abdominal pain can mimic appendicitis; hyperventilation can mimic pneumonia.

4. Administer insulin promptly to stop ketone and acid production.

5. Total body potassium is usually significantly diminished.

6. Cerebral edema is the most common cause of death.

7. If a normal or low sodium begins to fall with fluid replenishment, beware of secretion of antidiuretic hormone and possible cerebral edema.

8. Avoid excessive fluid therapy because of the risk of cerebral edema.

32. **Is continuous or bolus insulin better for the treatment of DKA?**
The choice of route of administration depends in part on the particular situation. In most centers, continuous insulin is preferred. Continuous insulin is given initially at a rate of 0.1 U/kg/h (after an initial bolus of 0.1 U/kg). This rate is adjusted to allow blood sugar to fall by 75–100 mg/dL/h. Alternatively, intramuscular insulin can be used with an initial dose of 0.25 U/kg and followed by 0.1 U/kg/h. Only regular insulin is used. Insulin lispro has not been evaluated for the management of DKA. Intermediate or long-acting insulins are not appropriate for the treatment of DKA

   Alternatively, hourly intramuscular injections may be easier to manage while a child is being transported between institutions. Continuous intravenous insulin is easier to titrate than intramuscular injections, although the differences may not be clinically significant. Most importantly, the injection of insulin subcutaneously is inappropriate until adequate hydration is established and the acidosis is resolving ($[HCO_3-]$ >15 mEq/L).

33. **How is the transition made to intermittent insulin therapy as DKA is resolving?**
The transition from insulin infusion to intermittent subcutaneous therapy is predicated on three factors:
   - **Normalization of biochemical parameters:** Insulin infusions should not be stopped until the blood sugar is <300 mg/dL, pH is >7.3, and HCO_3- is >15 mEq/L.
   - **Resumption of oral food intake:** As long as the patient is not eating and is receiving a constant supply of glucose by vein, it is easier to maintain a stable blood sugar using an insulin infusion rather than intermittent subcutaneous insulin. When oral intake is resumed, food is usually provided on an intermittent (bolus) basis; it is then reasonable to provide insulin in an intermittent fashion as well.
   - **Convenience/normal schedule:** Patients with diabetes generally are placed on a four-times-daily insulin regimen for the initial 24–36 hour period after an episode of ketoacidosis. Regular insulin is given before meals and before the bedtime snack. For the first dose of insulin after an episode of DKA, the child can be allowed to eat with the insulin drip running. If food is retained for 30 minutes without problems, a dose of subcutaneous insulin (0.25 U/kg) can be administered and the insulin infusion shut off. Subsequent doses of insulin should be given before meals.

34. **What risk factors are associated with the development of cerebral edema?**
Cerebral edema accounts for the majority of the 1–2% of case fatalities that occur in cases of DKA. It is unpredictable, often occurring as biochemical abnormalities are improving. It may be sudden in onset or occur gradually, but it typically occurs during the first 5–15 hours after therapy begins. Risk factors include the following:
   - <5 years of age
   - Newly diagnosed diabetics
   - Higher initial blood urea nitrogen level
   - Smaller increase in plasma sodium concentration during therapy

Glaser N, Barnett P, McCaslin I, et al; Pediatric Emergency Medicine Collaborative Research Committee of the American Academy of Pediatrics: Risk factors for cerebral edema in children with diabetic ketoacidosis. N Engl JMed 344:264–269, 2001.

Marcin JP, Glaser N, Barnett P, et al; American Academy of Pediatrics; The Pediatric Emergency Medicine Collaborative Research Commitee: Factors associated with adverse outcomes in children with diabetic ketoacidosis-related cerebral edema. J Pediatr 141:793–797, 2002.

35. **What signs and symptoms suggest worsening cerebral edema during the treatment of DKA?**
   - Decreasing sensorium
   - Combativeness, disorientation, and agitation
   - Sudden and severe headache

- Cranial nerve palsies
- Incontinence
- Pupillary asymmetry or sluggish responses
- Vomiting
- Papilledema
- Inappropriate slowing of heart rate
- Seizure

Early recognition is vital because intervention (e.g., intravenous mannitol, intubation, hyperventilation) can improve outcome in 50% of patients.

Maloney CP, Vicek BW, DelAguila M, Risk factors for developing brain herniation during diabetic ketoacidosis. Pediatr Neurol 21:721–727, 1999.

Rosenbloom AL, Schatz DA, Krischer JP, et al: Therapeutic controversy: Prevention and treatment of diabetes in children. J Clin Endo Metab 85:494–522, 2000.

DIABETES MELLITUS

36. **What are the risks of a child developing insulin-dependent diabetes mellitus (type 1) if one sibling is affected?**
- Identical twins: >50%
- HLA identical: 20%
- HLA haploidentical: 5%
- HLA nonidentical: 1%

Plotnick L: Insulin-dependent diabetes mellitus. Pediatr Rev 15:137–148, 1994.

37. **Can the development of diabetes in other siblings be predicted?**
In one series of 661 children who had a sibling with diabetes mellitus, 49 went on to develop type 1 diabetes. All but 6 cases were predicted on the basis of islet-cell autoantibody formation or an abnormal glucose tolerance test. If a sibling develops such an antibody *and* an abnormal glucose tolerance test, the risk for the development of diabetes mellitus increases 1,300-fold. Much research centers on ways of modulating the development of diabetes in those patients through the use of exogenous insulin or immunomodulators; however, no successful trials have yet been reported.

American Diabetes Association: www.diabetes.org

Mrena S, Savola K, Kulmala P, et al: Staging of preclinical type 1 diabetes in siblings of affected children. Childhood Diabetes in Finland Study Group. Pediatrics 104:925–930, 1999.

38. **How long does the "honeymoon" period last in newly diagnosed insulin-dependent diabetics?**
The "honeymoon" usually begins within 1–2 weeks after the initiation of insulin treatment. It is a period of falling or minimal exogenous insulin requirements that reflects continued residual endogenous insulin production. The duration of the honeymoon in a particular individual may last for a few weeks or months, but this is not predictable. However, evidence is accumulating that it may be prolonged by the maintenance of excellent control. Cessation of the honeymoon is often heralded by elevated fasting blood glucose levels before breakfast or by an increasing insulin requirement.

39. **How do the types of insulin vary in their timing and duration of action?**
See Table 6-3.

TABLE 6-3. INSULIN

Insulin*	Onset	Peak	Effective Duration (h)
Rapid-acting	5–15 min	30–90 min	3–5
Lispro (Humalog)			
Aspart (NovoLog)			
Short-acting	30–60 min	2–3 h	4–8
Regular U100			
Regular U500 (concentrated)			
Buffered regular (Velosulin)			
Intermediate-acting			
Isophane insulin (NPH, Humulin N/Novolin N)	2–4 h	4–10 h	10–16
Insulin zinc (Lente, Humulin L/Novolin L)	2–4 h	4–12 h	12–18
Long-acting			
Insulin zinc extended (Ultralente, Humulin U)	6–10 h	10–16 h	18–24
Glargine (Lantus)	2–4 h†	No peak	20–24

L = lente, NPH = neutral protamine Hagedorn, insulin lispro protamine (neutral protamine lispro).
*Assuming 0.1–0.2 U/kg per injection. Onset and duration vary significantly by injection site.
†Time to steady state.
Adapted from The American Diabetes Association: *Practical Insulin: A Handbook for Prescribing Providers,* 2002.

40. **What are the typical insulin dosages given after the "honeymoon" period?**
    Prepubertal children generally require about 0.5 U/kg/day. During the middle of puberty, dosages often exceed 1 U/kg/day, whereas postpubertal individuals require 0.75–1.0 U/kg/day. Athletes or those with a low caloric intake may require less insulin. For most children with type 1 diabetes, there are a variety of strategies and combinations of insulin that are currently used. There is a trend toward three or more doses of insulin each day. In addition, more children are on insulin pump therapy.

    DeWitt DE, Dugdale DC: Using new insulin strategies in the outpatient treatment of diabetes. JAMA 289: 2265–2269, 2003.

41. **When should the Somogyi phenomenon be suspected?**
    The Somogyi phenomenon is rebound hyperglycemia after an incident of hypoglycemia. This rebound is secondary to the release of counter-regulatory hormones, which is the natural response to hypoglycemia. As tighter diabetic control is maintained, there is an increased likelihood of hypoglycemia and, therefore, of the Somogyi phenomenon. If the hypoglycemia is recognized and treated promptly, rebound hyperglycemia is less likely to occur. Thus, the Somogyi is commonly reported more frequently at night because there is the greater likelihood of unrecognized and untreated hypoglycemia when the child is asleep. The Somogyi phenomenon should be suspected when a child whose blood sugar is in excellent control begins to have intermittent high blood glucoses in the morning. If that pattern is noted, blood glucose should be checked between 2:00 and 3:00 AM on several nights to determine

if hypoglycemia is occurring. If hypoglycemia can be documented, the dose or type of evening insulin may need to be altered, or the time that the dose is given may need to be changed.

42. **What causes the "dawn phenomenon"?**

The term *dawn phenomenon* describes a rise in blood glucose that occurs during the early morning hours (between 5:00 and 8:00 AM), particularly among patients who have normal glucose levels throughout most of the night. The rise in glucose is thought to be due to several factors, including the following:
- The normal increase in the morning cortisol level
- The cumulative effect of increased nocturnal growth hormone
- Insulinopenia as a result of the length of time since the last injection

Possible strategies for managing the dawn phenomenon include shifting the intermediate-acting insulin dose to a later time (before the bedtime snack), using a type of insulin with a longer duration of action (e.g., ultralente, insulin glargine), or initiating insulin pump therapy.

KEY POINTS: DIABETES MELLITUS TYPE 1

1. Destruction of pancreatic islet cells causes an absolute insulin deficiency.

2. Classic triad of symptoms: Polyuria, polydipsia, and polyphagia.

3. Tighter glucose control substantially lowers complication rates of retinopathy, nephropathy, and neuropathy.

4. Obtaining a hemoglobin A_{1C} (glycosylated) level is a way to assess average control over the previous 2–3 months.

5. Puberty is a time of increased insulin resistance, thereby requiring increased dosing.

43. **How rapidly can renal disease develop after the onset of diabetes mellitus?**

Microscopic changes in the glomerular basement membrane are present by 2 years after the diagnosis of diabetes. Microalbuminuria is often present within 10–15 years, and this is followed by a proteinuric period (>0.5 gm per 24 hours). Beyond this point, there is often a relentless decline in glomerular function. An azotemic period begins on average by the time the patient is 17 years old, and frank uremia occurs by the age of 20 years. Retrospective studies suggest that as many as 50% of patients with insulin-dependent diabetes mellitus diagnosed before the age of 30 years will develop end-stage renal disease. Patients with diabetic nephropathy account for 25% of those receiving long-term renal dialysis in the United States. Progression can be delayed by meticulous attention to glycemic control.

Joslin Diabetes Center: www.joslin.org

44. **How is hemoglobin A_1C helpful for monitoring diabetic control?**

Glycohemoglobin, also known as glycosylated hemoglobin or hemoglobin A_1C, is a hemoglobin-glucose combination formed nonenzymatically within the cell. Initially, an unstable bond is formed between glucose and the hemoglobin molecule. With time, this bond rearranges to form a more stable compound in which glucose is covalently bound to the hemoglobin molecule. The amount of the unstable form may rise rapidly in the presence of a high blood glucose level, while the stable form changes slowly and provides a time-average integral of the blood glucose concentration through the 120-day lifespan of the red blood cell. Thus, glycohemoglobin levels provide an objective measurement of averaged diabetic control over time. The American Diabetic Association recommends a level <7%.

45. Is tight control of diabetes better than conventional control?

The Diabetes Control and Complications Trial (DCCT) evaluated more than 1,400 diabetics (nearly 200 of whom were adolescents). Study subjects were randomized to receive either standard diabetic therapy (e.g., twice-daily insulin shots) or more intensive therapy (e.g., more frequent blood glucose monitoring and three or more shots daily). Intensive control reduced the risk of development of retinopathy by 53% and the occurrence of microalbuminuria by 55% as compared with conventional control. Subsequent follow-up 7–8 years after the end of the trial has revealed sustained renal benefits. The major adverse effect was a threefold increase in the rate of severe hypoglycemia. Whether the benefits of tighter control outweigh the potential risks of hypoglycemia in younger pediatric patients remains unknown.

DCCT Research Group: Retinopathy and nephropathy in patients with type 1 diabetes four years after a trial of intensive therapy. N Engl J Med 342:381–389, 2000.

Writing Team for the DCCT: Sustained effect of intensive treatment of type 1 diabetes mellitus on development and progression of diabetic nephropathy. JAMA 290:2159–2167, 2003.

46. What pathophysiologic process characterizes type 2 diabetes?

The key characteristic of type 2 diabetes is resistance to insulin action. There many also be insulin secretory defects.

47. Is the incidence of type 2 diabetes increasing?

Dramatically. Previously rare in pediatrics, it has increased 10-fold in the 1990s in some centers in the United States, and it accounts for half of new-onset diabetes cases. Some estimates expect that one of every three children born in the year 2000 will develop diabetes. The reason for the increase is unclear, but it is likely related to current trends of increasing childhood obesity, poor dietary habits, and sedentary behavior.

Fagot-Campagna A, Pettitt DJ, Engelgau MM, et al: Type 2 diabetes among North American children and adolescents: An epidemiologic review and a public health perspective. J Pediatr 136:664–672, 2000.

Narayan KM, Boyle JP, Thompson TJ, et al: Lifetime risk for diabetes mellitus in the United States. New Orleans, American Diabetes Association, 2003.

48. What historical and clinical features suggest type 2 rather than type 1 diabetes?

- **Obesity** is the hallmark of type 2 diabetes, whereas it is rare in children with type 1 diabetes at diagnosis.
- **Racial and ethnic minority groups,** particularly African Americans, Mexican Americans, and Pima Indians, are often affected.
- **Family history** is usually strongly positive; >50% of affected children have one or more first-degree relatives with type 2 diabetes.
- **Acanthosis nigricans** is present in 90% of cases.
- **Hyperandrogenism** is another disorder that is associated with insulin resistance and obesity.
- **Puberty** increases insulin resistance in all adolescents as a result of high levels of growth hormone.
- **Differing symptoms:** Unlike patients with type 1 diabetes, most youth with type 2 diabetes have little or no weight loss and absent or mild polyuria or nocturia, and the majority have glycosuria without ketonuria (although up to 33% can have ketonuria).

Liu L, Hironaka K, Pihoker C: Type 2 diabetes in youth. Curr Probl Pediatr Adolesc Health Care 34:254–272, 2004.

49. What is acanthosis nigricans?

Acanthosis nigricans is demonstrated by hyperpigmented, velvety patches that are found most prominently in intertriginous areas, especially on the nape of the neck (Fig. 6-1). These serve as a marker for insulin resistance.

50. **How is type 2 diabetes diagnosed?**
    - Random glucose concentration of ≥200 mg/dL
    - Fasting (>8 hours) glucose concentration of >126 mg/dL
    - Abnormal oral glucose tolerance test (glucose concentration >200 mg/dL after drinking 1.75 gm/kg of glucose)
      Although classification can usually be made on the basis of clinical characteristics, measurement of levels of fasting insulin and C-peptide (low in type 1; normal or elevated in type 2) or islet-cell autoantibodies (present in type 1; generally absent in type 2) can be useful.

    American Diabetes Association. Type 2 diabetes in children and adolescents. Pediatrics 105:671–680, 2000.

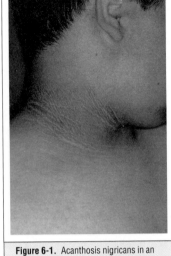

Figure 6-1. Acanthosis nigricans in an adolescent male. (From Schachner LA, Hansen RC (eds): Pediatric Dermatology, 3rd ed. Edinburgh, Mosby, 2003, p 915.)

51. **Which pediatric patients should be screened for type 2 diabetes?**
    Beginning at 10 years of age (or earlier if puberty initiates before age 10), a fasting blood sugar should be obtained for patients with any of the following:
    - Body mass index >85th percentile for age and sex
    - Any *two* of following risk factors:
      1. Positive family history in first- or second-degree relative
      2. Native American, African American, Hispanic, or Asian/Pacific Islander
      3. Presence of associated conditions (acanthosis nigricans, hypertension, dyslipidemia, polycystic ovarian syndrome)

    American Diabetes Association: Type 2 diabetes in children and adolescents. Diabetes Care 23:381–389, 2000

KEY POINTS: DIABETES MELLITUS TYPE 2

1. Tissue-level insulin resistance

2. Incidence: Rising rapidly as a result of the epidemic of obesity

3. Acanthosis nigricans: Rash found in 90% of cases

4. Diagnosis based on detecting hyperglycemia: Fasting (≥126 mg/dL), random (≥200 mg/dL), and postprandial glucose challenge (≥200 mg/dL)

5. Screen patients based on known risk factors (obesity, ethnicity, family history)

52. **When should oral hypoglycemic agents be considered as part of therapy?**
    If glucose control is not achieved with dietary adjustments and exercise within 2–3 months, oral hypoglycemic agents should be considered. Data in children and adolescents are

limited. Metformin (Glucophage) is the best studied and is recommended as initial therapy by many experts, but four category types of oral agents for use in type 2 diabetes are available.

Liu L, Hironaka K, Pihoker C: Type 2 diabetes in youth. Curr Probl Pediatr Adolesc Health Care 34:254–272, 2004.

GROWTH DISTURBANCES

53. **How do the growth rates of boys and girls differ?**
In both boys and girls, the rate or velocity of linear growth begins to decelerate at about 2 years of age. In girls, this deceleration continues until the age of approximately 11 years, at which time the adolescent growth spurt begins. For boys, the deceleration continues until the age of about 13 years. The peak rate of increase in males occurs at 14 years of age.

54. **What is the best predictor of a child's eventual adult height?**
Mid-parental height. This is an estimate of a child's expected genetic growth potential based on parental heights (preferably measured rather than by history).
- For girls: ([father's height – 13 cm] + [mother's height])/2.
- For boys: ([mother's height + 13 cm] + [father's height])/2.
This gives a rough range (±5 cm) of expected adult height. The predicted height can be compared with the present height percentile, and any significant deviation can be a clue of an abnormal growth pattern in a child. It is important to remember that some forms of growth hormone deficiency are inherited, so one should not automatically assume that the short child with short parents has familial short stature.

55. **When have most children achieved the height percentiles that are consistent with parental height?**
By the age of 2 years. Rough estimates of ultimate adult height can be obtained by taking a boy's length at age 2 years and a girl's length at age 18 months and doubling them.

56. **Name the major categories of causes of short stature.**
- Genetic
- Constitutional delay ("late bloomer")
- Chronic disease (e.g., inflammatory bowel disease, chronic renal failure, renal tubular acidosis, cyanotic congenital heart disease)
- Chromosomal/syndromic (e.g., Turner [45,X], 18q–, Down, achondroplasia)
- Endocrine (e.g., hypothyroidism, growth hormone deficiency, hypopituitarism, hypercortisolism [endogenous and exogenous])
- Psychosocial (e.g., chaotic social situation, orphanage)
- Intrauterine (e.g., small for gestational age)
Genetic patterns and constitutional delay account for the largest percentage of known causes.

57. **In a child with short stature, what rate of growth makes an endocrinologic cause unlikely?**
Rates of growth are age dependent. In general, a growth rate of ≥6 cm per year between the ages of 2 and 5 years or ≥5 cm per year in children between the age of 5 years and the adolescent growth spurt makes an endocrinologic cause of short stature less likely. The importance of sequential measurements using standard growth charts cannot be underestimated. Growth rates below the third percentile or crossing percentiles downward warrant further investigation.

58. **When evaluating a short child, why should you ask when the parents reached puberty?**

The age at which puberty occurred in other family members may help identify children with constitutional delay because this entity tends to run in families. Most women will remember their age at menarche, and this age can be used as a reference for the age at which other pubertal events occurred. The strongest association for pubertal delay is between father and son. The most useful reference point for adult males is the age at which they reached adult height because almost all normal males will have reached their adult height by the age of 17 years (around high-school graduation). Significant growth beyond this age suggests a history of pubertal delay.

59. **When does the pubertal growth spurt occur?**

For children with an average growth rate, pubertal growth begins earlier in girls. Mean age at the initiation of this spurt is 11 years for boys and 9 years for girls. Peak height velocity occurs at 13.5 years for boys and 11.5 years for girls. Peak velocity occurs at Tanner breast stage 2–3 for girls and Tanner testis stage 3–4 for boys. Girls generally stop growing at an average of 14 years of age, but boys continue to grow until 17 years of age.

Rogol AD, Roemmich JN, Clark PA: Growth at puberty. J Adolesc Health 31(6 Suppl):192–200, 2002.

60. **Are upper to lower body ratios helpful for the diagnosis of growth problems?**

Disproportionate short stature generally refers to an inappropriate ratio between truncal length and limb length (upper to lower segment ratio). Lower segment (limb length) is the distance from the superior border of the pubic bone to the floor surface. Height minus the lower segment gives the height of the upper segment (truncal length). In an infant, the head and trunk are quite long relative to the limbs, so the ratio of truncal length to limb length is about 1.7. Throughout childhood, this ratio declines, so that by 7–10 years of age this ratio is about 1.0. The adult ratio is 0.9.

An increased ratio is seen in bony dysplasias (e.g., achondroplasia, hypochondroplasia), hypothyroidism, gonadal dysgenesis, and Klinefelter syndrome (the patients are then tall in adolescence). Decreased ratios are seen in certain syndromes (e.g., Marfan syndrome), spinal disorders (e.g., scoliosis), and specific types of therapy (e.g., spinal irradiation).

Halac I, Zimmerman D: Evaluating short stature in children. Pediatr Ann 33:170–176, 2004.

61. **What laboratory studies should be obtained when evaluating short stature?**

Extensive laboratory tests are generally not indicated, unless the growth rate is abnormally low. Laboratory testing may include any or all of the following: complete blood count, urinalysis, chemistry panel, sedimentation rate, thyroxine, thyroid-stimulating hormone, insulin-like growth factor-I (IGF-I), and IGF-binding protein-3 (IGFBP-3).

Random growth hormone levels are of little value because they are generally low in the daytime, even in children of average height. IGF-I (or somatomedin C) mediates the anabolic effects of growth hormone, and levels correlate well with growth hormone status. However, IGF-I can also be low in nonendocrine conditions (e.g., malnutrition, liver disease).

IGFBP-3, which is the major binding protein for IGF-I in serum, is also regulated by growth hormone. IGFBP-3 levels generally indicate growth hormone status and are less affected by nutritional factors than IGF-I. Many endocrinologists now use IGF-I and IGFBP-3 as their initial screening tests for growth hormone deficiency.

Dattani M, Preece M: Growth hormone deficiency and related disorders: Insights into causation, diagnosis, and treatment. Lancet 363:1977–1987, 2004.

62. **In a very obese child, how does height measurement help to determine whether an endocrinopathy might be the cause?**

In children with simple obesity (e.g., familial), linear growth is enhanced; in children with endocrinopathies, it is usually impaired. If the height of a child is at or greater than the mid-parental height percentile, an endocrine cause of the obesity is unlikely. An exception is patients with Cushing syndrome, in which abnormal growth may not be a clue.

63. How does a growth chart help determine the diagnosis of failure to thrive?
If an infant is demonstrating deceleration of a previously established growth pattern or growth that is consistently less than the fifth percentile, the pattern of growth of head circumference, height, and weight can help establish the likely cause (Fig. 6-2). There are three main types of impaired growth:

- **Type I:** Retardation of weight with near-normal or slowly decelerating height and head circumference; most commonly seen in undernourished patients

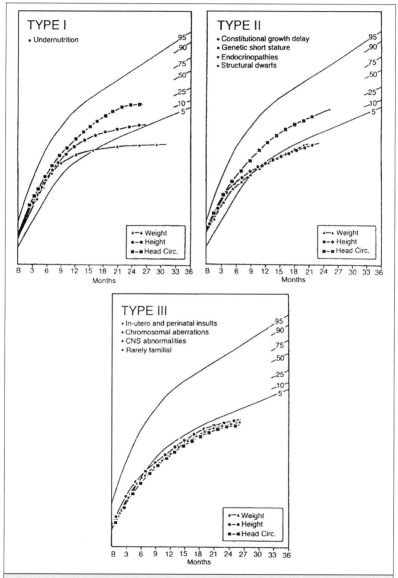

Figure 6-2. Types I, II, and III of impaired growth. (From Roy CC, Silverman A, Alagille DA: Pediatric Clinical Gastroenterology, 4th ed. St. Louis, Mosby, 1995, pp 4–8.)

- **Type II:** Near-proportional retardation of weight and height with normal head circumference; most commonly seen in patients with constitutional growth delay, genetic short stature, endocrinopathies, and structural dwarfism
- **Type III:** Concomitant retardation of weight, height, and head circumference; seen in patients with in utero and perinatal insults, chromosomal aberrations, and central nervous system abnormalities

64. **What is bone age?**

A measure of somatic maturity and growth potential. Standards of normal skeletal radiographic maturation are available, and these are based on the progression of ossification centers that occur with age. A radiograph of the hand and wrist is taken and compared with those standards to determine a patient's bone age. This result can be compared with chronologic age to gauge the remaining potential for growth.

65. **Why is a bone-age determination helpful for evaluating short stature?**

A single bone age is of value for differentiating familial short stature and genetic diseases, in which bone age is normal, from other causes of short stature. A **delayed bone age** (>2 standard deviations below the mean) that correlates with the child's height age (age on growth chart at which child's height would be at the 50th percentile) is suggestive of constitutional delay, whereas a **markedly delayed bone age** is suggestive of endocrinologic disease. Serial bone ages determined every 6–12 months are often helpful, because, in both the normal child and the child with constitutional delay, the bone age will advance in parallel with the chronologic age. In endocrinologic disease, the bone age falls progressively further behind the chronologic age. Bone age may be normal or delayed in patients with chronic disease, depending on the severity of disease, its duration, and the type of treatment used.

66. **What features suggest constitutional delay as a cause of short stature?**
- No signs or symptoms of systemic disease
- Bone age delayed up to 2–4 years but consistent with height age
- Period of poorest growth often occurring between the ages of 18 and 30 months, with steady linear growth thereafter (i.e., normal rate of growth for bone age)
- Parental or sibling history of delayed development
- Height predictions consistent with family characteristics

KEY POINTS: GROWTH DISTURBANCES

1. Bone age as a diagnostic key: Genetically determined short stature (bone age = chronologic age) versus constitutional delay (bone age < chronologic age.

2. Midline defects (e.g., single maxillary incisor, cleft lip/palate) and short stature suggest hypopituitarism.

3. Random growth hormone levels are usually not helpful (due to pulsatile delivery during sleep); provocative testing is more reliable.

4. Family history is key. Use growth data about family—especially siblings—to establish a pattern.

5. Short stature with overweight suggests endocrinopathy (adrenal, thyroid) and growth hormone deficiency.

6. Growth hormone deficiency that appears during the first year of life is associated with hypoglycemia; after the age of 5 years, it is associated with short stature.

67. **How is constitutional delay managed?**

    If the results of history, physical examination, and clinical laboratory evaluation are unremarkable, the child is seen once every 3–6 months for accurate height measurements and determination of growth rate. A bone age may be done yearly to assess the progression of bony maturation. In patients with constitutional delay, the rate of bone maturation should keep pace with the chronologic age. In children who are of mid to late pubertal ages (girls, >13 years; boys, >14 years) but showing minimal or no signs of puberty, selective use may be made of estrogen or testosterone supplementation to initiate puberty, or additional assessment may be indicated.

68. **Should growth hormone therapy be given to the normal short child?**

    This is one of the hotter areas of controversy in pediatric endocrinology. Opponents argue that short stature is not a disease, that current height velocity may not be predictive, and that what constitutes growth hormone sufficiency and insufficiency is not clearly defined. Long-term safety remains under study, and some recent studies suggest impairment of testicular function in treated males. Proponents counter that the treatment is safe and does improve height in 50% of treated patients to at least 5 cm greater than pretreatment predictions. Surveys have indicated that a majority of pediatric endocrinologists support growth hormone use in patients with short stature, normal growth-hormone stimulation tests, and subnormal growth velocity.

    Miller BS, Zimmerman D: Idiopathic short stature. Pediatr Ann 33:177–181, 2004.

    Saenger PJ: The case in support of growth hormone therapy. J Pediatr 136:106–109, 2000.

    Voss LD: Growth hormone therapy for the normal short child: Who needs it and who wants it? The case against growth hormone therapy. J Pediatr 136:103–106, 2000.

69. **What are the clinical manifestations of growth hormone excess?**

    Before puberty, the cardinal manifestations are an increase in growth velocity with minimal bone deformity and soft-tissue swelling—a condition called **pituitary gigantism.** Hypogonadotropic hypogonadism and delayed puberty often coexist with growth hormone excess, and affected children exhibit eunuchoid body proportions. If the growth hormone excess occurs after puberty (after epiphyseal closure), the more typical features of **acromegaly** occur, including coarsening of the facial features and soft-tissue swelling of the feet and hands. Growth hormone excess is rare in children.

HYPOGLYCEMIA

70. **How is hypoglycemia defined?**

    A serum glucose of <50 mg/100 mL is defined as hypoglycemia in childhood. Some argue for lower levels being used for term and preterm infants; however, these arguments are based on population sampling data rather than on physiology. Hypoglycemia is a laboratory finding, and its presence should always lead to a diligent search for the underlying pathology.

71. **Describe the clinical findings associated with hypoglycemia.**

    Neuroglycopenic symptoms include irritability, headache, confusion, unconsciousness, and seizure. **Adrenergic** signs include tachycardia, tremulousness, diaphoresis, and hunger. Any combination of the above signs and symptoms should lead to the measurement of the blood glucose level.

72. **What are the causes of childhood hypoglycemia?**

    No single cause predominates in any age group. Therefore, the entire differential diagnosis must be considered in any child who presents symptoms of hypoglycemia. Hypoglycemia often occurs as a result of a combination of two or more of the problems listed in Table 6-4 (e.g., prolonged fasting during an illness coupled with fever in medium-chain acyl-CoA dehydrogenase deficiency).

TABLE 6-4. DIFFERENTIAL DIAGNOSIS OF CHILDHOOD HYPOGLYCEMIA

Increased glucose utilization
Hyperinsulinism: Islet-cell adenoma or hyperplasia (nesidioblastosis), oral hypoglycemic
agents, exogenous insulin

Decreased glucose production
Inadequate glycogen reserves: Enzymatic defects in glycogen synthesis and glycogenolysis
Ineffective gluconeogenesis: Inadequate substrate (e.g., ketotic hypoglycemia), enzymatic
defects

Diminished availability of fats
Depleted fat stores
Failure to mobilize fats (e.g., hyperinsulinism)
Defective use of fats: Enzymatic defects in fatty-acid oxidation (e.g., medium-chain acyl
CoA dehydrogenase deficiency)

Decreased fuels and fuel stores
Fasting, malnutrition, prolonged illness, malabsorption

Increased fuel demand
Fever, exercise

Inadequate counterregulatory hormones
Growth hormone or cortisol deficiency, hypopituitarism

---

73. **An unconscious 3-year-old girl is brought to the emergency department with a
serum glucose concentration of 26 mg/dL. What other laboratory tests should
be performed?**
The principal laboratory evaluations should include the measurement of the following: (1) the
metabolic compounds associated with fasting adaptation; (2) the hormones that regulate these
processes; and (3) drugs that can interfere with glucose regulation.
A 3-mL red-top tube of **blood** can be sent for the measurement of the following:
- markers of the principal regulatory hormones: insulin, growth hormone, and cortisol;
- markers of fatty-acid metabolism: ketones (b-hydroxybutyrate and acetoacetate), free fatty
acids, and total and free carnitine; and
- markers of gluconeogenic pathways: lactate, pyruvate, and alanine.
  Urine can be tested for the following:
- ketones;
- metabolic byproducts associated with known causes of hypoglycemia (e.g., organic acids,
amino acids); and
- toxicology screen, especially for alcohol and salicylates.
   Taken together, these tests provide valuable clues as to the cause. For example, low
levels of ketones and free fatty acids suggest that fat was not appropriately mobilized. As a
consequence, ketones were not formed by the liver. Those biochemical abnormalities are seen

in hyperinsulinemic states and can be confirmed by documenting a high level of circulating insulin. Low urinary ketones also suggest an enzymatic defect in fatty acid oxidation.

Pershad J, Monroe K, Atchison J: Childhood hypoglycemia in an urban emergency department: Epidemiology and diagnostic approach to the problem. Pediatr Emerg Care 14:268–271, 1998.

74. **In patients with acute hypoglycemia, what are the treatment options?**
The principal acute treatment is the provision of glucose orally or intravenously. If the patient is alert, 4–8 ounces of a sugared beverage (e.g., orange juice, cola) may be given. If the patient is obtunded, intravenous glucose (2–3 mL/kg of $D_{10}W$ or 1 mL/kg of $D_{25}W$) should be administered rapidly. If venous access cannot be achieved promptly, glucose can be provided via a nasogastric tube because glucose is rapidly absorbed from the gut. The risk of prolonged hypoglycemia far outweighs the risk associated with the passage of a nasogastric tube in an obtunded patient. Subsequently, the blood sugar should be monitored closely and, if necessary, maintained by the constant infusion of glucose (6–8 mg/kg/min). D_{10} in an electrolyte solution given at about 1.5-times maintenance dose approximates that glucose rate. Larger quantities may be necessary, and the blood sugar should be closely followed. Glucagon promotes glycogen breakdown. In settings in which glycogen stores have not been depleted (e.g., insulin overdose), 1 mg of glucagon intramuscularly or subcutaneously will raise blood glucose levels.

Glucocorticoids should not be used routinely. Their only clear indication is in known primary or secondary adrenal insufficiency. In other settings, they have little acute value and may cloud the diagnostic process. The decision to use glucocorticoids is somewhat dependent on the child's medical history (e.g., reasonable to use in the context of a history of prior central nervous system irradiation).

HYPOTHALAMIC/PITUITARY DISORDERS

75. **What clinical signs or symptoms suggest hypothalamic dysfunction?**
The signs and symptoms of hypothalamic dysfunction are as variable as the processes controlled by the hypothalamus, ranging from disorders of hormonal production to disturbances of thermoregulation. Precocious or delayed sexual maturation represent the most common presentations of hypothalamic endocrine abnormality in childhood. Diabetes insipidus, psychic disturbances, and excessive sleepiness are found in about a third of all patients with hypothalamic dysfunction and may be the first manifestation of disease. Eating disorders (obesity, anorexia, bulimia) and convulsions are also reported. Dyshidrosis and disturbances of sphincteric control are occasionally seen.

76. **List the intracranial processes that can interfere with hypothalamic-pituitary function.**
- **Congenital:** Inherited deficiencies of gonadotropin-releasing factor, growth-hormone-releasing hormone; syndromic (Laurence-Moon-Diedl and Prader-Labhart-Willi syndromes); structural (craniopharyngioma, Rathke pouch cyst, hemangioma, hamartoma)
- **Infectious:** Meningitis and encephalitis
- **Tumors:** Glioma, dysgerminoma, and ependymoma
- **Idiopathic**

77. **What is the significance of an enlarged sella turcica on a skull film?**
The sella turcica derives its name from the Latin words for *Turkish saddle*. The name reflects the anatomic shape of the saddle-like prominence on the upper surface of the sphenoid bone in the middle cranial fossa, above which sits the pituitary gland. A variety of conditions can lead to sellar enlargement, including tumors of the pituitary or functional hypertrophy of the pituitary, which may occur in primary hypothyroidism or primary hypogonadism. Modern

imaging techniques have supplanted the skull series as a tool for searching for pituitary or hypothalamic disease; however, an enlarged sella may be noted on children in whom skull series are obtained for other reasons (e.g., head trauma).

78. **Which tests are useful for studying suspected hypothalamic and pituitary malfunction?**
Either magnetic resonance imaging or computed tomography scanning is required to rule out structural pathology before searching for functional abnormalities. Studies of the pituitary-hypothalamus may include any or all of the following:

- **Prolactin:** Random levels tend to be elevated in the presence of hypothalamic lesions. A normal level does not rule out structural abnormalities.
- **Thyrotropin-releasing hormone (TRH) provocative test:** TRH normally promotes the rapid release of thyroid-stimulating hormone (TSH) by the pituitary. In the presence of pituitary or hypothalamic dysfunction, the release of TSH is often blunted and delayed. TRH also promotes the release of prolactin. In patients with hypothalamic dysfunction, the prolactin response is often altered as well.
- **Growth hormone production tests** (*see* question 61): These tests are generally indicated only if the child's growth rate is subnormal. Growth hormone releasing factor is now available for testing pituitary responsiveness. It has proven useful, in some instances, for delineating pituitary causes of growth hormone underproduction from primary hypothalamic disease.
- **Gonadotropin-releasing hormone (GnRH) provocative test:** Random levels of leuteinizing hormone and follicle-stimulating hormone are not generally helpful if one is searching for pituitary hypofunction. The results of the GnRH test must be correlated with the age of the child, because there are developmental changes in the response to GnRH. GnRH is not currently available for use in testing.
- **Simultaneous urine and serum osmolalities:** A normal serum osmolality and a concentrated urine osmolality tend to rule out diabetes insipidus. If these results are equivocal, a water deprivation test may be required.

SEXUAL DIFFERENTIATION AND DEVELOPMENT

79. **An infant is born with ambiguous genitalia. What features of the history and physical examination are key in the evaluation?**
History: One should search for evidence of maternal androgen ingestion (rare now, but common in the 1960s with certain progestational agents), other hormonal use (e.g., for infertility or endometriosis), alcohol use, parental consanguinity, previous neonatal deaths, or a family history of previously affected children.
Physical examination: The presence of a gonadal structure in the labioscrotal fold strongly implies the presence of some Y chromosomal material. Gonads containing both ovarian and testicular components (ovotestes) have been found in the inguinal canal. However, it is rare to find an ovary in the inguinal canal. In the absence of a palpable gonad, no conclusions can be drawn regarding probable chromosomal sex. The size of the phallic structure and the location of the urethral meatus provide no information about genetic or chromosomal make up. However, phallic size and function are important considerations when determining the sex the child will be reared.

The presence of **midline abnormalities** (e.g., cleft palate) suggests hypothalamic or pituitary dysfunction, whereas congenital anomalies such as imperforate anus suggest structural derangements. A digital rectal examination will confirm the patency of the anus and may allow palpation of the uterus. Other anomalies should be noted because ambiguous genitalia can be a feature of numerous syndromes.

Sultan C, Paris F, Jeandel C, et al: Ambiguous genitalia in the newborn: Diagnosis, etiology and sex assignment. Endocr Dev 7:23–38, 2004.

80. **What are the causes of ambiguous genitalia?**
   1. **Undervirilized male** (XY karyotype)
      - *Androgen resistance:* Complete (testicular feminization), partial
      - *Defects of androgen synthesis:* 3beta-hydroxysteroid dehydrogenase deficiency, 5alpha-reductase deficiency
   2. **Virilized female** (XX karyotype)
      - *Excess androgen:* Congenital adrenal hyperplasia, 21-hydroxylase deficiency, 3beta-hydroxysteroid dehydrogenase deficiency
      - *Maternal androgen exposure:* Medication, virilizing adrenal tumor
   3. **Intersex** (mosaic karyotypes; e.g., XO/XY)
   4. **Structural abnormalities**

   MacLaughlin DT, Donahoe PK: Sex determination and differentiation. N Engl J Med 350:367–378, 2004.

81. **Which studies are essential for the evaluation of ambiguous genitalia?**
   - **Ultrasonography:** This test is the most helpful for identifying internal structures, particularly the uterus and occasionally the ovaries. The absence of a uterus suggests that testes were present early in gestation and produced Müllerian-inhibiting factor, thereby causing regression of the Müllerian-derived ducts and thus the uterus. The injection of contrast medium into the urethrovaginal opening(s) will often demonstrate a pouch posterior to the fused labioscrotal folds. Occasionally, the cervix and cervical canal will be highlighted by this study as well.
   - **Chromosomal analysis:** Obviously, this is useful for predicting gonadal content. Buccal smears searching for clumps of the nuclear membrane chromatin (Barr bodies, which represent the inactive X chromosome in girls) should not be used (even preliminarily) because of their high rates of inaccuracy.
   - **Measurement of adrenal steroids** (17-hydroxyprogesterone, 11-deoxycortisol, 17-hydroxypregnenolone): 17-Hydroxyprogesterone is the precursor that is elevated in the most common variety of congenital adrenal hyperplasia associated with ambiguous genitalia (21-hydroxylase deficiency).
   - **Measurement of testosterone and dihydrotestosterone**

   As important and useful as the testing is, it is also useful to have input from staff with expertise in this area, including a geneticist, a pediatric endocrinologist, and a pediatric urologist. It is also essential that information be synthesized by this group after all data are available and that it be communicated to the family by a single spokesperson.

   American Academy of Pediatrics, Committee on Genetics, Section on Endocrinology and Section on Urology: Developmental anomalies of the external genitalia in the newborn. Pediatrics 106:138–142, 2000.
   Rangecroft L; British Association of Paediatric Surgeons Working Party on the Surgical Management of Children Born with Ambiguous Genitalia: Surgical management of ambiguous genitalia. Arch Dis Child 88:799–801, 2003.

82. **What major criteria are used to define a micropenis?**
   To be classified as a micropenis, the phallus must meet two major criteria:
   1. The phallus must be normally formed, with the urethral meatus located on the head of the penis and the penis positioned in an appropriate relationship to the scrotum and other pelvic structures. If these features are not present, then the term *micropenis* should be avoided.
   2. The phallus must be >2.5 standard deviations below the appropriate mean for age. For a term newborn, this means that a penis <2 cm in stretched length is classified as a micropenis.
   It is essential that the phallus be measured appropriately. This entails the use of a rigid ruler pressed firmly against the pubic symphysis, depressing the suprapubic fat pad as much as possible. The phallus is grasped gently by its lateral margins and stretched. The measurement is taken along the dorsum of the penis. Note should also be made of the breadth of the phallic shaft. Micropenis must be recognized early in life so that appropriate diagnostic testing can be done.

   Lee PA, Mazur T, Danish R, et al: Micropenis. I. Criteria, etiologies and classification. Johns Hopkins Med J 146:156–163, 1980.

83. **What causes a micropenis?**
Regression of the Müllerian system, fusion of the labioscrotal folds, and migration of the urethral meatus occur during the first trimester of gestation. Further growth of the phallus during the second and third trimester is dependent on the production of testosterone by the fetal testis in response to fetal pituitary luteinizing hormone (LH). Growth hormone also enhances penile growth in utero. Thus, the following disorders can result in micropenis:
  - **Hypothalamic/pituitary dysfunction:** Isolated, Kallmann syndrome, Prader-Willi syndrome, septo-optic dysplasia
  - **Testicular dysfunction or failure:** Intrauterine testicular torsion (vanishing testes syndrome), testicular dysplasia
  - **Complex** (testicular and/or pituitary) **or idiopathic:** Robinow syndrome, Klinefelter syndrome, other X polysomies
  - **Partial androgen resistance**

84. **Outline the three main concerns to be addressed during the initial evaluation of a 1-month-old infant with micropenis.**
  1. **Is there a defect in the hypothalamic-pituitary-gonadal axis?** Specific tests include the measurement of testosterone, dihydrotestosterone, LH, and follicle-stimulating hormone. Because circulating levels of these hormones are normally quite high during the neonatal period, the measurement of random levels during the first 2 months of life may be useful for identifying diseases of the testes and pituitary. Beyond 3 months of age, the tests are generally not useful because the entire axis becomes quiescent and remains so until late childhood. Depending on the patient's age, provocative tests may be necessary, including the following: (1) repetitive testosterone injection to evaluate the ability of the penis to respond to hormonal stimulation; (2) the use of human chorionic gonadotropin as a stimulus for testosterone production by the testes; and (3) GnRH (this is not currently available) administration to examine the responsiveness of the pituitary to stimulation. The trial of testosterone therapy is especially important, because it indicates whether phallic growth is possible. If it is not, gender reassignment may become a consideration.
  2. **Does a possible pituitary deficiency involve other hormones?** Isolated growth hormone deficiency, gonadotropin deficiency, and panhypopituitarism have been associated with micropenis. The presence of hypoglycemia, hypothermia, or hyperbilirubinemia (e.g., associated with hypothyroidism) in a child with micropenis should lead one to search for other pituitary hormone deficits and structural abnormalities of the central nervous system (e.g., septo-optic dysplasia).
  3. **Is there a renal abnormality?** Because of the association of genital and renal abnormalities and nature's endless variations, it may be important in some cases to obtain an abdominal and pelvic ultrasound to better define the internal anatomy.

85. **If a 7.2-year-old girl develops breast buds and pubic hair, is this normal or precocious?**
Precocious puberty is the appearance of physical changes associated with sexual development earlier than normal. Traditionally this has been the development of secondary sexual characteristics along female lines in girls who are <8 years old and along male lines in boys who are <9 years old. In 1997, an office-based study of 17,000 healthy 3- to 12-year-old girls revealed that puberty was occurring on average 1 year earlier in white girls and 2 years earlier in black girls and suggested a revision of guidelines for the ages at which precocious puberty should be investigated. Many experts now recommend that an evaluation for precocious puberty of girls need not be undertaken for white girls >7 years old or black girls >6 years old with breast and/or pubic hair development. However, this remains controversial and a subject of ongoing debate and data collection. The recommendations for boys remain that

investigations for pathologic etiologies be undertaken if pubertal changes begin before the age of 9 years.

Kaplowitz PB, Oberfield SE: Reexamination of the age limit for defining when puberty is precocious in girls in the United States: Implications for evaluation and treatment. Pediatrics 104:936–941, 1999.

Herman-Giddens ME, Slora EJ, Wasserman RC, et al: Secondary sexual characteristics and menses in young girls seen in office practice: A study from the Pediatric Research in Office Settings network. Pediatrics 99:505–512, 1997.

86. **Breast buds are noted on a 2-year-old girl. Is this worrisome?**

Premature thelarche, or the development of breast buds, is the most common variation of normal pubertal development. A form of mild estrogenization, it typically occurs between the ages of 1 and 3 years. It is usually benign and should not be associated with the onset of other pubertal events. Precocious puberty, rather than simple premature thelarche, should be suspected if the following are present:

- breast, nipple, and areolar development reach Tanner stage III;
- androgenization with pubic and/or axillary hair begins; and
- linear growth accelerates.

Ongoing parental observation and periodic reexamination are all that are required if there are no signs of progression.

87. **Which aspects of the physical examination are particularly important when evaluating a patient with precocious puberty?**

- **Evidence of a central nervous system mass:** Examination of optic fundus for possible increased intracranial pressure; visual fields testing for evidence of optic nerve compression by a hypothalamic or pituitary mass
- **Evidence of androgenic influence:** Presence of acne and facial and axillary hair; increased muscle bulk and definition; extent of other body/pubic hair; in boys, increased scrotal rugation accompanied by thinning and pigmentation and penile elongation; in girls, clitoromegaly
- **Evidence of estrogenic influence:** Size of breast tissue and nipple/areolar contouring; vaginal mucosa color (increased estrogen causes cornification of vaginal epithelium with a color change from prepubertal shiny red to a more opalescent pink); labia minor (become more prominent and visible between the labia majora as puberty progresses)
- **Evidence of gonadotropic stimulation:** Testicular enlargement >2.5 cm in length or >4 mL in volume (preferably measured using a Prader orchidometer of labeled volumetric beads); pubertal development without testicular enlargement usually suggests adrenal pathology
- **Evidence of other mass:** Asymmetric testicular enlargement; hepatomegaly; abdominal mass

88. **Which radiologic and laboratory tests are indicated for the evaluation of precocious puberty?**

Radiologic evaluation

- *Bone age:* This study helps to determine the duration of exposure to the elevated sex hormone. A significantly advanced bone age as compared with the chronologic age suggests long-term exposure.
- *Abdominal and pelvic ultrasound:* In boys, this test identifies possible adrenal masses; in girls, it identifies adrenal masses, ovarian masses, or cysts. Increased uterine size and echogenicity suggest endometrial proliferation in response to circulating estrogen.

Laboratory evaluation

- *LH, follicle-stimulating hormone, estradiol, testosterone*
- *Adrenal steroid levels* (17-hydroxyprogesterone, androstenedione, cortisol): More extensive testing may be needed in a virilized child if the initial studies are normal.

- *Provocative testing* of the hypothalamic-pituitary axis (using a synthetic GnRH) or of the adrenal gland using a synthetic ACTH, especially in the child with slight but progressive pubertal changes

89. **Boys or girls: Who is more likely to have an identifiable cause for precocious puberty?**
Although precocious puberty occurs 80% of the time in girls, boys are more likely to have identifiable pathology. As a second general rule, the younger the child and the more rapid the onset of the condition, the greater the likelihood of detecting pathology.

90. **Discuss the terms that denote aspects of precocious sexual development.**
The terms used to describe precocious puberty reflect the fact that normal puberty is an orderly process by which female children are feminized and male children masculinized. The development of breast tissue without pubic hair is called *premature thelarche*. If pubic hair subsequently develops, the term *precocious puberty* is used. If pubic hair develops without breast tissue, it is *premature pubarche*. Because pubic hair development in the female is thought to be the result of adrenal androgens, the term *premature adrenarche* is commonly used. If the pubertal changes are early and appear to proceed in the orderly fashion of breast budding, pubic hair development, growth spurt, and, finally, menstruation, the term *true precocious puberty* is used. When some of the changes of puberty are present but their appearance is isolated or out of normal sequence (e.g., menses without breast development), the term *pseudoprecocious puberty* is used. When the changes of puberty are consistent with the child's sex, they are called *isosexual;* when they are discordant with the sex, they are *heterosexual*.

91. **When along the pubertal spectrum does the male voice begin to crack?**
Voice "breaking" has traditionally been regarded as one of the harbingers of puberty. However, sequential voice analysis reveals that it is usually a *late* event in puberty, usually occurring between Tanner stages III and IV.

Harries ML, Walker JM, Williams DM, et al: Changes in the male voice at puberty. Arch Dis Child 77:445–447, 1997.

THYROID DISORDERS

92. **Which thyroid function tests are "standard"?**
Diseases of the thyroid represent a heterogeneous group of disorders. As such, there are no "standard" thyroid function studies that are appropriate for all children with suspected thyroid disease. The choice of laboratory tests is based on the results of a careful history and physical examination.
Clinical findings that suggest hyperthyroidism: A TSH level and a thyroxine (T_4) level (or free T_4) should be obtained. TSH suppression is probably the most sensitive indictor of hyperthyroid status. If the patient is symptomatic and has a suppressed TSH level with a normal T_4 level, it will be necessary to obtain a triiodothyronine (T_3) radioimmunoassay because cases of T_3-thyrotoxicosis do occur. If the patient is asymptomatic but has an elevated T_4 level, then some measure of binding capacity should be obtained (e.g., a T_3 uptake).
Clinical findings that suggest hypothyroidism: The laboratory evaluation consists of the quantitation of T_4 and TSH. A low T_4 level and an elevated TSH level are diagnostic of hypothyroidism.

93. **What is the significance of antithyroid antibodies in children?**
In the pediatric population, **chronic lymphocytic thyroiditis** is the most common cause of hypothyroidism. The antibodies that are generally available as markers for this condition include antimicrosomal, antithyroglobulin, and antithyroidal peroxidase antibodies. Most

laboratories will run at least two of these assays. A titer of >1:2,000 on any assay provides strong evidence in favor of the diagnosis, but the absence of antibodies does not rule out chronic lymphocytic thyroiditis. High titers may also be seen in patients with Graves' disease. Low titers may be present with a wide range of systemic diseases, particularly autoimmune processes.

94. **Of what value is the T_3 resin uptake (T_3RU) test?**
The T_3RU test is a measure of **serum thyroid-binding capacity**. Because T_4 is primarily protein bound, only a small amount exists in the unbound (free) state. Physiologically, the free T_4 is the metabolically active compound, but it is technically complex to assay directly. In most cases, it has proved simpler to measure T_3RU and total T_4 and to calculate the amount of T_4 that is unbound. In patients with primary thyroidal disease, the T_3RU and the T_4 should go in the same direction (i.e., both increase or both decrease). If they go in opposite directions, it is probably a binding problem.

95. **What signs and symptoms in an infant suggest congenital hypothyroidism?**
See Table 6-5.

TABLE 6-5. SYMPTOMS AND SIGNS OF CONGENITAL HYPOTHYROIDISM	
Symptoms	Signs
Lethargy	Hypotonia, slow reflexes
Poor feeding	Poor weight gain
Prolonged jaundice	Jaundice
Constipation	Distended abdomen
Mottling	Acrocyanosis
Cold extremities	Coarse features
	Large fontanels/wide sutures
	Hoarse cry
	Goiter

96. **What causes congenital hypothyroidism?**
   - **Primary:** Agenesis/dysgenesis, ectopic, dyshormonogenesis
   - **Secondary:** Hypopituitarism, hypothalamic abnormality
   - **Other:** Transient, maternal factors (e.g., goitrogen ingestion, iodide deficiency)

97. **How common is goiter in newborns with congenital hypothyroidism?**
Congenital goiter is seen in only 20% of newborns with congenital hypothyroidism. Maternal ingestion of antithyroid medications, iodides, and goitrogens; congenital thyroid dyshormonogenic defects; and congenital hyperthyroidism are associated with palpable thyromegaly. Goiter in the newborn is difficult to recognize because of the infant's relatively short neck and increased subcutaneous fat. Palpation of the neck is often overlooked during newborn examinations.

98. **How effective are screening programs for congenital hypothyroidism?**
Screening programs correctly identify 90–95% of children who are affected with congenital hypothyroidism. Screening programs are most likely to miss infants with large ectopic glands, those with partial defects in thyroidal hormone biosynthesis, and those with secondary (pituitary or hypothalamic) disease. If an infant presents a clinical picture of

hypothyroidism and has had a normal newborn screen, it is important to realize that the false-negative rate of the screening is up to 10%.

99. **Discuss the risks of delaying treatment for congenital hypothyroidism.**
Therapy should begin as early as possible because outcome is related to the time treatment is started. Because <20% of patients will have distinctive clinical signs at 3–4 weeks of age, screening is now performed on all newborns in the United States at 2–3 days of age, and most affected children are started on therapy before they are 1 month old. The prognosis for intellectual development is directly related to the amount of time from birth to the initiation of therapy. Children begun on hormone replacement at <30 days of age have a mean intelligence quotient of 106, but those whose treatment started at 3–6 months have a mean intelligence quotient of 70.

100. **If goiter is noted during a routine examination of an asymptomatic 7-year-old boy, what should be the course of action?**
The evaluation of a child with goiter is generally simple. In the absence of signs of thyroidal disease, history should be obtained regarding recent exposure to iodine or other halogens. A family history should be obtained regarding thyroidal disease, because thyroiditis tends to run in families. The initial laboratory evaluation is typically T_4, TSH, and antithyroidal antibodies. If there is discrete nodularity within the thyroid or the gland is rock hard or tender, then further diagnostic evaluation (ultrasound, computed tomography scan) may be indicated. Parathyroid enlargement or lymphoma may be misdiagnosed as goiter.

101. **What are the causes of acquired hypothyroidism in childhood?**
The most common cause is **chronic lymphocytic thyroiditis**.

102. **What is the most common clinical presentation of symptoms of Hashimoto thyroiditis?**
Chronic lymphocytic thyroiditis (CLT), also called Hashimoto disease or autoimmune thyroiditis, is the most common thyroid problem in children and is thought to be caused by an autoimmune organ-specific process. Although symptoms of hypo- or hyperthyroidism may be present, the preponderance of pediatric patients are asymptomatic, and the condition is detected by the presence of goiter. The diagnosis of CLT is primarily based on the demonstration of antithyroglobulin and/or antimicrosomal antibody in high titers (>1:2,000).

Pearce EN, Farwell AP, Braverman LE: Thyroiditis. N Engl J Med 348:2646–2655, 2003.

103. **What should a parent be told about the prognosis of a child who has euthyroid goiter caused by chronic lymphocytic thyroiditis?**
About 50% of all children who present symptoms of euthyroid goiter will have resolution of the goiter over several years, regardless of whether or not thyroxine replacement is given. However, it is not possible to predict which children will recover completely, which will remain euthyroid with goiter, and which will become hypothyroid. Any child identified with thyroid disease should have T_4 and TSH values monitored every 4–6 months.

104. **What other autoimmune endocrine diseases are associated with chronic lymphocytic thyroiditis?**
Adrenal insufficiency (Schmidt syndrome), diabetes mellitus, and autoimmune polyendocrine syndrome (type II).

105. **What does a normal T_4 and an elevated TSH suggest?**
The diagnosis of hypothyroidism is based on finding both a low T_4 level and an elevated TSH level. However, on occasion the T_4 level can be maintained in a normal range by increased stimulation of the thyroid gland by TSH. This combination of laboratory values is suggestive of a failing thyroid and is referred to as **compensated hypothyroidism.** Because TSH is the most

useful physiologic marker for the adequacy of a circulating level of thyroid hormone, an elevated TSH level is an indication for thyroid replacement therapy. If the TSH level is only minimally elevated and the child is asymptomatic, it is worthwhile to wait 4–6 weeks and repeat the T_4 and TSH tests before instituting therapy.

106. What is the most common cause of hyperthyroidism in children?
Graves' disease is a multisystem disease that is characterized by hyperthyroidism, infiltrative ophthalmopathy, and, occasionally, an infiltrative dermopathy. The features of this disease may occur singly or in any combination. In the pediatric population, the ophthalmopathy seems to be less severe, and the dermopathy is rare; the full syndrome may never develop. There has been a tendency to use the terms *Graves' disease, thyrotoxicosis,* and *hyperthyroidism* interchangeably, but there are other causes of hyperthyroidism in childhood (e.g., factitious).

107. In addition to Graves' disease, what conditions may cause hyperthyroidism?
- **Excess TSH:** TSH-producing tumor
- **Abnormal thyroid stimulation:** TSH receptor antibody
- **Thyroid autonomy:** Adenoma, multinodular goiter
- **Thyroid inflammation:** Subacute thyroiditis, Hashimoto thyroiditis
- **Exogenous hormone:** Ingestion, ectopic thyroid tissue

108. Describe the typical features of hyperthyroidism that occurs as a result of Graves' disease.
History: The onset of symptoms is usually gradual, with increasing emotional lability and deteriorating school performance. Sleep disturbances, nervousness, and weight loss may be noted, as well as easy fatigability and heat intolerance. Observation of the child's behavior while the history is being obtained from the parent is often instructive.

Physical examination: Weight may be low for height, and many children will be tall for age and genetic potential. Some children will have experienced an acceleration in growth rate at the same time that their behavior began to deteriorate. The pulse rate is usually inappropriately high for age. A widened pulse pressure or an elevated blood pressure is often noted, although this is a more variable finding in children than in adults.

109. What causes Graves' disease?
Graves' disease is an autoimmune disorder in which TSH receptor antibodies bind to the TSH receptor, thereby resulting in the stimulation of thyroid hormone production and subsequent hyperthyroidism. Most thyroid receptor antibodies belong to the IgG class. The general name used for these antibodies is **human thyroid-stimulating immunoglobulins** (formerly called "long-acting thyroid stimulators").

110. How is the hyperthyroidism of Graves' disease distinguished from that occasionally found in patients with CLT?
Patients with hyperthyroidism as a result of CLT may be indistinguishable from those with Graves' disease. The presence of ophthalmologic findings points toward the latter entity, but the absence of exophthalmos does not rule out Graves' disease. The demonstration of human thyroid-stimulating antibodies is confirmatory of the Graves' disease diagnosis, but these tests may not be readily available. The best way to distinguish between these two entities is by determining the uptake of radioactive iodine at 6 and 24 hours after the administration of the isotope. Low or normal uptake supports the diagnosis of CLT, whereas elevated uptakes at 6 and 24 hours are more indicative of Graves' disease.

KEY POINTS: THYROID DISORDERS

1. Midline neck masses usually involve the thyroid gland or thyroid remnants, such as a thyroglossal duct cyst.

2. Neck extension improves visualization and palpation of thyroid masses, especially with swallowing.

3. Approximately 20–40% of solitary thyroid nodules in adolescents are malignant; expedited evaluation is needed.

4. Chronic lymphocytic thyroiditis is the most common cause of pediatric goiter in the United States.

5. Chronic lymphocytic thyroiditis most commonly appears as an asymptomatic goiter, thereby reinforcing the need for thyroid palpation (an often overlooked examination feature).

6. The best initial screening studies for hypo- or hyperthyroidism are total T_4 and thyroid-stimulating hormone.

---

111. Why does exophthalmos occur in Graves' disease?

The reason is unknown, but several facts suggest an autoimmune process:

- Histologic studies reveal lymphocytic infiltration of the retrobulbar muscles.
- Circulating lymphocytes are sensitized to an antigen that is unique to the retrobulbar tissues.
- The thyroglobulin-antithyroglobulin antibody complexes found in patients with Graves' disease bind specifically to the extraorbital muscles.

112. What treatment options are available for children with Graves' disease?

The three types of therapy are antithyroid medication, radioactive (^{131}I) ablation, and subtotal thyroidectomy.

Cheetham TD, Hughes IA, Barnes ND, Wraight EP: Treatment of hyperthyroidism in young people. Arch Dis Child 78:207–209, 1998.

113. Describe the principal modes of actions and the side effects of medications used to treat Graves' disease.

The thioamide derivatives—propylthiouracil and methimazole—are the keystones of long-term management. However, their effective onset of action is slow because they block the synthesis but not the release of thyroid hormone. Propranolol is useful for treating many of the beta-adrenergic effects of hyperthyroidism. It is used during the acute management of Graves' disease but should be discontinued when the thyroid disease is controlled. Iodide (which can transiently block thyroid hormone release) and glucocorticoids are useful "stopgap" medications while awaiting the inhibitory effects of the thioamide; they are generally used only when the patient is acutely symptomatic (i.e., thyroid storm).

Dotsch J, Rascher W, Dorr HG: Graves' disease in childhood: A review of the options for diagnosis and treatment. Paediatr Drugs 5:95–102, 2003.

114. Has radioactive iodide fallen into disfavor as a treatment option for Graves' disease?

On the contrary, radioactive iodide (^{131}I) is increasing in popularity. Concern had been voiced about the possible risk of thyroid carcinoma, leukemia, thyroid nodules, or genetic mutations, but as the individuals treated with ^{131}I during childhood have been followed for prolonged periods, experience suggests that children are *not* at a significantly increased risk of developing these conditions.

Rivkees SA, Sklar C, Freemark M: The management of Graves' disease in children, with special emphasis on radioiodine treatment. J Clin Endocrinol Metab 83:3767–3776, 1998.

115. **During a routine physical examination, a solitary thyroid nodule is palpated on an asymptomatic 10-year-old child. Can a "wait-and-see" approach be taken? Absolutely not.** In children with a solitary nodule, about 30–40% have a carcinoma, 20–30% have an adenoma, and the remainder will have thyroid abscess, thyroid cyst, multinodular goiter, Hashimoto thyroiditis, subacute thyroiditis, or nonthyroidal neck mass. Given the relatively high incidence of carcinoma, a thyroidal mass demands prompt evaluation. Previous irradiation to the head or neck is associated with a significantly increased incidence of thyroid carcinoma. A family history of thyroid disease increases the likelihood of chronic lymphocytic thyroiditis or Graves' disease. The presence of tenderness on palpation or high titers of antithyroid antibodies points away from a malignant process. However, in all cases, radiologic studies should be undertaken; in many cases, surgical exploration is required.

116. **How should this solitary thyroid nodule be investigated?**
The principal tools used in the investigation of a thyroid mass are ^{123}I scanning and ultrasound. **Ultrasound** is useful for delineating the size of the mass, its anatomic relationship to the rest of the thyroid, and the presence of cystic structures. **^{123}I imaging** that reveals a single nonfunctioning mass ("cold" nodule) suggests a carcinoma or adenoma and is a clear indication for surgery. Patchy uptake is more characteristic of chronic lymphocytic thyroiditis, whereas a poorly functioning lobe may be found in a subacute thyroiditis.

117. **How is the euthyroid sick syndrome diagnosed?**
This syndrome is an adaptive response to slow body metabolism. It is also called the **low T_3 syndrome** because the most consistent finding is a depression of serum T_3. Reverse T_3, a metabolically inactive metabolite, is increased, although this is rarely measured. T_4 and thyroid binding globulin (TBG) levels may be low or normal; free T_4 and TSH levels are normal. In sick preterm infants, the clinical picture is often confusing because levels of T_4, free T_4, and T_3 are naturally low. Infants and children with the euthyroid sick syndrome generally revert to normal as the primary illness resolves.

CHAPTER 7

GASTROENTEROLOGY

Douglas Jacobstein, MD, Peter Mamula, MD, Jonathan E. Markowitz, MD, MSCE, and Chris A. Liacouras, MD

CLINICAL ISSUES

1. **What are the causes of pancreatitis in children?**
   - **33%: Systemic disorders** (sepsis/shock, vasculitides, and viral infections, including mumps, influenza, and Epstein-Barr)
   - **25%: Idiopathic**
   - **15%: Trauma**
   - **10%: Anatomic/structural anomalies** (pancreatic divisum, duct anomalies, choledochal cyst, and cholelithiasis)
   - **5%: Metabolic disorders** (cystic fibrosis, hypercalcemia, hyperlipidemia, alpha$_1$-antitrypsin deficiency, and organic acidemias)
   - **5%: Drugs/toxins** (certain chemotherapeutic agents, valproic acid, thiazides, and alcohol)
   - **2%: Hereditary** (familial)

   Durie PR: Disturbances of exocrine pancreatic dysfunction. In Rudolph CD, Rudolph AM (eds): Rudolph's Pediatrics, 21st ed. New York, McGraw-Hill, 2003, p 1467.

2. **What are the potential pitfalls of relying solely on serum amylase to diagnose pancreatitis?**
   Although serum amylase is the most widely used test for diagnosis, it may not be the most sensitive or specific. It is usually elevated during the first 12 hours of the condition, but it may return to normal within 24–72 hours. A child can have severe pancreatitis with a normal serum amylase level.

   Falsely elevated serum amylase can occur if amylase is released from other injured areas (e.g., salivary glands in mumps, intestines in Crohn's disease, ovaries and fallopian tubes in salpingitis). Isoenzyme determinations can help to identify the source if the clinical picture is confusing.

   The serum lipase remains elevated for longer periods of time. Other blood tests that should be considered include cationic trypsinogen, hepatic transaminases, blood glucose, and calcium.

3. **How is ascites diagnosed by physical examination?**
   Severe ascites is commonly diagnosed by observation of the child in a supine and then an upright position. Bulging flanks, umbilical protrusion, and scrotal edema (in males) are generally evident. Three main techniques are used when the diagnosis is not obvious:
   - **Fluid wave:** This sign can be elicited in a cooperative patient by tapping sharply on one flank while receiving the wave with the other hand. The transmission of the wave through fatty tissue should be blocked by a hand placed on the center of the abdomen.
   - **Shifting dullness:** With the patient supine, percussion of the abdomen will demonstrate a central area of tympany at the top that is surrounded by flank percussion dullness. This dullness shifts when the patient moves laterally or stands up.
   - **"Puddle sign":** A cooperative and mobile patient may be examined in the knee-chest position. The pool of ascites is tapped while you listen for a sloshing sound or change in sound transmission with the stethoscope.

   Small amounts of ascites can be extremely difficult to detect with physical examination in children. Although ascites can be demonstrated on radiographs, the most sensitive and specific test is an abdominal-pelvic ultrasound, which can detect as little as 150 mL of ascitic fluid.

4. **How does the major cause of ascites in neonates differ from that of older children?**
Older children: Portal hypertension as a result of hepatic (e.g., chronic liver disease of multiple etiologies), prehepatic (e.g., portal vein thrombosis), or posthepatic (e.g., congestive heart failure, constrictive pericarditis) conditions.
Infants: Urinary ascites most commonly as a result of obstructive renal disease (e.g., posterior urethral valves).

5. **In what clinical settings is rectal prolapse most commonly seen?**
   - Constipation
   - Celiac disease
   - Malnutrition
   - Severe coughing (e.g., pertussis)
   - Cystic fibrosis
   - *Enterobius vermicularis* (pinworm) infestation
   - Myelomeningocele
   - Abnormalities of sacrum or coccyx
   - Ehlers-Danlos syndrome

6. **What is the likely diagnosis of an infant with excessive secretions and choking episodes in whom a nasogastric tube is unable to be passed into the stomach?**
Esophageal atresia with tracheoesophageal fistula. This congenital anomaly is usually diagnosed during the newborn period, often when a chest x-ray reveals the intended nasogastric tube coiled in the blind upper esophageal pouch with the stomach distended with air. Treatment is surgical. The three most common variations are shown in Fig. 7-1.

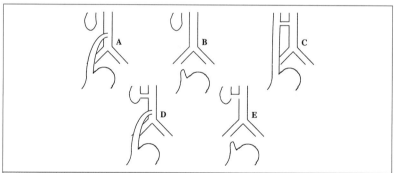

Figure 7-1. Esophageal atresia and tracheoesophageal fistula. *A,* Esophageal atresia with distal esophageal communications with the tracheobronchial tree. *B,* Esophageal atresia without a distal communication. *C,* "H"-type fistulas between otherwise intact trachea and esophagus. *D,* Esophageal atresia with both proximal and distal communication with the trachea. *E,* Esophageal atresia with proximal communication. (Katz DS, Math KR, Groskin SA: Radiology Secrets. Philadelphia, Hanley & Belfus, 1998, p 389.)

7. **How should the bowel be prepared before colonoscopy?**
Children <1 year old
   - Clear liquids for 24 hours
   - Pediatric Fleet enemas the night before and the morning of the examination

Children >1 year old
   - Clear liquids for 48 hours
   - X-prep (senna extract) or magnesium citrate orally on two successive nights before the examination
   - Adult Fleet enema the night before and the morning of the exam *or*

- GOLYTELY or CoLyte (2–4 liters over 3–4 hours) administered orally or via a nasogastric tube the night before the procedure may be substituted in children >5 years old; these must be used with caution in younger children.

8. **List the indications for lower gastrointestinal colonoscopy or endoscopy in children.**
   - Hematochezia in the absence of an anal source
   - History of familial polyposis
   - Chronic diarrhea of unclear etiology
   - Persistent severe unexplained lower abdominal pain
   - Colitis of unclear etiology
   - Diagnosis and management of inflammatory bowel disease
   - Removal of foreign body
   - Ureterosigmoidostomy, surveillance
   - Abnormality on barium enema
   - Dilation of a colonic stricture

9. **When is colonoscopy contraindicated?**
   - Suspected perforation
   - Toxic megacolon
   - Recent abdominal surgery
   - Unstable medical illness
   - Inadequate bowel preparation
   - Coagulopathy
   - Massive lower gastrointestinal bleeding

   Fox VL: Colonoscopy. In Walker WA, Durie PR, Hamilton JR, et al (eds): Pediatric Gastrointestinal Disease, 2nd ed. St. Louis, Mosby, 1996, pp 1533–1541.

10. **In children with recurrent abdominal pain, what historic features suggest a possible serious cause?**
    Recurrent abdominal pain is the most common chronic pain syndrome encountered in pediatrics. The vast majority of these cases have no identifiable organic basis. Features that suggest an identifiable cause include the following:
    - Pain localizing away from the umbilicus
    - Abnormalities in bowel function (i.e., constipation, diarrhea, incontinence)
    - Vomiting
    - Pain that awakens a child at night
    - Pain with radiation to the back, shoulder, or lower extremities
    - Dysuria
    - Rectal bleeding
    - Constitutional symptoms (i.e., fever, weight loss, altered rate of growth, rash, arthralgia)
    - Presentation of symptoms at the age of <4 years or >15 years
    - Family history of gastrointestinal or systemic illness (e.g., peptic ulcer disease, inflammatory bowel disease, lactose intolerance)

      Zeiter DK, Hyams JS: Recurrent abdominal pain in children. Pediatr Clin North Am 49:53–72, 2002.

11. **How does the average volume of the swallow of a child compare with that of an adult?**
    - Child (age 1¼–3½ years): 4.5 mL
    - Adult male: 21 mL
    - Adult female: 14 mL
    - Average: 0.27 mL/kg

      Jones DV, Work CE: Volume of a swallow. Am J Dis Child 102:427, 1961.

12. **What is intractable singultus?**
    Persistent hiccups.

13. **What is the most commonly ingested foreign body?**
   Coins account for more than 20,000 visits yearly to emergency rooms in the United States. Symptomatic patients are more likely to have the coin lodged in the esophagus, although a significant portion of these patients may be asymptomatic. Coins lodged in the esophagus should be removed endoscopically within 24 hours because of the risk of ulceration and perforation.

14. **Which is potentially more dangerous after ingestion: a penny made in 1977 or one made in 1987?**
   The penny from 1987. In 1982, the composition of pennies changed. Coins minted after that date have higher concentrations of zinc, which is more corrosive and potentially more harmful after prolonged contact with stomach acid.

15. **What is the difference radiographically between a coin in the esophagus and a coin in the trachea?**
   A coin in the esophagus appears *en face* in the anteroposterior view (sagittal plane), whereas a coin in the trachea appears *en face* on the lateral view (coronal plane). This occurs because the cartilaginous ring of the trachea is open posteriorly, but the opening of the esophagus is widest in the transverse position.

16. **A teenage girl has symptoms of swallowing difficulties improved by positional head and neck changes, nocturnal regurgitation, and halitosis. What is the likely diagnosis?**
   Achalasia. The cardinal symptom of this motility disorder of the esophagus is dysphagia. The diagnosis is made by barium swallow and esophageal manometry. The manometric findings are diagnostic, including elevated basal lower esophageal sphincter pressure with failure to relax and the absence of peristalsis throughout the esophageal body during the swallow.

CONSTIPATION

17. **When is the first stool of a neonate normally passed?**
   Ninety-nine percent of infants will pass a stool within the first 24 hours of life, and 100% will do so within 48 hours of birth. Failure to pass a stool can be an indication of intestinal obstruction or anatomic abnormality. Approximately 95% of patients with Hirschsprung's disease and 25% of patients with cystic fibrosis do not pass their first stool during the first 24 hours. The rule of early passage does not apply to premature babies, in whom delayed evacuation (>24 hours) is common, particularly with extreme prematurity.

18. **What constitutes constipation in childhood?**
   Strictly speaking, constipation is defined as infrequent stooling, difficulty passing feces, or chronic fecal retention. Normal stool frequency varies from several times a day to one stool every three days. In children, constipation should be considered when the normal stooling pattern becomes more infrequent, when stools become hard or are difficult to expel, or when the child exhibits withholding patterns or behavioral changes toward moving his or her bowels. Soiling (encopresis) can be a sign of constipation.

19. **How important is the rectal examination in patients with constipation?**
   Extremely important. The presence of large amounts of stool in the rectal vault almost always indicates functional constipation. If no stool is present, Hirschsprung's disease and abnormal anorectal anatomy should be considered. Failure to perform a rectal examination is a common omission during the evaluation of children, and impaction in chronic constipation often goes undetected. Abdominal radiographs can be used to show the degree of fecal retention and can be used to monitor treatment in children who have severe functional constipation.

   Lembo A, Camilleri M: Chronic constipation. N Engl J Med 149:1360–1368, 2003.
   Gold DM, Levine J, Weinstein TA, et al: Frequency of digital rectal examination in children with chronic constipation. Arch Pediatr Adolesc Med 153:377–379, 1999.

20. **Which clinical features differentiate chronic retentive constipation from Hirschsprung's disease?**
See Table 7-1.

TABLE 7-1. CLINICAL DISTINCTIONS BETWEEN CHRONIC RETENTIVE CONSTIPATION AND HIRSCHSPRUNG'S DISEASE	
Functional constipation	**Hirschsprung's disease**
Meconium passes within 24 hours	Meconium passes after 24 hours
Vomiting unusual	Vomiting common
Begins during toilet training	Begins shortly after birth
Soiling (encopresis) occurs	Soiling very rare
No enterocolitis	Enterocolitis
Palpable stool in rectal vault	No stool in rectal vault
Dilated anal canal	Narrow anal canal
Normal growth	Failure to thrive

21. **How is Hirschsprung's disease diagnosed?**
Hirschsprung's disease results from the failure of normal migration of ganglion cell precursors to their location in the gastrointestinal tract during gestation. The diagnosis can be made by obtaining an unprepped **barium enema,** which will demonstrate a change in the caliber of the large intestine at the site where normal bowel meets aganglionic bowel (transition zone). An unprepped barium enema is required because the use of cleansing enemas can dilate the abnormal portion of the colon and remove some of the distal impaction, thereby resulting in a false-negative result. After the study, the retention of barium for 24 or more hours is suggestive of Hirschsprung's disease or a significant motility disorder. **Rectal suction biopsies** or **full-thickness surgical biopsies** will confirm the absence of ganglion cells. Anal manometry is less reliable in children; in small infants, it requires specialized equipment.

22. **How is encopresis defined?**
Encopresis, or fecal soiling, may be defined as the involuntary passage of fecal material in an otherwise healthy and normal child. Children with encopresis typically sense no urge to defecate. Fecal soiling is almost always associated with severe functional constipation.

KEY POINTS: CONSTIPATION

1. Ninety-nine percent of full-term infants pass stool at <24 hours after birth. Failure to pass stool within the first 48 hours of life should be considered pathologic until proven otherwise.

2. The rectal examination is a common omission among patients undergoing an evaluation for constipation. Tone, the amount of stool, and the size of the rectal vault should be assessed.

3. Fecal soiling is almost always associated with severe functional constipation and not Hirschsprung's disease.

4. Treatment of functional constipation is multimodal and includes medications, dietary interventions, and behavioral modifications.

23. **How should children with chronic constipation and encopresis be managed?**
    - The rectosigmoid colon should be **aggressively cleansed** of fecal material. Multiple enemas over 2 or 3 days are commonly needed. Adult enemas should be used in children who are >2 years old.
    - Medications that act as an **osmotic laxative** by drawing fluid into the intestine to promote the passage of soft stools include lactulose (a nonabsorbable sugar) and polyethylene glycol powder. Lactulose is often the first choice in this category for children <1 year old.
    - An **oral lubricant**, such as mineral oil or Kondremul, is necessary to promote the continued passage of stool. In difficult cases, **stimulant medications**, such as milk of magnesia or Haley's MO, can be substituted. Although fecal soiling typically improves rapidly, a maintenance dose of mineral oil may be required for a prolonged period.
    - It is extremely important to **educate** patients and parents about the mechanics of the disorder. A high-fiber diet, possible limitation of cow milk, defined periods of toilet-sitting, and a behavior modification system that rewards normal bowel movements are essential for eventual success.

    Loening-BauckeV: Encopresis. Curr Opin Pediatr 14:570–575, 2002.
    Pashankar DS, Bishop WP, Loening-Baucke V: Long-term efficacy of polyethylene glycol 3350 for the treatment of chronic constipation in children with and without encopresis. Clin Pediatr 42:815–819, 2003.

24. **How does the use of mineral oil affect the absorption of fat-soluble vitamins?**
    Although several case reports have shown that the long-term use of mineral oil can potentially alter the absorption of fat-soluble vitamins (A, D, E, and K), vitamin deficiencies rarely occur. However, when mineral oil is prescribed, a multivitamin supplement (given at a different time than the mineral oil) is commonly added to the child's diet.

DIARRHEA/MALABSORPTION

25. **Which historic questions are key when seeking the cause of diarrhea?**
    - Recent medications, especially antibiotics
    - History of immunosuppression (e.g., recurrent major infections, history of malnutrition, acquired immunodeficiency syndrome, recent measles)
    - Illnesses in other family members or close contacts
    - Travel outside of the United States
    - Travel to rural or seacoast areas (i.e., involving the consumption of untreated water, raw milk, or raw shellfish)
    - Attendance in day care
    - Recent foods
    - Presence of family pets
    - Food preparation/water source

    Thielman NM, Guerrant RL: Acute infectious diarrhea. N Engl J Med 350:38–47, 2004.

26. **Which children should be seen for the medical evaluation of acute diarrhea?**
    - Young age (<6 months old or weighing <8 kg)
    - History of premature birth, chronic medical conditions, or concurrent illness
    - Fever ≥38°C for infants <3 months old or ≥39°C for children 3–36 months old
    - Visible blood in stool
    - High output, including frequent and substantial volumes of diarrhea
    - Persistent vomiting
    - Caregiver's report of signs that are consistent with dehydration
    - Change in mental status
    - Suboptimal response to oral rehydration therapy or inability of caregiver to administer this therapy

    King CK, Glass R, Bresee JS, Duggan C; Centers for Disease Control and Prevention: Managing acute gastroenteritis among children: Oral rehydration, maintenance, and nutritional therapy. MMWR Recomm Rep 52(RR-16):1–16, 2003.

27. **In what settings can diarrhea be a severe, life-threatening illness?**
    Severe diarrhea of any cause can lead to dehydration, which can cause significant morbidity and mortality. However, diarrhea can be a sign of a serious associated illness, which in itself can be life-threatening:
    - Intussusception
    - Salmonella gastroenteritis (neonatal or compromised host)
    - Hemolytic-uremic syndrome
    - Hirschsprung's disease (with toxic megacolon)
    - Pseudomembranous colitis
    - Inflammatory bowel disease (with toxic megacolon)

    Fleisher GR: Diarrhea. In Fleisher GR, Ludwig S (eds): Textbook of Pediatric Emergency Medicine, 4th ed. Baltimore, Lippincott Williams & Wilkins, 2000, p 204.

28. **Why is true diarrhea during the first few days of life especially concerning?**
    In addition to the greater potential for dehydration in a newborn, diarrhea in this age group is more commonly associated with major congenital intestinal defects involving electrolyte transport (e.g., congenital sodium- or chloride-losing diarrhea) or carbohydrate absorption (e.g., congenital lactase deficiency). Although viral enteritis can occur in the nursery, any newborn with true diarrhea warrants thorough evaluation and possible referral to a tertiary center.

29. **Which is a better predictor of bacteria as a cause of diarrhea: blood in the stool or neutrophils (PMNs) in the stool?**
    Stool PMNs are more reliable indicators of a bacterial etiology than positive stool guaiac tests for blood. Although about 30–50% of patients with blood in the stool will have a bacterial etiology, up to 70% will not. Thus, the presence of blood has a fair specificity but poor sensitivity. Stool PMNs, on the other hand, have a specificity and sensitivity of around 85%, with a positive predictive value of around 60%.

    DeWitt TG, Humphrey KF, McCarthy P: Clinical predictors of acute bacterial diarrhea in young children. Pediatrics 76:551–556, 1985.

30. **How is the stool examined for white blood cells?**
    Unlike dipstick testing for urine white blood cells, you must find stool PMNs the old-fashioned way. A thin smear of fresh stool is placed on a slide and air dried. The sample is covered with methylene blue for about 5 seconds, gently rinsed with tap water, and air dried again. The quantity of PMNs seen per high-power microscopic field can be classified as occasional, scattered, or diffuse.

31. **How do patterns of secretory/enterotoxigenic and inflammatory diarrhea vary?**
    Secretory/enterotoxigenic disease is characterized by watery diarrhea and the absence of fecal leukocytes. Inflammatory disease is characterized by dysentery (i.e., symptoms and blood stools) as well as fecal leukocytes and red blood cells.

    Northrup RS, Flanigan TP: Gastroenteritis. Pediatr Rev 15:461–472, 1994.

32. **What are the common causes of secretory/toxigenic diarrhea?**
    - Food poisoning (toxigenic)
    - *Staphylococcus aureus*
    - *Bacillus cereus*
    - *Clostridium perfringens*
    - Enterotoxigenic *Escherichia coli*
    - *Vibrio cholerae*
    - *Giardia lamblia*
    - *Cryptosporidium*

- Rotavirus
- Norwalk-like virus

33. **What are the common causes of inflammatory diarrhea?**
    - *Shigella* species
    - Invasive *Escherichia coli*
    - *Salmonella* species
    - *Campylobacter* species
    - *Clostridium difficile*
    - *Entamoeba histolytica*

34. **Why is *Salmonella* enteritis so concerning in a child who is <12 months old?**
    In older children with *Salmonella* gastroenteritis, secondary bacteremia and dissemination of disease rarely occur. In infants, however, 5–40% may have positive blood cultures for *Salmonella*, and, in 10% of these cases, *Salmonella* can cause meningitis, osteomyelitis, pericarditis, and pyelonephritis. Thus, in infants who are <1 year old, outpatient management of diarrhea assumes even greater significance, particularly if *Salmonella* is suspected.

35. **What is the most common cause of traveler's diarrhea?**
    Toxigenic *Escherichia coli* is clearly the most commonly identified cause. Depending on the location, however, other bacteria, viruses, or parasites can be present.

36. **How can traveler's diarrhea be prevented?**
    - **Avoidance:** In high-risk areas of developing countries, avoid previously peeled raw fruits and vegetables and any foods or beverages prepared with tap water.
    - **Bismuth subsalicylate:** Prophylactic bismuth subsalicylate (Pepto-Bismol) has been shown to minimize diarrheal illness in up to 75% of adults. Although some authorities recommend its use in children, others argue against it because of the risk of salicylate intoxication.
    - **Anti-infective drugs:** Prophylactic use of antimicrobial agents such as trimethoprim-sulfamethoxazole, neomycin, doxycycline, and ciprofloxacin can decrease the frequency of traveler's diarrhea in children and adults. However, routine use of antibiotics is not recommended because of potential risks of allergic drug reactions, antibiotic-associated colitis, and the development of resistant organisms.
    - **Immunization:** Although potentially an ideal solution, at present it is not an alternative.

37. **What is the most common treatment for traveler's diarrhea in children?**
    If symptoms develop, empirical therapy is indicated, and the regimen of trimethoprim-sulfamethoxazole and Imodium (for children >2 years old) is very effective. For adolescents, ciprofloxacin is an alternative.

38. **Which bacterial gastroenteritides may benefit from antimicrobial therapy?**
    See Table 7-2.

39. **List the differential diagnosis of chronic diarrhea by age group.**
    - **Newborns:** Congenital short gut, congenital lactose intolerance, malrotation with intermittent volvulus, ischemia, defective sodium/hydrogen exchange, congenital chloride diarrhea, microvillous disease
    - **Infants:** Protein sensitization, infection, parenteral diarrhea (during urinary or upper respiratory infection), immunoglobulin deficiency, diarrhea after gastroenteritis, cystic fibrosis, celiac disease, *Clostridium difficile* infection
    - **Toddlers:** Diarrhea after gastroenteritis, food allergy, excessive ingestion of fruit juice, toddler's diarrhea, hyperthyroidism, sucrase-isomaltase deficiency, constipation/impaction with overflow, teething

- **Older children:** Lactose intolerance, infection, inflammatory bowel disease, irritable bowel syndrome, laxative abuse

Gryboski J: The child with chronic diarrhea. Contemp Pediatr 10:71–97, 1993.
Keating JP: Chronic diarrhea. Pediatr Rev 26:5–14, 2005.

TABLE 7-2.	BENEFITS OF ANTIMICROBIAL THERAPY IN SPECIFIC BACTERIAL GASTROENTERITIDES
Enteropathogen	**Indication for or effect of therapy**
Shigella	Shortens duration of diarrhea
	Eliminates organisms from feces
Campylobacter jejuni	Shortens duration
	Prevents relapse
Salmonella	Indicated for infants <12 months old
	Bacteremia
	Metastatic foci (e.g., osteomyelitis)
	Enteric fever
	Immunocompromise
Escherichia coli	
Enteropathogenic	Use primarily in infants
	Intravenous use if invasive disease
Enterotoxigenic	Most illnesses brief and self-limited
Enteroinvasive	
Yersinia enterocolitica	None for gastroenteritis alone, but indicated if suspected septicemia or other localized infection
Clostridium difficile	10–20% relapse rate
Aeromonas hydrophila	Efficacy not clearly established

40. **How does osmotic diarrhea differ from secretory diarrhea?**
    See Table 7-3.

TABLE 7-3.	OSMOTIC DIARRHEA VERSUS SECRETORY DIARRHEA	
Stools	**Osmotic diarrhea**	**Secretory diarrhea**
Electrolytes	Na^+ <70 mmol/L	Na^+ >70 mmol/L
Osmotic gap*	>100 mOsm	<50 mOsm
pH	<5	>6
Reducing substance	Present	Absent
Volume	<20 mL/kg/day	>20 mL/kg/day
After fasting	<10 mL/kg/day	>20 mL/kg/day
Blood/pus/fat	Present or absent	Absent

*The osmotic gap is the osmolality of the fecal fluid minus the sum of the concentrations of the fecal electrolytes.
From Mehta DI, Lebenthal E: New developments in acute diarrhea. Curr Probl Pediatr 24:95–107, 1994.

41. **How should children with secretory diarrhea be managed?**
After the child is taken off feeds, a vigorous attempt must be initiated to maintain fluid and electrolyte balance. If this is successful, the child should be evaluated for proximal small bowel damage, enteric pathogens, and a baseline malabsorptive workup. If abnormalities of the mucosal integrity are suspected, a small bowel biopsy is performed; if the findings are significantly abnormal, the patient may be given parenteral alimentation and gradual refeeding. Electron microscopy may reveal congenital abnormalities of the microvillus membrane and the brush border. Hormonal causes of secretory diarrhea (e.g., a VIPoma, hypergastrinoma, or carcinoid syndrome) must be considered if initial studies are negative.

42. **What is the most common cause of antibiotic-associated colitis?**
Clostridium difficile. Fever, abdominal pain, and bloody diarrhea begin as early as a few days after starting antibiotics (especially clindamycin, ampicillin, and cephalosporins). Definitive diagnosis is made by sigmoidoscopy, which reveals pseudomembranous plaques or nodules (*see* Fig. 7-2).

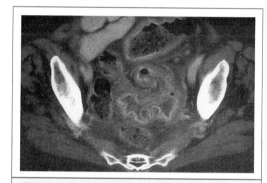

Figure 7-2. Pseudomembranous colitis. Note the multiple plaques characterizing the pseudomembranes; the plaques are characteristically yellow when viewed on endoscopy.

43. **How common is asymptomatic *C difficile* carriage?**
Neonates have a colonization rate of about 20%, infants of 30–40%, older children of 10%, and adolescents of 5%. Toxin assays are more indicative of *C difficile*-associated disease than culture. However, the toxin may be present without any symptoms, especially in infants.

Yassin SF, Young-Fadok IM, Zein NN, Pardi DS: *Clostridium difficile*-associated diarrhea and colitis. Mayo Clin Proc 76:725–730, 2001.

44. **What are the therapeutic alternatives for the treatment of pseudomembranous colitis?**
If the disease is not severe, children may be treated with the withdrawal of antibiotics and good supportive care. More severely ill children should be treated with oral vancomycin or metronidazole. Some clinicians have advocated cholestyramine to bind *C difficile* toxin.

45. **How helpful is eosinophilia as a diagnostic sign of parasitic disease?**
Normally, the total eosinophil count does not exceed $500/mm^3$. As a screening tool for suspected parasitic disease (e.g., in symptomatic patients returning from foreign travel), it has a very poor positive-predictive value (15–55%). Its negative-predictive value is better (73–96%), particularly if sequential eosinophil counts remain normal.

Mawhorter SD: Eosinophilia caused by parasites. Pediatr Ann 23:405–413, 1994.

46. **Name the three most common presenting symptoms of giardiasis.**
1. Asymptomatic carrier state
2. Chronic malabsorption with steatorrhea and failure to thrive
3. Acute gastroenteritis with diarrhea, weight loss, abdominal cramps, abdominal distention, nausea, and vomiting

47. **How reliable are the various diagnostic methods for detecting *Giardia*?**
    - Single stool examination for trophozoites or cysts: 50–75%
    - Three stool examinations (ideally 48 hours apart) for same: 95%
    - Single stool examination and stool enzyme-linked immunosorbent assay test for Giardia antigen: >95%
    - Duodenal aspirate or string test: >95%
    - Duodenal biopsy (gold standard): Closest to 100%

48. **Which patients are particularly susceptible to giardiasis?**
    Those with cystic fibrosis, chronic pancreatitis, achlorhydria, agammaglobulinemia, and hypogammaglobulinemia.

49. **What are the potential complications of amebiasis?**
    The parasite *Entamoeba histolytica* disseminates from the intestine to the liver in up to 10% of patients and to other organs less commonly.
    - Liver abscess
    - Pericarditis
    - Cerebral abscess
    - Empyema

    Haque R, Huston CD, Hughes M, et al: Amebiasis. N Engl J Med 348: 1565–1573, 2003.

50. **What is the triad of findings for acrodermatitis enteropathica?**
    Diarrhea, hair loss, and **dermatitis** are the presenting signs of this rare autosomal recessive disorder. The name nicely describes the disorder: there is a classic *acral* distribution of the rash. It is usually eczematous, often with a vesiculobullous or pustular component, and it involves skin around the body orifices as well. As for *enteropathica*, serum zinc levels are extremely low as a result of impaired gastrointestinal absorption. Dietary insufficiency of zinc may give an identical clinical picture. This has been found in children on long-term total parenteral nutrition without sufficient zinc and in very premature infants as a result of decreased stores and increased requirements.

51. **What features characterize "toddler's diarrhea"?**
    Toddler's diarrhea, which is also known as *chronic nonspecific diarrhea* and even *irritable bowel syndrome,* is a clinical entity of unclear etiology that occurs in infants between 6 and 40 months of age, often following a distinct identifiable enteritis and treatment with an antibiotic. Loose, nonbloody stools (at least two per day but usually more) occur without associated symptoms of fever, pain, or growth failure. Malabsorption is not a key feature.

    Multiple causes may be present: overconsumption of fruit juices, relative intestinal hypermotility, increased secretion of bile acids and sodium, and intestinal prostaglandin abnormalities. The diagnosis is one of exclusion, and toddlers should be evaluated for disaccharide intolerance, protein hypersensitivity, parasitic infestation, and inflammatory bowel disease. Treatment consists of reassurance, careful growth assessment, and psyllium bulking agents (as initial therapy). Other agents used with success have been cholestyramine and metronidazole.

52. **How does late-onset lactase deficiency vary by ethnicity?**
    See Table 7-4.

53. **Why is *lactate deficiency* a somewhat misleading term?**
    After high levels in infancy, lactase levels decline progressively; after the age of 5 years, most people have lactase levels of about 10% of those seen during infancy. Because it is statistically

more common to have these lower levels, the term *deficiency* may be a misnomer. Lactose intolerance may develop if excessive lactose loads are ingested.

TABLE 7-4. APPROXIMATE PERCENTAGE OF LOW LACTASE ACTIVITY BY ETHNIC GROUP			
United States		**Worldwide**	
White	20%	Dutch	0%
Hispanic	50%	French	32%
Black	75%	Filipino	55%
Native American	90%	Vietnamese	100%

54. **What conditions produce secondary lactose deficiency?**
Any disorder that alters the mucosa of the proximal small intestine may result in secondary lactose intolerance. For this reason, the lactose tolerance test is commonly used as a screening test for intestinal integrity, although this has the disadvantage of concomitantly identifying all primary lactose malabsorbers. Although a combination of factors is present in many disease processes, secondary lactose intolerance can be organized into lesions of the microsurface, total surface, transit time, and site of bacterial colonization in the small bowel.

At microvillus/brush border
Postenteritis
Bacterial overgrowth
Inflammatory lesions (Crohn's disease)
At level of the villus
Celiac disease
Allergic enteropathy
Eosinophilic gastroenteropathy

Bulk intestinal surface area
Short bowel syndrome
Altered transit with early lactose entry into colon
Hyperthyroidism
Dumping syndromes
Enteroenteral fistulas

55. **What is gluten?**
After starch has been extracted from wheat flour, *gluten* is the residue that is left. This residue is made up of multiple proteins that are distinguished by their solubility and extraction properties. For example, the alcohol-soluble fraction of wheat gluten is wheat gliadin; it is this protein component that is primarily responsible for the mucosal injury that occurs in the small bowel in patients with celiac sprue.

56. **What classic clinical features suggest celiac disease?**
Gluten-sensitive enteropathy (celiac disease) is a relatively common cause of severe diarrhea and malabsorption in infants and children. Children with celiac disease commonly present symptoms between the ages of 9 and 24 months with failure to thrive, diarrhea, abdominal distention, muscle wasting, and hypotonia. After several months of diarrhea, growth slows; weight typically decreases before height. Often, these children become irritable and depressed and display poor intake and symptoms of carbohydrate malabsorption. Vomiting is less common. On examination, the growth defect and distention are commonly striking. There may be a generalized lack of subcutaneous fat, with wasting of the buttocks, shoulder girdle, and thighs. Edema, rickets, and clubbing may also be seen.

Farrell RJ, Kelly CP: Celiac sprue. N Engl J Med 346:180–188, 2002.

57. **In what other ways may celiac disease present symptoms?**
Celiac disease can be a clinical mimic. Fifty percent of new cases have atypical forms, and patients present symptoms at older ages (5–6 years). Symptoms include the following:

- Dermatitis herpetiformis
- Iron-deficiency anemia
- Arthritis and arthralgia
- Dental enamel hypoplasias
- Chronic hepatitis
- Osteoporosis
- Pubertal delay

Fasano A, Catassi C: Current approaches to diagnosis and treatment of celiac disease: An evolving spectrum. Gastroenterology 120:636–651, 2001.

58. **How is the diagnosis of celiac disease confirmed?**
Definitive diagnosis of celiac disease requires **multiple small bowel biopsies**. In a typical sequence, the first biopsy on gluten should show villous atrophy, with increased crypt mitoses and disorganization and flattening of the columnar epithelium. This should resolve fully on the second biopsy after a strict gluten-free diet. To confirm the diagnosis and eliminate the possibility of a coincidental recovery after infectious enteritis, a third biopsy must be obtained after the patient has again been challenged with gluten. This biopsy again must show the manifestations of the disease.

Although biopsy remains the gold standard, two main screening **antibody tests**—antiendomysial and antitissue transglutaminase—can shorten the expense and invasiveness of this biopsy sequence. In many patients, the titer falls dramatically with treatment and increases again with challenge.

Baudon JJ, Johanet C, Absalon YB, et al: Diagnosing celiac disease: A comparison of human tissue transglutaminase antibodies with antigliadin and antiendomysium antibodies. Arch Ped Adolesc Med 158:154–188, 2004.

59. **Why might a 2-year-old child with typical clinical features of celiac disease, including classic small-bowel biopsy findings, have negative antibody studies?**
Antibodies found in patients with celiac disease—antigliadin immunoglobulin A (IgA), antiendomysial, antireticulin, and antitissue transglutaminase—are IgA antibodies. Selective IgA deficiency is the most common primary immunodeficiency in Western countries, with a prevalence of 1.5–2.5 per 1,000. Celiac disease is 10–20 times more common in individuals with selective IgA deficiency than in the general population. Therefore, in highly suspicious cases with negative antibody panels, a quantitative IgA level can be helpful to rule out IgA deficiency. Alternatively, one could measure antigliadin IgG antibodies, but these have the lowest specificity of the celiac antibodies.

Catassi C, Fabiani E: The spectrum of coeliac disease in children. Bailliere Clin Gastroenterol 11:485–507, 1997.

60. **In addition to celiac disease, what disorders are associated with a flat villous lesion?**

Acute enteritis
Bacterial disease
Viral disease
Protozoal (*Giardia*)
Radiation enteritis
Allergic enteropathy
Milk-soy protein allergy
Celiac disease
Eosinophilic gastroenteritis
Immunoregulatory abnormalities
Immunodeficiency
Graft-versus-host disease

Chronic enteritis
Tropical sprue, Whipple's disease
Intractable enterocolitis
Lymphoma
Malnutrition
Protein calorie
Folate deficiency
Iron deficiency
Congenital
Congenital villous atrophy

61. **How is fat malabsorption determined?**

The gold standard remains 72-hour fecal fat collections that measure both the dietary fat intake and the fecal fat excretion. This quantitative method can be difficult among younger infants. Other tests include Sudan staining of stool for fat globules (a qualitative test that, if positive, indicates gross steatorrhea), the steatocrit, and monitoring absorbed lipids after a standardized meal. Future methods may include breath testing (similar to carbohydrate testing). In an animal model, radioactively labeled mixed triglyceride (^{13}C-MTG) has been given by mouth and exhaled air measured. With normal lipolytic activity in the gastrointestinal tract, ^{13}CO$_2$ is split off and can be sampled in exhaled air.

Kalivianakis M, Elstrodt J, Havinga R, et al: Validation in an animal model of the carbon 13-labeled mixed triglyceride breath test for the detection of intestinal fat malabsorption. J Pediatr 135:444–450, 1999.

62. **How is the steatocrit measured?**

The steatocrit is a rapid measurement of the percentage of fat in a spot sample of stool. It is done by homogenizing stool with sand and water. From this slurry, a microhematocrit tube is filled and spun in a centrifuge. The lipid portion rises to the top, and the percentage that is the fat layer is calculated (much like a spun hematocrit). Newborns normally excrete up to 15% fat, and this percentage falls with age. A value of >5% is abnormal for any child >3 years old. This can be a crude estimate of fat malabsorption, but experts differ regarding its value.

Addison GM: Acid steatocrit. J Pediatr Gastroenterol Nutr 22:227, 1996.

Columbo C, Mairacca R, Ronchi M, et al: The steatocrit: A simple method for monitoring fat malabsorption in patients with cystic fibrosis. J Pediatr Gastroenterol Nutr 6:926–930, 1987.

63. **How is the degree of dehydration estimated in a child?**

See Table 7-5.

64. **What three individual clinical features are the most accurate for predicting 5% dehydration?**

1. Abnormal capillary refill
2. Abnormal skin turgor
3. Abnormal respiratory pattern

Steiner MJ, DeWalt DA, Byerley JS: Is this child dehydrated? JAMA 291:2746–2754, 2004.

65. **How accurate is blood urea nitrogen (BUN) as a means of assessing dehydration in children?**

Notoriously unreliable. The BUN does not begin to rise until the glomerular filtration rate falls to approximately one half of normal; it then rises by about 1% each hour, and it may rise even less in a fasting child with disease. In a prospective study, Bonadio and colleagues found that 80% of patients judged to be 5–10% dehydrated by common physical findings may have a normal BUN.

Bonadio WA, Hennes HH, Machi J, Madagame E: Efficacy of measuring BUN in assessing children with dehydration due to gastroenteritis. Ann Emerg Med 18:755–757, 1989.

66. **What is the physiologic basis for oral rehydration therapy?**

Intestinal solute transport mechanisms generate osmotic gradients by the movement of electrolytes and nutrients through the cell, and water passively follows. A coupled transport of sodium and glucose occurs at the intestinal brush border, and this is facilitated by the protein sodium glucose co-transporter 1. Oral replacement solutions are formulated with sufficient sodium, glucose, and osmolarity to maximize this cotransportation and to avoid problems of excessive sodium intake or additional osmotic diarrhea.

King CK, Glass R, Bresee JS, Duggan C; Centers for Disease Control and Prevention: Managing acute gastroenteritis among children: Oral rehydration, maintenance, and nutritional therapy. MMWR Recomm Rep 52(RR-16):1–16, 2003.

TABLE 7-5. CLINICAL FINDINGS TO ESTIMATE THE DEGREE OF DEHYDRATION

Signs and symptoms	Mild	Moderate	Severe
Body fluid lost (mL/kg)	<50	50–100	>100
Weight loss	<5%	5–10%	>10%
State of shock	Impending	Compensated	Uncompensated
General appearance	Thirsty, alert, restless	Thirsty, restless, or lethargic, irritable to touch	Drowsy; limp, cold, sweaty; older may be apprehensive; infants may be comatose
Vital signs			
Systolic blood pressure	Normal	Normal (orthostatic)	Very low or absent
Heart rate	Normal	Slight elevation (orthostatic)	Very elevated
Respiration	Normal	Deep, may be rapid	Deep and rapid (hyperpnea)
Other examinations			
Radial pulse	Normal rate and strength	Rapid and weak	Feeble, rapid, may be impalpable
Capillary refill	<2 seconds	2–3 seconds	>3 seconds
Skin elasticity	Retracts immediately	Retracts slowly (>3 seconds)	Retracts very slowly
Anterior fontanel	Flat	Depressed	Sunken
Mucous membranes	Normal/dry	Very dry	Very dry/cracked
Tears	Present	Absent	Absent
Skin color	Pale	Gray	Mottled
Laboratory tests			
Urine			
Volume	Decreased (<2–3 mL/kg/h)	Oliguric (1 mL/kg/h) (<1 mL/kg/h)	Anuric
Osmolarity (mOsm/L)	600	800	Maximal
Specific gravity	1.010	1.25	Maximal
Blood			
pH	7.40–7.22	7.30–6.92	7.10–6.80
Blood urea nitrogen	Upper normal	Elevated	High
HCO_3	Lower normal	Decreased (16–19 mEq/L)	Very decreased (<16 mEq/L)

From Shaw KN: Dehydration. In Fleisher GR, Ludwig S (eds): Textbook of Pediatric Emergency Medicine, 4th ed. Philadelphia, Lippincott Williams & Wilkins, 1999, p 198.

67. **How do the various oral rehydration solutions differ in composition from other liquids that are commonly used for rehydration?**

Each solution has some advantages and disadvantages. Many home remedies are either very deficient or very excessive in electrolytes or sugar. A main problem with recommended oral rehydration solutions is their low caloric content, but the development of cereal-based and polymer-based solutions—which increase calories without increasing osmolality—is in progress. Table 7-6 lists common oral rehydration solutions.

TABLE 7-6.	ORAL REHYDRATION SOLUTIONS					
Solution	Carbohydrate (gm/L)	Sodium (mEq/L)	Potassium (mEq/L)	Base (mEq/L)	Osmolality (mOsm/L)	Calories (cal/100 mL)
Diarrhea	—	50–100	25–35	25–40	250–300	—
WHO	G: 20	90	20	30	310	8
WHO/UNICEF	G: 20	75	20	25–35	245	8
Pedialyte	G: 25	45	20	30	250	10
Ricelyte	R: 30	50	25	34	210	12
Cereal-based oral rehydration solution	St: 50	60–90	20	30	315	42
Gatorade	G: 50	20	3	3	330	10
Chicken broth	0	250	5	0	450	0
Cola	F/G: 50–150	2	0.1	13	550	12–16
Apple juice	F/G/S: 100–150	3	30	0	700	15–18
Tea	0	0–1	0–1	0	0–5	0

WHO – World Health Organization, UNICEF = United Nations Children's Fund, G = glucose, R = rice syrup solids, St = starch, F = fructose, S = sucrose.

68. **How can the World Health Organization (WHO) oral electrolyte (rehydration) solution be duplicated?**

The WHO solution is 2% glucose, 20 mEq K^+/L, 90 mEq Na^+/L, 80 mEq Cl^-/L, and 30 mEq bicarbonate/L. This solution is approximated by adding 3/4 tsp of salt, 1 tsp of baking soda, 1 cup of orange juice (for KCl), and 8 tsp of sugar to a liter of water. In the United States, parental satisfaction with the WHO solution (reconstituted from packets) compares very favorably with more expensive, more readily-available commercial products. Packets are available in the United States from Cera Products (410-309-1000) and Jianas Brothers (816-421-2880).

Ladinsky M, Duggan A, Santosham M, et al: The World Health Organization oral rehydration solution in US pediatric practice: randomized trial to evaluate parent satisfaction. Arch Pediatr Adolesc Med 154:700–705, 2000.

69. **What are the basic principles guiding optimal treatment of children with diarrhea and mild dehydration?**

- Oral rehydration solution should be used for rehydration.
- Oral rehydration should be performed rapidly, ideally 50–100 mL/kg over 3–4 hours.

- For rapid realimentation, an age-appropriate, unrestricted diet is recommended as soon as dehydration is corrected.
- For breast-fed infants, nursing should be continued.
- For formula-fed infants, diluted formula is not recommended, and special formula is usually not necessary.
- Additional oral rehydration solution should be administered for ongoing losses through diarrhea.
- No unnecessary laboratory tests or medications should be administered.

King CK, Glass R, Bresee JS, Duggan C; Centers for Disease Control and Prevention: Managing acute gastroenteritis among children: Oral rehydration, maintenance, and nutritional therapy. MMWR Recomm Rep 52(RR-16):1–16, 2003.

70. **What traditional approaches to feeding during diarrhea are no longer recommended and should be voided?**
    - **Switching to lactose-free formula:** This is usually unnecessary because, for the majority of infants, clinical trials have not shown an advantage. Certain infants with severe malnutrition and dehydration may benefit from lactose-free formula.
    - **Diluted formula:** Half- or quarter-strength formula has been shown in clinical trials to be unnecessary and associated with prolonged symptoms and delays in nutritional recovery.
    - **Clear liquids:** Foods high in simple sugars (e.g., carbonated soft drinks, juice drinks, gelatin desserts) should be avoided because the high osmotic load might worsen diarrhea.
    - **Avoid fatty foods:** Fat may have a beneficial effect of reducing intestinal motility.
    - **BRAT diet:** The **b**ananas, **r**ice, **a**pplesauce, and **t**oast diet is unnecessarily restrictive and can provide suboptimal nutrition
    - **Avoid food ≥ 24 hours:** Early feeding decreases the intestinal permeability caused by infection, reduces illness duration, and improves nutritional outcome.

    Brown KH, Gastanaduy AS, Saavedra JM, et al: Effect of continued oral feeding on clinical and nutritional outcomes of acute diarrhea in children. J Pediatr 112:191–200, 1988.

    Brown KH, Peerson JM, Fontaine O: Use of nonhuman milks in the dietary management of young children with acute diarrhea: a meta-analysis of clinical trials. Pediatrics 93:17–27, 1994.

    King CK, Glass R, Bresee JS, Duggan C; Centers for Disease Control and Prevention: Managing acute gastroenteritis among children: Oral rehydration, maintenance, and nutritional therapy. MMWR Recomm Rep 52(RR-16):1–16, 2003.

71. **What are nonantimicrobial drug therapies for diarrhea?**
    In older children, adolescents, and adults, the following categories are used. Pediatric data are limited, and these medications are not typically approved or recommended for children <3 years old.
    - **Antimotility agents** (loperamide [Imodium], diphenoxylate and atropine [Lomotil], tincture of opium [Paregoric]): These can cause drowsiness, ileus, and nausea and potentiate the effects of certain bacterial enteritides (e.g., *Shigella, Salmonella*) or accelerate the course of antibiotic-associated colitis.
    - **Antisecretory drugs** (bismuth subsalicylate [Pepto-Bismol]): These involve the potential for salicylate overdose.
    - **Adsorbents** (attapulgite, kaolin-pectin [Donnagel, Kaopectate]): These can cause abdominal fullness and interfere with other medications.

72. **What is the role of probiotic organisms in the treatment of antibiotic-associated diarrhea?**
    Probiotics (which are the opposite of antibiotics) are living organisms that are believed to cause health benefits by replenishing some of the more than 500 species of intestinal bacteria

that antibiotics can suppress and by inhibiting the growth of more pathogenic flora. Among children receiving broad-spectrum antibiotics, about 20–40% are likely to experience some degree of diarrhea. *Lactobacillus GG* has been shown to limit the degree of diarrhea.

Markowitz JE, Bengmark S: Probiotics in health and disease in the pediatric patient. Pediatr Clin North Am 49:127–142, 2002.

KEY POINTS: DIARRHEA/MALABSORPTION

1. History is crucial to diagnosis and should include recent medications, ill family contacts, travel, attendance at school or day care, pets, and water sources.

2. The three keys to the assessment of dehydration are (1) capillary refill, (2) skin turgor, and (3) respiratory pattern.

3. The first line of therapy in infants and toddlers with mild dehydration from diarrhea is oral rehydration with a glucose- or electrolyte-containing solution.

4. Salmonella infection is more concerning among infants who are <1 year old because of the increased risk of dissemination (e.g., bacteremia, meningitis).

5. Toddler's diarrhea is a common cause of chronic diarrhea in children between the ages of 6 and 40 months.

6. Celiac disease (a sensitivity to gluten) is more widespread than previously thought.

FOOD ALLERGIES

73. **What are the most common food allergies in children?**
    Eggs, cow milk, and **peanuts** account for 75% of abnormal food challenges. Soy, wheat, fish, and chicken are also common allergens.

74. **Are food allergies in infants more or less common than generally perceived?**
    As the saying goes, "It depends on where your bread is buttered." Nearly a third of parents report that their infant has an adverse food reaction, and most equate this with allergy. In pediatric circles, the general perception is that true food allergies are relatively rare. The answer, as is custom, lies somewhere in between. A prospective study in Colorado of 489 infants followed from birth to the age of 3 years showed that 8% had allergies confirmed by food challenge. In Denmark, a prospective study of nearly 1,000 infants showed a prevalence of cow's milk allergy of 2.2%. The natural history of food allergies in infants is disappearance in nearly 90% of cases by the age of 3 years.

    Bock SA: Prospective appraisal of complaints of adverse reactions to foods in children during the first three years of life. Pediatrics 79:683–688, 1987.
    Host A, Halken S: A prospective study of cow's milk allergy in Danish infants during the first three years of life. Allergy 45:587–596, 1990.

75. **How are adverse food reactions characterized?**
    - **Food allergy:** Ingestion of food results in hypersensitivity reactions mediated most commonly by IgE

■ **Food intolerance:** Ingestion of food results in symptoms not immunologically mediated, and causes may include toxic contaminants (e.g., histamine in scombroid fish poisoning), pharmacologic properties of food (e.g., tyramine in aged cheeses), digestive and absorptive limitations of host (e.g., lactase deficiency), or idiosyncratic reactions

76. **What can be the acute manifestations of milk protein allergy in childhood?**
    ■ Angioedema
    ■ Urticaria
    ■ Acute vomiting and diarrhea
    ■ Anaphylactic shock
    ■ Gastrointestinal bleeding

77. **What is the most common chronic manifestation of milk protein allergy?**
    Diarrhea of variable severity. Histologic abnormalities of the small intestinal mucosa have been documented, with the most severe form seen as a flat villous lesion. Protein-losing enteropathy may result from disruption of the surface epithelium. The stools of children with primary milk protein intolerance often contain blood.

78. **What is Heiner syndrome?**
    Heiner syndrome is hematemesis and hemoptysis with failure to thrive. It is associated with milk allergy.

79. **Can laboratory tests confirm a diagnosis of milk allergy?**
    The laboratory tests available are *not* sensitive or specific enough to confirm the diagnosis fully. Tests of humoral or cellular immune function, radioallergosorbent tests, intradermal skin testing, and IgE levels have not been diagnostic. Specific assays for serum immunoglobulins directed against individual proteins in milk formulas may be useful. The peroral small-bowel biopsy may show signs of superficial damage, but postenteritis syndrome, celiac disease, and other diseases are also accompanied by this finding. The accurate diagnosis of milk protein allergy still relies on the clinical challenge test.

80. **Why is the DBPCFC a must for diagnosing food allergy?**
    The *double-blind, placebo-controlled food challenge*—while in need of a catchier acronym—is the gold standard for evaluating food allergies. The initial choice of food to be tested is usually based on history, skin tests, or radioallergosorbent testing. In a fasting patient without recent antihistamine use, small quantities of the chosen food (or placebo) are given in lyophilized form (i.e., food rapidly frozen and dehydrated under high vacuum) or as capsules or liquid. The quantities are doubled every 30–60 minutes as the patient is observed for up to 8 hours, depending on the anticipated reaction. Observers must be capable of responding to possible anaphylaxis, which usually occurs during the first 2 hours. If no reaction has occurred, the observer should knowingly give the food being tested to ensure that a false-negative test has not occurred.

81. **Why can children who are allergic to nuts usually eat peanuts without any problem?**
    Tree nuts (e.g., almonds, Brazil nuts, cashews, pecans, pistachios, or walnuts) are a relatively common cause of food allergy in adults and a less common one in children. Peanuts are a legume (like soy) and have no cross-reactivity with members of the nut family.

82. **Does delaying the introduction of solid foods until 4–6 months of age reduce the risk of food allergies?**
    This remains unclear and relatively unstudied, but it is usually recommended. The theoretical reason for the delay is to allow intestinal mucosal maturation with less "leakiness" so that fewer antigens can penetrate and initiate an immunologic response. One setting in which delay appears

to have proven benefit is in children with a strong family history of atopic dermatitis. Limiting solid foods during the first 4–6 months and also minimizing exposure to major allergenic foods (e.g., cow's milk, eggs, peanuts) diminish the prevalence and extent of atopic dermatitis.

Kajosaari M, Saarinen UM: Prophylaxis of atopic disease by six month's total solid food elimination. Arch Paediatr Scand 72:411–414, 1983.

GASTROESOPHAGEAL REFLUX/PEPTIC ULCER DISEASE

83. **How rapidly do infants outgrow gastroesophageal reflux (GER)?**
Forty percent of healthy infants regurgitate more than once a day, and mild reflux does not represent disease. As a rule, in those infants who have more significant primary GER, 50% resolve by 6 months of age, 75% by 12 months of age, and 95% by 18 months of age. GER in older children may be more widespread than appreciated. In a survey of parents of children and adolescents (3–17 years), frequent symptoms of heartburn regurgitation were found to be relatively common (2–8% of patients).

Nelson SP, Chen EH, Syniar GM, Christoffel KK: Prevalence of symptoms of gastroesophageal reflux during childhood. Arch Pediatr Adolesc Med 154:150–154, 2000.

Orenstein SR: Gastroesophageal reflux. Pediatr Rev 20:24–28, 1999.

84. **Which test is most reliable for the diagnosis of GER?**
The diagnosis can be made either clinically or by diagnostic testing. Clinically, reflux should be suspected in any child who demonstrates frequent, effortless vomiting or regurgitation without evidence of gastrointestinal obstruction. With regard to diagnostic testing, the upper gastrointestinal barium study is not sensitive for identifying reflux because it is seen in only 50% of affected patients. The "milk scan" is a more physiologic test, but it detects only postprandial reflux. Unfortunately, significant damage occurs during nocturnal reflux, which cannot be modeled by a "milk scan." Endoscopically, the presence of histologic esophagitis is suggestive but not diagnostic of reflux. Scintigraphy, a noninvasive test that uses radiolabeled meal, is very specific but only moderately sensitive for predicting reflux. The **24-hour pH probe** continues to be the most reliable test for the diagnosis of GER.

Orenstein SR: Tests to assess symptoms of gastroesophageal reflux in infants and children. J Pediatr Gastro Nutr 37:S29–S32, 2003.

85. **How are the complications of GER treated?**

Simple GER	**Failure to thrive**
Counseling	Nutritional rehabilitation
Thickened feeding	Nasogastric feeding
Positional therapy	**Apnea**
Esophagitis	Monitoring
Antacids	Fundoplication, if severe
Cimetidine, ranitidine,	**Recurrent aspiration**
or famotidine	Fundoplication
Sucralfate	Jejunal feeding
Prokinetic agents (bethanecol,	**Failure of medical and nutritional therapy**
metoclopramide)	Fundoplication

Cezard JP: Managing gastroesophageal reflux in children. Digestion 69:S3–S8, 2004.

86. **An infant with known GER who periodically arches his or her back likely has what syndrome?**
Sandifer syndrome is paroxysmal dystonic posturing with opisthotonus and unusual twisting of the head and neck (resembling torticollis) in association with GER. Typically, an esophageal hiatal hernia is also present.

87. **How effective are milk-thickening agents as a treatment for GER?**

    Although not as effective as once thought, thickened feedings do alleviate GER in 40–50% of infants, especially when the child is placed in the prone position, with the head elevated approximately 30°.

    Hassall E: Decisions in diagnosing and managing chronic gastroesophageal reflux disease in children. J Pediatric 146: S3–S12, 2005.

88. **What is the Nissen fundoplication?**

    The Nissen fundoplication is the most commonly performed antireflux surgical procedure. It involves wrapping a portion of the gastric fundus 360° around the distal esophagus in an effort to tighten the gastroesophageal junction.

89. **Which infants are candidates for fundoplication?**

    The vast majority of infants with developmental GER do not require fundoplication. It is indicated in patients with recurrent aspiration, refractory or Barrett's esophagitis, reflux-associated apnea, and reflux-associated failure to thrive that is refractory to medical therapy. Patients with severe reflux and psychomotor retardation should be evaluated for fundoplication if a feeding gastrostomy is contemplated.

90. **What are the signs and symptoms of primary peptic ulcer (PUD) in childhood?**

    Abdominal pain is the most common symptom of primary PUD; it is present in 90% of patients. Although the quality and character of the pain can be variable, it is usually localized to the epigastric region. Classically, ulcer pain is temporally related to meals; however, in children, this association occurs only about half the time. **Nocturnal pain** occurs in about 60% of patients and is a key feature for distinguishing organic from nonorganic pain. **Melena** is a feature in about a third of cases. Vomiting, hematemesis, and perforation are uncommon features.

91. **How do the presenting symptoms of secondary ulcer disease differ from primary PUD?**

    Secondary ulcers in association with other conditions are often silent until very acute symptomatology develops. **Pain** occurs only in about 25% of patients, but 80% develop **melena**, 60% have **hematemesis**, and 30% have **perforation**, often with severe bleeding and shock. The secondary ulcers involve much higher mortality and morbidity, and they require surgical intervention. In patients with primary PUD, symptoms are often recurrent and protracted. Delays in diagnosis can last for up to 2–4 years.

92. **What conditions are associated with secondary ulcers in children?**

    - **Systemic diseases:** Sepsis, acidosis, sickle cell anemia, cystic fibrosis, systemic lupus erythematosus, renal failure, severe hypoglycemia
    - **Traumatic injury:** Head trauma, burns, major surgery
    - **Drugs/toxins:** Corticosteroids, nonsteroidal anti-inflammatory drugs, theophylline, tolazoline, aspirin

93. **What treatments are available for PUD in children?**

    - **Acid-neutralizing antacids:** Effective for promoting ulcer healing; used more commonly for symptomatic pain relief because of poor compliance as a result of the large volumes (0.5 mL/kg/dose) required for therapy and potential side effects (e.g., diarrhea, constipation)
    - **H_2-receptor antagonists:** Include cimetidine, ranitidine, and famotidine; well-tolerated in children, with few side effects

- **Proton-pump inhibitors:** Inhibit the gastric acid pump
- **Sucralfate:** Chemical complex of sucrose octasulfate and aluminum hydroxide that binds to the ulcer base and acts as a barrier; adsorbs pepsin and neutralizes hydrogen ions
- **Anticholinergics:** Decrease acid secretion; at effective doses, side effects (e.g., dry mouth, blurred vision) may be significant
- **Antibiotics:** As treatment for *Helicobacter pylori* infection; most effective treatment remains unclear, but combination therapy with amoxicillin, bismuth subsalicylate (Pepto-Bismol), and metronidazole has an eradication rate of 60–90%

94. **What is the relationship of *Helicobacter pylori* infection to antral gastritis, PUD, and recurrent abdominal pain in children?**

This is an area of considerable interest, debate, and research. In adults, *H. pylori* has been associated with duodenal ulceration in >90% of patients and with gastric ulceration in 70% of patients. However, asymptomatic colonization complicates the picture. In asymptomatic adult volunteers, 20–25% of patients have *H. pylori* colonization as compared with only 4% of asymptomatic children. Studies seem to indicate that, among children, there is a strong relationship between *H. pylori* and antral gastritis (Fig. 7-3) and primary duodenal ulcer disease but a weak relationship between *H. pylori* and gastric ulcers and recurrent abdominal pain.

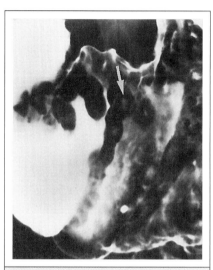

Figure 7-3. Antral gastritis. Note the thickened folds in the gastric antrum and the punctate lesions (arrow). (From Katz DS, Math KR, Groskin SA: Radiology Secrets. Philadelphia, Hanley & Belfus, 1998, p 106.)

Czinn SJ: Helicobacter pylori infection: Detection, investigation, management. J Pediatr 146:S21–S26, 2005.

Hassall E: Peptic ulcer disease and current approaches to *Helicobacter pylori*. J Pediatr 138:462–468, 2001.

95. **What methods are available for detecting the presence of *Helicobacter pylori* in the stomach or the duodenum?**

Noninvasive tests
- Stable isotope ^{13}C-urea breath test
- Serology (serum enzyme-linked immunosorbent assay test for IgG and IgA titers)
- Stool antigen test

Invasive tests
- Culture of biopsy specimen
- Polymerase chain reaction testing of biopsy specimen
- Identification of histologic gastritis
- Special stains for *H. pylori*

KEY POINTS: GASTROESOPHAGEAL REFLUX/PEPTIC ULCER DISEASE

1. More than 40% of healthy infants regurgitate effortlessly >1 time per day. This does *not* represent significant gastroesophageal reflux.

2. Tests to consider when evaluating significant reflux include the 24-hour pH probe (most reliable), an upper gastrointestinal barium study, nuclear scintigraphy, and esophagogastroduodenoscopy.

3. By the age of 18 months, the symptoms of 95% of infants with significant reflux have resolved.

4. The most common presenting symptom of peptic ulcer disease is abdominal pain that is generally localized to the epigastric region.

96. **What is the basis for the C-urea breath test for *Helicobacter*?**
    H. pylori produces urease, which can metabolize urea and produce CO_2; this is then exhaled by the patient. ^{13}C-labeled urea given orally to the patient exploits this peculiar metabolic step. If *H. pylori* is present in the proximal gastrointestinal tract, labeled CO_2 is released. This is a reliable test, but it requires (nonradioactive) labeled substrate and a mass-spectroscopy center for the assay.

97. **Which patients should be evaluated for Zollinger-Ellison syndrome (ZES)?**
    ZES, a rare diagnosis in children, is an ulcer disease caused by a gastrin-secreting tumor (gastrinoma). Patients usually present with symptoms resulting from peptic ulcer disease, and nearly all patients with ZES develop ulcers at some time during the course of the disease. In general, these ulcers are more persistent and progressive and commonly less responsive to treatment. Although the duodenal bulb is the most common location for both ZES- and non-ZES-associated ulcers, atypical ulcers in the distal duodenum or jejunum are more common in patients with ZES. In children, any ulcer that does not heal after the first course of therapy should be investigated, as should patients with gastric acid hypersecretion and prominent gastric rugae.

GASTROINTESTINAL BLEEDING

98. **What features on physical examination can help identify an unknown cause of gastrointestinal bleeding?**

Skin	Signs of chronic liver disease (e.g., spider angiomas, venous distension, caput medusae, jaundice)
	Signs of coagulopathy (e.g., petechiae, purpura)
	Signs of vascular dysplasias (e.g., telangiectasia, hemangiomas)
	Signs of vasculitis (e.g., palpable purpura on legs and buttocks suggests Henoch-Schönlein purpura)
Head and neck	Signs of epistaxis (especially before placing a nasogastric [NG] tube, which can induce bleeding)
	Hyperpigmented spots on the lips and gums (suggests Peutz-Jeghers syndrome, which is associated with multiple intestinal polyps)
	Webbed neck (suggests Turner syndrome, which is associated with gastrointestinal vascular malformations and inflammatory bowel disease)

Cardiac	Murmur of aortic stenosis (in adults, associated with vascular malformations of the ascending colon, although this association not certain in children)
Abdomen	Splenomegaly or hepatomegaly (suggests portal hypertension and possible esophageal varices)
	Ascites (suggests chronic liver disease and possible varices)
Rectum	Perianal ulcerations and skin tags (suggest inflammatory bowel disease)
	Presence of polyps, melena, or hematochezia

Mezoff AG, Preud'homme DL: How serious is that GI bleed? Contemp Pediatr 11:60–92, 1994.

99. **In patients with acute gastrointestinal bleeding, how may vital signs indicate the extent of volume depletion?**

It is important to remember that, when acute bleeding occurs in children, it may take from 12–72 hours for full equilibration of a patient's hemoglobin to occur. Vital signs are much more useful for patient management in the acute setting (Table 7-7).

Mezoff AG, Preud'homme DL: How serious is that GI bleed? Contemp Pediatr 11:60–92, 1994.

TABLE 7-7. VITAL SIGNS AND BLOOD VOLUME LOSS

Vital signs	Blood volume loss
Tachycardia without orthostasis	5–10% loss
Orthostatic changes:	>10% loss
Pulse increases by 20 beats per minute	
Blood pressure decreases by 10 mmHg	
Hypotension and resting tachycardia	30% loss
Nonpalpable pulses	>40% loss

100. **What is the simplest way of differentiating upper gastrointestinal from lower gastrointestinal bleeding?**

Nasogastric lavage. After the insertion of a soft NG tube (12 Fr in small children, 14–16 Fr in older children), 3–5 mL/kg of room-temperature normal saline is instilled. If bright red blood or coffee ground material is aspirated, the test is positive. A pink-tinged effluent is not a positive test, because it can simply denote the dissolution of a clot and not active intestinal bleeding. By definition, upper gastrointestinal bleeding occurs proximal to the ligament of Treitz. If the lavage is negative, it is unlikely that the bleeding is above this ligament, and this rules out gastric, esophageal, or nasal sources. However, bleeding from duodenal ulcers and duodenal duplications may sometimes be missed by these aspirates.

101. **How does the type of bloody stool help pinpoint the location of a gastrointestinal bleed?**

Hematochezia (bright red blood): Normal stool spotting on toilet tissue likely suggests distal bleeding (e.g., anal fissure, juvenile colonic polyp). Mucous or diarrheal stools (especially if painful) indicate left-sided or diffuse colitis.

Melena (black, tarry stools): Indicates blood denatured by acid and usually implies a lesion, likely before the ligament of Treitz. However, melena can be seen in patients with Meckel's diverticulum as a result of denaturation by anomalous gastric mucosa.

Currant jelly (dark maroon) stools usually come from the distal ileum or colon and often are associated with ischemia (e.g., intussusception).

Because blood is a cathartic, intestinal transit time can be greatly accelerated and makes defining the site of bleeding by the magnitude and color of the blood difficult. This difficulty underscores the importance of the initial NG tube insertion.

102. **What can cause false-negative and false-positive results when stool testing for blood?**

Hemoglobin and its various derivatives (e.g., oxyhemoglobin, reduced hemoglobin, methemoglobin, carboxyhemoglobin) can serve as catalysts for the oxidation of guaiac (Hemoccult) or benzidine (Hematest) when a hydrogen peroxide developer is added, thereby producing a color change.

False negatives: Ingestion of large doses of ascorbic acid; delayed transit time or bacterial overgrowth, allowing bacteria to degrade the hemoglobin to porphyrin

False positives: Recent ingestion of red meat or peroxidase-containing fruits and vegetables (e.g., broccoli, radishes, cauliflower, cantaloupes, turnips)

103. **How do the causes of *lower* gastrointestinal bleeding vary by age group?**

- **Newborns** (in order of frequency): Anal fissure, allergic proctocolitis, infectious diarrhea, Hirschsprung's disease, necrotizing enterocolitis, volvulus, stress ulcer, vascular malformation, gastrointestinal duplication
- **Infants** (in order of frequency): Anal fissure, infectious diarrhea, allergic proctocolitis, Meckel's diverticulum, intussusception, gastrointestinal duplication, peptic ulcer, foreign body
- **Older children** (in order of frequency): Anal fissure, polyp, infectious diarrhea, lymphonodular hyperplasia, inflammatory bowel disease, Henoch-Schönlein purpura, Meckel's diverticulum, peptic ulcer, hemolytic uremic syndrome, vascular malformations

Mezoff AG, Prud'homme DL: How serious is that GI bleed? Contemp Pediatr 11:60–92, 1994.

104. **A previously asymptomatic 18-month-old child has large amounts of painless rectal bleeding (red but mixed with darker clots). What is the likely diagnosis?**

Although juvenile polyps can also cause painless rectal bleeding, the more likely diagnosis is a **Meckel's diverticulum.** This outpouching occurs from the failure of the intestinal end of the omphalomesenteric duct to obliterate. Up to 2% of the population may have a Meckel's diverticulum, and about half contain gastric mucosa; most are usually silent throughout life. Meckel's diverticulum is twice as common in males and usually appears during the first 2 years of life as massive painless bleeding that is red or maroon in color. Tarry stools are observed in about 10% of cases. A history of previous minor episodes may be obtained. The presentation can range from shock to intussusception with obstruction, volvulus, or torsion. Meckel diverticulitis, which occurs in 10–20% of cases, may be indistinguishable from appendicitis.

105. **In a child with a juvenile polyp, how common are polyposis syndromes?**

Juvenile polyps are the most common type of intestinal tumor in children, usually presenting with hematochezia. Up to a third of these patients can have chronic blood loss with microcytic anemia. Juvenile polyposis is common (up to 12%) in patients with symptomatic polyps, especially with right-colonic polyps, anemia, and adenomas. The importance of establishing a diagnosis of a polyposis syndrome is that some syndromes (i.e., Peutz-Jeghers [Fig. 7-4] and juvenile polyposis coli) are associated with a risk of developing adenocarcinoma as high as 30% in as few as 10 years following diagnosis.

Hoffenberg EJ, Sauaia A, Maltzman T, et al: Symptomatic colonic polyps in childhood: Not so benign. J Pediatr Gastroenterol Nutr 28:175–181, 1999.

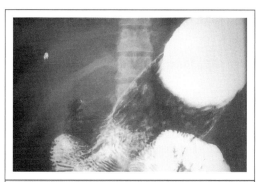

Figure 7-4. Image from a double-contrast upper gastrointestinal series reveals multiple gastric polyps in a patient with Peutz-Jeghers syndrome. (From Katz DS, Math KR, Groskin SA: Radiology Secrets. Philadelphia, Hanley & Belfus, 1998, p 139.)

106. **Worldwide, what is the most common cause of gastrointestinal blood loss in children? Hookworm infection.**
Caused by the parasites *Necator americanus* or *Ancylostoma duodenale*, this infection is often asymptomatic. Progressive microscopic blood loss often leads to anemia as a result of iron deficiency.

Crompton DW: The public health importance of hookworm disease. Parasitology 121:S39–S50, 2000.

107. **Describe the management for massive upper gastrointestinal bleeding.**
This type of hemorrhage is a life-threatening emergency, and initial therapy precedes the specific diagnostic evaluation. Management includes the following:
- Brief history and character of bleeding, previous episodes, and bleeding disorders
- Vital signs
- Intravascular access and serologic studies (complete blood cell count, liver function tests, coagulation profile, crossmatch)
- Nasogastric tube insertion
- Full history and physical examination
- Transfusion and intravascular support
- Determination of probable etiology
1. *Peptic disease:* Diagnostic endoscopy; Therapeutic endoscopy; H_2-blockers, antacids, sucralfate
   If no resolution: Surgical repair of ulcer, Partial resection
2. *Variceal bleeding:* Diagnostic endoscopy; Therapeutic endoscopy; Vasopressin, octreotide
   If no resolution: Sengstaken-Blakemore tube, Emergency portosystemic shunt, Esophageal devascularization
3. *Mallory-Weiss tear*
4. *Superficial vascular anomaly:* Endoscopic ablation

108. **How do the causes of upper gastrointestinal bleeding vary by age group?**
- **Newborns** (in order of frequency): Swallowed maternal blood, hemorrhagic gastritis, stress ulcer, idiopathic bleeding, coagulopathy, gastric outlet obstruction, gastric volvulus, pyloric stenosis, antral or pyloric webs

- **Infants** (in order of frequency): Epistaxis, gastritis, esophagitis, stress ulcer, gastric/duodenal ulcer, foreign body, gastric volvulus, esophageal varices
- **Children** (in order of frequency): Epistaxis, tonsillitis/sinusitis, gastritis, gastric/duodenal ulcer, medication, Mallory-Weiss tears, tumors, hematologic disorders, esophageal varices, Münchausen/Münchausen-by-proxy syndrome

Mezoff AG, Preud'Homme DL: How serious is that GI bleed? Contemp Pediatr 11:60–92, 1994.

KEY POINTS: GASTROINTESTINAL BLEEDING

1. Hemoglobin measurement is a much less reliable indicator of volume depletion than vital signs during the assessment of acute gastrointestinal bleeding.

2. Nasogastric lavage is a simple method for differentiating upper gastrointestinal bleeding from lower gastrointestinal bleeding and should always be performed in all patients suspected of having a significant gastrointestinal bleed.

3. The two most common causes of painless rectal bleeding in children are juvenile polyps and Meckel's diverticula.

109. **Why is the buffering of gastric acid important for controlling upper gastrointestinal bleeding?**
    - Acid is ulcerogenic and can cause and propagate erosions.
    - Coagulation is better in a neutral or alkaline environment than in an acidic one.
    - Platelet plugs are disrupted by gastric pepsins, but these pepsins function less well in a neutral or alkaline environment.

    Mezoff AG, Preud'Homme DL: How serious is that GI bleed? Contemp Pediatr 11:60–92, 1994.

110. **Name the six most common causes of massive gastrointestinal bleeding in children.**
    1. Esophageal varices
    2. Meckel's diverticulum
    3. Hemorrhagic gastritis
    4. Crohn's disease with ileal ulcer
    5. Peptic ulcer (mainly duodenal)
    6. Arteriovenous malformation

    Treem WR: Gastrointestinal bleeding in children. Gastrointest Endosc Clin North Am 5:75–97, 1994.

HEPATIC/BILIARY DISEASE

111. **What laboratory tests are commonly used to evaluate liver disease?**
    See Table 7-8.

112. **What conditions are associated with elevations of aminotransferases?**
    - Hepatocellular inflammation (hepatitis)
    - Drug- or toxin-associated hepatic injury
    - Hypoperfusion or hypoxia

- Passive congestion (right-sided congestive heart failure, Budd-Chiari syndrome, constrictive pericarditis)
- Nonhepatic disorders (muscular dystrophy, celiac disease, macroenzyme of aspartate aminotransferase [AST])

Teitelbaum JE: Normal hepatobiliary function. In Rudolph CD, Rudolph AM (eds): Rudolph's Pediatrics, 21st ed. New York, McGraw-Hill, 2003, pp 1479.

TABLE 7-8.   LABORATORY TESTS COMMONLY USED TO EVALUATE LIVER DISEASE

Test	Clinical Significance
Alanine aminotransferase (ALT, SGPT)	Increased with damaged hepatocytes
Aspartate aminotransferase (AST, SGOT)	Less sensitive than ALT for hepatic injury
Alkaline phosphatase (AP)	Increased in cholestatic disease; determine source by isoenzyme
γ-Glutamyltransferase (GGT)	More sensitive marker for cholestasis than AP
Bilirubin	Differential diagnosis different for conjugated versus unconjugated
Albumin	Can indicate chronic impairment in hepatic synthetic function
Prealbumin	Shorter half-life; may reflect more acute synthetic capabilities
Prothrombin time (PT)	Reflects synthetic function as a result of short half-life of factors
Ammonia	Impaired removal in patients with chronic liver disease

Data from Teitelbaum JE: Normal hepatobiliary function. In Rudolph CD, Rudolph AM (eds): Rudolph's Pediatrics, 21st ed. New York, McGraw-Hill, 2003, pp 1473–1481.

113. **What distinguishes conjugated from unconjugated bilirubin?**
Bilirubin released from erythrocytes (unconjugated) is taken up by the liver and enzymatically converted (conjugated) to a more water-soluble form. On the basis of laboratory methodology, measurements of unconjugated bilirubin are referred to as *indirect-reacting* and those of conjugated bilirubin as *direct-reacting*.

114. **When are levels of conjugated bilirubin considered abnormal?**
When they are >30% of total bilirubin. In significant indirect (unconjugated) hyperbilirubinemia, direct (conjugated) levels usually do not exceed 15%. The levels between 15% and 30% are thus somewhat indeterminate.

115. **When should conjugated hyperbilirubinemia be suspected?**
Conjugated hyperbilirubinemia requires the evaluation of patients at all ages. The physician will try to identify if the cause is obstruction of the biliary tract, intrahepatic cholestasis, or poorly-functioning hepatocytes. The differential diagnosis is long, including congential anomalies

(biliary atresia, choledochal cyst), gallstones, hepatic fibrosis, infections (e.g., viral, parasitic, syphilitic, bacterial [particularly urinary tract infection]) and genetic and metabolic abnormalities.

116. **What is the likelihood of chronic hepatic disease developing after acute infections with hepatitis viruses A–G?**
    - **Hepatitis A:** 95% recover within 1–2 weeks of illness; chronic disease is unusual
    - **Hepatitis B:** >90% of perinatally infected infants develop chronic hepatitis B infection; 25–50% of children who acquire the virus between 1 and 5 years of age develop chronic infection; in older children and adults, only 6–10% develop chronic infection
    - **Hepatitis C:** 50–60% develop persistent infection
    - **Hepatitis D:** Occurs only in patients with acute or chronic hepatitis B infection; 80% develop viral persistence
    - **Hepatitis E:** Does not cause chronic hepatitis
    - **Hepatitis G:** Unknown

    American Academy of Pediatrics: Hepatitis A-G. In Pickering LK (ed): 2003 Red Book, Report of the Committee on Infectious Diseases, 26th ed. Elk Grove Village, IL, American Academy of Pediatrics, 2003, pp 309–343.

117. **In addition to viral hepatitis, what are other causes of chronic hepatitis in children?**
    - **Metabolic/genetic disorders:** Wilson's disease, alpha$_1$-antitrypsin deficiency, cystic fibrosis, steatohepatitis
    - **Toxic hepatitis:** Drugs, hepatotoxins, radiation
    - **Autoimmune hepatitis:** Anti-smooth-muscle, antibody-positive, anti-liver-kidney microsomal, antibody-positive

118. **In children with alpha$_1$-antitrypsin deficiency, which organ system is initially involved: lung or liver?**
    alpha$_1$-Antitrypsin is a major inhibitor of several proteolytic enzymes, primarily leukocyte elastase. Because leukocyte elastase functions relatively unchecked, elastic fibers in the lung are digested, with the resultant destruction of alveolar walls and eventual panacinar emphysema. However, because the pulmonary effects take years to evolve, this condition rarely presents with pulmonary disease in children. More common presenting symptoms are neonatal cholestasis, hepatomegaly, chronic hepatitis, or, rarely, cirrhosis with liver failure.

    Primhak RA, Tanner MS: Alpha-1 antitrypsin deficiency. Arch Dis Child 85:2–5, 2001.

119. **How is Pi typing useful for the evaluation of alpha$_1$-antitrypsin deficiency?**
    Pi typing (short for **p**rotease **i**nhibitor typing) takes advantage of the fact that there are >70 variants of the alpha$_1$-antitrypsin protein, each with a different electrophoretic mobility. Alleles are inherited in a codominant fashion, and thus a gene from each parent is expressed in one individual. MM is the normal phenotype and has the highest activity; ZZ has the lowest activity and the most common association with liver disease. PiMM is the most common Pi type, with a distribution of about 87%; PiMS represents 8%, and PiMZ 2%. The incidence of PiZZ ranges between 1 in 2,000 and 1 in 5,000.

120. **What is the metabolic defect in patients with Wilson's disease?**
    Wilson's disease is an autosomal recessive **defect of copper metabolism** that results in markedly increased levels of copper in many tissues, most notably the liver, basal ganglia, and cornea (Kayser-Fleischer rings). The combination of markedly increased copper levels in a liver biopsy specimen, low serum ceruloplasmin, and increased urinary copper excretion strongly suggests Wilson's disease.

121. **Is there a treatment of choice for Wilson's disease?**

    D-**Penicillamine**, a copper-chelating agent, is the drug of choice. Another copper-chelating drug, trientine, has been used successfully in patients who have discontinued penicillamine because of hypersensitivity reactions. Zinc sulfate, which inhibits intestinal copper absorption, has also been used. Patients require a low copper diet for life.

122. **An infant with cholestasis, triangular facies, and a pulmonic stenosis murmur is likely to have what syndrome?**

    Alagille syndrome (arteriohepatic dysplasia). Also called **syndromic bile duct paucity**, this condition consists of a constellation of conjugated hyperbilirubinemia and cholestasis, typical triangular facies, cardiac lesions of pulmonic stenosis, peripheral pulmonic stenosis, or, occasionally, more significant lesions, butterfly vertebrae, and eye findings of posterior embryotoxon and Axenfeld's anomaly or iris processes. The patient may have extreme cholestasis, with pruritus and marked hypercholesterolemia. Although some patients have developmental delay, most develop appropriately. The usual mode of inheritance of Alagille syndrome is autosomal dominant.

123. **A 3-year-old child who experiences mild fluctuating jaundice in times of illness "just like his Uncle Kevin" is likely to have what condition?**

    Gilbert syndrome, which is due primarily to a decrease in hepatic glucuronyl transferase activity. Normally, bilirubin is disconjugated to glucuronic acid. In patients with Gilbert syndrome, the defective total conjugation results in the increased production of monoglucuronides in bile and mild elevation in serum unconjugated (indirect) bilirubin. The syndrome is inherited in an autosomal dominant fashion with incomplete penetrance (boys outnumber girls by 4 to 1). Frequency of this gene in the population is estimated at 2–6%. Elevations of bilirubin are noted during times of medical and physical stress, particularly fasting.

124. **Describe the clinical findings of portal hypertension.**

    Obstruction of portal flow is manifested by two physical signs: **splenomegaly** and **increased collateral venous circulations**. Collaterals are evident on physical examination in the anus and abdominal wall and by special studies in the esophagus. Hemorrhoids may suggest collaterals, but, in older patients, these are present in high frequency without liver disease, and thus their presence has no predictive value. Dilation of the paraumbilical veins produces a rosette around the umbilicus (the caput medusae), and the dilated superficial veins of the abdominal wall are visible. A venous hum may be present in the subxiphoid region from varices in the falciform ligament.

125. **How do the clinical presentations of acute and chronic liver failure vary?**

    Acute hepatic failure: This appears as worsening of the hyperbilirubinemia and a decreased synthetic capacity that is evidenced by a worsening coagulation profile (vitamin-K resistant) and decreasing concentrations of fibrinogen, urea, and serum albumin. Encephalopathy (with concomitant increases in serum ammonia) may develop. As the liver mass shrinks, hepatic transaminases (a markor of liver damage) may paradoxically fall toward normal. These patients are at high risk for hypoglycemia.

    Chronic hepatic failure: This is caused by a wide variety of infectious, toxic, and metabolic abnormalities, and it is characterized by jaundice and cutaneous manifestations (e.g., spider angiomas, caput medusae, palmar erythema). Fluid retention, the development of ascites, renal hypoperfusion, and metabolic acidosis may occur. Mental status alterations and tremulous asterixis are chronic neurologic features. Ominous signs are gastrointestinal bleeding, renal failure, cerebral edema, and coma.

126. **A patient with liver failure develops confusion. Why worry?**

    Hepatic encephalopathy can appear as either a rapid progression to coma or as mild fluctuations in mental status over an extended amount of time. A single underlying cause has not been established, but suspected toxins include ammonia, other neurotoxins, and a relatively increased gamma-aminobutyric acid (GABA) activity. Management requires the limitation of protein intake, the use of lactulose to promote mild diarrhea, antibiotics to reduce ammonia production, intracranial pressure monitoring in advanced cases, and possible peritoneal dialysis for patients in severe coma and before liver transplantation.

KEY POINTS: HEPATIC/BILIARY DISEASE

1. Portal hypertension manifests clinically as splenomegaly and increased collateral venous circulation.

2. Conjugated hyperbilirubinemia in any child is abnormal and deserves further investigation.

3. Extrahepatic biliary atresia is the most common pediatric indication for liver transplantation.

4. The younger the patient, the more likely it is that acute hepatitis B infection will become chronic.

127. **In children with liver failure, how should gastrointestinal hemorrhage be managed?**
   - Pass an NG tube to monitor upper gastrointestinal hemorrhage in patients with portal hypertension
   - Daily vitamin K intravenously (0.2 mg/kg) for 3 days, and continue if response is seen
   - Judicious administration of fresh frozen plasma for clinical bleeding
   - Have cross-matched blood available at all times; for children with variceal bleeding, have 40 mL/kg whole blood and 0.2 U/kg platelets available
   - For gastritis or peptic ulceration, treat with ranitidine (2–6 mL/kg/day) and maintain a gastric pH level of >5

128. **What is the most common indication for pediatric liver transplantation?**
   The most common indication is **extrahepatic biliary atresia** with chronic liver failure after a Kasai hepatoportoenterostomy. Other common indications include inborn errors of metabolism (e.g., alpha$_1$-antitrypsin deficiency, hereditary tyrosinemia, Wilson's disease) and idiopathic fulminant hepatic failure.

129. **Which patients are at risk for cholelithiasis?**
   See Table 7-9.

INFLAMMATORY BOWEL DISEASE

130. **How do ulcerative colitis and Crohn's disease vary in intestinal distribution?**
   Ulcerative colitis is limited to the superficial mucosa of the colon. It always involves the rectum and extends proximally to a variable extent. Limited distal ulcerative colitis has also been called *ulcerative proctitis* and in children may have a better prognosis. Regional enteritis, or **Crohn's disease**, is a transmural inflammation of the bowel that may affect the entire tract from the mouth to the anus. The syndrome of limited Crohn's colitis may be difficult to differentiate from ulcerative colitis. Differentiation is often based on the findings of significant inflammation seen on upper endoscopy. The typical cobblestone appearance of Crohn's disease is produced by criss-crossing ulcerations (Fig. 7-5).

TABLE 7-9.   PATIENTS AT RISK FOR CHOLELITHIASIS

	Pigment stone	Cholesterol stone
Demography		
Race	—	Native American
Sex	—	Females
Age	—	Adolescence
Diet	—	Obesity
Total parenteral nutrition	+++	—
Hemolytic disease (especially sickle cell disease, thalassemia, hereditary spherocytosis)	+++	—
Cystic fibrosis	—	+++
Ileal disease	—	+++
Defects in bile salt synthesis	—	+++
Hypertriglyceridemia	—	+++
Diabetes mellitus	—	+++

Adapted from Shaffer EA: Gallbladder disease. In Walker WA, Watkins JB (eds): Pediatric Gastrointestinal Disease. Philadelphia, B.C. Decker, 1991, p 1154.

131. **What features differentiate ulcerative colitis from Crohn's disease?**
See Table 7-10.

132. **As the severity of ulcerative colitis increases, how does the treatment vary?**
Treatment varies according to the age of the patient and the duration and severity of disease. Mesalamine (5-aminosalicylic acid) is the usual first therapy in all cases of ulcerative colitis. Steroid or 5-aminosalicylic acid enemas may control distal-limited disease. In more severe cases, prednisone (or any of the steroid group) is used to induce remission. When outpatient therapy is unsuccessful, elemental diets or parenteral alimentation are instituted. Long courses of intake restriction and aggressive intravenous nutritional therapy are likely to be efficacious. Immunosuppressive therapy (6-mercaptopurine or azathioprine) has a

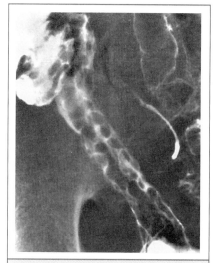

Figure 7-5. Criss-crossing ulcerations produce a cobblestone appearance in patients with Crohn's disease. (From Katz DS, Math KR, Groskin SA: Radiology Secrets. Philadelphia, Hanley & Belfus, 1998, p 150.)

TABLE 7-10. FEATURES THAT DIFFERENTIATE ULCERATIVE COLITIS FROM CROHN'S DISEASE

	Ulcerative colitis	Crohn's disease
Incidence (age range, 10–19 years)	2 in 100,000	4.5 in 100,000
Onset during childhood	15–20%	20–25%
Clinical presentation	Diarrhea: 50%	Diarrhea: 80%
	Rectal bleeding: > 90%	Rectal bleeding: 50%
	Weight loss: 65%	Weight loss: 85%
	Growth failure: 10%	Growth failure: 35%
	Pain with defecation	Anorexia, postprandial pain; extraintestinal signs may predominate
Site of disease at presentation	Rectal involvement: 100%	Ileum ± colon: 50–70%
	Left-sided colitis: 50–60%	Colon alone: 10–20%
	Severe pancolitis: 10%	Proximal small bowel: 10–15%
		Gastroduodenal: <5%
Endoscopic findings	Continuous inflammation	Focal or segmental inflammation
	100% rectal involvement	Rectal sparing
	Erythema, edema, friability, ulceration on abnormal mucosa	Aphthous or linear ulcerations on normal-appearing mucosa
		Cobblestoning
		Abnormal terminal ileum: >50%
Histologic findings	Mucin depletion	Epithelioid granulomas
	Villous mucosal surface pattern	Histiocytic infiltrates
		Pericryptitis
	Crypt abscesses	Submucosal extension of inflammation
	Epithelial atypia	
	Continuous disease	Discontinuous disease

From Hofley PM, Piccoli DA: Inflammatory bowel disease in children. Med Clin North Am 78:1281–1302, 1994.

role in the maintenance of remission. Infliximab, a chimeric antibody, has been used to treat ulcerative colitis with some degree of success, although its use remains controversial. When medical therapy fails or when toxic megacolon is present, surgical therapy is necessary.

Kim SC, Ferry GD: Inflammatory bowel diseases in pediatric and adolescent patients: Clinical, therapeutic, and psychosocial considerations. Gastroenterology 126:1550–1560, 2004.

Mamula P, Mascarenhas MR, Baldassano RN: Biological and novel therapies for inflammatory bowel disease. Pediatr Clin North Am 49:1–26, 2002.

133. **In a child diagnosed who has been with inflammatory bowel disease (IBD), what are the potential long-term complications?**
    - **Severe perianal disease** can be a debilitating complication. More prevalent in patients with Crohn's disease, it may range from simple skin tags to total devastation of the perineum.

- In patients with Crohn's disease, **enteroenteral fistulas** may occur and "short circuit" the absorptive process. The thickened bowel may obstruct or perforate, thus requiring operation. The recurrence rate is high after surgery, repeated operations are often necessary, and short bowel syndrome may result. In many cases a permanent ostomy is placed, although pouch construction and continent ileostomies have become more common.
- In cases of ulcerative colitis, the patient may require **surgery** because of the severity or duration of disease. In the past, most patients had total colectomy and ileostomy, but the current recommended procedure is a subtotal colectomy and an endorectal pull-through with rectal mucosal stripping. This procedure maintains intestinal continuity, and the patient develops normal rectal continence, although with increased stool frequency.
- **Toxic megacolon** is more common among patients with ulcerative colitis. After a progressive course, fever and a decrease in diarrhea usually herald a distended, tender, and tympanitic abdomen. The profound dilation of the bowel may be segmental or total, and massive hemorrhage or perforation may ensue. Mortality is high if toxic megacolon is not identified and treated aggressively.
- **Growth retardation and delayed puberty** are seen in both diseases but are more common in patients with Crohn's disease. The insidious onset may result in several years of linear growth failure before the correct diagnosis is made. With epiphyseal closure, linear growth is terminated, and short adult stature will be permanent.
- **Hepatic complications** of IBD include chronic active hepatitis and sclerosing cholangitis, which may require liver transplantation.
- **Nephrolithiasis** may occur in patients with resections or steatorrhea as a result of the increased intestinal absorption of oxalate.
- Chronic reactive and restrictive **pulmonary disease** has been noted.
- Arthralgias are common, but destructive **joint disease** is uncommon.

KEY POINTS: INFLAMMATORY BOWEL DISEASE

1. Ulcerative colitis is limited to the superficial mucosa of the large intestine, always involves the rectum, and demonstrates no skip lesions.

2. Crohn's disease can occur anywhere in the gastrointestinal tract (from the mouth to the anus) and demonstrates transmural inflammation with skip lesions; noncaseating granulomas may be found on microscopic pathology.

3. Potential long-term complications of inflammatory bowel disease include chronic growth failure, abscesses, fistulas, nephrolithiasis, and toxic megacolon.

4. Patients with inflammatory bowel disease have an increased lifetime risk of malignancy.

134. Are children with IBD at increased risk for malignancy?

The risk of malignancy has not been studied systematically among pediatric populations with IBD. The risk in adults depends both on the disease and its duration. After 10 years of ulcerative colitis, the risk rises dramatically (1–2% increased incidence of malignancy per year). The risk is felt to be higher in patients with pancolitis as compared with those with limited left-sided disease. The carcinomas associated with ulcerative colitis are often poorly differentiated and metastasize early; they have a poorer prognosis and are more difficult to identify by radiographic and colonoscopic examinations. Most authors indicate that carcinoma of the bowel is much less common among patients with Crohn's disease, although this has been disputed.

The risk of lymphoma is increased in patients with Crohn's disease. Immunosuppressive therapy (e.g., azathioprine) may also increase the risk of neoplasia.

135. **When is surgery indicated for children with IBD?**

Crohn's disease		Ulcerative colitis
Perforation with abscess formation	*Urgent:*	Hemorrhage
		Perforation
Obstruction with or without stenosis		Toxic megacolon
Uncontrolled massive bleeding		Acute fulminant colitis unresponsive to maximal medical therapy
Draining fistulas and sinuses	*Elective:*	Chronic disease with recurrent severe
Toxic megacolon		exacerbations
Growth failure in patients with localized despite		Continuous incapacitating disease
areas of resectable disease		adequate medical treatment
		Growth retardation with pubertal delay
		Disease of >10 years' duration with evidence of epithelial dysplasia

From Hofley PM, Piccoli DA: Inflammatory bowel disease in children. Med Clin North Am 78:1293–1295, 1994.

136. **Which has a better prognosis: Crohn's disease or ulcerative colitis?**
The outcome for patients with ulcerative colitis is better unless toxic megacolon or carcinoma develops. In these patients, surgery is curative, and the chronic morbidity depends on the type of surgery employed. Patients with Crohn's disease can be expected to lead a functional and productive life. However, as many as three fourths require surgery within 5 years of diagnosis, and only half of those with growth failure achieve significant catch-up growth.

LIPID DISORDERS

137. **How are lipoproteins categorized?**
The three major lipoprotein groups are classified by their density or electrophoretic properties: **very-low-density lipoproteins** (VLDL or pre-beta), **low-density lipoproteins** (LDL or beta), and **high-density lipoproteins** (HDL or alpha$_1$). In addition, chylomicrons and an intermediate-density lipoprotein (IDL or "floating beta") can be found in plasma, although their quantities are typically much less, except in children with disorders of lipid metabolism.

138. **What are normal cholesterol levels for children and adolescents?**
Total cholesterol (mg/dL)
- Acceptable: <170
- Borderline: 170–199
- High: >200

LDL cholesterol (mg/dL)
- Acceptable: <110
- Borderline: 110–129
- High: >130

American Academy of Pediatrics, Committee on Nutrition: Cholesterol in childhood. Pediatrics 101(1 Pt 1):141–147, 1998.

139. How is LDL cholesterol calculated?
LDL cholesterol = total cholesterol − (HDL cholesterol + [total triglyceride/5])

140. Which children should have their cholesterol measured?
This is a controversial issue that involves both proponents and opponents of universal screening. Current recommendations, which were developed by the National Cholesterol Education Committee and the American Academy of Pediatrics, adopt a middle ground: to screen all children aged ≥2 years old if is the following are present:

- Family history of parents or grandparents aged 55 years or younger with documented premature cardiovascular disease
- History of a parent with elevated total cholesterol (>240 mg/dL)
- Parental and/or family history is unobtainable (e.g., adoption)
  Proponents of universal screening have since argued that the guidelines are not sufficiently sensitive and may miss up to 50% of children with elevated lipids.

American Academy of Pediatrics, Committee on Nutrition: Cholesterol in childhood. Pediatrics 101(1 Pt 1):141–147, 1998.

O'Loughlin J, Lauzon B, Paradis G, et al: Usefulness of the American Academy of Pediatrics recommendations for identifying youths with hypercholesterolemia. Pediatrics 113:1723–1727, 2004.

141. Outline arguments against universal screening for elevated cholesterol.
- Instrumentation for cholesterol measurement is not standardized, and some children will be mislabeled.
- If pediatric dietary recommendations (e.g., total fat <30% of calories) are routinely followed, many children with hypercholesterolemia will achieve normal levels.
- Serum cholesterol may not be the most sensitive indicator of future atherosclerotic heart disease.
- Tracking (persistence of high or low levels over time) is not precise for serum cholesterol.
- Although fatty arterial plaques occur in children, atherosclerotic events are rare before the third decade, and present evidence suggests reversibility at that age with treatment.
- The cost of universal screening is large as compared with its benefits.

Newman TB, Garber AM: Cholesterol screening in children and adolescents. Pediatrics 105:637–638, 2000.

Newman TB, Garber AM, Holtzman NA, Hulley SB: Problems with the report of the Expert Panel on blood cholesterol levels in children and adolescents. Arch Pediatr Adolesc Med 149:241–247, 1995.

142. How are the primary genetic hyperlipidemias classified?
See Table 7-11.

143. What is the most common hyperlipidemia in childhood?
Familial hypercholesterolemia, type IIA, with elevated cholesterol and LDL. This condition results from a lack of functional LDL receptors on cell membranes as a result of various mutations. When LDL cannot attach and release cholesterol to the cell, feedback suppression of hydroxymethylglutaryl coenzyme A reductase (the rate-limiting enzyme of cholesterol synthesis) does not occur, and cholesterol synthesis continues excessively. In the homozygous form of type IIa, xanthomas may appear before the age of 10 years and vascular disease before the age of 20 years. However, the homozygous form is very rare, with an incidence of 1 in 1,000,000 births. The *heterozygous variety* has a much higher incidence of 1 in 500, but it is less likely to produce clinical manifestations in children.

TABLE 7-11. CLASSIFICATION OF PRIMARY GENETIC HYPERLIPIDEMIAS

Frederickson type	Lipids increased	Lipoproteins increased	Prevalence	Clinical findings
I	Triglyceride	Chylomicrons	Very rare	Eruptive xanthomas, pancreatitis, recurrent abdominal pain, lipemia retinalis, hepatosplenomegaly
IIa	Cholesterol	LDL	Common	Tendon xanthomas, PVD
IIb	Cholesterol, triglyceride	LDL + VLDL	Common	PVD, no xanthomas
III	Cholesterol, Triglyceride	VLDL remnants (IDL)	Rare	PVD, yellow palm creases
IV	Triglyceride	VLDL	Uncommon	PVD, xanthomas, hyperglycemia
V	Triglyceride, cholesterol	VLDL + chylomicrons	Very rare	Pancreatitis, lipemia retinalis, xanthomas, hyperglycemia

LDL = low-density lipoproteins, PVD = premature vascular disease, VLDL = very-low-density lipoproteins, IDL = intermediate-density lipoproteins.

144. **What are the treatment options for familial hypercholesterolemia?**
    - **Nonpharmacologic therapy:** Dietary restriction of cholesterol and fat; exercise and weight loss
    - **Lipid-lowering resins:** Cholestyramine and the related resin, colestipol, lower plasma cholesterol by trapping bile acids in the gut, thereby causing more cholesterol to be shunted to bile acid synthesis.
    - **Niacin** (nicotinic acid): Reduces LDL synthesis
    - **Gemfibrozil:** Enhances VLDL breakdown
    - **Hydroxymethylglutaryl coenzyme A reductase inhibitors** ("statins"): Inhibitors of the rate-limiting enzyme of cholesterol synthesis

    Obarzanek E, Kimm SY, Barton BA, et al; DISC Collaborative Research Group: Long-term safety and efficacy of a cholesterol-lowering diet in children with elevated low-density lipoprotein cholesterol: seven year results of the Dietary Intervention Study in Children (DISC). Pediatrics 107:256–264, 2001.
    Weigman A, Hutten BA, de Groot E, et al: Efficacy and safety of statin therapy in children with familial hypercholesterolemia: A randomized controlled trial. JAMA 292:331–337, 2004.

NUTRITION

145. **What are various requirements for protein, fat, and carbohydrates?**
    Protein should account for 7–15% of caloric intake and should include a balance of the 11 essential amino acids. Protein requirements range from 0.7–2.5 gm/kg/day. **Fats** should

provide 30–50% of caloric intake. Although most of these calories are derived from long-chain triglycerides, sterols, medium-chain triglycerides, and fatty acids may be important in certain diets. Linoleic acid and arachidonic acid are essential for tissue membrane synthesis, and approximately 3% of intake must be composed of these triglycerides. The remaining 50–60% of calories should come from **carbohydrates**. About half of these are contributed by mono- and disaccharides (e.g., sucrose, lactose) and the remainder by starches.

146. **If recommended caloric intakes are maintained, what is normal daily weight gain of young children?**
See Table 7-12.

TABLE 7-12.	NORMAL DAILY WEIGHT GAIN IN YOUNG CHILDREN*	
Age	Weight gain recommended (grams)	Caloric intake (kcal/kg/day)
0–3 months	26–31	100–120
3–6 months	17–18	105–115
6–9 months	12–13	100–105
9–12 months	9	100–105
1–3 years	7–9	100
4–6 years	6	90

*It should be noted that, when babies are primarily breast fed, growth during months 3–18 is less than that indicated by the table. On average, breast-fed babies gain 0.65 kg less than formula-fed infants during the first year of life.
Data from Dewey KG, Heinig MJ, Nommsen LA, et al: Growth of breast-fed and formula-fed infants from 0 to 18 months: The DARLING Study. Pediatrics 89:1035–1041, 1992; and National Research Council, Food and Nutrition Board: Recommended Daily Allowances. Washington, DC, National Academy of Sciences, 1989.

147. **What are the recommended bottle feedings by age?**
See Table 7-13.

TABLE 7-13.	RECOMMENDED BOTTLE FEEDINGS BY AGE	
Age	Number of feedings	Fluid ounces per feeding
Birth–1 week	6–10	1–3
1 week–1 month	7–8	2–4
1–3 months	5–7	4–6
3–6 months	4–5	6–7
6–9 months	3–4	7–8
10–12 months	3	7–8

148. **Why is honey not recommended for infants during the first year of life?**
Honey has been associated with infantile botulism (so have some commercial corn syrups). *Clostridium botulinum* spores contaminate the honey and are ingested. In infants, intestinal colonization and multiplication of the organism may result in toxin production and lead to symptoms of constipation, listlessness, and weakness.

149. **How is nutritional status objectively assessed in children?**
   - **Growth chart:** Anthropometric data give an estimate of the height, weight, and head circumference of a child as compared with a population standard. A change in the child's percentile months may signify the presence of a nutritional problem or systemic disease.
   - **Compare actual with ideal body weight** (average weight for height age): The ideal body weight is determined by plotting the child's height on the 50th percentile and recording the corresponding age. The 50th percentile weight for that age is obtained, and this ideal body weight is divided by the actual weight. The result is expressed as a percentage—the percent ideal body weight—that gives a better stratification of patients with significant malnutrition. An ideal body weight percentage of >120% is obese, 110–120% is overweight, 90–110% is normal, 80–90% is mild wasting, 70–80% is moderate wasting, and <70% is severe wasting.
   - **Measurement of midarm circumference:** This provides information about the subcutaneous fat stores, and the midarm-muscle circumference (calculated from the triceps skinfold thickness) estimates the somatic protein or muscle mass.
   - **Laboratory assessment:** Vitamin and mineral status can be directly assayed. Measurements of *albumin* (half-life, 14–20 days), *transferrin* (half-life, 8–10 days), and *prealbumin* (half-life, 2–3 days) can provide information about protein synthesis, but each may be affected by certain diseases. The ratio of albumin to globulin may decrease in patients with protein malnutrition.

150. **What features on examination of the scalp, eyes, and mouth suggest problems of malnutrition?**
   See Table 7-14.

151. **How do marasmus and kwashiorkor differ clinically?**
   - **Kwashiorkor** is edematous malnutrition as a result of low serum oncotic pressure. The low serum proteins result from a disproportionately low protein intake as compared with the overall caloric intake. These children appear replete or fat, but they have dependent edema, hyperkeratosis, and atrophic hair and skin. They generally have severe anorexia, diarrhea, and frequent infections, and they may have cardiac failure.
   - **Marasmus** is severe nonedematous malnutrition caused by a mixed deficiency of both protein and calories. Serum protein and albumin levels are usually normal, but there is a marked decrease in muscle mass and adipose tissue. Signs are similar to those noted in hypothyroid children, with cold intolerance, listlessness, thin sparse hair, dry skin with decreased turgor, and hypotonia. Diarrhea, anorexia, vomiting, and recurrent infections may be noted.

152. **What are the major complications of intravenous hyperalimentation?**
   - **Mechanical:** Local or distant site thrombosis, perforation of the vasculature or heart, and accidental breakage or infiltration of the infusate into the subcutaneous, pleural, or pericardial space
   - **Infectious:** Particularly line-associated sepsis
   - **Metabolic:** Congestive heart failure and pulmonary edema from excessive infusate; hyper- and hypoglycemia; electrolyte, mineral, and vitamin disorders; hyperlipidemia; metabolic acidosis; hyperammonemia; hepatic disorders (e.g., cholestasis, cholelithiasis, hepatitis)

SURGICAL ISSUES

153. **What is the natural history of an umbilical hernia?**
   Most umbilical hernias <0.5 cm spontaneously close before a patient is 2 years old. Those between 0.5 cm and 1.5 cm take up to 4 years to close. If the umbilical hernia is >2 cm, it may

still close spontaneously but may take up to 6 years or more to do so. Unlike an inguinal hernia, incarceration and strangulation are very rare with an umbilical hernia.

Yazbeck S: Abdominal wall developmental defects and omphalomesenteric remnants. In Roy CC (ed): Pediatric Clinical Gastroenterology, 4th ed. St. Louis, Mosby–Year Book, 1995, pp 134–135.

TABLE 7-14. EFFECTS OF MALNUTRITION ON SCALP, EYES, AND MOUTH	
Clinical sign	Nutrient deficiency
Epithelial	
Skin	
Xerosis, dry scaling	Essential fatty acids
Hyperkeratosis, plaques around hair follicles	Vitamin A
Ecchymoses, petechiae	Vitamin K
Hair	
Easily plucked, dyspigmented, lackluster	Protein calorie
Mucosal	
Mouth, lips, and tongue	B vitamins
Angular stomatitis (inflammation at corners of the mouth)	B_2 (riboflavin)
Cheilosis (reddened lips with fissures at angles)	B_2, B_6 (pyridoxine)
Glossitis (inflammation of tongue)	B_6, B_3 (niacin), B_2
Magenta tongue	B_2
Edema of tongue, tongue fissures	B_3
Spongy, bleeding gums	Vitamin C
Ocular	
Conjunctival pallor due to anemia	Vitamin E (premature infants), iron, folic acid, vitamin B_{12}, copper
Bitot's spots (grayish, yellow, or white foamy spots on the whites of the eyes)	Vitamin A
Conjunctival or corneal xerosis, keratomalacia	Vitamin A
Periorbital edema	Protein

154. Which umbilical hernias warrant surgical repair?

Because of the high probability of self-resolution, indications for surgery are controversial. Some authorities argue that a hernia of >1.5 cm at the age of 2 years warrants closure as a result of its likely persistence for years. Others argue that, because the likelihood of incarceration is small for umbilical hernias, surgical closure is warranted before puberty only for persistent pain, history of incarceration, or associated psychologic disturbances.

155. When should an infant with inguinal hernia have it electively repaired?

After the diagnosis of inguinal hernia is made, it should be repaired as soon as possible. In a large study of children with incarcerated hernia, 40% of patients had a known inguinal hernia before incarceration, and 80% were awaiting elective repair. Eighty percent of the children with incarceration of a hernia were infants <1 year old. Delay of repair should be minimized, especially in this age group.

Stylianos S, Jacir NN, Harris BH: Incarceration of inguinal hernia in infants prior to elective repair. J Pediatr Surg 18:582–583, 1993.

156. Does surgical repair of one hernia warrant intraoperative exploration for another?

This is a controversial topic. Surveys have shown that, during the repair of a clinical unilateral inguinal hernia, 65–90% of pediatric surgeons routinely explore the contralateral side in boys, and 84–90% report that they do so routinely in girls. Proponents of bilateral exploration argue that there is a high incidence of later contralateral hernia, particularly in children <2 years old and in those in whom the initial appearance is on the left. In one study, 548 children with unilateral hernia repair without contralateral exploration were followed prospectively: 28% with incarcerated hernia later developed a contralateral hernia, and 9% overall developed a contralateral hernia at a median interval of 6 months. Whether or not this 10% recurrence rate mandates contralateral exploration forms much of the basis of the controversy.

Tackett LD, Breuer CK, Luks FI, et al: Incidence of contralateral inguinal hernia: A prospective analysis. J Pediatr Surg 34:684–688, 1999.

157. How are incarcerated inguinal hernias reduced?

Incarceration occurs most commonly during the first year of life. Because the infant will likely need to be admitted, nothing should be given to eat or drink. Reduction is most easily accomplished if the infant is calm (preferably asleep), warm, and, if possible, in a slightly reverse Trendelenburg's position. Analgesia (e.g., 0.1 mg/kg of intravenous morphine) may facilitate the relaxed state. With one hand, the examiner stabilizes the base of the hernia by the internal inguinal ring and, with the other hand, milks the sac distally to progressively force fluids and/or gas through the ring to eventually allow complete reduction. If unsuccessful, immediate surgery is indicated.

158. Under what clinical settings should manual reduction of an inguinal hernia not be attempted?

When the patient has clinical findings of shock, perforation, peritonitis, gastrointestinal bleeding or obstruction, or evidence of gangrenous bowel (bluish discoloration of the abdominal wall).

159. How do causes of intestinal obstruction vary by age?

Infant/young child
- Pyloric stenosis
- Intussusception
- Inguinal hernia
- Appendicitis
- Malrotation
- Intestinal duplication
- Intestinal atresia or stenosis
- Omphalomesenteric remnants
- Intraluminal web
- Hirschsprung's disease
- Adhesions

Older child
- Appendicitis (perforated)
- Intussusception (lead-point)

- Adhesions
- Malrotation
- Inguinal hernia
- Omphalomesenteric remnants
- Inflammatory bowel disease

Caty MG, Azizhan RG: Acute surgical conditions of the abdomen. Pediatr Ann 23:192–194, 199–201, 1994.

160. **What is the significance of green vomiting during the first 72 hours of life?**

During the neonatal period, green vomiting should always be interpreted as a sign of potential intestinal obstruction requiring surgical intervention. In one study of 45 infants with green vomiting, 20% had surgical conditions (e.g., malrotation, jejunal atresia, jejunal stenosis), 10% had nonsurgical obstruction (e.g., meconium plug, microcolon), and 70% had idiopathic vomiting that self-resolved. If plain radiographs are equivocal or abnormal, upper or lower gastrointestinal contrast studies should be done.

Lilien LD, Srinivasan G, Pyati SP, et al: Green vomiting in the first 72 hours in normal infants. Am J Dis Child 140:662–664, 1986.

161. **What are the clinical findings of malrotation of the intestine?**

Malrotation of the intestine is the result of the abnormal rotation of the intestine around the superior mesenteric artery during embryologic development. Arrest of this counterclockwise rotation may occur at any degree of rotation. The lesion may display in utero volvulus, or it may be asymptomatic throughout life. Infants may display intermittent vomiting or complete obstruction. Any infant with bilious vomiting should be considered emergent and requires careful evaluation for volvulus and other high-grade surgical obstructions. Recurrent abdominal pain, distention, or lower gastrointestinal bleeding may result from intermittent volvulus. Full volvulus with arterial compromise results in intestinal necrosis, peritonitis, perforation, and an extremely high incidence of mortality. Because of the extensive nature of the lesion, postoperative short gut syndrome is present in many patients who require resection.

162. **Describe the x-ray findings associated with malrotation.**

The upper gastrointestinal series will show malposition and malfixation of the ligament of Treitz. The proximal small bowel may be located in the right upper quadrant, but this is not always true. The cecum as viewed from either the upper gastrointestinal series or a barium enema may be unfixed or malpositioned. In both malrotation and volvulus, the plain films may be entirely normal. There may be proximal obstruction with gastroduodenal distention. In volvulus, the barium studies may show an obstruction near the gastroduodenal junction, often with a twisted appearance.

163. **In an asymptomatic child with an incidental finding of malrotation, is surgery indicated?**

Because of the persistent possibility of acute volvulus and intestinal obstruction, surgery is *always* indicated when intestinal malrotation is diagnosed.

164. **In what settings should intussusception be suspected?**

Intussusception (when one portion of the bowel invaginates into the other) usually occurs before the second year of life; half of all cases occur between the ages of 3 and 9 months. Colicky pain is seen in >80% of cases, but it may be absent. It typically lasts 15–30 minutes, and the baby usually sleeps between attacks. In about two thirds of cases, there is blood in the stool (currant jelly stools). Other presenting symptoms include massive lower gastrointestinal bleeding or blood streaking on the stools. The infant may appear quite toxic, dehydrated, or in shock; fever and tachycardia are common. A right lower quadrant mass may be palpable, or the area may feel surprisingly empty. Distention may accompany decreased bowel sounds.

165. **How commonly does intussusception appear with the classic findings?**
The classic triad of intussusception (colicky pain, vomiting, and passage of bloody stool) is the exception; overall, 80% of patients do not have this triad of symptoms. About 30% have blood in the stool, and this percentage may drop to about 15% if the abdominal pain was present for <12 hours. Palpation of a mass can suggest the diagnosis, but generally a high degree of suspicion is important.

Klein EJ, Kapoor D, Shugerman RP: The diagnosis of intussusception. Clin Pediatr 43:343–347, 2004.

166. **What causes intussusception?**
Intussusception is caused by one proximal segment of the bowel being invaginated and progressively drawn caudad and encased by the lumen of distal bowel. This causes obstruction and may occlude the vascular supply of the bowel segment. There is commonly a lead point on the proximal bowel that initiates the process. Lead points have included juvenile polyps, lymphoid hyperplasia, hypertrophied Peyer's patches, eosinophilic granuloma of the ileum, lymphoma, lymphosarcoma, leiomyosarcoma, leukemic infiltrate, duplication cysts, ectopic pancreas, Meckel's diverticulum, hematoma, Henoch-Schönlein syndrome, worms, foreign bodies, and appendicitis.

Navarro O, Dugougeat F, Kornecki A, et al: The impact of imaging in the management of intussception owing to pathologic lead points in children, a review of 43 cases. Pediatr Radiol 30:594–603, 2000.

167. **What is the most common type of intussusception?**
Ileocolic intussusception. It is also the most common cause of intestinal obstruction during infancy. Cecocecal and colocolic intussusceptions are less common. Gastroduodenal intussusception is rare and is usually associated with a gastric mass lesion such as a polyp or a leiomyoma. Enteroenteral intussusception is seen after surgery and in patients with Henoch-Schönlein syndrome.

168. **How is intussusception diagnosed?**
Radiographs typically demonstrate a small bowel obstruction pattern, but the diagnostic study of choice is a **barium enema**, which should be performed in all children with symptoms of <48 hours' duration. In 80% of cases, the barium enema under fixed hydrostatic pressure will reduce the intussusception. If this is unsuccessful, surgical reduction is necessary.

169. **How frequently does intussusception recur?**
Idiopathic ileocolic intussusception recurs in about **3–9%** of all cases. Intussusceptions in older children tend to recur at a higher frequency if the causative lesion is not removed. It is important to investigate cases of recurrent intussusception for an underlying lesion.

Daneman A, Alton DJ, Lobo E, et al: Patterns of recurrence of intussusception in children: A 17-year review. Pediatr Radiol 28:913–919, 1998.

170. **Rotavirus vaccine and intussusception: how are they intertwined?**
The oral rotavirus vaccine, licensed in the United States in 1998, was suspended from use when increased rates of intussusception were noted.

Murphy TV, Gargiullo PM, Massoudi MS, et al; Rotavirus Intussusception Investigation Team: Intussusception among infants given an oral rotavirus vaccine. N Engl J Med 344:564–572, 2001.

171. **Duodenal or jejunoileal atresia: which is associated with other embryonic abnormalities?**
Duodenal atresia. Duodenal atresia is caused by a persistence of the proliferative stage of gut development and a lack of secondary vacuolization and recanalization. It is associated with a high incidence of other early embryonic abnormalities. Extraintestinal anomalies occur in two thirds of patients with this condition.

Jejunoileal atresia occurs after the establishment of continuity and patency as evidenced by distal meconium seen in these patients. The etiology is postulated to be a vascular accident, volvulus, or mechanical perforation. Jejunoileal atresias are usually not associated with any other systemic abnormality.

172. **What is the classic radiographic finding in duodenal atresia?**
The **double bubble.** Swallowed air distends the stomach and the proximal duodenum (Fig. 7-6).

173. **How does the infant with biliary atresia classically appear?**
In classic cases, a term infant develops a recognizable jaundice by the third week of life, with increasingly dark urine and acholic stools. Usually the child appears well, with acceptable growth. The skin color sometimes appears somewhat greenish yellow. The spleen becomes palpable after the third or fourth week, at which time the liver is usually hard and enlarged. In other cases, the jaundice is clearly present in the conjugated form during the first week of life. There is also a strong association between the polysplenia syndrome and biliary atresia.

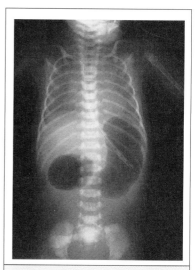

Figure 7-6. Duodenal atresia. (From Zitelli BJ, Davis HW: Atlas of Pediatric Physical Diagnosis, 4th ed. St. Louis, Mosby, 2002, p 573.)

174. **What is the surgical procedure for biliary atresia?**
The **Kasai procedure** (hepatoportoenterostomy). The remnants of the extrahepatic biliary tree are identified, and a cholangiogram is performed to verify the diagnosis. An intestinal limb is attached to drain bile from the porta hepatitis.

175. **When should a Kasai procedure be performed?**
As soon as possible. Earlier operation results in a dramatically improved outcome. Patients operated on when they are <70 days old have an increased likelihood of a successful procedure, although exceptions at both ends of this spectrum are common. Some surgeons now suggest that infants diagnosed late in the course of disease should have a primary liver transplant rather than a hepatoportoenterostomy, because, after 3 months of age, sufficient liver injury has occurred to make the Kasai procedure unlikely to be successful.

176. **Which is accompanied by more complications: high or low imperforate anus?**
High-type imperforations. The distinction is based on whether the blind end of the terminal bowel or rectum ends above (high-type) or below (low-type) the level of the pelvic levator musculature. The patients with high-type imperforations will have ectopic fistulae (rectourinary, rectovaginal), urologic anomalies (hydronephrosis or double collecting system), and lumbosacral spine defects (sacral agenesis, hemivertebrae). The surgical repair in these patients is much more extensive, and future problems of incontinence, fecal impaction, and strictures are much more likely.

177. **What is the classic presentation of pyloric stenosis?**

An infant 3–6 weeks old has progressive nonbilious projectile vomiting leading to dehydration with hypochloremic, hypokalemic, metabolic alkalosis. On physical examination, a pyloric "olive" is palpable, and peristaltic waves are visible.

178. **How is pyloric stenosis diagnosed?**

If the classic signs and symptoms are present in association with the typical blood chemistry findings (hypochloremia, hypokalemia, metabolic alkalosis) and a mass is palpated, the diagnosis can be made on **clinical** grounds. If the diagnosis is in doubt, **ultrasound** can be used to visualize the hypertrophic pyloric musculature (Fig. 7-7). **Upper gastrointestinal contrast** studies demonstrate pyloric obstruction with the characteristic "string sign" and enlarged "shoulders" bordering the elongated and obstructed pyloric channel.

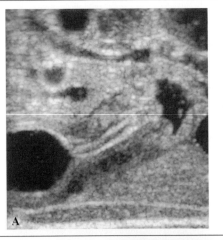

Figure 7-7. *A,* Ultrasound of pyloric stenosis. Note the elongated and curved pyloric channel with parallel walls and the thickened muscle with a "shoulder" projecting into the antrum. *B,* Longitudinal sonograph of the pylorus in a patient with pyloric stenosis. 1, canal length = 1.7 cm; 2, muscle wall thickness = 0.6 cm. (From Glick PL, Pearl RH, Irish MS, Caty MG: Pediatric Surgery Secrets. Philadelphia, Hanley & Belfus, 2001, p 203.)

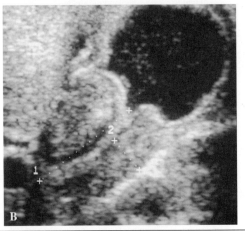

179. **What is the mechanism of hyperbilirubinemia in babies with pyloric stenosis?**

Unconjugated hyperbilirubinemia has been noted in 10–25% of babies with pyloric stenosis. Although an enhanced enterohepatic circulation for bilirubin probably plays a role in the pathogenesis of the hyperbilirubinemia, hepatic glucuronyl transferase activity is markedly depressed in these jaundiced infants. The mechanism of diminished glucuronyl transferase activity is not known, although inhibition of the enzyme by intestinal hormones has been suggested.

180. **In a patient with suspected pyloric stenosis, why is an acidic urine very worrisome?**

As vomiting progresses in infants with pyloric stenosis, a worsening hypochloremic metabolic alkalosis develops. Multiple factors (e.g., volume depletion, elevated aldosterone levels) result in maximal renal efforts to reabsorb sodium. In the distal tubule, this is typically achieved by exchanging sodium for potassium and hydrogen. When total body potassium levels are very low, hydrogen is preferentially exchanged, and a paradoxic aciduria develops (in the setting of an alkaline plasma). This acidic urine is an indication that intravascular volume expansion and electrolyte replenishment (especially chloride and potassium) are urgently needed.

181. **What is the connection between pyloric stenosis and erythromycin?**

In studies of infants who have received erythromycin (primarily as prophylaxis after exposure to pertussis), the incidence of pyloric stenosis is significantly increased.

Honein MA, Paulozzi LJ, Himelright IM, et al: Infantile hypertrophic pyloric stenosis after pertussis prophylaxis with erythromycin: A case review and cohort study. Lancet 354:2102–2105, 1999.

182. **What is the short bowel syndrome?**

The short bowel syndrome results from extensive resection of the small intestine. Normally, the majority of carbohydrates, proteins, fats, and vitamins are absorbed in the jejunum and the proximal ileum. The terminal ileum is responsible for the uptake of bile acids and vitamin B_{12}. Short bowel syndrome results in failure to thrive, malabsorption, diarrhea, vitamin deficiency, bacterial contamination, and gastric hypersecretion.

183. **Why are infants with short bowel syndrome prone to renal calculi?**

Chronic intestinal malabsorption results in an increase of intraluminal fatty acids, which saponify with dietary calcium. Thus, nonabsorbable calcium oxalate does not form, excessive oxalate is absorbed, and hyperoxaluria with crystal formation results.

184. **In extensive small bowel resection, how much is "too much"?**

Infants who retain 20 cm of small bowel as measured from the ligament of Treitz can survive *if the ileocecal valve is intact*. If the ileocecal valve has been removed, the infant usually requires a minimum of 40 cm of bowel to survive. The importance of the ileocecal valve appears to relate to its ability to retard transit time and minimize bacterial contamination of the small intestine.

185. **What conditions may mimic appendicitis?**

- Gastroenteritis
- Ruptured ovarian follicle/ovarian torsion
- Mesenteric adenitis
- Inflammatory bowel disease
- Constipation
- Henoch-Schönlein purpura
- Pelvic inflammatory disease
- Primary peritonitis
- Pyelonephritis
- Perforated peptic ulcer
- Right lower lobe pneumonia
- Pancreatitis

Caty MG, Azizhan RG: Acute surgical conditions of the abdomen. Pediatr Ann 23:192–194, 199–201, 1994.

KEY POINTS: SURGICAL ISSUES

1. Bilious (dark green) emesis in a newborn is a true gastrointestinal emergency; it is a sign of potential obstruction.

2. Malrotation is diagnosed on the basis of the malposition/malfixation of the ligament of Treitz, as seen on an upper gastrointestinal series. Malrotation can lead to acute volvulus and should always be repaired.

3. The classic triad of intussusception consists of the following: (1) colicky abdominal pain, (2) vomiting, and (3) bloody stools with mucous. However, it occurs in fewer than 20% of patients.

4. Pyloric stenosis typically appears with progressive, nonbilious, projectile vomiting and a hypochloremic, hypokalemic metabolic alkalosis in an infant between the ages of 3 and 6 weeks old.

5. The classic picture of appendicitis is anorexia followed by pain followed by nausea and vomiting, with subsequent localization of findings to the right lower quadrant. However, there is a large degree of variability, particularly among younger patients.

---

186. **Appendicitis in children: clinical, laboratory, or radiologic diagnosis?**
The diagnosis of appendicitis has traditionally been a clinical one. The classic picture in children is a period of **anorexia followed by pain, nausea, and vomiting.** Abdominal pain begins periumbilically and then shifts after 4–6 hours to the right lower quadrant. Fever is low grade. Peritoneal signs are detected on examination. In unequivocal cases, experienced surgeons would argue that no laboratory tests are needed.

　　Laboratory studies have limited value in equivocal cases. *White blood cell count* of >18,000/mm³ or a marked left shift is unusual in uncomplicated cases and suggests perforation or another diagnosis. A *urinalysis* with many white blood cells suggests a urinary tract infection as the primary pathology.

　　Limited computed tomography (CT) scanning with rectal contrast is emerging as a powerful tool for diagnosis with sensitivities and specificities between 98–100% in children. Three-percent diatrizoate meglumine saline solution is instilled into the colon in a slow controlled drip; oral and intravenous contrast are not needed. Diagnosis is based on the visualization of an abnormal appendix or pericecal inflammation or abscess with or without the presence of an appendicolith. This type of imaging can supplement or supplant abdominal ultrasound studies; plain abdominal films are of limited value.

Garcia Pena BM, Cook EF, Mandl KD: Selective imaging strategies to diagnose pediatric appendicitis. Pediatrics 113:24–28, 2004.

Kosloske AM, Love CL, Rohrer JE, et al: The diagnosis of appendicitis in children: Outcomes of a strategy based on pediatric surgical evaluation. Pediatrics 113(1 Pt 1):29–34, 2004.

Kwok MY, Kim MK, Gorelick MH: Evidence-based approach to the diagnosis of appendicitis in children. Pediatr Emerg Care 20:690–698, 2004.

187. **How specific is the diagnosis of appendicitis if an appendicolith is noted on x-ray?**
Although an appendicolith (or fecalith) on x-ray studies (plain film or CT scan) is significantly associated with appendicitis, it is not sufficiently specific to be the sole basis for the diagnosis. On CT scanning, these can be noted in 65% of patients with appendicitis and in up to 15% of patients without appendicitis. The positive predictive value of finding an appendicolith is about 75%; in its absence, the negative predictive value is only 26%.

Lowe LH, Penney MW, Scheker LE, et al: Appendicolith revealed on CT in children with suspected appendicitis: How specific is it in the diagnosis of appendicitis? Am J Roentgenol 175:981–984, 2000.

188. **Should a digital rectal examination be performed on all children with possible appendicitis?**

Tradition says yes, but reviews of studies of the practice indicate that in children it can be emotionally and physically traumatic and associated with a high false-positive interpretation. It may be most helpful in equivocal cases involving pelvic or retrocecal appendicitis (about a third of cases), suspected abscess formation, or for attempted palpation of adnexal/cervical tissues when vaginal examination is not indicated. Thus, many clinicians now view it as "investigatory" rather than "routine" and only when results will change management.

Brewster GS, Herbert ME: Medical myth: A digital rectal examination should be performed on all individuals with possible appendicitis. West J Med 173:207–208, 2000.

189. **In children taken to surgery for suspected appendicitis, how often is perforation of the appendix present?**

It depends to a large extent on the age of the child (and, of course, on the skill of the clinician). Unfortunately, as a result of the variable location of the appendix, the clinical presentation of pain in appendicitis is often very different from the classical case. The younger the child, the more difficult the diagnosis. In infants <1 year old, nearly 100% of patients who come to surgery have a perforation. Fortunately, appendicitis is rare in this age group because the appendiceal opening at the cecum is much larger than the tip, and obstruction is unusual. In children <2 years old, 70–80% are perforated; in those ≤5 years old, 50% are perforated. Particularly in younger children, a high index of suspicion is necessary, and rapid diagnosis is critical. If the onset of symptoms can be pinpointed (usually anorexia related to a meal), 10% of patients will have perforation during the first 24 hours, but >50% will perforate by 48 hours.

ACKNOWLEDGMENT

The editors gratefully acknowledge contributions by Dr. David A. Piccoli that were retained from the first three editions of *Pediatric Secrets*.

CHAPTER 8

GENETICS

Kwame Anyane-Yeboa, MD

DOWN SYNDROME

1. **What are the common physical characteristics of children with Down syndrome?**
   - Upslanted palpebral fissures with epicanthal folds
   - Small, low-set ears with overfolded upper helices
   - Short neck with excess skin folds in newborns
   - Prominent tongue
   - Flattened occiput
   - Exaggerated gap between first and second toe
   - Hypotonia

2. **Are Brushfield spots pathognomonic for Down syndrome?**
   No. Brushfield spots are speckled areas that occur in the periphery of the iris. They are seen in about 75% of patients with Down syndrome but also in up to 7% of normal newborns.

3. **What is the chance that a newborn with a simian crease has Down syndrome?**
   A single transverse palmar crease is present in 5% of normal newborns. Bilateral palmar creases are found in 1%. These features are twice as common in males as they are in females. However, about 45% of newborn infants with Down syndrome have a single transverse crease. Because Down syndrome occurs in 1 in 800 live births, the chance that a newborn with a simian crease has Down syndrome is only **1 in 60**.

4. **Why is an extensive cardiac evaluation recommended for newborns with Down syndrome?**
   About 40–50% have congenital heart disease, but most infants are asymptomatic during the newborn period. Defects include atrioventricular canal (most common, 60%), ventriculoseptal defect, and patent ductus arteriosus.

5. **What proportion of infants with Down syndrome have congenital hypothyroidism?**
   About 2% (1 in 50) as compared with 0.025% (1 in 4,000) for all newborns. This emphasizes the importance of the state-mandated newborn thyroid screen.

6. **What other conditions of increased risk should not be overlooked during early infancy?**
   - **Gastrointestinal malformations,** including duodenal atresia and tracheoesophageal fistula
   - **Cryptorchidism**
   - **Lens opacities/cataracts**
   - **Strabismus**
   - **Hearing loss,** both sensorineural and conductive

7. **What is the expected intelligence quotient (IQ) of a child with Down syndrome?**
   The IQ range is generally 25–50, with a mean reported IQ of 54; occasionally, the IQ may be higher. Intelligence deteriorates during adulthood, with clinical and pathologic findings consistent with advanced Alzheimer disease. By age 40, the mean IQ is 24.

KEY POINTS: INCREASED RISKS FOR PATIENTS WITH DOWN ✓ SYNDROME DURING THE NEWBORN PERIOD AND EARLY INFANCY

1. Congenital heart disease: A-V canal defects, ventriculoseptal defects

2. Gastrointestinal malformations: Duodenal atresia, tracheoesophageal atresia

3. Congenital hypothyroidism

4. Lens opacities/cataracts

5. Hearing loss

6. Cryptorchidism

8. **Down syndrome is a risk factor for what malignancy?**
   Leukemia. Its frequency in these individuals is fiftyfold higher for younger children (0–4 years old) and tenfold higher for individuals 5–29 years old, for a twentyfold increase in lifetime risk. Before leukemia becomes apparent, children with Down syndrome are at increased risk for other unusual white-cell problems, including *transient myeloproliferative disorder* (a disorder of marked leukocytosis, blast cells, thrombocytopenia, and hepatosplenomegaly, which spontaneously resolves) and a *leukemoid reaction* (markedly elevated white blood cell count with myeloblasts without splenomegaly, which also spontaneously resolves).

   Olney HJ, Gozzetti A, Rowley JD: Chromosomal abnormalities in childhood hematologic malignant disease. In Nathan DG, Orkin SD, Ginsburg D, Look AT (eds): Nathan and Oski's Hematology of Infancy and Childhood, 6th ed. Philadelphia, W.B. Saunders, 2003, p 1120–1121.

9. **What is the genetic basis for Down syndrome?**
   The syndrome can be caused by trisomy of all or part of chromosome 21:
   - Full trisomy 21: 94%
   - Mosaic trisomy 21: 2.4%
   - Translocation: 3.3%

10. **What chromosomal abnormalities are related to maternal age?**
    All trisomies and some sex chromosomal abnormalities (except 45X and 47, XYY).

11. **How does the risk of having an infant with Down syndrome change with advancing maternal age?**

Maternal Age	Approximate Risk of Down Syndrome
30	1:1,000
35	1:365
40	1:100
45	1:50

    Most cases of Down syndrome involve nondisjunction at meiosis I in the mother. This may be related to the lengthy stage of meiotic arrest between oocyte development in the fetus until ovulation, which may occur as much as 40 years later.

12. **What percentage of all babies with Down syndrome are born to women over the age of 35?**
    Only 20%. Although their individual risk is higher, women in this age bracket account for only 5% of all pregnancies in the United States.

    Haddow JE, Palomaki GE, Knight GJ, et al: Prenatal screening for Down syndrome with use of maternal serum markers. N Engl J Med 327:588–593, 1992.

13. **Does advanced paternal age increase the risk of having a child with trisomy 21?**
There does not appear to be an increased risk of Down syndrome associated with paternal age until after age 55. Some studies have noted an increased risk of having children with Down syndrome after this age, although others have not. The reports are controversial, and the statistical analysis needed to perform such a study is cumbersome. It is known that approximately 10% of all trisomy 21 cases derive the extra chromosome 21 from the father.

14. **Which is technically correct: Down's syndrome or Down syndrome?**
In 1866, John Langdon Down, physician at the Earlswood Asylum in Surrey, England, described the phenotype of a syndrome that now bears his name. However, it was not until 1959 that it was determined that this disorder is caused by an extra chromosome 21. The correct designation is *Down syndrome.*

CLINICAL ISSUES

15. **What genetically inherited disease has the highest known mutation rate per gamete per generation?**
Neurofibromatosis. The estimated mutation rate for this disorder is 1.3×10^{-4} per haploid genome. The clinical features are café-au-lait spots and axillary freckling in childhood followed by the development of neurofibromas in later years. There is approximately a 10% risk of malignancy with this condition, and mental deficiency is common.

16. **Which disorders with ethnic and racial predilections most commonly warrant maternal screening for carrier status?**
See Table 8-1.

TABLE 8-1. MATERNAL SCREENING ACCORDING TO ETHINC AND RACIAL PREDILECTIONS

Disorder	Ethnic or racial group	Screening test
Tay-Sachs disease	Ashkenazi Jewish, French, French Canadian	Decreased serum hexos-aminidase A concentration, DNA studies
Familial dysautonomia	Ashkenazi Jewish	DNA
Gaucher disease	Ashkenazi Jewish	DNA
Canavan disease	Ashkenazi Jewish	DNA
Bloom syndrome	Ashkenazi Jewish	DNA
Fanconi anemia	Ashkenazi Jewish	DNA
Nieman-Pick disease (type A)	Ashkenazi Jewish	DNA
Mucolipidosis IV	Ashkenazi Jewish	DNA
Cystic fibrosis	Panethnic	DNA
Sickle cell anemia	Black, African, Mediterranean, Arab, Indian, Pakistani	Presence of sickling in hemolysate followed by confirmatory hemoglobin electrophoresis
Alpha- and beta-thalassemia	Mediterranean, Southern and Southeast Asian, Chinese	Mean corpuscular volume $<80\mu m^3$, followed by confirmatory hemoglobin electrophoresis

17. **Why are mitochondrial disorders transmitted from generation to generation by the mother and not the father?**
Mitochondrial DNA abnormalities (e.g., many cases of ragged red fiber myopathies) are passed on from the mother because mitochondria are present in the cytoplasm of the egg and not the sperm. Transmission to males or females is equally likely; however, expression is variable because mosaicism with normal and abnormal mitochondria in varying proportions is very common.

>   Johns DR: Mitochondrial DNA and disease. N Engl J Med 333:638–644, 1995.

18. **Which syndromes are associated with advanced paternal age?**
Advanced paternal age is well documented to be associated with **new dominant mutations.** The assumption is that the increased mutation rate is the result of the accumulation of new mutations from many cell divisions. The more cell divisions, the more likely an error (mutation) will occur. The mutation rate in fathers who are >50 years old is five times higher than the mutation rate in fathers who are <20 years old. Autosomal dominant new mutations that have been mapped and identified, including **achondroplasia**, **Apert syndrome**, and **Marfan syndrome**.

19. **What is the most common genetic lethal disease?**
Cystic fibrosis (CF). A genetic lethal disease is one that interferes with a person's ability to reproduce as a result of early death (before childbearing age) or impaired sexual function. CF is the most common autosomal recessive disorder in whites, occurring in 1 in 1,600 infants (1 out of every 20 individuals is a carrier for this condition). CF is characterized by widespread dysfunction of exocrine glands, chronic pulmonary disease, pancreatic insufficiency, and intestinal obstructions. Males are azoospermic. The median survival is approximately 29 years.

20. **Assuming that the husband is healthy and that no one in the wife's family has cystic fibrosis, what is the risk that a couple will have a child with cystic fibrosis if the husband's brother has the disease?**
See Fig. 8-1.

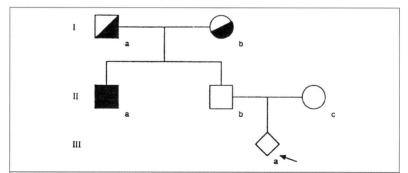

Figure 8-1. Risk of cystic fibrosis (CF) in offspring of a mother with no family history of CF and a healthy father whose brother has CF. (1) Because IIa is affected with CF, both his parents must be carriers. (2) The chance of IIb being a carrier is two out of three, since we know that he is not affected by CF. (3) The risk of IIc being a carrier is 1 in 20 (the population risk). (4) The chance of IIIa being affected is calculated as follows: father's carrier risk × mother's carrier risk × chance that both will pass on their recessive CF gene to their child = $\frac{2}{3} \times \frac{1}{20} \times \frac{1}{4} = \frac{1}{120}$.

21. **What are the "fat baby" syndromes?**
    - **Prader-Willi** (obesity, hypotonia, small hands and feet)
    - **Beckwith-Wiedemann** (macrosomia, omphalocele, macroglossia, ear creases)
    - **Sotos** (macrosomia, macrocephaly, large hands and feet)
    - **Weaver** (macrosomia, accelerated skeletal maturation, camptodactyly)
    - **Bardet-Biedl** (obesity, retinal pigmentation, polydactyly)
    - **Infants of diabetic mothers**

22. **What is the "H_3O" of Prader-Willi syndrome?**
    Hyperphagia, hypotonia, hypopigmentation, and **obesity**. About 70% of Prader-Willi patients will have a deletion of an imprinted gene *SNPRN* on the long arm of paternally derived chromosome 15; in about 20% of these patients, both copies of the chromosome are maternally derived. The phenomenon in which a child inherits two complete or partial copies of the same chromosome from only one parent is referred to as *uniparental disomy*. The maternal uniparental disomy for chromosome 15 results in Prader-Willi syndrome, just as does a deletion of the paternal copy of the chromosome.

23. **What syndrome is associated with unprovoked outbursts of laughter?**
    Angelman syndrome. In 1965, Harry Angelman described a syndrome in three "puppet children," as he called them. Other characteristics include severe mental retardation, lack of speech, unsteady gait, microcephaly, and seizures. Facial features include maxillary hypoplasia, large mouth (often with protruding tongue), and prognathism (large chin).

24. **What is the genetic basis of Angelman syndrome?**
    About 70% of cases are due to deletions of an imprinted gene, UBE3A (E6-associated protein ubiquitin-protein ligase gene), which resides on the long arm of the maternally-derived chromosome 15. About 25% of cases are due to UBE3A mutations, and a small percentage of cases is due to paternal disomy of chromosome 15. (Both copies of chromosome 15 are derived from the father.)

25. **Name the two most common forms of dwarfism that are recognizable at birth.**
    - **Thanatophoric dwarfism:** This is the most common, but it is a *lethal* chondrodysplasia that is characterized by flattened, U-shaped vertebral bodies; telephone-receiver-shaped femurs; macrocephaly; and redundant skinfolds that cause a pug-like appearance. *Thanatophoric* means death-loving (an apt description). The incidence is 1 in 6,400 births.
    - **Achondroplasia:** This is the most common *viable* skeletal dysplasia, occurring 1 in 26,000 live births. Its features are small stature, macrocephaly, depressed nasal bridge, lordosis, and a trident hand.

26. **What chromosomal abnormality is found in cri-du-chat syndrome?**
    This syndrome is the result of a deletion of material from the short arm of chromosome 5 (i.e., 5p–), which causes many problems, including growth retardation, microcephaly, and severe mental retardation. Patients have a characteristic *cat-like cry* during infancy, from which the syndrome derives its name. In 85% of cases, the deletion is a de novo event. In 15%, it is due to malsegregation from a balanced parental translocation.
    www.geneclinics.org

27. **What syndrome is associated with CATCH22?**
    This acronym has been used to describe the salient features of **DiGeorge/velocardiofacial syndrome:**

C = **C**ongenital heart disease
A = **A**bnormal face
T = **T**hymic aplasia/hypoplasia
C = **C**left palate
H = **H**ypocalcemia
22: Microdeletion of chromosome **22**q11
The cardiovascular lesions frequently encountered are tetralogy of Fallot, truncus arteriosis, interrupted aortic arch, right-sided aortic arch, and double-outlet right ventricle. Any infant with any of these cardiovascular lesions should be screened for DiGeorge/velocardiofacial syndrome.

28. List the syndromes and malformations associated with congenital limb hemihypertrophy.

- Beckwith-Wiedemann syndrome
- Conradi-Hünermann syndrome
- Klippel-Trenaunay-Weber syndrome
- Proteus syndrome
- Neurofibromatosis
- Hypomelanosis of Ito
- CHILD syndrome (**c**ongenital **h**emidysplasia, **i**chthyosiform erythroderma, **l**imb **d**efects)

29. For what condition are these patients with isolated limb hypertrophy at risk?

Embryonal cell tumors, including Wilms tumor, adrenal tumors, and hepatoblastoma. The risk for patients with isolated hemihypertrophy is about 6%; for patients with Beckwith-Wiedemann syndrome, it is 7.5%. Surveillance with abdominal ultrasound and alphafetoprotein measurements every 3 months are recommended until the child is at least 7 years old. In patients with Beckwith-Wiedemann syndrome, facial appearance is also affected (Fig. 8-2).

30. What is confined placental mosaicism (CPM)?

The abnormal cell line in this condition is "confined" either to the cytotrophoblast or chorionic stroma cells of the placenta and is not present in the fetus itself. This situation may be discovered when, on chorionic villous sampling, there is an abnormal chromosome result (reflecting the placenta); however, the fetus appears to be healthy, and amniocentesis is normal. The diagnosis of CPM postnatally is usually made retrospectively by follow-up studies on the infant or on the fetus, placenta, and membranes. The clinical significance of CPM is not yet clear.

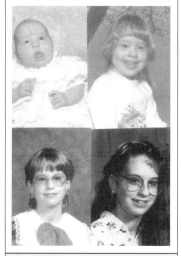

Figure 8-2. Facial shape in Beckwith-Wiedemann syndrome, illustrated from birth to adolescence in a single person. In infancy and early childhood, the face is round with prominent cheeks and relative narrowing of the forehead. Note that by adolescence the trend is toward normalization. (From Allanson JE: Pitfalls of genetic diagnosis in the adolescent: The changing face. Adolesc Med State Art Rev 13:257–268, 2002.)

31. What are the most common microchromosome deletion syndromes?

- DiGeorge/velocardiofacial syndrome (DGS/VCF)
- Prader-Willi syndrome (PWS)
- Angelman syndrome (AS)
- William syndrome (WS)
- Alagille syndrome

- Rubinstein-Taybi syndrome (RTS)
- Wilms' tumor-aniridia-ambiguous genitalia-mental retardation syndrome (WAGR)
- Miller-Dieker syndrome

Ensenauer RE, Michels VV, Reinke SS: Genetic testing: practical, ethical, and counseling considerations. Mayo Clin Proc 80:63–73, 2005.

32. **What are the cardinal features of Alagille syndrome?**
    - In about 90% of cases, a history of prolonged neonatal jaundice due to paucity of intrahepatic ducts (and occasionally extrahepatic ducts)
    - Cardiac lesions occur in 85% of cases and are predominantly peripheral pulmonic stenosis, but might include pulmonary valve stenosis, partial anomalous venous drainage, ASD, or VSD
    - In about 90% of cases, anterior ocular segment dysgenesis, particularly posterior embryotoxon
    - Bilateral or unilateral optic disc drusen in 80–90% of cases
    - Hemivertebrae or butterfly vertebrae in about 90% of cases
    - Autosomal dominant mode of inheritance, with incomplete penetrance
    - Mutations detected in the Jagged1 gene in the majority of patients
    - Deletion of chromosome 20p11 in a small percentage of patients

33. **What are the reasons that a disease might be genetically determined but the family history would be negative?**
    - Autosomal recessive inheritance
    - X-linked recessive inheritance
    - Genetic heterogeneity (e.g., retinitis pigmentosa may be transmitted as autosomal recessive or dominant or X-linked recessive)
    - Spontaneous mutation
    - Nonpenetrance
    - Expressivity (i.e., variable expression)
    - Extramarital paternity
    - Phenocopy (i.e., an environmentally determined copy of a genetic disorder)

    Juberg RC: . . . but the family history was negative. J Pediatr 91:693–694, 1977.

DYSMORPHOLOGY

34. **How are structural dysmorphisms categorized?**
    - **Malformation:** A problem of poor formation (likely genetically based) in which the abnormality is present at the onset of development (e.g., hypoplastic thumbs of Fanconi syndrome)
    - **Disruption:** An extrinsic destructive process interferes with previously normal development (e.g., thalidomide causing limb abnormalities)
    - **Deformation:** An extrinsic mechanical force causes abnormalities that are usually asymmetrical (e.g,. breech position causing tibial bowing and positional club feet)
    - **Dysplasia:** An abnormal cellular organization or function that generally affects only a single tissue type (e.g., cartilage abnormalities that result in achondroplasia)

35. **What are the principal kinds of morphologic defects in infants with multiple anomalies?**
    - **Developmental or polytopic field defect:** A pattern of anomalies derived from the disturbance of a single region or part of an embryo that responds as a coordinated unit to extrinsic or intrinsic influences. Field defects are believed to be derivatives of a single malformative or disruptive process. For example, if the rostral mesoderm is disturbed early during development, multiple anomalies of the head and face can occur.
    - **Sequence:** A pattern of multiple anomalies derived from a single known (or presumed) prior anomaly or mechanical factor. For example, the entity of micrognathia, glossoptosis, and cleft soft palate is more properly called the Pierre Robin sequence (rather than syndrome),

because the small mandible likely causes the developing tongue to be pushed posteriorly, which does not allow the posterior palatal shelves to close properly.

- **Syndrome:** The nonrandom occurrence of multiple anomalies with such an increased frequency that a pathogenetically causal relationship (often of unknown cause) is felt to be involved. For example, chromosomal syndromes (e.g., Down) have characteristic clinical features.
- **Association:** The nonrandom occurrence of multiple anomalies without a known field defect, sequence initiator, or causal relationship but with such a frequency that the malformations have a statistical connection.

36. **How common are major and a minor malformations in newborns?**
Major malformations are unusual morphologic features that cause medical, cosmetic, or developmental consequences to the patient. **Minor anomalies** are features that do not cause medical or cosmetic problems. Approximately 14% of newborn babies will have a minor anomaly, whereas only 2–3% will have a major malformation.

37. **Identify the most common major congenital anomalies in the United States.**
Anencephaly and spina bifida. The combined prevalence is 0.5–2.0 per 1,000 live births.

38. **What is the clinical significance of a minor malformation?**
The recognition of minor malformations in a newborn may serve as an indicator of altered morphogenesis or as a valuable clue to the diagnosis of a specific disorder. The presence of several minor malformations is unusual and often indicates a serious problem in morphogenesis. For example, when three or more minor malformations are discovered in a child, there is a >90% risk of a major malformation also being present. The most common minor malformations involve the face, ears, hands, and feet. Almost any minor defect may occasionally be found as an unusual familial trait.

39. **How common are minor anomalies in newborns?**
See Table 8-2.

TABLE 8-2. COMMON MINOR ANOMALIES

Physical feature	Black infants (%)	White infants (%)
Palpable metopic suture	42	64
Third sagittal fontanel	10	3
Double hair whorl	6	7
Overfolded ear helix	51	38
Preauricular sinus	5	0.8
Preauricular tag	0.7	0.3
Epicanthal folds, bilateral	1	1.4
Brushfield spots, bilateral	0.2	7
Anteverted nostrils	2	2.6
Supernumerary nipple	2.2	0.2
Umbilical hernia	6	0.7
Sacral dimple	0.6	4.8
Clinodactyly of both 5th fingers	4.5	5.2
Syndactyly, 2nd–3rd toes	0.5	0.6

Adapted from Holmes LB: Congenital malformations. In Behrman BE (ed): Nelson Textbook of Pediatrics, 14th ed. Philadelphia, W.B. Saunders, 1992, p 295.

40. **Describe the most common anomaly associations.**
   CHARGE: Coloboma of the eye, **h**eart defects, **a**tresia of the choanae, **r**etardation (mental and growth), **g**enital anomalies (in males), and **e**ar anomalies
   MURCS: Müllerian duct aplasia, **r**enal aplasia, and **c**ervicothoracic **s**omite dysplasia
   VATER: Vertebral, **a**nal, **t**racheo**e**sophageal, and **r**enal or **r**adial anomalies
   VACTERL: VATER anomalies plus **c**ardiac and **l**imb anomalies

41. **What malformations are associated with oligohydramnios and polyhydramnios?**
   During later pregnancy, the bulk of amniotic fluid arises as a product of fetal urination. Any malformation that leads to impaired urine production will cause **oligohydramnios**, including renal dysplasia, renal agenesis, and bladder outlet obstruction. Oligohydramnios is often associated with intrauterine growth retardation.
   The etiology of **polyhydramnios** may be broken down into maternal causes (30%), fetal causes (30%), and idiopathic causes (40%). Maternal disorders such as diabetes, erythroblastosis fetalis, and preeclampsia are often associated with excess amniotic fluid. Fetal disorders that commonly predispose a mother to polyhydramnios are central nervous system anomalies (e.g., anencephaly, hydrocephaly, neurologic disorders), gastrointestinal disorders (e.g., tracheoesophageal fistula, duodenal atresia), fetal circulatory disorders, and multiple gestation. The etiology for polyhydramnios in fetuses with central nervous system and upper gastrointestinal anomalies is presumed to be impaired fetal swallowing ability.

42. **How do clinodactyly, syndactyly, and camptodactyly differ?**
   - **Clinodactyly:** Curvature of a toe or finger (usually the fifth) as a result of hypoplasia of the middle phalanx, which is the last fetal bone to develop in the hands and feet. Normal curvature can consist of up to 8° of inward turning; curvature beyond this is considered a minor anomaly.
   - **Syndactyly:** An incomplete separation of the fingers (usually 3rd and 4th) or toes (usually 2nd or 3rd).
   - **Camptodactyly:** Abnormal persistent flexion of fingers or toes.

43. **What is the proper way to test for low-set ears?**
   This designation is made when the upper portion of the ear (helix) meets the head at a level below a horizontal line drawn from the lateral aspect of the palpebral fissure. The best way to measure is to align a straight edge between the two inner canthi and determine whether the ears lie completely below this plane (Fig. 8-3). In normal individuals, approximately 10% of the ear is above this plane.

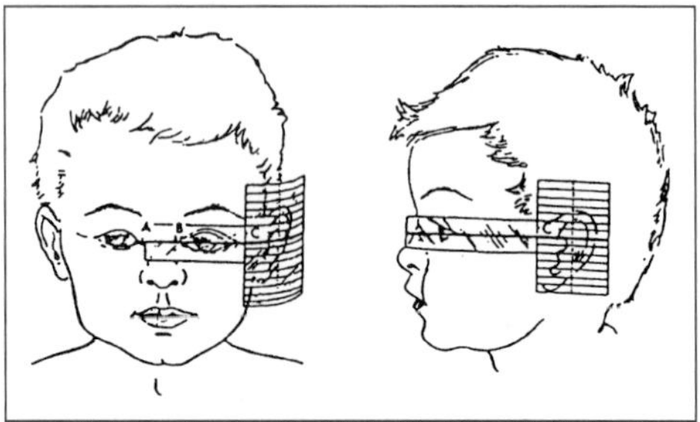

Figure 8-3. How to test for low-set ears. (From Feingold M, Bossert WH: Normal values for selected physical parameters: An aid to syndrome delineation. In Bergsma D [ed]: The National Foundation–March of Dimes Birth Defects Series 10:9, 1974.)

44. **Where is the Darwinian tubercle located?**
   Also called the *auricular tubercle*, this is a cartilaginous bump on the upper part of the outer ear below and posterior to the helix. It is a minor variant that should not be considered an anomaly.

45. **What is the inheritance pattern of cleft lip and palate?**
   Most cases of cleft lip and palate are inherited in a polygenic or multifactorial pattern. The male-to-female ratio is 3:2, and the incidence in the general population is approximately 1 in

1,000. Recurrence risk after one affected child is 3–4%; after two affected children, it is 8–9%.

46. How can hypertelorism be rapidly assessed?
If an imaginary third eye would fit between the eyes, hypertelorism is possible. Precise measurement involves measuring the distance between the center of each eye's pupil. This is a difficult measurement in newborns and uncooperative patients because of eye movement. In practice, the best way to determine hypotelorism or hypertelorism is to measure the inner and outer canthal distances and to then plot these measurements on standardized tables of norms.

47. Which syndromes are associated with iris colobomas?
Colobomas of the iris (Fig. 8-4) are the result of abnormal ocular development and embryogenesis. They are frequently associated with chromosomal syndromes (most commonly trisomy 13, 4p–, 13q–) and triploidy. In addition, they may be commonly found in patients with the CHARGE association, Goltz syndrome, and Rieger syndrome. Whenever iris colobomas are noted, chromosome analysis is recommended. The special case of complete absence of the iris (aniridia) is associated with the development of Wilms

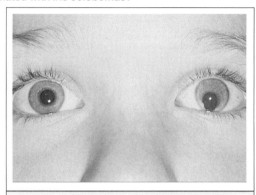

Figure 8-4. Left iris coloboma. (From Zitelli BJ, Davis HW: Atlas of Pediatric Physical Diagnosis, 4th ed. St. Louis, Mosby, 2002, p 674.).

tumor and may be caused by an interstitial deletion of the short arm of chromosome 11.

GENETIC PRINCIPLES

48. What is the risk of having a child with a recessive disorder when the parents are first or second cousins?
First cousins may share more than one deleterious recessive gene. They have ⅛ of their genes in common, and their progeny are homozygous at 1/16 of their gene loci. Second cousins have only 1/32 of their genes in common. The risk that consanguineous parents will produce a child with a severe or lethal abnormality is 6% for first-cousin marriages and 1% for second-cousin marriages.

49. Identify the common symbols used in the construction of a pedigree chart.
See Fig. 8-5.

50. How can the same genotype lead to different phenotypes?
In **parental imprinting** (an area of the regulation of gene expression that is incompletely understood), the expression of an identical gene is dependent on whether the gene is inherited from the mother or the father. For example, in patients with Huntington's disease, the clinical manifestations occur much earlier if the gene is inherited from the father rather than the mother. Modification of the genes by methylation of the DNA during development has been hypothesized as one explanation of the variability.

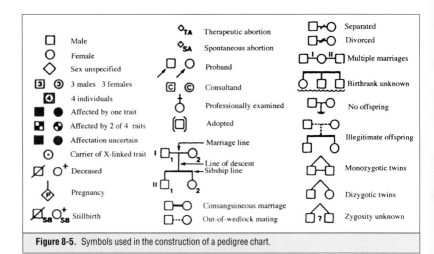

Figure 8-5. Symbols used in the construction of a pedigree chart.

51. **What is FISH?**
    Fluorescence **in s**itu **h**ybridization (FISH) is a molecular cytogenetic technique that is used to identify abnormalities of chromosome number or structure using a single-stranded DNA probe (for a known piece of DNA or chromosome segment). The probe is labeled with a fluorescent tag and targeted to a single-strand DNA that has been denatured in place on a microscope slide. The use of fluorescent microscopy enables the detection of more than one probe, each of which is labeled with a different color. An example of the use of FISH is for the rapid prenatal diagnosis of trisomies with the use of amniotic fluid or chorionic villi testing using interphase cells from cultured specimens and probes for the most common chromosomal abnormalities (13, 18, 21, X, and Y). Although interphase FISH for prenatal diagnosis has low false-positive and false-negative rates, it is considered investigational and is used only in conjunction with standard cytogenetic analysis.

52. **46, XY, t(4:8), (p21;q22)—What does it all mean?**
    46: Normal number of chromosomes
    XY: Genetic male
    t(4:8): The first set of parentheses refers to the chromosomes. The symbol in front indicates the change: **t** stands for reciprocal translocation, **del** for deletion, **dup** for duplication, and **inv** for inversion.
    (p21;q22): The second set of parentheses refers to the bands on the chromosomes. The short arm symbol is **p**; the long arm symbol is **q**.
    In this case, a genetic male with a normal number of chromosomes has a reciprocal translocation between the short arm of chromosome 4 at band 21 and the long arm of chromosome 8 at band 22.

SEX-CHROMOSOME ABNORMALITIES

53. **What are the features of the four most common sex-chromosome abnormalities?**
    See Table 8-3.

TABLE 8-3.	MOST COMMON SEX CHROMOSOME DISORDERS			
	47,XXY (Klinefelter)	47,XYY	47,XXX	45,X (Turner)
Frequency of live births	1 in 2,000	1 in 2,000	1 in 2,000	1 in 8,000
Maternal age association	+	−	+	−
Phenotype	Tall, eunuchoid habitus, under-developed secondary sexual charac-teristics, gynecomastia	Tall, severe acne, indistingui-shable from normal males	Tall, indistin-guishable from normal females	Short stature, webbed neck, shield chest, pedal edema at birth, coarctation of the aorta
IQ and behavior problems	80–100; behav-ioral problems;	90–110; behavioral problems; aggressive behavior	90–110; behavioral problems	Mildly deficient to normal intelligence; spatial-perceptual difficulties
Reproductive function	Extremely rare	Common	Common	Extremely rare
Gonad	Hypoplastic testes, Leydig cell hyperplasia, Sertoli cell hypoplasia, seminiferous tubule dys-genesis, few spermatogenic precursors	Normal-size testes, normal testicular histology	Normal size ovaries, normal ovarian histology	Streak ovaries with deficient follicles

From Donnenfeld AE, Dunn LK: Common chromosome disorders detected prenatally. Postgrad Obstet Gynecol 6:5, 1986.

54. **What did Lyon hypothesize?**
   The *Lyon hypothesis* is that, in any cell, only one X chromosome will be functional. Any other X chromosomes present in that cell will be condensed, late replicating, and inactive (called the *Barr body*). The inactive X may be either paternal or maternal in origin, but all descendants of a particular cell will have the same inactive parentally derived chromosome.

55. **Is it possible to get identical twins of different sexes?**
   Yes. If anaphase lag (loss) of a Y chromosome occurs at the time of cell separation into twin embryos, a female fetus with karyotype 45,X (Turner syndrome) and a normal male fetus (46,XY) result.

56. **Of the four most common types of sex-chromosome abnormalities, which is identifiable at birth?**
Only infants with **Turner syndrome** have physical features that are easily identifiable at birth.

Sybert VP, McCauley E: Turner's syndrome. N Engl J Med 351:1227-1238, 2004.

57. **What are the similarities between Noonan syndrome and Turner syndrome?**
    - Dorsal hand and pedal edema
    - Low posterior hairline
    - Web neck (pterygium colli)
    - Congenital elbow flexion (cubitus valgus)
    - Broad chest with wide-spaced nipples
    - Narrow, hyperconvex nails
    - Prominent ears
    - Short fourth metacarpal and/or metatarsal

58. **Describe the differences between Noonan syndrome and Turner syndrome.**

Turner syndrome	Noonan syndrome
Affects females only	Affects both males and females
Chromosome disorder	Normal chromosomes
(45,X)	Autosomal dominant disorder
Near-normal intelligence	Mental deficiency
Coarctation of aorta is the most common cardiac defect	Pulmonary stenosis is the most common cardiac defect
Amenorrhea and sterility due to ovarian dysgenesis	Normal menstrual cycle in females

KEY POINTS: TURNER SYNDROME

1. Majority: 45,X

2. Newborn period: Only sign may be lymphedema of feet and/or hands

3. Adolescence: Primary amenorrhea due to ovarian dysplasia

4. Short stature often prompts initial work-up

5. Normal mental development

6. Classic features: Webbed neck with low hairline, broad chest with wide-spaced nipples

7. Increased risk for congenital heart disease: Coarctation of the aorta

59. **What is the most common inherited form of mental retardation?**
Fragile X syndrome. It affects an estimated 1 in 1,000 males and 1 in 2,000 females. Approximately 2–6% of male subjects and 2–4% of female subjects with unexplained mental retardation will carry the full fragile X mutation.

60. **What is the nature of the mutation in fragile X syndrome?**
Expansion of trinucleotide repeat sequences. When the lymphocytes of an affected male are grown in a folate-deficient medium and the chromosomes examined, a substantial fraction of X chromosomes demonstrate a break near the distal end of the long arm. This site—the fragile X mental retardation-1 gene (FMR-1)—was identified and sequenced in 1991. At the center of the gene is a repeating trinucleotide sequence (CGG) that, in normal individuals, repeats 6–45 times.

However, in carriers, the sequence expands to 50–200 times (called a premutation). In fully affected individuals, it expands to 200–600 copies.

61. **What are the associated medical problems of fragile X syndrome in males?**
Flat feet (80%), macroorchidism (80% after puberty), mitral valve prolapse (50–80% in adulthood), recurrent otitis media (60%), strabismus (30%), refractive errors (20%), seizures (15%), and scoliosis (>20%).

Lachiewicz AM, Dawson DV, Spiridigliozzi GA: Physical characteristics of young boys with fragile X syndrome: Reasons for difficulties in making a diagnosis in young males. Am J Med Genet 92:229–236, 2000.

62. **What is the outcome for girls with fragile X?**
Heterozygous females who carry the fragile X chromosome have more behavioral and developmental problems (including attention deficit hyperactivity disorder), cognitive difficulties (50% with an IQ in the mentally retarded or borderline range), and physical differences (prominent ears, long and narrow face). Cytogenetic testing is recommended for all sisters of fragile X males.

Hagerman RJ, Jackson C, Amiri K, et al: Girls with fragile X syndrome: Physical and neurocognitive status and outcome. Pediatrics 89:395–400, 1992.

KEY POINTS: FRAGILE X SYNDROME

1. Most common cause of inherited mental retardation

2. Prepubertal: Elongated face, flattened nasal bridge, protruding ears

3. Pubertal: Macroorchidism

4. Heterozygous females: 50% with IQ in the borderline or mentally retarded range

5. First recognized trinucleotide repeat disorder

TERATOLOGY

63. **Which drugs are known to be teratogenic?**
Most teratogenic drugs exert a deleterious effect in a minority of exposed fetuses. Exact malformation rates are unavailable because of the inability to perform a statistical evaluation on a randomized, controlled population. Known teratogens are summarized in Table 8-4.

64. **Describe the characteristic features of the fetal hydantoin syndrome.**
Craniofacial: Broad nasal bridge, wide fontanel, low-set hairline, broad alveolar ridge, metopic ridging, short neck, ocular hypertelorism, microcephaly, cleft lip/palate, abnormal or low-set ears, epicanthal folds, ptosis of eyelids, coloboma, and coarse scalp hair
Limbs: Small or absent nails, hypoplasia of distal phalanges, altered palmar crease, digital thumb, and dislocated hip
Approximately 10% of infants whose mothers took phenytoin (Dilantin) during pregnancy have a major malformation; 30% have minor abnormalities.

65. **Does cocaine cause fetal malformations?**
Yes. Several malformations are associated with maternal cocaine use. All are believed to be due to a disruption in normal organ growth and development as a result of vascular insufficiency. Intestinal atresias due to mesenteric artery vasoconstriction or thrombosis and urinary tract anomalies, including urethral obstruction, hydronephrosis, and hypospadias, are most commonly reported. Limb reduction defects, which are often described as transverse terminal defects of the forearm or amputation of the digits of the hands and feet, have also been identified.

TABLE 8-4. KNOWN TERATOGENS

Drug	Major Teratogenic Effect
Thalidomide	Limb defects
Lithium	Ebstein tricuspid valve anomaly
Aminopterin	Craniofacial and limb anomalies
Methotrexate	Craniofacial and limb anomalies
Phenytoin	Facial dysmorphism, dysplastic nails
Trimethadione	Craniofacial dysmorphism, growth retardation
Valproic acid	Neural tube defects
Diethylstilbestrol	Müllerian anomalies, clear cell adenocarcinoma
Androgens	Virilization
Tetracycline	Teeth and bone maldevelopment
Streptomycin	Ototoxicity
Warfarin	Nasal hypoplasia, bone maldevelopment
Penicillamine	Cutis laxa
Accutane (retinoic acid)	Craniofacial and cardiac anomalies
Propylthiouracil	Goiter
Radioactive iodine	Hypothyroidism

66. **What amount of alcohol is safe to ingest during pregnancy?**
    This is unknown. The full dysmorphologic manifestations of fetal alcohol syndrome are associated with heavy intake. However, most infants will not display the full syndrome. For infants born to women with lesser degrees of alcohol intake during pregnancy and who demonstrate more subtle abnormalities (e.g., cognitive and behavioral problems), it is more difficult to ascribe risk because of confounding variables (e.g., maternal illness, pregnancy weight gain, other drug use [especially marijuana]). Furthermore, for reasons that are unclear, it appears that infants who are prenatally exposed to similar amounts of alcohol are likely to have different consequences. Because current data do not support the concept that any amount of alcohol is safe during pregnancy, the American Academy of Pediatrics recommends abstinence from alcohol for women who are pregnant or who are planning to become pregnant.

    Committee on Substance Abuse and Committee on Children with Disabilities: Fetal alcohol syndrome and fetal alcohol effects. Pediatrics 91:1004–1006, 1993.

67. **What are the frequent facial features of the fetal alcohol syndrome?**
    Skull: Microcephaly, midface hypoplasia
    Eyes: Short palpebral fissures, epicanthal folds, ptosis, strabismus
    Mouth: Hypoplastic philtrum, thin upper lip, prominent lateral palatine ridges, retrognathia in infancy, micrognathia or relative prognathia in adolescence
    Nose: Flat nasal bridge, short and upturned nose (see Fig. 8-6.)

    Hoyme HE, May PA, Kalberg WO, et al: A practical clinical approach to diagnosis of fetal alcohol spectrum disorders: Clarification of the 1996 Institute of Medicine criteria. Pediatrics 115:39–47, 2005.

68. **What happens to children with fetal alcohol syndrome when they grow up?**
    A follow-up study of 61 adolescents and adults revealed that relative short stature and microcephaly persisted, but facial anomalies became more subtle. Academic functioning, particularly in arithmetic, was delayed to the early-grade-school level. Intermediate or significant maladap-

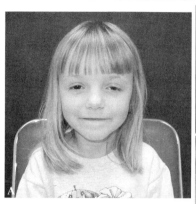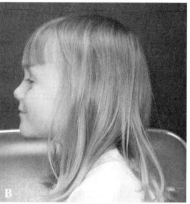

Figure 8-6. Patient with fetal alcohol syndrome. *A,* Note bilateral ptosis, short palpebral fissures, smooth philtrum, and thin upper lip. *B,* Short palpebral fissures are sometimes more noticeable in profile. Head circumference is second percentile.(From Seaver LH: Adverse environmental exposures in pregnancy: Teratology in adolescent medicine practice. Adolesc Med State Art Rev 13:269–291, 2002.)

KEY POINTS: FETAL ALCOHOL SYNDROME

1. Growth deficiencies: Prenatal and postnatal

2. Microcephaly with neurodevelopmental abnormalities

3. Short palpebral fissures

4. Smooth philtrum

5. Thin upper lip

tive behavior was present in 100% of patients. Severely unstable family environments were common.

Streissguth AP, Aase JM, Clarren SK, et al: Fetal alcohol syndrome in adolescents and adults. JAMA 265:1961–1967, 1991.

ACKNOWLEDGMENT

The editors gratefully acknowledge contributions by Drs. Elain H. Zackai, JoAnn Bergoffen, Alan E. Donnenfeld, and Jeffrey E. Ming that were retained from the first three editions of *Pediatric Secrets*.

CHAPTER 9

HEMATOLOGY

Steven E. McKenzie, MD, PhD

BONE MARROW FAILURE

1. **What are the types of bone marrow failure?**
    Bone marrow failure is manifested by **pancytopenia** or, at times, by **cytopenia of a single cell type**. It can be **acquired** (acquired aplastic anemia) or **inherited/genetic** (e.g., Fanconi anemia, Kostmann syndrome, Diamond-Blackfan anemia, amegakaryocytic thrombocytopenia, thrombocytopenia-absent radius).

    Alter BP: Bone marrow failure syndromes in children. Pediatr Clin North Am 49:973–988, 2002.

2. **What are the causes of acquired aplastic anemia?**
    After careful exclusion of the known causes listed below, >80% of cases remain classified as idiopathic. A variety of associated conditions include the following:

Radiation	**Immune diseases**
Drugs and chemicals	Eosinophilic fasciitis
Regular: Cytotoxic, benzene	Hypogammaglobulinemia
Idiosyncratic: Chloramphenicol, anti-	**Thymoma**
inflammatory drugs, antiepileptics, gold	**Pregnancy**
Viruses	**Paroxysmal nocturnal hemoglobinuria**
Epstein-Barr virus	**Preleukemia**
Hepatitis (primarily B)	
Parvovirus (in immunocompromised hosts)	
Human immunodeficiency virus	

    Shimamura A, Guinana EC: Acquired aplastic anemia. In Nathan DG, Orkin SD, Ginsburg D, Look AT (eds): Nathan and Oski's Hematology of Infancy and Childhood, 6th ed. Philadelphia, W.B. Saunders, 2003, p 257.

3. **What is the definition of severe aplastic anemia?**
    Severe disease includes a hypocellular bone marrow biopsy (<30% of the normal hematopoietic cell density for age) and decreases in at least two out of three peripheral blood counts: neutrophil count <500 cells/mm^3, platelet count <20,000 cells/mm^3, or reticulocyte count <1% after correction for the hematocrit. Categorization has important prognostic and therapeutic implications.

4. **What are the treatments and prognosis for children with aplastic anemia?**
    In the absence of definitive treatment, <20% of children with severe acquired aplastic anemia survive for >2 years. When bone marrow transplantation is performed using a human leukocyte antigen (HLA)-identical sibling donor, the 2-year survival rate exceeds 85%. The usual approach to the newly diagnosed child with severe acquired aplastic anemia is to perform bone marrow transplantation if there is an HLA-identical sibling to serve as the donor.

    Approximately 80% of children with severe aplastic anemia do not have a sibling donor for bone marrow transplantation. These children receive medical therapy, usually the combination of antithymocyte, cyclosporine, and hematopoietic growth factors, such as granulocyte–macrophage colony-stimulating factor or granulocyte colony-stimulating factor. Two-year response and survival rates for combination medical therapy now exceed 80% in children.

Locasciulli A: Acquired aplastic anemia in children: Incidence, prognosis and treatment options. Paediatr Drugs 4:761–766, 2002.

Trigg ME: Hematopoietic stem cells. Pediatrics 113:S1051–S1057, 2004.

5. **What is the probable diagnosis of a 6-year-old child with pancytopenia, short stature, abnormal thumbs, and areas of hyperpigmentation?**

Fanconi anemia, or constitutional aplastic anemia, is a genetic disorder in which numerous physical abnormalities are often present at birth, and aplastic anemia occurs around the age of 5 years. The more common physical abnormalities include hyperpigmentation, anomalies of the thumb and radius, small size, microcephaly, and renal anomalies (e.g., absent, duplicated, or pelvic horseshoe kidneys). Patients with Fanconi anemia are also susceptible to leukemia and epithelial carcinomas.

6. **How is the diagnosis of Fanconi anemia made?**

Chromosomal breakage analysis can be used to make the diagnosis, and molecular diagnosis can confirm the diagnosis and be used to test relatives. In studies of peripheral blood lymphocytes, a high percentage of patients with Fanconi anemia will have chromosomal breaks, gaps, or rearrangements.

Tischkowitz M, Dokal I: Fanconi anaemia and leukemia—clinical and molecular aspects. Br J Haematol 126:176–191, 2004.

7. **What is transient erythroblastopenia of childhood (TEC) and Diamond-Blackfan anemia?**

Both are disorders of red-cell production that occur during early childhood. Both disorders are characterized by a low hemoglobin level and an inappropriately low reticulocyte count. The bone marrows of patients with these conditions may be indistinguishable, showing reduced or absent erythroid activity in both cases.

8. **Why is distinguishing between the two conditions extremely important?**

TEC is a self-limited disorder, whereas Diamond-Blackfan syndrome usually requires lifelong treatment.

9. **How are the two conditions diagnosed?**

Although there is an overlap in the age of presentation, Diamond-Blackfan syndrome commonly causes anemia during the first 6 months of life, whereas TEC occurs more frequently after the age of 1 year. The red cells in patients with Diamond-Blackfan syndrome have fetal characteristics that are useful for distinguishing this disorder from TEC, including increased mean cell volume, elevated level of hemoglobin F, and presence of i antigen. The level of adenine deaminase may be elevated in patients with Diamond-Blackfan syndrome but normal in children with TEC. Twenty-five percent of Caucasian patients with Diamond-Blackfan anemia have been found to have mutations in the gene for ribosomal protein S19, and molecular diagnosis for these mutations is very helpful when positive.

Drpatchinskaia N, Gustavsson P, Andersson B, et al: The gene encoding ribosomal protein S19 is mutated in Diamond-Blackfan anaemia. Nat Genet 21:169–175, 1999.

Willig TN, Niemeyer CM, Leblanc T, et al: Identification of new prognosis factors from the clinical and epidemiologic analysis of a registry of 229 Diamond-Blackfan anemia patients. DBA group of Societe d'Hematologie et d'Immunologie Pediatrique (SHIP), Gesellshaft fur Padiatrische Onkologie und Hamatologie (GPOH), and the European Society for Pediatric Hematology and Immunology (ESPHI). Pediatric Res 46:553–561, 1999.

10. **What is Kostmann syndrome?**

Kostmann syndrome is severe congenital neutropenia. At birth or shortly thereafter, very severe neutropenia (absolute neutrophil count of 0–200/mm^3) is noted, often at the time of significant bacterial infection (e.g., deep skin abscess, pneumonia, sepsis). Even with antibiotic treatment, there is a high mortality during infancy unless granulocyte colony-stimulating factor therapy is used to elevate the neutrophil count. An alternative treatment is bone marrow transplantation from an HLA-identical sibling donor.

CLINICAL ISSUES

11. **What is the hemoglobin value below which children are considered to be anemic (lower limit of normal)?**

Newborn (full term)	13.0 gm/dL
3 months	9.5 gm/dL
1–3 years	11.0 gm/dL
4–8 years	11.5 gm/dL
8–12 years	11.5 gm/dL
12–16 years	12.0 gm/dL

Dallman P, Siimes MA: Percentile curves for hemoglobin and red-cell volume in infancy and childhood. J Pediatr 94:26–31, 1979.

12. **In patients with severe chronic anemia, how rapidly can transfusions be given?**

When anemia is chronic, there has been cardiovascular adaptation and a relatively normal blood volume. Excessively rapid transfusions can lead to congestive heart failure. For patients with a hemoglobin level of <5 gm/dL who exhibit no signs of cardiac failure, a safe regimen is to transfuse packed red blood cells at a rate of 1–2 mL/kg per hour by continuous infusion until the desired target is reached. In most patients, 1 mL/kg will raise the hematocrit level by 1%. Judicious use of a diuretic like furosemide (or automated erythrocytapheresis, in larger children) can be considered.

Jayabose S, Tugal O, Ruddy R, et al: Transfusion therapy for severe anemia. Am J Pediatr Hematol Oncol 15:324–327, 1993.

13. **When does the physiologic anemia of infancy occur?**

Physiologic anemia occurs at 8–12 weeks in full-term infants and at 6–8 weeks in premature infants. Full-term infants may exhibit hemoglobin levels as low as 9 gm/dL at this time, and very premature infants may have levels as low as 7 gm/dL.

14. **Why does the physiologic anemia of infancy occur?**

The mechanisms responsible for physiologic anemia are not completely understood. Red blood cell (RBC) survival time is decreased in both premature and full-term infants. Furthermore, the ability to increase erythropoietin production in response to ongoing tissue hypoxia is somewhat blunted, although the response to exogenous erythropoietin is normal.

15. **In what settings of shortened RBC survival can the reticulocyte count be normal or decreased?**

As a rule, the reticulocyte count is elevated in conditions of shortened RBC survival (e.g., hemoglobinopathies, membrane disorders, immune hemolysis) and decreased in anemias that are characterized by impaired RBC production (e.g., iron deficiency, aplastic anemia). The reticulocyte count may be unexpectedly low in a setting of shortened RBC survival in the following conditions:

- **Aplastic or hypoplastic crisis** is occurring at the same time, as is seen in patients with human parvovirus B19 infection.
- An autoantibody in **immune-mediated hemolysis** reacting with antigens that are present on reticulocytes leads to increased clearance of these cells.
- In patients in chronic states of hemolysis, the marrow may become unresponsive as a result of **micronutrient deficiency** (e.g., iron, folate) or because of a reduction in erythropoietin production, as is seen in patients with chronic renal failure.

16. **How does the pathophysiology of anemia differ in chronic and acute infection?**
Chronic infection and other inflammatory states impair the release of iron from reticuloendothelial cells, thereby decreasing the amount of this necessary ingredient that are available for RBC production. The lack of mobilizable iron may be to the result of the action of proinflammatory cytokines (e.g., IL-1, TNF-alpha). Giving additional iron under these circumstances further increases reticuloendothelial iron stores and does little to help the anemia.
Acute infection may cause anemia through a variety of mechanisms, including bone marrow suppression, shortened RBC lifespan, red-cell fragmentation, and immune-mediated RBC destruction.

17. **Describe the differential diagnosis for children with splenomegaly and anemia.**
Key question: Is the anemia the cause of the splenomegaly, or is the splenomegaly the cause of the anemia?

Anemia causing splenomegaly	Splenomegaly causing anemia
Membrane disorders	Cirrhotic liver disease
Hemoglobinopathies	Cavernous transformation of portal vessels
Enzyme abnormalities	Storage diseases
Immune hemolytic anemia	Persistent viral infections

18. **A 14-month-old child presents symptoms including marked cyanosis, lethargy, and normal oxygen saturation by pulse oximetry after drinking from a neighbor's well. What is the likely diagnosis?**
Methemoglobinemia should always be considered when a patient presents symptoms of cyanosis without demonstrable respiratory or cardiac disease. Methemoglobin is produced by the oxidation of ferrous iron in hemoglobin into ferric iron. Methemoglobin cannot transport oxygen. Normally, it constitutes <2% of circulating hemoglobin. Oxidant toxins (e.g., antimalarial drugs, nitrates in food or well water) can dramatically increase the concentration. Patients with cyanosis as a result of methemoglobinemia can have normal oxygen saturation as measured by pulse oximetry because the oximeter operates by measuring only hemoglobin that is available for saturation.

19. **How can the diagnosis of methemoglobinemia be made at the bedside?**
In patients with methemoglobinemia, the inability of the red cell to maintain hemoglobin iron in the ferrous (Fe^{2+}) state leads to a loss of oxygen-carrying capacity. When a drop of blood from a patient with methemoglobinemia is placed on a piece of filter paper, it generally has a brownish color. When the filter paper is waved in the air, the color of the blood remains brown because the hemoglobin is unable to bind oxygen. By contrast, blood from a normal individual turns from brown to red when the filter paper is waved in the air.

20. **What is the treatment for methemoglobinemia?**
In an acute situation in which levels of methemoglobin are >30%, treatment consists of 1–2 mg/kg of 1% methylene blue administered intravenously over 5 minutes and repeated in 1 hour if levels have not fallen to normal. Failure to respond to therapy should raise the possibility of glucose-6-phosphate-dehydrogenase (G6PD) deficiency, which prevents the conversion of

methylene blue to the metabolite that is active in the treatment of methemoglobinemia. In these cases, hyperbaric oxygen therapy or exchange transfusion may be necessary.

21. **Why are infants at greater risk for the development of methemoglobinemia?**
    - **Antioxidant defense mechanisms** (e.g., soluble cytochrome b_5 and NADH-dependent cytochrome b_5 reductase) are 40% lower in infants than teenagers.
    - An infant's **intestinal pH** is relatively alkaline as compared with older children's. If nitrates are ingested (e.g., from fertilizer-contaminated well water), this higher pH more readily allows bacterial conversion of nitrate to nitrite, which is a potent oxidant.
    - Infants are more susceptible to various **oxidant exposures:** nitrate reductase from foods such as undercooked spinach, menadione (vitamin K_3) for the prevention of neonatal hemorrhage, over-the-counter teething preparations with benzocaine, and metoclopramide for gastroesophageal reflux.

    Bunn HF: Human hemoglobins: Normal and abnormal. In Nathan DG, Orkin SH (eds): Nathan and Oski's Hematology of Infancy and Childhood, 5th ed. Philadelphia, W.B. Saunders, 1998, pp 729–751.

22. **What are the indications for the use of leukoreduced red blood cells?**
    When packed red cells are prepared from whole blood and then filtered, most of the remaining white cells are removed from the product. Because febrile transfusion reactions are usually the result of leukocytes, filtered products should be used for patients who have experienced such reactions to previous blood transfusions. Filtered red cells are also effective for reducing the transmission of cytomegalovirus in at-risk individuals. In addition, the use of filtered blood components reduces the risk of HLA alloimmunization, which is desirable for patients who have undergone repeated transfusions and for those who may need stem cell or solid organ transplants. Currently, many red-cell products are leukoreduced at the time of collection (i.e., prestorage). Other products can be leukoreduced at the time of administration.

COAGULATION DISORDERS

23. **What features on history or physical examination help pinpoint the cause of a bleeding problem?**
    Although there can be considerable overlap, in general, platelet problems result in petechiae, especially on dependent parts of the body and mucosal surfaces. Additional manifestations of platelet disorders include epistaxis, hematuria, menorrhagia, and gastrointestinal hemorrhages. Ecchymoses are suspicious for coagulation factor deficiencies or platelet problems when they occur in unusual areas, are out of proportion with the extent of described trauma (also seen in child abuse), or are present in different stages of healing. Delayed bleeding from old wounds and extensive hemorrhage (particularly into joint spaces or after immunizations) are also suggestive of coagulation protein disorders. Bleeding from multiple sites in an ill patient is worrisome for disseminated intravascular coagulation. If a patient has tolerated tonsillectomy and/or adenoidectomy or extraction of multiple wisdom teeth without major hemorrhage, a significant inherited bleeding disorder is unlikely.

24. **What do the aPTT and PT measure?**
    Activated partial thromboplastin time (aPTT) measures the clotting ability of the intrinsic phase of coagulation; isolated prolongation in a patient with clinical bleeding likely means a problem with factor VIII, IX, or XI. **Prothrombin time (PT)** monitors components of the extrinsic pathway; isolated prolongation is most commonly seen with severe factor VII deficiency.

25. **What are the inheritance patterns of common bleeding and clotting disorders?**
    - **von Willebrand disease:** This is the most common coagulopathy and it is autosomal dominant in the majority of cases.

- **Factor VIII deficiency** (hemophilia A) and **factor IX deficiency** (hemophilia B): These conditions are inherited in an X-linked pattern so that females are carriers and males are affected. Inquiry about affected maternal male first cousins or uncles is appropriate. In general, heterozygotes for clotting factor deficiencies are not clinically affected.
- **Factor V Leiden, protein C, and antithrombin III:** These are not sex-linked disorders; heterozygosity for factor V mutation is present in 3–6% of Caucasian children, and evidence indicates that some of these heterozygous individuals may have problems related to hypercoagulation (e.g., venous thrombosis).

Journeycake JM, Buchanan GR: Coagulation disorders. Pediatr Rev 24:83–91, 2003.

26. **Why is the lack of a family history of bleeding problems only moderate evidence against the likelihood of hemophilia A in a patient?**

The abnormal factor VIII gene responsible for hemophilia A exhibits marked heterogeneity, and up to a third of cases (either the immediate-carrier mother or the son himself) may have developed a **spontaneous mutation**. Molecular diagnosis of the most common mutation in severe factor VIII deficiency—a gene inversion in the distal portion of the gene in the affected male, the mother, and maternal relatives—may help the physician with understanding the family history.

27. **Which is most common: von Willebrand disease, factor VIII deficiency, or factor IX deficiency?**

von Willebrand disease. Frequency is estimated to be between 1 in 100 to 1 in 500. Factor VIII deficiency (hemophilia A) is more common (1 in 5,000) than factor IX deficiency (hemophilia B), affecting 80–85% of all patients with clinically diagnosed factor deficiency.

28. **How are the doses of replacement factor calculated for a hemophiliac with or without life-threatening hemorrhage?**

For moderate (1–5% of normal factor levels) to severe (<1% of normal) hemophilia, recombinant factor VIII or factor IX concentrates are the treatments of choice. Each unit of factor VIII or factor IX is equivalent to the activity of 1 mL of normal plasma. With the recombinant products, a dose of 1 unit/kg should increase the factor VIII level by 1.5–2% and the factor IX level by 1%. If there is an antibody inhibitor of the replacement factor, correction will not be achieved. Under these circumstances, alternate therapies are needed, such as porcine factor VIII, factor VIII inhibitor bypassing activity complexes, or recombinant factor VIIa.

For minor hemorrhages (e.g., knee and elbow bleeds), factor levels should be increased to 20–30% of normal.

For major bleeding episodes (e.g., hip bleeds, intracranial hemorrhage, bleeding around the airway), factor levels should be raised to 70–100% and repeat dosing strongly considered under close medical supervision.

Kelly KM, Butler RB, Farace L, et al: Superior in vivo response of recombinant factor VIII concentrate in children with hemophilia A. J Pediatr 130:537–540, 1997.

Lee C. Recombinant clotting factors in the treatment of hemophilia. Thromb Haemostasis 82:516–524, 1999.

29. **What are the half-lives of exogenously administered factors VIII and IX?**

The half-lives for the *first* doses of factors VIII and IX are 6–8 hours and 4–6 hours, respectively. With *subsequent* doses, factor VIII has a half-life of 8–12 hours, whereas factor IX has a half-life of 18–24 hours. Thus, for serious bleeding, the second dose of factor VIII should be given 6–8 hours after the first, whereas the second dose of factor IX should be given 4–6 hours after the first. Subsequent doses are usually given every 12 hours for factor VIII replacement and every 24 hours for factor IX replacement, but the measurement of actual factor levels may be necessary to guide therapy in life-threatening situations.

Gill JC: Transfusion principles for congenital coagulation disorders. In Hoffman R, Benz EJ, Shattil SJ, et al (eds): Hematology: Basic Principles and Practice, 3rd ed. New York, Churchill Livingstone, 2000, pp 2282–2290.

30. **Can someone with isolated factor XII deficiency causing an elevated aPTT undergo surgery?**

    The aPTT test requires functional factor XII in the test tube to activate factor XI, and, in patients with factor XII deficiency, the aPTT is prolonged. However, because there is an alternative for activation of factor XI in the body via the FVII/TF (extrinsic pathway) that leads to the generation of thrombin, the risk of perioperative bleeding with isolated factor XII deficiency is considered to be that of the average patient. It is prudent to know the personal and family bleeding histories in an individual with a prolonged aPTT; to rule out factor XI, IX, VIII, and von Willebrand factor deficiencies; and to rule out the presence of an inhibitor of coagulation before the diagnosis of isolated factor XII deficiency can be made.

31. **What can cause an elevation of the PT when other coagulation testing is normal?**

    Factor VII deficiency. PT measures the function of the common pathway factors (including X, V, II, and fibrinogen) as well as the extrinsic pathway (tissue factor and factor VII). The aPTT measures the common pathway plus the function of the intrinsic pathway (including factors XII, XI, IX, and VIII). Isolated factor VII deficiency selectively elevates the PT. Other causes of elevated PT (e.g., liver disease, vitamin K deficiency, warfarin toxicity) are not selective for lowering factor VII activity.

32. **Who gets hemophilia C?**

    More commonly called *factor XI deficiency*, this is an uncommon type of hemophilia (<5% of total hemophilia patients). Unlike the X-linked nature of hemophilias A and B, it is an autosomal recessive disease that occurs most frequently in Ashkenazi Jews.

    Asadai R, et al: Factor XI deficiency in Ashkanazi Jews in Israel. N Engl J Med 325: 153-58, 1991.

KEY POINTS: HEMOPHILIA

1. X-linked recessive disorder

2. Hemophilia A: Factor VIII abnormalities (75–85% of total cases)

3. Hemophilia B: Factor IX abnormalities

4. Severity based on factor levels: Severe (<1%), moderate (1–5%), mild (5–25%)

5. Common initial presentation: Bleeding after circumcision

33. **Why is factor IX deficiency also called "Christmas disease"?**

    In 1952, investigators in England noted that, when blood from one group of hemophiliacs was added to the blood of another group of hemophiliacs, the clotting time was shortened. This provided the basis for the discovery of plasma substances in addition to what was then called "antihemophilic globulin" (and now called factor VIII), which is responsible for normal clotting. The name was derived because the first patient examined in detail with the unusual clotting deficiency (later designated as factor IX) was a boy named Christmas. The publication of the landmark article in fact occurred during the last week of December in 1952.

    Biggs R, Douglas AS, Macfarlane RG, et al: Christmas disease: A condition previously mistaken for haemophilia. Br Med J 262:1378–1382, 1952.

34. **What is the von Willebrand factor (vWF)?**
Synthesized in megakaryocytes and endothelial cells, vWF is a large multimeric protein that binds to collagen at points of endothelial injury. It serves as a bridge between damaged endothelium and adhering platelets, and it facilitates platelet attachment. It also serves as a carrier protein for factor VIII in circulation; it minimizes the clearance of factor VIII from plasma and accelerates its cellular synthesis.

35. **What are the coagulation abnormalities in von Willebrand disease?**
von Willebrand disease is actually a group of disorders caused by qualitative or quantitative abnormalities in vWF. Coagulation abnormalities in children with severe disease can include a prolonged bleeding time, prolonged PTT, decreased factor VIII coagulant activity, decreased factor VIII antigen, and decreased ability of patient plasma to induce aggregation of normal platelets in the presence of ristocetin (the so-called "ristocetin cofactor activity").

36. **What are the common variants of von Willebrand disease?**
See Table 9-1.

TABLE 9-1. COMMON VARIANTS OF VON WILLEBRAND DISEASE	Type I	Type IIA	Type IIB
Frequency	65–80%	10–12%	3–5%
Genetic transmission	Autosomal dominant	Autosomal dominant	Autosomal dominant
Ristocetin cofactor activity	Low	Low	Low
Low-dose ristocetin-induced platelet aggregation	Normal	Normal	Increased
Multimeric electrophoretic pattern	Normal mix (various sizes)	Large, intermediate forms absent	Large multimers absent
Response to desmopressin	Good	Poor	Decreases platelets

Adapted from Montgomery RR, Gill JC, Scott JP, et al: Hemophilia and von Willebrand disease. In Nathan DG, Orkin SD, Ginsburg D, Look AT (eds): Hematology of Infancy and Childhood, 6th ed. Philadelphia, W.B. Saunders, 2003, p 1561.

37. **What are the best screening diagnostic tests for suspected von Willebrand disease?**
- Activated partial thromboplastin time
- Ristocetin cofactor assay
- Bleeding time

More than 90% of patients with von Willebrand disease demonstrate at least one abnormality. The diagnosis can be difficult because test results can vary widely among patients. Stress, pregnancy, or medications (e.g., oral contraceptives) can cause variation even in an individual patient. Although the bleeding time and PTT are often abnormal, in milder disease they are frequently normal. More extensive (and expensive) testing, including vWF antigen, factor VIII clotting activity, ristocetin-induced platelet aggregation, and multimer analysis, can be done to determine subtype or to eliminate false negatives if clinical suspicion remains high.

38. What does the ristocetin cofactor assay measure?

vWF activity. vWF will bind to the glycoprotein IB receptor on platelets in the presence of the antibiotic ristocetin. A patient's plasma is serially diluted and mixed with platelets. The presence of vWF allows for platelet agglutination, which can then be quantified on the basis of the dilutions.

39. How is von Willebrand disease treated?

Treatment depends on the variant of vWD disease that is identified:

- If protein is normal but diminished in quantity, desmopressin is given to stimulate endogenous release.
- If protein is abnormal but bleeding is mild, desmopressin may also be of value.
- If protein is abnormal but bleeding is severe, licensed vWF concentrates may be administered.

   Mannucci PM: Treatment of von Willebrand's disease. N Engl J Med 351:683–694, 2004.

40. What is the role of vitamin K in coagulation?

Vitamin K is essential for the gamma-carboxylation of both procoagulants (including factors II, VII, IX, and X) and anticoagulants (proteins C and S). Gamma-carboxylation occurs in the liver and converts the proteins to their functional forms. Vitamin K is obtained in three ways: (1) as dietary fat-soluble K_1 (phytonadione) from leafy vegetables and fruits; (2) as K_2 (menaquinone) from synthesis by intestinal bacteria, and (3) as water-soluble K_3 (menadione) from commercial synthesis.

41. In what settings outside the newborn period can vitamin K abnormalities contribute to a bleeding diathesis?

- **Malabsorptive intestinal disorders** (e.g., cystic fibrosis, Crohn's disease, short-bowel syndrome)
- **Prolonged antibiotic therapy** (this diminishes intestinal bacteria)
- **Prolonged hyperalimentation without supplementation**
- **Malnutrition**
- **Chronic hepatic disorders** (hepatitis, alpha$_1$-antitrypsin deficiency) that can diminish both the absorption of fat-soluble vitamin K (as a result of diminished bile salt production) and the use of vitamin K in factor conversion
- **Drugs** that can disrupt vitamin K include phenobarbital, phenytoin, rifampin, and warfarin

42. What is the best test for distinguishing coagulation disturbances resulting from hepatic disease, disseminated intravascular coagulation (DIC), and vitamin K deficiency?

Factors II, V, VII, IX, and X are made in the liver, and all of these factors (except factor V) are vitamin K dependent. Therefore, the measurement of **factor V** is a useful test to distinguish liver disease from vitamin K deficiency because this factor is reduced in the former and normal in the latter disorder. Factor VIII is reduced in patients with DIC because of the consumptive process, but this factor is normal or increased in patients with liver disease and vitamin K deficiency. Therefore, the **factor VIII** level is a good test to distinguish DIC from the other two disorders (*see* Table 9-2).

43. What is DIC?

DIC is an acquired syndrome that is precipitated by a variety of diseases and characterized by diffuse fibrin deposition in the microvasculature; consumption of coagulation factors; and endogenous generation of thrombin and plasmin. The process is uncontrolled, and the result can be significant microthrombus formation with ischemic injury to multiple organ systems.

TABLE 9-2. COAGULATION ABNORMALITIES IN LIVER DISEASE, VITAMIN K DEFICIENCY, AND DISSEMINATED INTRAVASCULAR COAGULATION

	Factor V	Factor VII	Factor VIII
Liver disease	Low	Low	Normal or increased
Vitamin K deficiency	Normal	Low	Normal
Disseminated intravascular coagulation	Low	Low	Low

44. **What tests are valuable for the diagnosis of suspected DIC?**
See Table 9-3.

TABLE 9-3. TESTS FOR DIAGNOSIS OF DIC

Test	Usual Results
Prothrombin time; activated partial thromboplastin time	Prolonged
Fibrinogen	<100 mg/dL*
Platelet count	Low
D-dimer	>2 µg/mL
Factors II, V, and VIII	Usually low*

*These results may be normal, however, especially in patients with mild disseminated intravascular coagulation because synthesis increases with accelerated consumption.
From Nathan DG, Orkin SH, Ginsburg D, Look AT (eds): Nathan and Oski's Hematology of Infancy and Childhood, 6th ed. Philadelphia, W.B. Saunders, 2003, p 1524.

45. **What is the treatment of choice for DIC?**
DIC occurs most commonly in the context of bacterial sepsis and hypotension. The best treatment is reversal of the underlying cause through treatment of the infection and appropriate fluid and pressor management. If bleeding is severe or if hemorrhage is occurring in a life-threatening location, platelets and fresh frozen plasma should be given to make up for the loss of these elements, which is occurring from consumption. Heparin has not been proved to be effective for increasing survival in patients with sepsis and DIC. The replenishment of depleted antithrombin III levels with antithrombin III concentrate may decrease the risk of new thromboses.

46. **What are the common hereditary disorders that predispose a child to thrombosis?**
   - **Factor V Leiden:** This is an abnormal factor V protein that is resistant to the normal antithrombotic effect of activated protein C.
   - **Protein C deficiency:** Protein C inactivates factors V and VIII and stimulates fibrinolysis.
   - **Protein S deficiency:** Protein S serves as a cofactor for the activity of protein C.
   - **Antithrombin III deficiency:** Antithrombin III is involved in the inhibition of thrombin, factor X, and, to a lesser extent, factor IX.
   - **Prothrombin variation** (gene position 20210 AT).
   - **Hyperhomocysteinemia** is often the result of a mutation of the MTHFR gene.
   - **Antiphospholipid antibodies.**

Hoppe C, Matsunaga A: Pediatric thrombosis. Pediatr Clin North Am 49:1257–1283, 2002.
Beck MJ, Berman B: Review of thrombophilic states. Clin Pediatr 44:193-199, 2005.

HEMATOLOGY LABORATORY

47. **Of the seven red-cell parameters given by a Coulter counter, which are measured and which are calculated?**
The Coulter counter, which is the most commonly used automated electronic cell counter, uses the impedance principle. A precise volume of blood passes through a narrow aperture and impedes an electrically charged field, and each "blip" is counted as a cell. The larger the red cell, the greater the electric displacement. In a separate chamber, the same volume is hemolyzed and colorimetrically analyzed to determine the hemoglobin concentration.

Measured values
- Red blood cell (RBC) count
- Mean corpuscular volume (MCV)
- Hemoglobin (Hb)

Calculated values
- Mean corpuscular hemoglobin (MCH, measured in pg/cell) = $(10 \times [Hb/RBC])$
- Mean corpuscular hemoglobin concentration (MCHC, measured in gm/dL) = $(100 \times [Hb/Hct])$
- Hematocrit (Hct, given as a percentage) = $(RBC \times [MCV/10])$
- Red-cell distribution width (RDW) = coefficient of variation in RBC size

48. **How does the mean corpuscular volume help provide a quick screen of the possible causes of anemia?**
- **Microcytic:** Iron deficiency, thalassemias, sideroblastic anemia
- **Normocytic:** Autoimmune hemolytic anemia, hemoglobinopathies, enzyme deficiencies, membrane disorders, anemia of chronic inflammation
- **Macrocytic:** Disorders of B_{12} and folic acid metabolism, bone marrow failure

49. **What is a quick rule of thumb for approximating MCV?**
70 + (age in years). This number (in mm^3) approximates the lower limit of MCV in children <12 years old, below which microcytosis is present. After the age of 12 years, the lower limit for normal MCV is 82 mm^3.

50. **In addition to an elevated reticulocyte count, what laboratory studies suggest increased destruction (rather than decreased production) of RBCs as a cause of anemia?**
- **Increased serum erythrocyte lactate dehydrogenase:** More commonly seen in patients with hemolytic diseases, it can be greatly elevated in patients with ineffective erythropoiesis (e.g., megaloblastic anemia).
- **Decreased serum haptoglobin:** When RBCs lyse, serum haptoglobin binds the released hemoglobin and is excreted. However, up to 2% of the population has congenitally absent haptoglobin.
- **Hyperbilirubinemia (indirect):** This is usually increased with RBC lysis. However, it may also be elevated in patients with ineffective erythropoiesis (e.g., megaloblastic anemia). Additionally, 2% of the population has Gilbert disease. In these patients, acute infection can cause a transient elevation of bilirubin as a result of liver enzymatic dysfunction rather than hemolysis.

51. **What is the difference between the direct and indirect Coombs' tests?**
Coombs' serum is rabbit antihuman immunoglobulin.
- **Direct test:** Coombs' serum is added directly to a patient's washed RBCs. The occurrence of agglutination means that the patient's RBCs have been sensitized in vivo by the antibody. Direct Coombs' testing is vital for diagnosing autoimmune hemolytic anemias.

- **Indirect test:** This involves incubating a patient's serum with RBCs of a known type and adding Coombs' serum. If in vitro sensitization occurs, agglutination will result, which indicates that antibodies are present against the known blood type. Indirect testing is key for blood crossmatching.

52. **How is the corrected reticulocyte count calculated?**

Because the reticulocyte count is expressed as a percentage of total RBCs, it must be corrected according to the extent of anemia with the following formula: reticulocyte % × (patient Hct/normal Hct) = corrected reticulocyte count. For example, a very anemic 10-year-old patient with a hematocrit level of 7% (in contrast with an expected normal hematocrit of 36%) and a reticulocyte count of 5% has a corrected reticulocyte count of 1.0%: 5% × (7%/36%) = 1%. This is not appropriately elevated, as might be seen in patients with severe iron deficiency. The key concept is the appropriateness of the reticulocyte response to anemia. The corrected "retic count" should be elevated if the bone marrow is working properly and has all the right nutrients for making RBCs, including iron, folate, and vitamin B_{12}.

53. **What is the significance of targeting on an RBC smear?**

Red-cell targets on a peripheral smear are caused by excessive membrane relative to the amount of hemoglobin. Therefore, *target cells* are found when the membrane is increased (e.g., in patients with liver disease) or when the intracellular hemoglobin is diminished (e.g., in patients with iron deficiency or thalassemia trait). Target cells may also be found in patients with certain hemoglobinopathies (e.g., hemoglobins C and SC). In these instances, the target cells are caused by aggregation of the abnormal hemoglobin.

54. **In what conditions are Howell-Jolly bodies found?**

Howell-Jolly bodies are nuclear remnants that are found in the red cells of patients with **reduced or absent splenic function** and in patients with **megaloblastic anemias.** They are occasionally present in the red cells of premature infants. Howell-Jolly bodies are dense, dark, and perfectly round, and their characteristic appearance makes them easily distinguishable from other red-cell inclusions and from platelets overlying red cells.

55. **What is the cause of Heinz bodies?**

Heinz bodies represent **precipitated denatured hemoglobin** in the red cell. Heinz bodies occur when the hemoglobin is intrinsically unstable (e.g., as in hemoglobin Koln) or when the enzymes that normally protect hemoglobin from oxidative denaturation are abnormal or deficient (e.g., as in G6PD deficiency). These inclusions are not visible with a routine Wright-Giemsa stain but can be seen readily with methyl violet or brilliant cresyl blue stains.

56. **Of what clinical value is the sedimentation rate?**

An elevated erythrocyte sedimentation rate (ESR) is a nonspecific marker for inflammatory disease. The rate of sedimentation increases when inflammatory paraproteins bind to the RBC surface. The test may be of some value for suggesting the presence of deep-seated infection or collagen vascular disease, particularly in patients with fever of unknown origin. A better use of the ESR may be for the monitoring of the response to therapy in particular infections (e.g., bacterial endocarditis, osteomyelitis). In these conditions, a falling ESR is considered to be a reliable indicator of the resolution of the inflammatory process.

HEMOLYTIC ANEMIA

57. **What clinical features are suspicious for hemolytic anemia?**
   - Discolored urine (dark, brown, red)
   - Jaundice

- Pallor
- Tachycardia
- Splenic and/or liver enlargement
- If very severe, hypovolemic shock or congestive heart failure

58. **What two types of RBC forms are commonly seen on the peripheral smear in patients with hemolytic anemia?**
    - **Spherocytes or microspherocytes:** These forms can be seen in any hemolytic anemia that results from a loss of RBC membrane surface area (e.g., Coombs'-positive hemolytic anemia, DIC, or hereditary spherocytosis).
    - **Schistocytes:** These various forms of fragmented RBCs can be seen in patients with microangiopathic hemolytic anemia, which is a form of intravascular hemolysis caused by mechanical disruption (e.g., prosthetic heart valves, hemolytic-uremic syndrome, cavernous hemangioma).

59. **Name the two most common inherited disorders of red-cell membranes.**
    Hereditary spherocytosis is characterized by hemolysis (anemia, reticulocytosis, jaundice, splenomegaly), spherocytosis, and, in most cases, a family history of hemolytic anemia. The diagnosis can be made by establishing the presence of the clinical findings and by the finding of increased osmotic fragility of the RBCs. Hereditary spherocytosis is inherited as an autosomal dominant disorder about 75% of the time.

    Hereditary elliptocytosis is characterized by variable hemolysis, with a predominance of elliptocytes on the blood smear. It is usually inherited in an autosomal dominant pattern.

60. **Which disorder is most commonly associated with an elevated MCHC?**
    Hereditary spherocytosis. The hyperchromic appearance of spherocytes and microspherocytes is the result of the loss of surface membrane, an excess of hemoglobin, and mild cellular dehydration. In other hemolytic anemias that are associated with spherocytosis, the percentage of spherocytes is usually insufficient to raise the MCHC.

61. **What is the osmotic fragility test?**
    This is a test to confirm the diagnosis hereditary spherocytosis. A normal red blood cell is discoid in shape as a result of its relative excess of surface area per cell volume from the redundancy of its cell membrane. In increasingly hypotonic solutions, more and more red cells will swell and burst at a standard rate. In spherocytosis, because there is less surface area to cell volume, more cells burst as compared with normal in these hypotonic solutions, particularly after incubating at 37°C for 24 hours. This tendency toward earlier lysis makes them osmotically fragile (Fig. 9-1).

    Shah S, Vega R: Hereditary spherocytosis. Pediatr Rev 25:166–171, 2004.

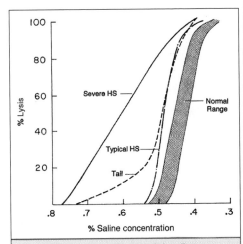

Figure 9-1. Osmotic fragility curves in hereditary spherocytosis. (From Nathan DG, Orkin SH, Ginsburg D, Look AT (eds): Nathan and Oski's Hematology of Infancy and Childhood, 6th ed. Philadelphia, W.B. Saunders, 2003, p 610.)

62. **What is the difference between alloimmune and autoimmune hemolytic anemia?**
   - **Alloimmune hemolytic anemia:** Antibodies responsible for hemolysis are directed against another's red blood cells.
   - **Autoimmune hemolytic anemia:** Antibodies are directed against the host's red cells.

63. **In which settings do alloimmune and autoimmune hemolytic anemia most commonly appear?**
   Isoimmune: Red-cell antigen incompatibility between mother and fetus transfusion of incompatible blood
   Autoimmune: *Primary:* Autoimmune hemolytic anemia (AIHA)
   - Secondary infections (e.g., *Mycoplasma pneumoniae*, Epstein-Barr virus, varicella, viral hepatitis)
   - Drugs (e.g., antimalarials, penicillin, tetracycline)
   - Systemic autoimmune disorders (e.g., systemic lupus erythematosus, dermatomyositis)

64. **How does the cause of AIHA vary by age?**
   AIHA in children <10 years old is more likely to be *primary*. In children >10 years old, AIHA is more likely to be *secondary* to an underlying disease.

65. **What is the most important test to establish the diagnosis of AIHA?**
   The Coombs' test. The diagnosis of AIHA requires the presence of autoantibodies that bind to erythrocytes. However, approximately 10% of patients with AIHA are Coombs' negative. Thus, patients should be treated for AIHA if the disease is strongly suspected, even if the direct Coombs' test is negative.

66. **What are the differences between autoimmune hemolytic anemias caused by "warm" and "cold" erythrocyte autoantibodies?**
   Warm (usually immunoglobulin G antibodies with maximum activity at 37°C): These are most commonly directed against the Rh antigens and generally do not require complement for in vivo hemolysis. Hemolysis is predominantly *extravascular*—consumption occurs primarily in the spleen. Warm antibody-mediated hemolytic anemia is more likely to be associated with underlying disease (especially systemic lupus erythematosus in females) and to become chronic. Splenectomy and/or immunosuppression (e.g., with steroids) are often effective therapies.
   Cold (immunoglobulin M antibodies with maximum activity between 0–30°C): These are most commonly directed against I or i antigen. Hemolysis is most commonly *intravascular*, via complement activation. Extravascular hemolysis that does occur primarily involves hepatic consumption. Cold antibody-mediated hemolytic anemia is more commonly associated with acute infection (e.g., *Mycoplasma pneumoniae*, cytomegalovirus). Patients are less likely to develop chronic hemolysis, and therapy (e.g., splenectomy, immunosuppression) is often ineffective.

67. **An 8-year-old black male developed jaundice and very dark urine 24–48 hours after beginning nitrofurantoin for a urinary tract infection. What is the likely diagnosis?**
   G6PD deficiency is the most common hemolytic anemia caused by an RBC enzymatic defect. The enzyme G6PD is a key component of the pentose phosphate pathway, which ordinarily generates sufficient nicotinamide adenine dinucleotide phosphate hydrogen to maintain glutathione in a reduced state (and to make it available for combating oxidant stresses). The deficiency is inherited in an X-linked recessive fashion. In patients who are deficient (most commonly those of African, Mediterranean, or Asian ancestry), oxidant stresses (particularly certain drugs) can result in hemolysis.

68. **In a patient with G6PD deficiency, why is the initial diagnosis often difficult in the acute setting?**

The amount of G6PD enzymatic activity depends on the age of the RBC. Older RBCs have the least, and reticulocytes have the most. In an acute hemolytic episode, the older cells are destroyed first; younger ones may remain, and reticulocytes may increase. If erythrocytic G6PD levels are measured at this point, the result may be misleadingly near or above the normal range. If clinical suspicions remain, repeating the test when the reticulocyte count is reduced will give a more accurate measurement.

69. **What is favism?**

Favism refers to the clinical syndrome of acute hemolytic anemia from the ingestion of fava beans as an oxidative challenge in patients with G6PD deficiency. This is particularly common in portions of the Mediterranean and Asia, where fava beans are a dietary staple.

IRON-DEFICIENCY ANEMIA

70. **At what age do exclusively breast-fed infants become at risk for iron deficiency?**

Healthy term infants who are exclusively breast fed are at risk for iron deficiency after they are 6 months old. The age of risk for exclusively breast-fed premature infants can be more complicated, particularly for the smaller and sicker infants, and recommendations vary. The lower iron stores of premature infants are more rapidly depleted as compared with term babies.

Leung AK, Chan KW: Iron deficiency anemia. Adv Pediatr 48:385–408, 2001.

71. **Why are infants who begin consuming cow milk at an early age susceptible to iron-deficiency anemia?**

Lower bioavailability. Although breast milk and cow milk contain about the same amount of iron (0.5–1.0 mg/L), nonheme iron is absorbed at 50% efficiency from breast milk but at only 10% from cow milk. In addition, cow milk may cause microscopic gastrointestinal bleeding in younger infants as a result of mucosal injury, possibly from sensitivity to bovine albumin. In older infants, cow milk may interfere with iron absorption from other sources.

Fuchs G, DeWier M, Hutchinson S, et al: Gastrointestinal blood loss in older infants: Impact of cow milk versus formula. J Pediat Gastroenterol Nutr 16:4–9, 1993.

Sullivan P: Cow's milk-induced intestinal bleeding in infancy. Arch Dis Child 68:240–245, 1993.

72. **For which pediatric groups should screening for iron-deficiency anemia be considered?**

- Low birth weight
- Consumption of whole cow milk before the age of 7 months
- Use of formula not fortified with iron
- Low socioeconomic status
- Exclusive breast feeding (without solid or formula supplementation) beyond the age of 6 months
- Perinatal blood loss
- Teenage females (if menstruation is heavy or if pregnant)

Oski F: Iron deficiency in infancy and childhood. N Engl J Med 329:190–193, 1993.

73. **How common is anemia in teenage athletes?**

Significant anemia is uncommon. However, iron deficiency without anemia may be found in approximately half of adolescent female athletes and up to one eighth of male athletes, particularly long-distance runners. However, an adverse effect of this iron deficiency on athletic performance in the absence of anemia has never been conclusively demonstrated. On the other hand, iron depletion (with or without anemia) may be associated with lassitude, decreased concentration ability, and mood swings.

Ballin A, Berar M, Rubinstein U, et al: Iron state in female adolescents. Am J Dis Chil 146:803–805, 1992.

Rowland TW: Iron deficiency in the young athlete. Pediatr Clin North Am 37:1153–1162, 1990.

74. **As iron becomes depleted from the body, what is the progression at which laboratory tests change?**

    The left end of the line for each test indicates the point at which the result deviates from its baseline. As shown in Fig. 9-2, in general, the depletion of marrow, liver, and spleen reserves (as represented by ferritin) occurs first. This is followed by a decrease in transport iron (as represented by transferrin saturation) and finally a fall in hemoglobin and mean corpuscular volume (MCV). The figure illustrates that the absence of anemia does not exclude the possibility of iron deficiency and that iron depletion is relatively advanced before anemia develops. Tests of soluble transferrin receptor have become of interest in patients with iron-deficiency anemia because the elevated levels are very sensitive indicators.

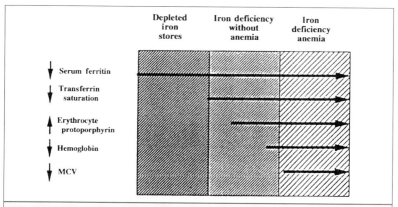

Figure 9-2. Progression of laboratory test changes with iron depletion. (From Dallman PR, Yip R, Oski FA: Iron deficiency and related nutritional anemias. In Nathan DG, Oski FA (eds): Hematology of Infancy and Childhood, 4th ed. Philadelphia, W.B. Saunders, 1993, p 427.)

75. **How might the reticulocyte hemoglobin content be helpful for the diagnosis of iron deficiency?**

    Because the reticulocyte is the most recently produced red blood cell in circulation, the earliest sign of iron deficiency may be a fall in the concentration of hemoglobin in reticulocytes. This number can be calculated from automated counting equipment and may be a reliable and inexpensive alternative to ferritin. Studies have indicated that patients with a concentration of ≥30 pg per cell have virtually no chance of iron deficiency.

Brugnara C, Zurakowski D, DiCanzio J, et al: Reticulocyte hemoglobin content to diagnose iron deficiency in children. JAMA 281:2225–2230, 1999.

Cohen AR: Choosing the best strategy to prevent childhood iron deficiency. JAMA 281:2247–48, 1999.

76. **Why are tests for iron stores more difficult to interpret during acute inflammatory states?**
The *ferritin* level, which is used to monitor body iron stores, is exquisitely sensitive to inflammation, increasing even with mild upper respiratory infections. Elevations of ferritin may persist for some time. By contrast, *serum iron, transferrin level,* and *percent transferrin saturation* may decrease with infection or inflammation. *Free erythrocyte protoporphyrin* should not be affected by acute inflammation but may increase in chronic inflammatory states.

77. **Why is the RDW helpful for diagnosing microcytic anemia?**
The RDW is a quantification of anisocytosis (variation in red-cell size). It is derived from the RBC size histogram that is measured by automated cell counters, and it is reported as a percentage. In children, normal values range from about 11.5–14.5% but can vary among instruments. Statistically, it is the coefficient of variation of red-cell volume distribution.

78. **How is the RDW useful for distinguishing causes of microcytic anemia?**
When elevated in a patient with microcytosis, it suggests that iron deficiency is a more likely cause of anemia than the thalassemia trait. Children with the thalassemia trait tend to have values that overlap with normal RDW values. The combination of an RDW above the normal range with a free erythrocyte protoporphyrin level of >35 µg/dL is more sensitive and specific for iron-deficiency anemia.

79. **What is the Mentzer index?**
MCV/RBC. This is one of the formulas that is used to distinguish the hypochromic, microcytic anemias of the thalassemia trait from iron deficiency. As a general rule, iron deficiency causes alterations in RBCs that tend to be variable, whereas thalassemia generally results in more uniformly smaller cells. In patients with the beta-thalassemia trait, the Mentzer index is usually <13; in patients with iron deficiency, it is usually >13.

80. **In a child with suspected iron-deficiency anemia, is a therapeutic trial with iron an acceptable diagnostic approach?**
Yes. If an infant or child is otherwise well, a therapeutic trial of 4–6 mg/kg/day of elemental iron can substitute for additional diagnostic testing (e.g., ferritin, transferrin saturation, free erythrocyte protoporphyrin), because dietary iron deficiency is the most likely cause of microcytic anemia. If the child is iron deficient, compliant with therapy, and there is not ongoing undetected blood loss, the hemoglobin should rise by >1 gm/dL in about 2 weeks. If the hemoglobin does rise, therapy should be continued for an additional 2 months to replenish iron stores.

81. **After iron therapy is initiated, how early can a response be detected?**
2–5 days: Increase in reticulocyte count
7–10 days: Increase in hemoglobin level
For patients with mild iron-deficiency anemia, the hemoglobin level should be checked after several weeks of therapy. For patients with more severe anemia, it may be useful to check the hemoglobin and reticulocyte levels after several days to make certain that the hemoglobin has not declined to dangerous levels and that the reticulocyte response is beginning.

82. **What foods affect the bioavailability of nonheme iron?**
It is **decreased** by phosphates, tannates, polyphenols, and oxalates found in cereal, eggs, milk, cheese, tea, and complex carbohydrates. It is **increased** by fructose, citrate, and especially ascorbic acid found in red kidney beans, cauliflower, and bananas. In children with iron deficiency, the administration of replacement iron with a vitamin-C-fortified fruit juice 30 minutes before a meal makes physiologic sense.

KEY POINTS: IRON-DEFICIENCY ANEMIA

1. The introduction of whole cow's milk before the age of 1 year increases risk as a result of occult gastrointestinal bleeding.
2. Red-cell distribution width is increased, because deficiency results in uneven red-cell size (anisocytosis).
3. Low levels of ferritin indicate diminished tissue iron stores.
4. This condition impairs cognitive development in infants.

83. **What are the differences between pica, geophagia, and pagophagia?**
All are clinical markers that suggest the diagnosis of iron deficiency. **Pica** is a more general term that indicates a hunger for material that is not normally consumed as food. **Geophagia** refers to the consumption of dirt or clay, and **pagophagia** refers to the excessive consumption of ice. These are distinguished from *cissa*, which is the physiologic craving during pregnancy for unusual food items or combinations.

84. **Discuss the relationship between iron deficiency and development in infants and toddlers.**
Multiple studies have shown an association between iron deficiency in infants between 9 and 24 months old and lower motor and cognitive scores and increased behavioral problems as compared with nonanemic controls. Some longer-term studies suggest that the developmental impairments may be long lasting. Debate remains about whether this relationship is causal and, if so, whether the correction of anemia leads to a reversal of the problems.

Buchanan GR: The tragedy of iron deficiency during infancy and childhood. J Pediatr 135:413–415, 1999.

85. **Why are iron-deficient children at increased risk for lead poisoning?**
- Pica associated with iron deficiency increases the likelihood of ingestion of lead-contaminated items.
- Gastrointestinal absorption of lead may be increased in patients who consume less iron-containing nutrients.

Watson WS, Morrison J, Bethel MI, et al: Food iron and lead absorption in humans. Am J Clin Nutr 44:248–256, 1986.

MEGALOBLASTIC ANEMIA

86. **What is megoblastic anemia?**
Megaloblastic anemia is a macrocytic anemia that is characterized by large red-cell precursors (megaloblasts) in the bone marrow and that is usually caused by nutritional deficiencies of either folic acid (folate) or vitamin B_{12} (cobalamin).

87. **Is megaloblastic anemia the most common cause of macrocytic anemia?**
No. Macrocytic anemia can be found in conditions associated with a high reticulocyte count (e.g., hemolytic anemia, hemorrhage), bone marrow failure (e.g., Fanconi's anemia, aplastic anemia, Diamond-Blackfan anemia), liver disease, Down syndrome, and hypothyroidism.

88. **What findings on a complete blood count are suggestive of megaloblastic anemia?**
    - **Red cells:** Elevated MCH and mean cell volume (often 106 fl or more), with normal MCHC; marked variability in cell size (anisocytosis) and shape (poikilocytosis)
    - **Neutrophils:** Hypersegmentation (>5% of neutrophils with five lobes or a single neutrophil with six lobes)
    - **Platelets:** Usually normal; thrombocytopenia in more severe anemia

89. **What are the causes of vitamin B_{12} (cobalamin) deficiency in children?**

Decreased intake	Decreased absorption
May occur in vegetarians who consume no animal products	Ileal mucosal abnormalities (e.g., Crohn's disease)
	Surgical resection of terminal ileum
Seen in exclusively breast-fed infants of B_{12}-deficient mothers	Competition for cobalamin in bacterial overgrowth syndromes or infection with the fish tapeworm *Diphyllobothrium latum*)
General malnutrition	Congenital abnormalities of the receptor for vitamin B_{12}–intrinsic factor complex
	Gastric mucosal defects that interfere with the secretion of intrinsic factor

90. **What are the best dietary sources of folate and B_{12}?**
    - **Folate:** Folate-rich foods include liver, kidney, and yeast. Good sources also include green vegetables (particularly spinach) and nuts. Moderate sources include fruits, bread, cereals, fish, eggs, and cheese. Pasteurization or boiling destroys folate.
    - **Vitamin B_{12}:** Humans do not manufacture B_{12}; bacteria and fungi do. Animals require it, whereas plants do not. Consequently, our major dietary source of vitamin B_{12} is the consumption of animal tissue, milk, or eggs. Seafood, which live on bacterial diets, are also a good dietary source. Of note is that B_{12} is required for normal folate metabolism.

91. **What is pernicious anemia?**
    Pernicious anemia is a megaloblastic anemia that is caused by a *lack of intrinsic factor*. Intrinsic factor is a glycoprotein that is released from the gastric parietal cells that binds to vitamin B_{12} to form a complex that is ultimately absorbed in the terminal ileum.

92. **A 10-month-old child who was exclusively fed goat milk is likely to develop what type of anemia?**
    Megaloblastic anemia as a result of folic acid deficiency. Goat milk contains very little folic acid compared to cow milk. Infants who are consuming large amounts of goat milk—especially if they are not receiving significant supplemental solid foods—are susceptible to this type of anemia. In addition, the diagnosis can be complicated by the higher risk of coexistent iron-deficiency anemia in this age group.

PLATELET DISORDERS

93. **How can a platelet count be estimated from a peripheral smear?**
    As a rule, each platelet that is visible on a high-power microscopic field (100× objective) represents 15,000–20,000 platelets/mm³. If platelet clumps are observed, the count is usually >100,000/mm³.

94. **How much does a platelet transfusion raise the platelet count?**
    In general, 0.1–0.2 unit/kg of transfused platelets should raise the platelet count by 40,000/mm³ (or 1.0 unit/m² should raise the count by 10,000/mm³). In normal patients,

platelet survival time is 7–10 days, but this is often considerably shorter in thrombocytopenic patients as a result of a variety of causes.

95. **A previously healthy 3-year-old child develops mucosal petechiae, multiple ecchymoses, and a platelet count of 20,000/mm^3 2 weeks after a bout of chickenpox. What is the most likely diagnosis?**
Acute idiopathic (immune) thrombocytopenic purpura (ITP). ITP is one of the most common bleeding disorders of childhood, and the presentation of symptoms occurs after infection in about 50% of cases.

Cines DB, Blanchette VS: Immune thrombocytopenic purpura. N Engl J Med 346:995–1008, 2002.

96. **What is the natural history of acute childhood ITP?**
With or without medical treatment, 50–60% of patients with acute ITP will have normal platelet counts within 1–3 months of diagnosis, and 75% are well after 6 months. By 1 year, only 10% of children with ITP remain thrombocytopenic, and some of the children with chronic ITP still improve as long as 5–10 years after diagnosis. About 5% of patients have recurrent ITP. Because of this predominantly benign natural course of ITP, careful consideration is necessary before instituting treatment that is hazardous or irreversible.

97. **In a toddler with suspected ITP, what is the significance of a palpable spleen on examination?**
Although patients with ITP may rarely have a palpable spleen tip, the presence of splenomegaly in a patient with thrombocytopenia warrants more aggressive evaluation for an associated problem (e.g., collagen-vascular disease, hypersplenism).

98. **In patients with suspected ITP, should a bone marrow evaluation be done?**
This is a topic of much debate. A major concern is that, without a bone marrow aspiration, the diagnosis of leukemia may be delayed or the course of illness worsened by treatment (typically corticosteroids) that is begun for presumed ITP. However, it is very rare that patients with leukemia present with symptoms of isolated thrombocytopenia. Local custom will likely prevail regarding the need for bone marrow examination in the setting of "classic" acute ITP, but heightened consideration should be given if the following are present: (1) other cell lines are involved; (2) history and physical examination have atypical features (e.g., weight loss, hepatosplenomegaly); and (3) steroid therapy is to be used.

Blanchette VS, Carcao M: Childhood acute immune thrombocytopenic purpura: 20 years later. Semin Thromb Hemost 29:605–617, 2003.

99. **When should medical treatment be given for acute ITP without active bleeding?**
Because the long-term prognosis of ITP does not appear to be influenced by medical treatment, the management of a newly-diagnosed child with ITP and no serious bleeding remains controversial. The principal concern is susceptibility to intracranial bleeding, which occurs in <1% of affected patients (but can have 30–50% mortality), almost always when the platelet count is <10,000/mm^3. Local custom will prevail, but some authorities will treat medically when the platelet count is <10,000/mm^3 and/or there is active mucous membrane hemorrhage; this minimizes the chance of intracranial catastrophe and avoids the excessive limitations of physical activity that might otherwise be imposed on a child with ITP.

100. **How do treatments for ITP compare?**
Intravenous immune globulin (IVIG): 0.8–1.0 gm/kg/day, raises the platelet count in approximately 85% of patients. The response usually occurs within 48 hours and persists for 3–4 weeks. Up to 75% of patients will have some degree of limited adverse reaction (e.g., nausea, vomiting, headaches, fever). IVIG is more expensive than steroids.

Corticosteroids: Corticosteroids are similarly effective, but oral steroids take about twice as long (4 days) to raise the platelet count significantly. The steroid effect may be multifactorial because signs of hemorrhage tend to decrease before the increase in platelets occurs. This may include microvascular endothelial stability. Side effects of long-term frequent steroid use are multiple.

Anti-D immunoglobulin: Anti-D immunoglobulin (immunoglobulin with antibody rto (D)) should be given intravenously to individuals with adequate hemoglobin count, (Rh)D-positive RBCs, and intact splenic function. It is more rapidly given than IVIG, with a slightly smaller proportion of responders.

101. **Which children with ITP are candidates for splenectomy?**
Splenectomy improves the platelet count in up to 90% of patients. Because spontaneous remission is common in acute ITP, splenectomy is usually limited to bleeding that is life threatening and unresponsive to medical therapies. Patients with ITP lasting >1 year with continued bleeding, severe thrombocytopenia, or unacceptable restrictions may be reasonable candidates for splenectomy.

102. **In what conditions of children is thrombocytosis most commonly seen?**
   - Acute infections (e.g., upper and lower respiratory tract infections)
   - Chronic infections (e.g., tuberculosis)
   - Iron-deficiency anemia
   - Hemolytic anemia
   - Medications (e.g., vinca alkaloids, epinephrine, corticosteroids)
   - Inflammatory disease (e.g., Kawasaki disease)
   - Malignancy (e.g., chronic myelogenous or megakaryocytic leukemia)

   Schafer AI: Thrombocytosis. N Engl J Med 350:1211–1219, 2004.
   Yohannan MD, Higgy KE, al-Mashhadani SA, Santhosh-Kumar CR: Thrombocytosis. Etiologic analysis of 663 patients. Clin Pediatr 33:340–343, 1994.

103. **What level of thrombocytosis requires treatment?**
A high platelet count in most children does not appear to be a cause of significant morbidity because it is often transient. In some centers, aspirin in doses of 81 mg daily are administered when the platelet count exceeds $1.5 \times 10^6/mm^3$. The early introduction of aspirin therapy may be more important if the patient has other problems that might contribute to hyperviscosity, such as a high white blood cell count or hemoglobin level.

SICKLE CELL DISEASE

104. **What is the mutation that results in sickle cell disease?**
On the beta chain, valine is substituted for glutamic acid at position 6. The alpha chain is normal. The result is sickle hemoglobin (HbS).

105. **Why is sickle cell disease often asymptomatic during the first months of life?**
During the neonatal period, the presence of large amounts of fetal hemoglobin reduces the rate of polymerization of HbS and the sickling of RBCs that contain this abnormal hemoglobin. As the amount of fetal hemoglobin decreases after age 3–6 months, patients with sickle cell disease are increasingly likely to experience their first clinical manifestations.

106. **What are the two major pathophysiologic mechanisms in sickle cell anemia that cause the morbidities associated with the disease?**
   - **Hemolysis:** Sickled RBCs undergo both intravascular and extravascular hemolysis, which leads to anemia, reticulocytosis, jaundice, gallstones, and occasional aplastic crisis.

- **Vaso-occlusion:** Intermittent and chronic vaso-occlusion result in both acute exacerbations (e.g., painful crisis, stroke) and chronic disease manifestations (e.g., retinopathy, renal disease). The adhesion of sickled erythrocytes to inflamed vascular endothelium is a principal pathologic component.

107. **A 6-month-old black male has painful swelling of both hands. What is the most likely diagnosis?**
Hand-foot syndrome, or **dactylitis.** This common early manifestation of sickling disorders in infants and young children is characterized by painful swelling of the hands, feet, and proximal fingers and toes caused by symmetric infarction in the metacarpals, metatarsals, and phalanges (Fig. 9-3). A lack of systemic signs, the presence of symmetric

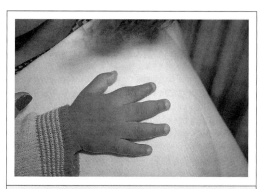

Figure 9-3. Swelling of the fingers from dactylitis. (From Lissauer T, Clayden G: Illustrated Textbook of Pediatrics. London, Mosby, 1997, p 238.)

involvement, and young patient age help distinguish hand-foot syndrome from the much less common osteomyelitis, which may also complicate sickle cell disease.

108. **When does functional asplenia occur in children with sickle cell disease?**
It may begin as early as 5 or 6 months of age, and it may precede the presence of Howell-Jolly bodies in the peripheral smear. Most children with HbSs who are >5 years old have functional asplenia, with a small, atrophied spleen. Clinical experience indicates that the period of increased risk for serious bacterial infection parallels the development of functional asplenia. Consequently, in addition to routine vaccinations, antibiotic prophylaxis with penicillin is recommended beginning at 2 months of age. Loss of splenic function usually occurs later in patients with HbSC or HbS beta+-thalassemia.

Claster S, Vichinsky EP: Managing sickle cell disease. BMJ 327:1151–1155, 2003.

109. **What are the three main categories of crises in patients with sickle cell disease?**
- **Aplastic crisis:** Hemoglobin may fall as much as 10-15% per day without reticulocytosis
- **Vaso-occlusive crisis:** Includes painful crises (most common), acute chest syndrome, acute central nervous system events (stroke), and priapism
- **Acute splenic sequestration:** May occur rapidly, with profound hypotension and cardiac decompensation

Dover GJ, Platt OS: Sickle cell disease. In Nathan DG, Orkin SH, Ginsburg D, Look AT (eds): Nathan and Oski's Hematology of Infancy and Childhood, 6th ed. Philadelphia, W.B. Saunders, 2003, pp 802–811.

110. **What is the most common cause of death in children with sickle cell disease?**
Infection. Splenic dysfunction causes increased susceptibility to meningitis and sepsis (particularly pneumococcal).

111. **How should a child with a vaso-occlusive (painful) crisis be managed?**
For outpatients with an acute painful crisis, ibuprofen or acetaminophen and codeine are reasonable choices. Patients with intensely painful crises require day unit or inpatient hospitalization for opioid (including morphine and meperidine) analgesics, ideally given intravenously.

Patient-controlled analgesia offers the dual benefit of a constant infusion and intermittent boluses of an analgesic. Other supplementary agents, including nonsteroidal analgesics (e.g., ketorolac), vasodilators/membrane active agents (e.g., cetiedil citrate), and high-dose methylprednisone, are under study. For severe crises, blood transfusions to reduce the percentage of sickle cells to <30% may be beneficial.

Jacob E, Miaskowski C, Savedra M, et al: Management of vaso-occlusive pain in children with sickle cell disease. J Ped Hematol Onco 25:307–311, 2003.

Melzer-Lange MD, Walsh-Kelly CM, Lea G, et al: Patient-controlled analgesia for sickle cell pain crisis in a pediatric emergency department. Pediatr Emerg Care 20:2–4, 2004.

112. **How should children with sequestration crisis be managed?**
Acute sequestration crisis represents a true emergency in sickle cell disease and is the second leading cause of death in young children with sickle cell disease. The clinical problem is primarily one of hypovolemic shock as a result of the pooling of blood in the acutely enlarged spleen. The hemoglobin level may drop to as low as 1–2 gm/dL. The major therapeutic effort should be directed toward **volume replacement** with whatever fluid is handy. In most instances, normal saline or colloid solutions will be adequate until properly cross-matched blood is available. Acute sequestration crisis is one of the few instances for patients with sickle cell disease in which **transfusion with whole blood** is appropriate because the problem is one of hypovolemia and anemia rather than anemia alone. If whole blood is not available, packed RBCs alone or packed RBCs plus plasma may be an alternative therapy.

113. **What is the "acute chest syndrome" in sickle cell patients?**
Acute chest syndrome refers to the constellation of findings (e.g., fever, cough, chest pain, pulmonary infiltrates) that can resemble pneumonia or pulmonary infarction. The exact mechanism is unknown, and the cause is likely multifactorial. Various infections (e.g., viral, chlamydial, mycoplasmal) may initiate respiratory inflammation, which ultimately causes localized hypoxia; increased pulmonary sickling may then result. Rib and other bone infarcts can also occur, and hypoventilation may result from chest splinting. Pulmonary fat embolism has been seen to occur, particularly in the setting of a preceding bony painful crisis (e.g., the thigh).

Zar HJ: Etiology of sickle cell chest. Pediatr Pulmon 26:S188–S190, 2004.

114. **How should the acute chest syndrome in sickle cell patients be treated?**
- **Aggressively,** because rapid progression to respiratory failure is possible.
- **Optimization of ventilation** is vital, including supplemental oxygen, analgesics adequate to minimize splinting, incentive spirometry, and other possible measures (e.g., bronchodilators, nitrous oxide).
- **Judicious hydration:** Overly vigorous hydration can lead to pulmonary edema.
- **Antibiotics:** These should typically be given to cover *Chlamydia, Mycoplasma* and *Streptococcus pneumoniae.*
- **Blood transfusion,** including erythrocytapheresis (automated RBC exchange transfusion), has been shown to improve the status of patients with acute chest syndrome; this should be considered for patients with severe or worsening disease.

Graham LM: Sickle cell disease: Pulmonary management options. Pediatr Pulmonol 26:S191–S193, 2004.

115. **How often is priapism a problem in children with sickle cell disease?**
Priapism is an unwanted, painful erection that is usually unrelated to sexual activity. It is an underappreciated morbidity in adolescents with sickle cell disease, usually occurring at least once by the age of 20 years and typically by the age of 12 years. Most patients are unaware of the term and the consequences; early intervention may prevent irreversible penile fibrosis and impotence.

Maples BL, Hagemann TM: Treatment of priapism in pediatric patients with sickle cell disease. Am J Health Sys Pharm 61:355–363, 2004.

KEY POINTS: SICKLE CELL DISEASE

1. A genetic mutation leads to abnormal beta-globin chain.

2. Eight percent of African Americans have the sickle cell trait.

3. Crises: Hemolytic, vaso-occlusive, sequestration, and aplastic.

4. The risk of serious bacterial infection is increased among these patients as a result of functional asplenia.

5. Dactylitis (painful hand/foot swelling) is often the earliest manifestation.

116. **What are the long-term morbidities associated with sickle cell disease?**
     - Chronic lung disease
     - Renal failure
     - Congestive heart failure
     - Retinal damage
     - Leg ulcers
     - Aseptic necrosis of the hip or shoulder
     - Poor growth

117. **How common is the sickle cell trait in the United States?**
     Heterozygosity for the sickle gene occurs in about 8% of blacks in the United States, 3% of Hispanics in the eastern United States, and a much smaller percentage of individuals of Italian, Greek, Arabic, and Veddah Indian heritage. Of note is that 2% of blacks in the United States have the hemoglobin C trait.

118. **Does sickle cell trait have any significant morbidity?**
     Under normal physiologic conditions, no. RBCs in individuals with sickle cell trait contain only 30–40% sickle hemoglobin, which is insufficient to cause sickling. However, in hypoxic settings, sickling may occur. Portions of the kidney may have physiologically low oxygen concentrations that can interfere with function and lead to an inability to concentrate urine (hyposthenuria) and hematuria (usually microscopic and asymptomatic). At high altitudes (e.g., when mountain climbing or in an unpressurized aircraft), splenic infarction is possible.

119. **What is the second most common worldwide hemoglobin variant?**
     Hemoglobin E. This variant is particularly high in the southeast Asian population (especially those of Laotian, Thai, and Cambodian heritage). Heterozygotes are asymptomatic; homozy gotes can have a mild microcytic anemia. The most common abnormal findings on a peripheral smear are microcytosis and target cells.

THALASSEMIA

120. **What are the thalassemias?**
     The thalassemias are a heterogeneous group of disorders of hereditary anemia due to *diminished* or *absent normal globin chain production*. Normally, four alpha-globin genes and two beta-globin genes are expressed to make the tetrameric globin protein, which then combines with a heme moiety to make the predominant hemoglobin that is found in red cells, HbA (sub-

units $\alpha_2 \beta_2$). Depending on the number of genes that are deleted, the production of polypeptide chains is diminished. In patients with alpha-thalassemia, alpha-globin production is lowered; in patients with beta-thalassemia, beta-globin production is lowered. When one class of polypeptide chains is diminished, this leads to a relative excess of the other chain. The result is ineffective erythropoiesis, precipitation of unstable hemoglobins, and hemolysis as a result of intramedullary RBC destruction.

121. **What accounts for the variability in the clinical expression of the thalassemias?**
Clinical heterogeneity results from variability in the number of gene deletions (particularly in alpha-thalassemia). As a rule, the greater the number of deletions, the more severe the symptoms. A large number of point mutations have been identified in various populations; this can contribute to the phenotypic diversity. In addition, the inheritance of other thalassemia genes (e.g., delta-thalassemia) or the persistence of fetal hemoglobin can modify the clinical course.

122. **How is the diagnosis of thalassemia made in most clinical laboratories?**
Homozygous beta-thalassemia is detected by the absence (β^0) or reduction (β^+) of the amount of HbA ($\alpha_2 \beta_2$) relative to HbF ($\alpha_2 \gamma_2$ or fetal hemoglobin) on hemoglobin electrophoresis. The carrier state for beta-thalassemia is characterized by a low mean cell volume and, in most instances, an increased level of HbA$_2$ ($\alpha_2 \delta_2$) or HbF. The levels of these two hemoglobins are most accurately measured by column chromatography. Estimation or quantitation from electrophoretic patterns is frequently misleading.

The alpha-thalassemia trait remains a diagnosis of exclusion (low mean cell volume in the absence of an identifiable cause) in the clinical laboratory, although the enumeration of missing alpha genes for the most common deletions in specific ethnic populations is accomplished by molecular techniques. Newer polymerase chain reaction-based DNA tests for the common variants have become very useful.

123. **Describe the clinical features of the alpha-thalassemia syndromes.**
When all four alpha-globin genes are missing or nonfunctional, this results in severe intrauterine anemia and hydrops fetalis. Extraordinary therapy such as in utero transfusion may result in survival. Absence of three functional alpha-globin genes results in HbH disease, which is a chronic moderate to severe anemia with jaundice and splenomegaly that may necessitate RBC transfusion therapy. Absence of two alpha-globin genes is associated with mild microcytic anemia. Absence of one alpha-globin gene is clinically silent (*see* Table 9-4).

TABLE 9-4.   CLINICAL FEATURES OF ALPHA-THALASSEMIA

Syndrome	Usual genotype	Alpha gene number	Clinical features
Normal	$\alpha\alpha/\alpha\alpha$	4	Normal
Silent carrier	$\alpha-/\alpha\alpha$	3	Normal
Alpha-thalassemia trait	$\alpha-/\alpha-$	2	Mild microcytic anemia
HbH disease	$--/\alpha\alpha$	1	Moderate microcytic anemia
			Splenomegaly
			Jaundice
Homozygous alpha-thalassemia	$--/--$	0	Fetal hydrops as a result of severe anemia

124. **What are the clinical features of the beta-thalassemia syndromes?**
- **Thalassemia minor:** Minimal or no anemia (hemoglobin 9–12 gm/dL); microcytosis; elevated RBC count
- **Thalassemia intermedia:** Microcytic anemia with hemoglobin usually >7 gm/dL; growth failure; hepatosplenomegaly; hyperbilirubinemia; thalassemic facies (i.e., frontal bossing, mandibular malocclusion, prominent malar eminences due to extramedullary hematopoiesis) develop between the ages of 2 and 5 years
- **Thalassemia major** (Cooley's anemia): Severe anemia (hemoglobin 1–6 gm/dl) usually during the first year of life; hepatosplenomegaly; growth failure

  Olivieri NF: The beta-thalassemias. N Engl J Med 341:99–109, 1999.

125. **How can coexistent iron deficiency increase the difficulty of diagnosing beta-thalassemia?**
The beta-thalassemia trait is usually diagnosed by hemoglobin electrophoresis, with quantitative hemoglobins revealing elevated HbA_2 and/or HbF levels. Iron deficiency can cause a lowering of HbA_2, thereby masking the diagnosis. With iron replacement, the hemoglobin A_2 will rise to the expected elevated levels seen in patients with the beta-thalassemia trait.

KEY POINTS: THALASSEMIA

1. Normal hemoglobin (HbA): Tetramer of two alpha and two beta chains

2. Associated with quantitative reduction in globin synthesis

3. Homozygous beta-thalassemia is most severe form, with pallor, jaundice, hepatosplenomegaly, growth retardation

4. Expansion of facial bones resulting from extramedullary hematopoiesis

5. Severity of alpha-thalassemia depends on number of genes deleted (1–4)

6. Alpha-thalassemia: More common among people of Southeast Asian ethnicity

7. Beta-thalassemia: More common in people of Mediterranean ethnicity

126. **What are the adverse effects of chronic transfusional iron overload in children with thalassemia?**
- **Cardiac:** Congestive heart failure, dysrhythmias, and, less frequently, pericarditis
- **Endocrine:** Delays in growth and sexual development, hypoparathyroidism, hypothyroidism; diabetes as a result of iron overload is irreversible, even with intensive chelation
- **Hepatic:** Progressive liver fibrosis and cirrhosis

127. **What are the two most common diseases that are associated with transfusion-related iron overload?**
Thalassemia major and sickle cell disease.

128. **How do you reduce iron accumulation in children who require repeated transfusions?**
- **Chelation therapy:** Subcutaneous or intravenous deferoxamine has been the standard therapy for transfusional overload.
- **Splenectomy:** This is used primarily in patients with thalassemia (and a small subgroup of sickle cell patients) who have hypersplenism, which results in the premature destruction of RBCs and increased transfusion requirements.

- **Diet:** Drinking tea with meals reduces dietary iron absorption and may be most helpful in patients with diseases such as thalassemia intermedia, in which the bulk of excessive iron is dietary in origin.
- **Erythrocytapheresis:** Automated erythrocytapheresis rather than repeated simple transfusions may markedly reduce transfusional iron loading in patients with sickle cell disease.

Lo L, Singer ST: Thalassemia: Current approach to an old disease. Pediatr Clin North Am 49:1165–1192, 2002.

ACKNOWLEDGMENT

The editors gratefully acknowledge contributions by Dr. Anne F. Reilly that were retained from the prior edition of *Pediatric Secrets*.

IMMUNOLOGY

Georg A. Holländer, MD, and Anders Fasth, MD, PhD

CHAPTER 10

CLINICAL ISSUES

1. **What are the immunoglobulin G (IgG) subclasses?**
   IgG can be classified according to structural, chemical, and biologic differences into four subclasses: IgG1, IgG2, IgG3, and IgG4. The relative contribution of each to total IgG is 70%, 20%, 7%, and 3%, respectively. In response to protein antigens, IgG1 and IgG3 subclasses predominate, whereas IgG2 and IgG4 are typically noted with polysaccharide antigens.

2. **What is an IgG subclass deficiency?**
   A disproportionately low level of one subclass with normal levels of total IgG. In the mid 1970s, reports began to appear describing children with recurrent infections (primarily sinopulmonary) who had selective subclass deficiencies. Most common was IgG2 deficiency, but multiple other combinations have since been described.

3. **Why is there controversy about the diagnostic significance of subclass deficiencies?**
   - IgG values have a very wide and age-dependent range.
   - Methodologic variability among laboratories is widespread.
   - Specific antibody responses may be more important than absolute subclass quantities.
   - Coexistent immunologic problems (e.g., IgA deficiency) may be present.
   - Subclass deficiencies can be the presenting abnormality in more serious immunologic disorders (e.g., ataxia-telangiectasia, common variable immunodeficiency, chronic mucocutaneous candidiasis, adenosine deaminase deficiency).
   - Some younger patients with subclass deficiencies have immunoglobulin levels that return to normal with maturation.

     Shackelford PG: IgG subclasses: Importance in pediatric practice. Pediatr Rev 14:291–296, 1993.

4. **What are the immunologic risks for asplenic patients?**
   Overwhelming bacterial infections have been noted in children and adults with anatomic or functional asplenia. The incidence of mortality from septicemia is increased by fifty fold in individuals after the traumatic loss of splenic function. The risk of bacteremia is higher in younger (versus older) children and may be greater during the first few years after splenectomy. *Streptococcus pneumoniae, Haemophilus influenzae* type B, and *Neisseria meningitidis* are the most frequent pathogens observed in asplenic children.

5. **What is the significance of a leukemoid reaction?**
   A leukemoid reaction usually refers to a white-cell count >50,000/mm^3 and an accompanying shift to the left. (i.e., the differential count shows an increase in immature cells). Causes include bacterial sepsis, tuberculosis, congenital syphilis, congenital or acquired toxoplasmosis, and erythroblastosis fetalis. Infants with Down syndrome may also have a leukemoid reaction that is often confused with acute leukemia during the first year of life.

6. **Name the three most common causes of eosinophilia in children in the United States.**

   Eosinophilia, which is usually defined as >10% eosinophils or an absolute eosinophil count of $\geq 1000/mm^3$, is most commonly seen in three atopic conditions: **atopic dermatitis, allergic rhinitis,** and **asthma**.

7. **What conditions are associated with extreme elevations of eosinophils in children?**
   - Visceral larval migrans (toxocariasis)
   - Other parasitic disease (trichinosis, hookworm, ascariasis, strongyloidiasis)
   - Eosinophilic leukemia
   - Hodgkin's disease
   - Drug hypersensitivity
   - Idiopathic hypereosinophilic syndrome

   Lukens JN: Eosinophilia in children. Pediatr Clin North Am 19:969–981, 1972.

8. **What is the first immune disorder to involve a congenital defect in programmed cell death (apoptosis)?**

   Autoimmune lymphoproliferative syndrome (also known as Canale-Smith syndrome). Patients display a nonmalignant, noninfectious lymphoproliferation with splenomegaly, chronic lymphadenopathy, and, often, hepatomegaly. Lymphocytes persist that normally would die. Diagnosis rests on increases in alpha/beta T-cell antigen receptor positive, CD4$^-$CD8$^-$ (i.e., double negative) T cells, and defective in vitro Fas-mediated lymphocyte apoptosis.

DEVELOPMENTAL PHYSIOLOGY

9. **How do immunoglobulin levels change during the first years of life?**
   - **IgG** levels in a full-term baby are equal or higher (5–10%) than maternal levels as a result of active placental transport. With an IgG half-life of 21 days, this transported maternal IgG reaches a nadir after 3–5 months. As the infant begins to make IgG, the level begins to rise slowly; it is 60% of adult level at 1 year of age, and it achieves the adult level by 6–10 years of age.
   - **IgM** concentrations are normally very low at birth, and 75% of normal adult concentrations are usually achieved by about 1 year of age.
   - **IgA** is the last immunoglobulin produced and approaches 20% of adult value by 1 year; however, full adult levels are not reached until adolescence. Because delays in the production of IgA are not unusual, the diagnosis of IgA deficiency is difficult to make with certainty in a child who is <2 years old.
   - **IgD** and **IgE,** both of which are present in low concentrations in the newborn, reach 10–40% of adult concentrations by 1 year of age.

10. **Which are the characteristics of immunoglobulin transport across the placenta?**

    IgG is the only isotype that is transferred across the placenta. All IgG subclasses cross the placenta, and their relative concentrations in the cord serum are comparable with those of the maternal serum. Transfer of IgG can first be detected as early as 8 weeks of gestation, and levels rise steadily between 18 and 22 weeks. By 30 weeks, the serum concentrations of IgG are approximately 50% of those observed in neonates born at term. IgG concentrations comparable with those of the mother are achieved by 34 weeks of gestation, and values at term can be higher by approximately 10% as compared with maternal serum levels as a result of the active transport across the placenta.

11. **How does the complement system of the neonate compare with that of an adult?**

The alternative and the classical complement pathway activity are moderately (50% lysis of target cells via the alternative pathway [AP_{50}]: 50–65% of adult values) to slightly (the quantity of dilution of serum required to lyase 50% of red blood cells in a standard hemolytic complement assay [CH_{50}]: 55–90% of adult values) diminished in the term neonate. In preterm neonates, these activities may be further decreased. Most notably, the serum concentrations for factors C8 and C9 are approximately 20% of those seen in adults.

12. **What determines immunoglobulin levels during infancy?**

Immunoglobulin serum concentrations are determined by the amount of maternal IgG transported across the placenta, by catabolism of maternal IgG, and by the rate of synthesis of the infant's own IgM, IgG, and IgA. The development of specific antibodies is dependent on antigen exposure, antigen presentation, and the availability of T-cell help and T-cell maturation. Newborns readily produce antibodies against (vaccine) proteins, whereas polysaccharides fail to induce an adequate response during the first 2 years of life.

13. **Why are antibodies not produced by the fetus in appreciable quantities?**

- The fetus is in a sterile environment and is not exposed to foreign antigens.
- The active transport of maternal IgG across the placenta may suppress fetal antibody synthesis.
- Fetal and neonatal monocyte/macrophages may not process foreign antigens normally.

14. **What is the role of the thymus?**

The thymus is the primary lymphoid organ for the production and generation of T cells bearing the alpha/beta T-cell antigen receptor. The thymus is responsible for the central selection of the T-cell repertoire, which allows for the establishment of tolerance toward self-antigens and responsiveness to nonself (i.e., foreign) antigens.

15. **At what age does thymic function cease?**

At birth, the thymus is at two thirds of its mature weight and reaches its peak mass at around 10 years of age. Subsequently, thymic size declines, but substantial function (as measured by the output of new T cells) persists into very late adulthood (70–80 years of age).

Douek DC, McFarland RD, Keiser PH, et al: Changes in thymic function with age and during the treatment of HIV infection. Nature 396:690–695, 1998.

16. **What are the advantages of breast milk for the immune system of infants?**

Several studies have reported that human milk enhances the development of the immune system, especially with regard to measuring antibody formation. For example, antibody levels in response to immunization with conjugate *Haemophilus influenzae* type B vaccine are significantly higher in breast-fed babies than in formula-fed babies; this suggests that breast feeding enhances the active immune response during the first year of life.

Pabst HF, Spady DW: Effect of breast-feeding on antibody response to conjugate vaccine. Lancet 336:269–270, 1990.

17. **How does neutrophil function in the neonate compare with that of adults?**

There is a diminished neutrophil storage in the neonate, and the cells display a reduced adhesion and migration capacity in response to chemotactic stimuli. By contrast, the efficiency for the ingestion and killing of bacteria is normal for these cells. Under suboptimal conditions, however, these effector functions may be diminished, and neutrophils from sick and stressed neonates can display a decreased microbicidal activity.

NEUTROPENIA

18. **How is neutropenia defined?**

Neutropenia is arbitrarily defined as an absolute neutrophil count (ANC) of <1,500/mm^3. The ANC is determined by multiplying the percentage of bands and neutrophils by the total white blood cell count. An ANC of <500/mm^3 is severe neutropenia. A granulocytosis is defined as ANC <100/mm^3. As a rule, the lower the ANC, the greater the risk of infectious complications. During the first 2 years of life (outside of the neonatal period), when normal white blood counts are generally lower, an ANC <1000/mm^3 is considered neutropenic.

KEY POINTS: INFECTIONS IN IMMUNODEFICIENCIES

1. Increased frequency

2. Increased and prolonged severity

3. Unusual organisms (frequently opportunistic microorganisms)

4. Unexpected or severe complications of infection

5. Repeated infections without a symptom-free interval

19. **How do children with neutrophil disorders present?**

Neutrophil disorders include those that affect quantity (e.g., various neutropenias) and those that affect function (e.g., chemotaxis, phagocytosis, bactericidal activity). These defects should be considered part of the differential diagnosis in patients with delayed separation of the umbilical cord, recurrent infections with bacteria or fungi of low virulence (but minimal problems with recurrent viral or protozoal infections), poor wound healing, and specific locales of infection (e.g., recurrent furunculosis, perirectal abscesses, gingivitis).

20. **What is the most common cause of transient neutropenia in children?**

Viral infections, including influenza, adenovirus, coxsackie virus, respiratory syncytial virus, hepatitis A and B, measles, rubella, Epstein-Barr virus, cytomegalovirus, and varicella. The neutropenia usually develops during the first 2 days of illness and may persist for up to a week. Multiple factors likely contribute to the neutropenia, including a redistribution of neutrophils (increased margination rather than circulation), sequestration in reticuloendothelial tissue, increased use in injured tissues, and marrow suppression. In general, otherwise healthy children with transient neutropenia as a result of viral infections are at low risk for serious infectious complications.

21. **Excluding intrinsic defects in myeloid stem cells, what conditions are associated with neutropenia in children?**

- **Bone marrow infiltration:** Leukemia, myelofibrosis
- **Drugs**
- **Immunologic factors:** Neonatal alloimmune (secondary to maternal IgG directed against fetal neutrophils) and autoimmune (e.g., autoimmune neutropenia of childhood) conditions
- **Metabolic factors:** Hyperglycinemia, isovaleric acidemia, propionic acidemia, methylmalonic acidemia, glycogen storage disease type IB
- **Nutritional deficiencies:** Anorexia nervosa, marasmus, B$_{12}$/folate deficiency, copper deficiency
- **Sequestration:** Splenic enlargement

Dinauer MC: The phagocyte system and disorders of granulocyte function and granulopoiesis. In Nathan DG, Orkin SH, Look AT, Ginsburg D (eds): Hematology of Infancy and Childhood, 5th ed. Philadelphia, W.B. Saunders, 2003, pp 948–958.

22. **Which drugs are frequently associated with neutropenia?**
Many drugs can cause neutropenia, and this is frequently the result of either a dose-dependent bone-marrow suppression or a hapten-induced generation of antineutrophil antibodies. Neutropenia is also relatively frequently observed in patients treated with phenothiazine, sulfonamides, semisynthetic penicillins, nonsteroidal anti-inflammatory agents, and antithyroid medications. Within days after stopping the drug, immature neutrophils usually reappear in the peripheral blood.

23. **Which is the most common form of chronic childhood neutropenia?**
Autoimmune neutropenia of infancy (ANI). This disorder displays a 3:2 female predominance and is caused by a chronic depletion of mature neutrophils. Approximately 90% of all cases are detected within the first 14 months of life. The median duration of neutropenia is 20 months, and 95% of patients with this condition have fully recovered by the time they are 4 years old. The ANC of infants with ANI is usually below 500/mm^3, and the bone marrow displays normal cellularity despite an arrest at late stages of metamyelocytes or at the band stage. Antineutrophil antibodies are occasionally detected, but their presence is not necessary for the diagnosis of ANI.

24. **Which primary immune deficiencies that affect lymphocytes are typically associated with neutropenia?**
   - **X-linked agammaglobulinemia:** One third of patients will have neutropenia at some point during the course of their disease.
   - **Hyper-IgM syndrome:** This is typically is associated with cyclic or persistent neutropenia.
   - Several **T-cell defects** as well as the rare **NK-cell deficiencies** can be associated with neutropenia

25. **Which hematologic disorder is frequently observed in neonates delivered from mothers with severe pregnancy-induced hypertension?**
Approximately half of all neonates born to women with severe pregnancy-induced hypertension display **neutropenia**. Because the neutrophils are only transiently depressed, an increased risk for infection is not observed.

PRIMARY IMMUNODEFICIENCIES

26. **How common are primary immunodeficiencies?**
Primary immunodeficiencies: 1:10,000 (excluding asymptomatic IgA deficiency)
   - B-cell defects: 50%
   - Combined cellular and antibody deficiencies: 20%
   - T-cell–restricted deficiencies: 10%
   - Phagocytic disorders: 18%
   - Complement component disorders: 2%

   Immune Deficiency Foundation: www.primaryimmune.org

27. **What are the typical clinical findings of the various primary immunodeficiencies?**
See Table 10-1.

28. **What are the typical features of transient hypogammaglobulinemia of infancy (THI)?**
THI is characterized by diminished concentrations of one or more classes of Ig. This deficiency is most commonly understood as an age-related delay in the acquisition of the ability to produce normal Ig isotype concentrations, and it can be also understood as a rare physiologic event. The frequency of THI has been estimated to be lower than 1 in 1,000, and it represents less than 5% of all of the diagnoses of primary immunodeficiencies. Typically, no consistent immunologic

defects are observed among individuals with THI. None of the infections noted in these patients are usually life threatening. In sharp contrast with patients with X-linked agammaglobulinemia, children with THI respond to immunizations with tetanus and diphtheria toxoids; they also have isohemagglutinin titers and a normal number of T and B cells.

TABLE 10-1. CLINICAL FINDINGS OF PRIMARY IMMUNODEFICIENCIES

	Predominant B-cell deficiency	Predominant T-cell deficiency	Phagocytic defects	Complement defects
Age at onset	After maternal antibodies have disappeared (usually >6 months)	Early infancy	Early infancy	Any age
Type of infection	Gram-positive or gram-negative (encapsulated) bacteria; *Mycoplasma; Giardia; Cryptosporidium; Campylobacter;* enteroviruses	Viruses, particularly CMV_1 and CBV; systemic BCG after vaccination; fungal; *Pneumocystis carinii*	Gram-positive or gram-negative bacteria; catalase-positive organisms in CGD, especially *Aspergillus*	*Streptococcus; Neisseria*
Clinical findings	Recurrent respiratory tract infections; diarrhea; malabsorption; ileitis; colitis; cholangitis; arthritis; dermatomyositis; meningoencephalitis	Poor growth and failure to thrive; oral candidiasis; skin rashes; sparse hair; opportunistic; infections; graft-versus-host disease; bony abnormalities; hepatosplenomegaly	Poor wound healing; skin diseases (e.g., seborrheic dermatitis, impetigo, abscess); cellulitis without pus; suppurative adenitis; periodontitis; liver abscess; Crohn disease; osteomyelitis; bladder outlet obstruction	Rheumatoid disorders; angioedema; increased susceptibility to infection

CMV_1 = cytomegalovirus 1, CBV = coxsackie B virus, BCG = Bacillus calmette guerin, CGD = chronic granulomatous disease.

29. **Why are male children more likely to suffer from a primary immunodeficiency?**
Several primary immunodeficiency disorders are linked to the X-chromosome: agammaglobulinemia, hyper-IgM syndrome, severe combined immunodeficiency (the common cytokine-

receptor gamma-chain deficiency), lymphoproliferative syndrome, Wiskott-Aldrich syndrome, one form of chronic granulomatous disease, and properidine deficiency. This fact accounts for the observation that the male-to-female ratio is 4:1 among patients with a primary immunodeficiency that are younger than 16 years old.

30. **Which is the most common type of primary immunodeficiency?**
    Selective IgA deficiency is the most common primary immunodeficiency. The prevalence of selective IgA deficiency has been calculated to range from 1 in 220 to 1 in 3,000, depending on the population studied. However, most IgA-deficient subjects remain healthy, which has been attributed to a compensatory increase of IgM in bodily secretions. A minority of these patients demonstrate normal levels of secretory IgA and normal numbers of IgA-bearing mucosal plasma cells. Although IgA represents <15% of total immunoglobulin, it is predominant on mucosal surfaces. Therefore, most patients with symptoms have recurrent diseases involving mucosal surfaces, including otitis media, sinopulmonary infections, and chronic diarrhea. Systemic infections are rare.

31. **What are the diagnostic criteria for IgA deficiency?**
    Serum concentrations of IgA <0.05 gm/L are diagnostic and almost invariably associated with a concomitant lack of secretory IgA. Serum levels for IgM are normal, and concentrations for IgG (particularly IgG1 and IgG3) may be increased in a third of all IgA-deficient patients.

32. **What is the association of autoimmune disorders and IgA deficiency?**
    Autoimmune disorders have been described in up to 40% of patients with selective IgA deficiency. These include systemic lupus erythematosus, rheumatoid arthritis, thyroiditis, celiac disease, pernicious anemia, Addison disease, idiopathic thrombocytopenic purpura, and autoimmune hemolytic anemia.

33. **Why is immunoglobulin therapy not used as a treatment for selective IgA deficiency?**
    Unless a patient has a concurrent IgG subclass deficiency (even in this setting, therapy is controversial), gamma-globulin therapy is not indicated and is in fact relatively contraindicated because of the following:
    - The short half-life of IgA makes frequent replacement therapy impractical.
    - Gamma-globulin preparations have insufficient IgA quantities to restore mucosal surfaces.
    - Patients can develop anti-IgA antibodies with the potential for hypersensitivity complications, including anaphylaxis.

34. **In an infant with panhypogammaglobulinemia, how can the quantitation of B and T lymphocytes in peripheral blood help distinguish the diagnostic possibilities?**
    - Normal numbers of T lymphocytes, no detectable B lymphocytes: X-linked agammaglobulinemia (Bruton's disease)
    - Normal numbers of T and B lymphocytes: Transient hypogammaglobulinemia of infancy, common variable immunodeficiency
    - Decreased numbers of T lymphocytes, normal or decreased numbers of B lymphocytes: Severe combined immunodeficiency
    - Decreased CD4 lymphocytes: Human immunodeficiency virus (HIV) infection

35. **What are the criteria for the diagnosis of X-linked agammaglobulinemia (XLA)?**
    - Onset of recurrent bacterial infections at <5 years of age
    - Serum immunoglobulin values for IgG, IgM, and IgA well below 2 standard deviations of the normal for age

- Absent isohemagglutinins
- Poor to absent response to vaccines
- Less than 2% peripheral B cells (CD19⁺)

36. **What are the typical clinical manifestations of XLA?**
Newborns with XLA have normal serum levels of IgG at birth and few—if any—symptoms. Typically, symptoms begin at the age of 4–12 months, although as many as 20% of patients with XLA present with clinical symptoms as late as 3–5 years of age. Infections are the most common clinical manifestation and frequently occur as a result of encapsulated bacteria, *Staphylococcus aureus*, *Salmonella*, *Campylobacter*, *Mycoplasma*, and *Giardia lamblia*. Infections may be localized to the respiratory tract (e.g., otitis media, sinusitis, pneumonia), the skin (e.g., pyoderma), or the gastrointestinal tract (e.g., diarrhea), or they may spread hematogenously (e.g., sepsis, meningitis, septic arthritis).

37. **To which viral infections are patients with XLA most susceptible?**
Enteroviral infections (polio, ECHO, and coxsackie). It has been calculated that the vaccine-associated poliomyelitis after inoculation with the live polio virus is increased in patients with XLA by a factor of 10,000. More than half of patients with XLA with long-standing enteroviral infections will show weakness, hearing loss, headache, seizures, ataxia, paresthesias, and lethargy or coma. The major causes of death in these patients are enteroviral infections.

KEY POINTS: WARNING SIGNS OF IMMUNODEFICIENCY

1. Six or more new ear infections within 1 year

2. Two or more serious sinus infections within 1 year

3. Two or more months on antibiotics with little effect

4. Two or more severe pneumonias within 1 year

5. Failure of an infant to gain weight and grow normally

6. Recurrent deep skin or organ abscesses

7. Persistent thrush in mouth or elsewhere on skin after 1 year of age

8. Need for intravenous antibiotics to clear infections

9. Two or more deep-seated infections such as meningitis, osteomyelitis, cellulitis, or sepsis

10. A family history of primary immune deficiency

38. **How frequently is the mother not the carrier of the disease in XLA?**
Approximately one third of all XLA cases are thought to be caused by new mutations.

39. **Which are the typical immunologic laboratory findings in patients with the complete form of XLA?**
Low to absent concentrations of all immunoglobulin isotypes; absent or low B cells; lack of germinal centers in lymph nodes; absence of tonsils; a complete or almost complete block at the developmental pre-B-cell stage; normal T-cell and NK-cell numbers and functions.

40. **What are the typical laboratory findings of common variable immunodeficiency (CVID)?**

Laboratory evaluations in patients with CVID typically demonstrate low IgG levels and low to absent IgA and IgM serum concentrations. Similarly, specific antibodies to previously encountered pathogens and to vaccines and isohemagglutinins are low to absent. A large proportion of patients with CVID exhibit a depressed switch from IgM to IgG. Although lymphocyte subsets are normal in the majority of patients with CVID, standard T-cell function tests (e.g., in vitro proliferation in response to mitogens, nominal antigens, and allogeneic cells) are subnormal in approximately half of all patients.

41. **What are the clinical features of CVID?**

Symptoms of CVID may first occur during childhood, but they more often occur after puberty and include increased infections, particularly in the respiratory tract; involvement of the gastrointestinal tract (e.g., chronic malabsorption, nodular lymphoid hyperplasia, gastric atrophy with achlorhydria); and autoimmune disorders (e.g., rheumatoid arthritis, autoimmune hemolytic anemia, pernicious anemia, neutropenia, thrombocytopenia, chronic active hepatitis, vitiligo, parotitis).

42. **Which is the treatment of choice for CVID?**

The treatment of CVID includes Ig substitution, antibiotics, and physiotherapy for chest disease. The effect of a higher dose of immunoglobulin to maintain trogh levels of IgG at low-normal levels may be beneficial with regard to a decrease in the incidence of infections and the frequency of hospitalization.

43. **What is the underlying disorder in an 8-year-old girl with atypical eczema, pneumatoceles, and bouts of severe furunculosis?**

Hyper-IgE syndrome is the most likely diagnosis. This disease is clinically characterized by the following:

- Recurrent infections (almost invariably caused by *Staphylococcus aureus*) of the skin, lungs (causing frequently persistent pneumatoceles), ears, sinuses, eyes, joints, and viscera
- Atypical eczema with lichenified skin
- Coarse facial features, especially the nose
- Osteopenia of unknown cause
- Delayed tooth exfoliation (i.e., prolonged retention of primary teeth)

The laboratory evaluation of the hyper-IgE syndrome reveals massively elevated IgE levels associated with IgG subclass and specific antibody deficiencies; variable dysfunctions of neutrophils; and an imbalance of cytokine production as a result of a Th2 predominance (IL-4, IL-5).

Grimbacher B, Holland SM, Gallin JI, et al: Hyper-IgE syndrome with recurrent infections—an autosomal dominant multisystem disorder. N Engl J Med 340:697–702, 1999.

44. **Which is the medical treatment of choice for the hyper-IgE syndrome?**

Continuous antimicrobial therapy is usually necessary to control the deep-seated infections. No specific immunotherapeutic regimen has been successful; in particular, intravenous substitution of immunoglobulins and interferon are of no proven benefit for patients with this disorder.

45. **What are the proven indications for intravenous immunoglobulin therapy?**

- Humoral and combined primary immune deficiencies with low to absent levels of IgM and/or IgG (XLA, CVID, hyper-IgM syndrome, severe combined immune deficiency [SCID], Wiskott-Aldrich syndrome, ataxia telangiectasia, antibody deficiencies with normal serum immunoglobulins, selected cases of symptomatic IgG subclass deficiencies despite antibiotic treatment)
- Kawasaki disease
- Idiopathic thrombocytopenic purpura

- Guillain-Barré syndrome (acute inflammatory demyelating polyradiculopathy)
- Chronic inflammatory demyelinating polyradiculoneuropathy
- Dermatomyositis (adults)
- Multifocal motor neuropathy

Ballow M: Intravenous immune serum globulin therapy. In Leung DYM, Sampson HA, Geha RS, Szefler SJ (eds): Pediatric Allergy: Principles and Practice. St. Louis, Mosby, 2003, p 188.

46. **What is the recommended dosage for intravenous immunoglobulin (IVIG) substitution in Ig-deficient patients?**
An individual dose of IVIG is chosen that maintains a trough level >500 mg/dL. This is achieved within 4–8 months using an IVIG dosage of 400–600 mg/kg/month. Trough serum IgG levels should be determined every 3 months until a steady-state concentration is achieved and every 6–8 months thereafter to monitor the adequacy of the IVIG dosage. Individuals with a high catabolism of IgG, however, will need a more frequent infusion of smaller doses to maintain the appropriate serum levels. Moreover, periods of active infections may necessitate either higher dosages or shorter intervals between IVIG treatments.

47. **What are the pharmacologic characteristics of IVIG?**
After the infusion, 100% of the IgG stays in the intravascular compartment. Over the course of the next 3–4 days, IgG equilibrates with the extra cellular space, with 85% of the infused IgG still situated in the circulation. By the end of the first week, half of the IgG given has left the circulation, and by 4 weeks after the infusion, the serum levels have returned to baseline. However, these data apply to healthy individuals with a regular catabolism, and they have to be adjusted for both patients with a higher metabolic rate and for individuals transfused with increased IgG concentrations.

48. **What are the adverse reactions to IVIG?**
Approximately 10% of patients receiving IVIG treatment experience mild side effects including headaches, myalgias, nausea, vomiting, and facial flushing. The majority of these side effects are related to the presence of acute or chronic infections, the rate of infusion, and/or the temperature of the IVIG solution. Uncommon reactions are chest tightness and bronchospasm. Aseptic meningitis with rapid onset of severe headaches and photophobia has been noted, especially in patients with a history of migraines.

49. **Which viral infections can result in hypogammaglobulinemia in the immunocompetent individual?**
Epstein-Barr virus, HIV, and **congenital rubella.** Single cases of hypogammaglobulinemia have also been described among children infected with cytomegalovirus and parvovirus B19.

50. **What is the classic triad of Wiskott-Aldrich syndrome?**
Thrombocytopenia with small platelets volume, eczema, and **immunodeficiency.** This syndrome is an X-linked disorder, and the initial manifestations are often present at birth and consist of petechiae, bruises, and bloody diarrhea as a result of thrombocytopenia. The eczema is similar in presentation to classical atopic eczema (antecubital and popliteal fossa). Infections are common and include (in decreasing frequency): otitis media, pneumonia, sinusitis, sepsis, and meningitis. The severity of immunodeficiency may vary but usually affects both T- and B-cell functions. It is important to note that this immunodeficiency is progressive and associated with a high risk of developing cancer; a teenager with this condition has a 10–20% statistical risk of developing a lymphoid neoplasm. Only about a third of patients with Wiskott-Aldrich syndrome present with this classic triad.

Sullivan KE, Mullen CA, Blaese RM, Winkelstein JA: A multi-institutional survey of the Wiskott-Aldrich syndrome. J Pediatr 125(6 Pt 1):876–885, 1995.

51. **What is the likely diagnosis of a patient presenting with a progressive ataxia and recurrent bacterial sinopulmonary infections?**
   Ataxia-telangiectasia (A-T). In patients with A-T, primarily progressive cerebella ataxia develops during infancy and is typically associated with other neurologic symptoms (e.g., the loss or decrease of deep tendon reflexes, choreoathetosis, apraxia of eye movements). The signs of telangiectasia occur usually after the onset of ataxia, generally between 2 and 8 years of age. The telangiectasias are primarily at the bulbar conjunctivae. Recurrent infections (as a consequence of a humoral and cellular immunodeficiency) are observed in 80% of patients with A-T and are typically localized to the middle ear and the upper airways.

KEY POINTS: SUSPECT IMMUNODEFICIENCY IN INFANTS WITH THESE CONDITIONS

1. Failure to thrive

2. Persistent cough

3. Persistent candidiasis

4. Absolute lymphocyte count <2000/mm^3

52. **Which laboratory tests support the diagnosis of A-T?**
   Although the diagnosis of A-T chiefly relies on the clinical presentation, several laboratory findings support the diagnosis. The peripheral blood count usually reveals lymphopenia and eosinophilia. There is often a reduction of IgA (70% of all cases), IgG2/IgG4, and IgE; a poor antipolysaccharide response; and an increased frequency of autoantibodies, including antibodies to IgA and IgG. T-cell immunity is abnormal in about 60% of patients.

53. **What is the single most important laboratory test if severe combined immunodeficiency (SCID) is suspected?**
   A full blood count to document **lymphopenia** (2,000/mm^3) is the single most important laboratory test during the initial evaluation of a patient for suspected SCID. However, a minority of patients with SCID (approximately 20%) may have a normal absolute lymphocyte count.

54. **What are the typical clinical features of SCID?**
   - Recurrent bacterial infections (typically pneumonia, otitis media, and sepsis)
   - Persistent viral infections (respiratory syncytial virus, enterovirus, parainfluenza, cytomegalovirus)
   - Opportunistic infections (*Pneumocystis carinii, jerovici* fungi)
   - Failure to thrive
   - Diarrhea (enterovirus, rotavirus)
   - May include skin rash (due to maternal-fetal engraftment with graft-versus-host disease, Omenn syndrome (associated with RAG-deficiency, interleukin-7 receptor alpha-chain deficiency, and Artemis deficiency), and hepatosplenomegaly (due to maternal-fetal engraftment, transfusion of nonirradiated blood, or after generalized BCG infection after immunization)
   www.scid.net

55. **In children with SCID, how often is a family history positive for affected relatives?**
   Between 50% and 60% of the time. SCID can be inherited in both an autosomal-recessive and an X-linked form.

   Stephan JL, Vlekova V, Le Deist F, et al: Severe combined immunodeficiency: A retrospective single-center study of clinical presentation and outcome in 117 patients. J Pediatr 123:564–572, 1993.

56. **What disease did the "bubble boy" have?**
Adenosine deaminase (ADA) deficiency. In this form of SCID, the lack of ADA results in abnormalities of B- and T-cell function and increased susceptibility to infection. The bubble served as a means of minimizing contagion but also promoted social isolation. Although bone marrow transplantation has been curative as a treatment of this condition, ADA deficiency is the first disease (by initial reports) to be treated by gene therapy (i.e., insertion of functional ADA genes into the patient's autologous cells and followed by infusion).

57. **What are the clinical phenotypes of adenosine deaminase deficiency?**
   - **Neonatal/infantile onset** (80–90%): Clinically and immunologically virtually indistinguishable from all forms of classical SCID; lymphopenia with absent humoral and cellular immune functions; failure to thrive; severe infections with fungal, viral, and opportunistic pathogens. Half of these patients have skeletal abnormalities at the costochondral junction (flared ribs).
   - **Delayed onset** (15–20%): Recurrent infections, particularly sinopulmonary infections and septicemia, with a frequent failure to generate specific antibodies. Increased IgE levels, IgG subclass deficiencies, and autoimmunity (hypoparathyroidism, type 1 diabetes, hemolytic anemia, and idiopathic thrombocytopenia) provide evidence of immune dysregulation.

   Shovlin CL, Simmonds HA, Fairbanks LD, et al: Adult onset immunodeficiency caused by inherited adenosine deaminase deficiency. J Immunol 153:2331–2339, 1994.

58. **Describe the molecular defect of chronic granulomatous disease (CGD).**
CGD is characterized by a profound defect in the oxygen metabolic burst in myeloid cells following the phagocytosis of microbes. The molecular mechanisms responsible for this disease are heterogenous, as any defect of the four subunits that constitute the nicotinamide adenine dinucleotide phosphate hydrogen–oxidase can cause CGD. As a consequence, superoxide, oxygen radicals, and peroxide production are lacking, and patients with CGD cannot kill catalase-positive pathogenic bacteria and fungi (e.g., *Staphylococcus aureus, Nocardia, Serratia, Aspergillus*).

59. **Which laboratory tests are used for the diagnosis of CGD?**
Patients suspected to have CGD can be diagnosed as a result of their failure to generate reactive oxygen species during the respiratory burst or, alternatively, as a result of their inability to kill catalase-positive bacteria (*Staphylococcus aureus, Escherichia coli*) in vitro with their phagocytes. The screening tests for the production of superoxide are the slide nitroblue tetrazolium reduction test and the flow cytometric 2′,7′-dichlorofluorescein test.

60. **What types of infections are commonly seen in children with CGD?**
Superficial staphylococcal skin infections, particularly around the nose, eyes, and anus, are common. Severe adenitis, recurrent pneumonia, indolent osteomyelitis, and chronic diarrhea are frequent. A male child with a liver abscess should be considered to have chronic granulomatous disease until it is proven otherwise.

61. **What are the cornerstones of CGD treatment?**
   - Prevention of infections through immunization and prophylactic antibiotic and anti-*Aspergillus* treatment; avoidance of certain sources of pathogens
   - Use of prophylactic recombinant human interferon-gamma (the use is questioned by some clinicians)
   - Early and aggressive use of parenteral antibiotics
   - Surgical treatment of recalcitrant infections

   Bemiller LS, Roberts DH, Starko KM, Curnutte JT: Safety and effectiveness of long-term interferon gamma therapy in patients with chronic granulomatous disease. Blood Cells Mol Dis 21:239–247, 1995.

62. **Which disorder has to be considered in a newborn patient with delayed separation of the umbilical cord?**
Patients with **leukocyte adhesion deficiency type I** suffer from a profound impairment of leucocyte mobilization into extravascular sites. The hallmark of this disorder is the complete absence of neutrophils at the site of infection and inflammation (e.g., wound healing).

63. **An infant with hypocalcemic tetany, a loud cardiac murmur, and dysmorphic facies probably has what syndrome?**
DiGeorge syndrome (also called DiGeorge sequence or anomaly and 22q11 syndrome). The clinical pattern results from microdeletions of the long arm of chromosome 22q11 with maldevelopment of the third and fourth pharyngeal pouches during embryogenesis. This results in a spectrum of malformations and clinical findings, including the following:
   - **Cardiac defects:** Aortic arch and conotruncal anomalies, especially truncus arteriosus
   - **Parathyroid absence** or **hypoplasia** with abnormal calcium homeostasis
   - **Abnormal facies,** including round/broad low-set ears with folded helix, short philtrum, hypertelorism, notched ear pinna, hooped eyelids, malar flatness, micrognathia, and down-slanting palpebral fissures
   - **Mild mental retardation** (IQ~70)
   - **Language/speech problems**
   - **Behavior disorder**
   - **Thymic hypoplasia:** Degree of thymic maldevelopment is variable and usually results in diminished numbers of T cells; clinically significant immunologic abnormalities often absent

64. **What are the two main phenotypes associated with complement component deficiencies?**
Generally, deficiencies of the *early* complement components (C1, C2, C3, and C4; factor I and factor H) are associated with autoimmune diseases (glomerulonephritis, systemic lupus erythematosus, dermatomyositis, scleroderma, and vasculitis) or with a predisposition to infections with encapsulated organisms. Deficiencies of the *terminal* components (C5, C6, C7, C8, and possibly C9) are associated with recurrent neisserial diseases.

65. **Which potential life-threatening disorder of the complement system is associated with nonpruritic swelling and occasional recurrent abdominal pain?**
Hereditary C1 inhibitor deficiency. Angioedema of any part of the body—including the airway and the intestine—can occur as a consequence of failure to inactivate the complement and kinin systems. The condition has also been called hereditary angioneurotic edema. Infections, oral contraceptives, pregnancy, minor trauma, stress, and other variable have been noted to precipitate this autosomal-dominant disease. Diagnosis is confirmed by direct assay of the inhibitor level. Clinical presentations include the following:
   - **Recurrent facial and extremity swelling:** Acute, circumscribed edema that is not painful, red, or pruritic, thereby clearly distinguished from urticaria; usually self-resolves in 72 hours
   - **Abdominal pain:** Recurrent and often severe, colicky pain as a result of interstitial wall edema with vomiting and/or diarrhea; may be misdiagnosed as an acute abdomen
   - **Hoarseness, stridor:** A true emergency because death by asphyxiation may occur as a result of laryngeal edema; epinephrine, hydrocortisone, and antihistamines often of only limited benefit, and tracheostomy needed if there is progression of symptoms

LABORATORY ISSUES

66. **Which are the initial screening tests for a suspected immunodeficiency?**
The basic screening tests should include complete blood count (including hemoglobin, morphology, and absolute cellularity); quantification of immunoglobulin levels (IgM, IgG, IgE, and

IgA); antibody responses to previous antigen exposures (e.g., vaccines, pathogen-defined infections); determination of isohemagglutinin titers; assessment of the classical complement pathway by determining the CH_{50}; and work-up of infections, including determination of C-reactive protein, blood cultures, and appropriate radiography. The choice of the laboratory tests is generally dependent on the clinical findings and the immunodeficiency suspected, and the results have to be compared with age-matched controls. It is important to note that there is no justification for a blanket screening; tests should only be ordered if their results will affect either the diagnosis or management of the patient.

67. **Which laboratory tests allow for a broad evaluation of the humoral immune system?**
    1. **Serum immunoglobulin levels, quantitative:** IgM, IgG, IgA, and IgE. A combined IgG, IgA, and IgM level <400 mg/dL suggests immunoglobulin deficiency; >5000 IU/mL for IgE suggests hyper-IgE syndrome.
    2. **IgG subclasses:** These immunoglobulins should generally be measured primarily in patients >6 years old, in certain circumstances (e.g., in patients with selective IgA deficiency and normal to low IgG concentrations but demonstrated functional antibody deficiency), and in patients with recurrent sinopulmonary infections.
       - *Specific antibody titers:* In response to documented infections and vaccinations
       - *Isohemagglutinin titer (anti-A, anti-B):* ≤1:4 after the age of 1 year suggests specific IgM deficiency
       - *Tetanus/diphtheria* (IgG1)
       - *Pneumococcal polysaccharide antigens* (IgG2)
       - *Viral respiratory agents* (IgG3)
    3. **Determination of B-cell numbers:** In the peripheral blood with the use of flow cytometry (CD19, CD20)
    4. **B-cell proliferation and immunoglobulin production:** With the use of in vitro assays

68. **Which diagnostic tests allow for the specific evaluation of T-cell functions?**
    - **Total lymphocyte count:** Although most T-cell immunodeficiencies are not associated with a decreased lymphocyte count, a total count of <1,500/mm^3 suggests a deficiency.
    - **T-cell subpopulations:** Total T cells with <60% mononuclear cells, helper (CD4) cells <200/μl, or CD4/CD8 <1.0 suggest T-cell deficiency.
    - **Delayed-type hypersensitivity skin testing**
    - **Proliferative responses** to mitogens, antigens, and allogeneic cells
    - **Acquisition of activation markers** on T cells (using flow cytometry)
    - **Cytotoxic assay**
    - **Cytokine synthesis.**
    - **Adenosine deaminase** and **purine nucleoside phosphorylase** determination in red blood cells
    - **Molecular biologic studies** (including karyotyping and fluorescent in situ hybridizations)
    - **Histology** of thymic and lymph-node biopsies

69. **What are the principle cell-surface antigens to be used to identify cells of the human immune system by flow cytometry?**
    - **Pan-T-cell markers:** CD2 (leukocyte-function-associated Antigen-3 [LFA-3] receptor) and CD3ε (part of the T-cell receptor complex)
    - **T-cell subpopulations:** CD4, CD8, αβ, and γδ T-cell antigen receptors
    - **Activated T cells:** CD25 (alpha-chain of interleukin-2 [IL-2] receptor), human leukocyte antigen-D related (HLA-DR)
    - **Pan-B-cell markers:** CD19, CD20
    - **NK cells:** CD16 (Fc receptor), CD56 (N-CAM isoform)
    - **Monocytes:** CD11b (C3bi receptor), CD14 (LPS coreceptor)

70. What is the value of skin testing for the diagnosis of T-cell deficiencies?

Skin tests for the assessment of delayed-type hypersensitivity are difficult to evaluate. A positive test is useful for eliminating the diagnosis of severe T-cell deficiency, whereas a negative test may reflect a T-cell defect, or it may result from the lack of an anamnestic response to the antigens used. Seventy-five percent of normal children between the ages of 12 and 36 months will respond to *Candida* skin testing at 1:10 dilution, and, by 18 months, approximately 90% of normal children will respond to one of a panel of recall antigens (tetanus toxoid, trichophyton, and *Candida*); the younger the child, the less likely the reactivity. The cell-mediated reaction may be obscured by a humoral (Arthus) reaction as a result of previous priming.

71. What is the importance of the CD4/CD8 ratio?

The CD4/CD8 ratio is an index of helper to suppressor/cytotoxic cells and may be significantly altered in patients with a variety of immunodeficiencies. In normal individuals, the ratio ranges from 1.4–1.8/1.0. In patients with viral infections (particularly HIV), the ratio can be reduced; in patients with bacterial infections, it can be increased.

72. How is white cell function evaluated in children with suspected disorders?

Neutrophils and monocyte/macrophages are enumerated and examined morphologically after histochemical staining. Monoclonal antibodies directed against CD14 (a surface antigen on monocytes) are used in conjunction with flow cytometry to quantify the number of monocytes/macrophages. Suspected abnormalities in hexose monophosphate activity (as seen in children with chronic granulomatous disease) can be investigated with either nitroblue tetrazolium dye reduction or a dichlorofluorescein assay. Chemotaxis is commonly assayed in agarose, and in vitro quantitative microbicidal assays can be used to assess the bactericidal capacity of isolated neutrophils and monocytes.

73. How is the classic complement cascade evaluated?

The primary screening test is the CH_{50}. This test assesses the ability of an individual's serum (in varying dilutions) to lyse sheep red blood cells after those cells are sensitized with rabbit IgM anti-sheep antibody. The CH_{50} is an arbitrary unit that indicates the quantity of complement necessary for 50% lysis of the red blood cells in a standardized setting. Test results are usually expressed as a derived reciprocal of the test dilution needed for 50% lysis. The test is relatively insensitive because major reductions in individual complement components are necessary before the CH_{50} is altered. Therefore, determination **C3** and **C4 levels** are often included in the initial screening of a child with a suspected complement deficiency.

CHAPTER 11

INFECTIOUS DISEASES

Alexis M. Elward, MD, David A. Hunstad, MD, and Joseph W. St. Geme, III, MD

ANTI-INFECTIVE THERAPY

1. **What medications are used for the treatment of influenza in children?**
   Older agents include amantadine and rimantadine, both of which block the entry of influenza into host cells and inhibit a viral assembly protein called M2. Because the M2 protein of influenza B strains is unaffected by these agents, the drugs are effective only against influenza A strains.
   Newer agents inhibit viral neuraminidase, which is necessary for the detachment of new virions from the surface of infected cells. Oseltamivir (Tamiflu) is available as a capsule or suspension and is useful for the prophylaxis or treatment of both influenza A and B infection. It can be used for the treatment of children as young as 1 year old and for prophylaxis in adolescents ≥13 years old. Zanamivir (Relenza) is an inhaled powder that can be used for the treatment of influenza A and B infections in otherwise healthy patients ≥7 years old.

2. **What are the differences among classes of penicillins?**
   - **Penicillins** (penicillins G [intravenous] and V [oral]): Penicillin G is the drug of choice for *Treponema pallidum* infection (syphilis) and is useful for the treatment of certain other infections (e.g., group A streptococcal pharyngitis and some anaerobic infections).
   - **Aminopenicillins** (ampicillin and amoxicillin): The spectrum is similar to that of penicillin but includes additional activity against aerobic gram-negative bacteria.
   - **Penicillinase-resistant penicillins** (methicillin, oxacillin, nafcillin, and dicloxacillin): These have excellent activity against sensitive strains of *Staphylococcus aureus*.
   - **Antipseudomonal penicillins** (piperacillin and ticarcillin): These have an expanded gram-negative spectrum and can be used to treat susceptible strains of *Pseudomonas aeruginosa*.
   The spectrum of certain penicillins can be increased by the addition of a beta-lactamase inhibitor. Beta-lactamases are a common basis for penicillin resistance in some bacteria (e.g., *Staphylococcus aureus*) but not in other species (e.g., *Streptococcus pneumoniae*). Available combinations include amoxicillin-clavulanate, ampicillin-sulbactam, piperacillin-tazobactam, and ticarcillin-clavulanate.

3. **Is methicillin-resistant *Staphylococcus aureus* (MRSA) only a problem in hospitals and nursing homes?**
   Recent years have seen a sharp increase in the proportion of bone, joint, skin, and soft-tissue infections caused by community-acquired strains of MRSA. Infectious disease specialists in a number of metropolitan areas now report that 10–70% of community-acquired *S. aureus* isolates are resistant to methicillin. These strains have been uniformly susceptible to vancomycin, and some specialists advocate the empiric use of vancomycin for such infections in high-prevalence areas until culture results are known. Fortunately, many community-acquired MRSA strains retain susceptibility to clindamycin, trimethoprim-sulfamethoxazole, minocycline, rifampin, and other agents that may be useful for the eradication of these infections.

4. **How should infections with vancomycin-resistant enterococci be managed?**

   Resistance to vancomycin has been observed in both *Enterococcus faecium* and *Enterococcus faecalis*. Many patients have succumbed to bacteremia or other invasive infections with vancomycin-resistant enterococci (VRE). Most of these infections are acquired nosocomially, which reflects the fact that the organism can survive on inanimate surfaces (including medical equipment) for weeks. Basic tenets of anti-infective therapy apply: foreign bodies should be removed, infected fluid collections should be drained, and patients should be placed on contact isolation to prevent spread. The combination streptogramin agent quinupristin-dalfopristin (Synercid) and the oxazolidinone antibiotic linezolid (Zyvox) have shown promise in early use. Of note is that quinupristin-dalfopristin has activity against *E. faecalis* but not *E. faecium*

5. **Is vancomycin still effective against all staphylococci?**

   Within a few years of the emergence of VRE, isolates of *S. aureus* with reduced susceptibility to vancomycin were reported. In some of these isolates, acquisition of resistance genes from VRE has been demonstrated. Fortunately, these isolates have retained susceptibility to a variety of other antibiotics.

6. **Is amphotericin B the drug of choice for invasive aspergillosis?**

   Invasive aspergillosis in immunocompromised patients (e.g., transplant recipients) is fatal if left untreated, and amphotericin B remains a mainstay of therapy. However, cure rates are only in the range of 60–70%. In addition, long-term therapy with traditional amphotericin B often leads to renal toxicity, including wasting of electrolytes (especially potassium and magnesium) and decreased glomerular filtration rate. The use of lipid-based amphotericin B products (AmBisome or Abelcet) has reduced the frequency of these adverse effects without compromising treatment efficacy. The newer antifungal voriconazole has demonstrated equal-to-superior cure rates for invasive aspergillosis with very few side effects, either alone or in combination with another new agent called caspofungin. This latter agent is the only currently available echinocandin, which is a new class of sterol-inhibiting antifungals.

7. **Are quinolones safe to use in children?**

   Members of the quinolone class of antibiotics act against bacterial DNA gyrase and topoisomerase II, two enzymes that are required for bacterial DNA replication. No member of the class is approved by the U.S. Food and Drug Administration (FDA) for use in patients <18 years old, and part of the basis for this recommendation is the occurrence of arthropathy in immature beagle dogs treated with ciprofloxacin or other quinolones. However, there is growing anecdotal experience with the use of these antibiotics in adolescents and children, primarily those with cystic fibrosis in whom endogenous *Pseudomonas aeruginosa* strains may display high-level resistance to other antibiotic classes (e.g., antipseudomonal penicillins, carbapenems, aminoglycosides). No significant joint disability has been reported among adolescents treated with quinolones.

8. **What are the differences among first-, second-, third-, and fourth-generation cephalosporins?**

   First-generation cephalosporins (e.g., cefazolin, cephalexin, cefadroxil)
   - Alternative drugs for patients allergic to penicillins, although there is a 5–10% risk of cross reactivity
   - Prophylaxis for orthopedic and cardiovascular surgery
   - Better *S. aureus* coverage as compared with second- and third-generation cephalosporins
   - Lack of efficacy against *Haemophilus influenzae*

   Second-generation cephalosporins (e.g., cefaclor, cefuroxime, cefprozil, cefpodoxime)
   - Increased spectrum of activity, including many gram-negative organisms
   - Prophylaxis for intra-abdominal and pelvic surgery (e.g., cefoxitin)
   - Improved compliance with oral medications (most with twice-daily dosing)

- Poor penetration into the cerebrospinal fluid
- No antipseudomonal activity

Third-generation cephalosporins (e.g., ceftriaxone, cefotaxime, cefixime, cefdinir)
- Broadest spectrum, including excellent activity against gram-negative bacteria
- Generally less activity against gram-positive organisms than earlier generations
- Very high blood and cerebrospinal fluid levels achievable in relation to minimal inhibitory concentration for bacterial strains
- Wide therapeutic index with generally minimal toxicity (similar to previous generations)
- Some offer single-daily dosing
- More expensive

Fourth-generation cephalosporins (e.g., ceftazidime, cefepime, cefoperazone)
- Spectrum similar to third-generation agents, with the addition of antipseudomonal activity

Darville T, Yamauchi T: The cephalosporin antibiotics. Pediatr Rev 15:54–62, 1994.

9. **Are antibiotic-resistant pneumococci more virulent than sensitive strains?**
    Up to 50% of pneumococcal isolates from sterile body sites are *nonsusceptible* (i.e., *intermediate-* or *high-level resistant*) to penicillin (minimum inhibitory concentration, ≥0.12 µg/mL), and, of these, 50% are also nonsusceptible to cefotaxime and ceftriaxone. The strongest risk factors for infection as a result of nonsusceptible strains include day-care attendance and recent treatment with antibiotics. It does *not* appear that the nonsusceptible strains are more virulent or that they present symptoms that form a different clinical picture than susceptible strains. For central nervous system infection with nonsusceptible strains, treatment requires the use of cefotaxime or ceftriaxone plus vancomycin. In some cases, the addition of rifampin may be useful for eradication.

    American Academy of Pediatrics: Pneumococcal infections. In Pickering LK (ed): 2003 Red Book: Report of the Committee on Infectious Diseases, 26th ed. Elk Grove Village, IL, American Academy of Pediatrics, 2003, p 491.
    Friedland IR, McCracken GH, Jr.: Management of infections caused by antibiotic-resistant *Streptococcus pneumoniae*. N Engl J Med 331:377–382, 1994.

10. **Which organisms are particularly dangerous to clinical microbiology laboratory workers?**
    The laboratory should be alerted when highly transmissible bacterial agents are suspected in specimens that have been submitted for culture. These bacteria include *Francisella tularensis* (the causative agent of tularemia), *Bacillus anthracis* (anthrax), and *Coxiella burnetii* (Q fever). In addition, the laboratory may process fungal cultures that contain molds and dimorphic fungi (e.g. *Histoplasma, Blastomyces*) in a biosafety cabinet to prevent exposure to spores.

11. **In which patients should trimethoprim-sulfamethoxazole (TMP-SMX) be avoided or used with caution?**
    TMP-SMX acts by inhibiting the folic acid pathway of bacteria. Disruption of human folate metabolism may occur, thereby affecting rapidly replicating cells, especially in the bone marrow and skin. Avoidance or cautious use is suggested in the following settings:
    - Patients who have not received folate supplementation and who are known or expected to be deficient in folate because of phenytoin use, therapy with another folate antagonist, protein-calorie malnutrition, or prematurity
    - Pregnancy
    - Fragile X syndrome
    - Known sensitivity to any sulfonamide
    - Age of ≤2 months
    - History of skin rash while receiving TMP-SMX
    - G6PD deficiency

Gutman LT: The use of trimethoprim-sulfamethoxazole in children: A review of adverse reactions and indications. Pediatr Infect Dis J 3:349–357, 1984.

12. **Which antibiotic is associated with the "red man syndrome"?**
The red man syndrome is a frequent occurrence with the rapid infusion of **vancomycin** and is characterized by flushing of the neck, face, and thorax. The histamine release underlying this reaction is directly caused by vancomycin. It is not mediated by IgE and therefore does not represent a true hypersensitivity reaction. Generally, the reaction can be avoided by slowing the rate of drug infusion. Administration of an H_1-receptor antagonist (e.g., diphenhydramine) before vancomycin is given is also effective for preventing this reaction.

13. **How can the emergence of antibiotic-resistant pathogens be minimized?**
   - Appropriate hand hygiene, contact isolation, and environmental decontamination to reduce the transmission of resistant organisms to other patients
   - Use of the most potent, narrowest-spectrum antibiotic possible for an appropriate length of time
   - Minimization of the empiric use of broad-spectrum antibiotics
   - Avoidance of antibiotic treatment of illnesses that are likely viral
   - Awareness of local antibiotic resistance patterns

Woodin KA, Morrison SH: Antibiotics: Mechanisms of action. Pediatr Rev 15:440–447, 1994.

14. **Why is chicken soup so helpful for upper respiratory infections (URIs)?**
The benefits of chicken soup have been of lore for hundreds of years, beginning in the 12th century, when physician and philosopher Maimonides extolled its virtue. The precise mechanisms of its anecdotal therapeutic benefits remain elusive. One recent study at the University of Nebraska found that the nonparticulate component of chicken soup in vitro inhibited neutrophil migration in a concentration-dependent manner. This anti-inflammatory effect may be one mechanism by which chicken soup mitigates the symptoms of URIs.

Rennard BO, Ertl RF, Gossman GL, et al: Chicken soup inhibits neutrophil chemotaxis in vitro. Chest 118:1150–1157, 2000.

CLINICAL ISSUES

15. **Name the three stages of pertussis infection (whooping cough).**
   1. **Catarrhal** (1–2 weeks): Low-grade fever, upper respiratory infection symptoms
   2. **Paroxysmal** (2–4 weeks): Severe cough occurring in paroxysms, onset of inspiratory "whoop"
   3. **Convalescent** (1–2 weeks): Resolution of symptoms

16. **What is the most common cause of death in children with whooping cough?**
Ninety percent of deaths are attributable to **pneumonia**, which most often develops as a secondary bacterial infection. These cases can be easily missed during the paroxysmal phase, when respiratory symptoms are so prominent and usually attributed solely to pertussis. A new spiking fever should prompt a careful search for an evolving pneumonia.

17. **Is erythromycin of value in pertussis infection?**
If used during the first 14 days of illness or before the paroxysmal stage, erythromycin can decrease the severity of symptoms during the paroxysmal stage. If the diagnosis is established later in the course, erythromycin should still be administered to eliminate the nasopharyngeal carriage of *Bordetella pertussis* and limit the spread of disease. The dose is 50 mg/kg/day (divided into four daily doses) for 14 days, with a maximum total daily dose of 1 gm. Recent evidence suggests that treatment with azithromycin (10–12 mg/kg/day in one dose) or

clarithromycin (15–20 mg/kg/day divided into two doses) for 5–7 days is also effective for eradicating carriage and preventing transmission.

18. **Do antibiotics prevent the development of pneumonia after a URI?**
Over 90% of URIs are caused by viruses, and children <5 years old (especially those in day-care environments) can experience 6–8 URI episodes per year. Multiple studies have shown that antibiotic treatment of URIs does *not* shorten their course or prevent the development of pneumonia.

  Gadomski AM: Potential interventions for preventing pneumonia among young children: Lack of effect of antibiotic treatment for upper respiratory infections. Pediatr Infect Dis J 12:115–120, 1993.

19. **Sternal edema is classically the sign of what infection?**
Mumps.

20. **How does Hatchcock's sign help distinguish swelling as a result of mumps from swelling caused by adenitis?**
Upward pressure applied to the angle of the mandible produces tenderness with mumps (*Hatchcock's sign*); this maneuver produces no tenderness with adenitis.

21. **Summarize the distinguishing features of staphylococcal scalded skin syndrome, staphylococcal toxic shock syndrome, and streptococcal toxic shock syndrome.**
See Table 11-1.

22. **What percentage of cases of staphylococcal toxic shock syndrome are nonmenstrual?**
Over the past two decades, the epidemiology of toxic shock syndrome has changed, reflecting changes in tampon composition and a decrease in absorbency. In 1996, >50% of reported cases were nonmenstrual. The syndrome occurs in the setting of focal staphylococcal colonization or focal infections, including empyema, osteomyelitis, soft-tissue abscess, surgical infections, and burns.

23. **Which diseases are transmitted by ticks?**

Disease	Agent
Lyme disease	*Borrelia burgdorferi*
Relapsing fever	*Borrelia* species
Tularemia	*Francisella tularensis*
Rocky Mountain spotted fever	*Rickettsia rickettsii*
Queensland tick typhus	*Rickettsia australis*
Boutonneuse fever	*Rickettsia conorii*
Asian tick typhus	*Rickettsia sibirica*
Colorado tick fever	Arbovirus
Tick-borne encephalitis	Arbovirus
Ehrlichiosis	*Ehrlichia chaffeensis, Ehrlichia equi, Ehrlichia phagocytophila, Ehrlichia ewingii*
Babesiosis	*Babesia microti, Babesia divergens, Babesia bovis*

  Drutz JE: Arthropods. In Feigin RD, Cherry JD (eds): Textbook of Pediatric Infectious Diseases, 5th ed. Philadelphia, W.B. Saunders, 2004, p 2836.

24. **What are the two primary types of human ehrlichiosis?**
Human monocytic ehrlichiosis and **human granulocytic ehrlichiosis**. Both are febrile illnesses that are caused by different agents but that have similar clinical pictures of significant systemic symptoms (e.g., intense headache, chills, myalgia) and, sometimes, rash. The presentation of

symptoms can mimic Rocky Mountain spotted fever. Laboratory features include anemia, lymphopenia, leukopenia, thrombocytopenia, hyponatremia, elevated liver function tests, and cerebrospinal fluid (CSF) abnormalities (e.g., lymphocytic pleocytosis, elevated total protein).

Jacobs RF, Schultze GE: Ehrlichiosis in children. J Pediatr 131:184–192, 1997.

TABLE 11-1. DISTINGUISHING FEATURES OF STAPHYLOCOCCAL SCALDED SKIN SYNDROME, STAPHYLOCOCCAL TOXIC SHOCK SYNDROME, AND STREPTOCOCCAL TOXIC SHOCK SYNDROME

Clinical features	Staphylococcal scalded skin syndrome	Staphylococcal toxic shock syndrome	Group A streptococcal toxic shock-like syndrome
Organism	Staphylococcus aureus Usually phage group 11, type 71	Staphylococcus aureus Usually phage group 1, type 29	Group A streptococci Usually type 1, 3, or 18 Exotoxin A production
Site of infection	Usually focal Mucocutaneous border: nose, mouth, diaper area Sometimes inapparent	Mucous membranes Infected wound or furuncle Sometimes inapparent	Blood, abscess, pneumonia, empyema, cellulitis, necrotizing fasciitis Sometimes inapparent
Skin rash	Tender erythroderma: face/neck, generalized Bullae, no petechiae	Tender erythroderma: trunk, hands, feet Edema of hands, feet	Erythroderma: trunk, extremities
Desquamation	Early, first 1–2 days, generalized	Late, 7–10 days, mostly hands and feet Hyperemia of oral and vaginal mucosa	Late, 7–10 days, mostly hands and feet Hyperemia of oral and vaginal mucosa
Mucous membranes	Normal	Hypertrophy of tongue papillae	Hypertrophy of tongue papillae
Conjunctivae	Normal	Markedly injected	Injected
Course	Insidious, 4–7 days Benign, <1% mortality	Fulminant, shock with secondary multiple organ failure, 10% mortality	Fulminant, shock with early primary multiple organ failure, 30–50% mortality

Adapted from Bass JW: Treatment of skin and skin structure infections. Pediatr Infect Dis J 11:152–155, 1992.

25. **What is the preferred treatment for human ehrlichiosis?**

Doxycycline is the drug of choice to treat human ehrlichiosis. Early clinical experience suggested that chloramphenicol may also be effective, but in vitro susceptibility testing of E. chaffeensis and the human granulocytic ehrlichiosis agent revealed resistance to chloramphenicol.

Although tetracyclines are generally contraindicated in children <8 years old because of associated dental staining, short courses of treatment with these agents—especially doxycycline—are unlikely to cause dental abnormalities.

26. **What the heck are the HACEKs?**
    The *HACEK* organisms include *Haemophilus aphrophilus, Haemophilus paraphrophilus, Actinobacillus actinomycetemcomitans, Cardiobacterium hominis, Eikenella corrodens,* and *Kingella kingae.* These organisms share the property of slow growth in culture and have a predilection for producing endocarditis. They should be considered in cases of apparent culture-negative endocarditis.

27. **In the setting of clinical signs and symptoms of encephalitis, what electroencephalogram pattern is suggestive of herpes simplex virus disease?**
    Periodic lateralized epileptiform discharges. These may be seen in other, rarer forms of encephalitis, such as Epstein-Barr virus encephalitis, Creutzfeldt-Jakob disease, and subacute sclerosing panencephalitis.

28. **What is the best approach to diagnosing herpes simplex virus (HSV) encephalitis in children?**
    In the past, no single noninvasive method could simply and reproducibly diagnose HSV encephalitis; definitive diagnosis relied on brain biopsy. In recent years, a number of studies have demonstrated that analysis of CSF using the polymerase chain reaction (PCR) allows for rapid and accurate diagnosis. According to Lakeman and colleagues, PCR detects >98% of cases and may be more sensitive than brain biopsy. Nowadays, brain biopsy should be considered only when PCR is negative and the diagnosis remains obscure or PCR is positive but the clinical course is atypical for HSV encephalitis and the response to antiviral therapy is slow.

    Lakeman FD, Whitley RJ: Diagnosis of herpes simplex encephalitis: Application of polymerase chain reaction to cerebrospinal fluid from brain-biopsied patients and correlation with disease. National Institute of Allergy and Infectious Diseases Collaborative Antiviral Study Group. J Infect Dis 171:857–863, 1995.

    Whitley RJ, Lakeman FD. Herpes simplex virus infections of the central nervous system: Therapeutic and diagnostic considerations. Clin Infect Dis 20:414–420, 1995.

29. **Can acyclovir be used to prevent or treat oral HSV infections?**
    In immunocompetent hosts, oral acyclovir offers significant therapeutic benefit in primary HSV gingivostomatitis but has limited efficacy for the treatment of recurrent herpes labialis. Topical acyclovir has not shown consistent benefit in either of these settings. Prophylaxis with oral acyclovir can reduce the number of recurrences in adults with herpes labialis, but it has not been studied in children.

30. **How quickly do central lines become colonized?**
    The timing and rate of central line colonization depend on a number of factors. Manipulation of the catheter (e.g., for blood drawing, medication administration, or flushing) and poor hand-washing by health care providers are probably the most important factors that increase the risk of colonization. In general, the likelihood of colonization increases with the length of time that the catheter has been in place. Colonization rates have been reported to be <10% for catheters <3 days old, approximately 15% for catheters 3–7 days old, and about 20% for catheters in place for >7 days.

31. **What is the most proper medical term for oral thrush?**
    Acute pseudomembranous candidiasis. Quite a mouthful. Although thrush is sometimes confused with residual formula in the mouth in infants, formula is more easily removed with a tongue blade. When thrush is scraped, small bleeding points often occur on the underlying mucosa.

CONGENITAL INFECTIONS

32. Which congenital infections cause cerebral calcifications?
Cerebral calcifications are most frequently observed in congenital *Toxoplasma* and cytomegalovirus (CMV) infections. They are seen occasionally in patients with congenital herpes simplex virus infection and rarely in patients with congenital rubella infection.

33. What are the late sequelae of congenital infections?
The late sequelae of chronic intrauterine infections are relatively common and may occur in infants who are asymptomatic at birth. Most sequelae present symptoms later in childhood rather than infancy.

- CMV: Hearing loss,* minimal to severe brain dysfunction* (motor, learning, language, and behavioral disorders)
- Rubella: Hearing loss,* minimal to severe brain dysfunction* (motor, learning, language, and behavioral disorders), autism,* juvenile diabetes, thyroid dysfunction, precocious puberty, progressive degenerative brain disorder*
- Toxoplasmosis: Chorioretinitis,* minimal to severe brain dysfunction,* hearing loss, precocious puberty
- Neonatal herpes: Recurrent eye and skin infection, minimal to severe brain dysfunction
- Hepatitis B virus: Chronic subclinical hepatitis, rarely fulminant hepatitis

  *Seen with infections that are subclinical during early infancy.
  Plotkin SA, Alpert G: A practical guide to the diagnosis of congenital infections in the newborn infant. Pediatr Clin North Am 33:465–479, 1986.

34. What is the most common congenital infection?
Congenital CMV infection, which in some large screening studies occurs in up to 1.3% of newborns. However, 90–95% of infected neonates are asymptomatic. Some infants who are asymptomatic at birth later develop hearing loss.

35. How is CMV transmitted from mother to infant?
CMV can be transmitted by the transplacental route or through contact with cervical secretions or breast milk. On occasion, transmission may occur by contact with saliva or urine.

36. Should congenital CMV be treated?
Treatment is recommended for infants with life- or vision-threatening disease, such as severe retinitis, interstitial pneumonitis, hepatitis, or thrombocytopenia.

37. How do complications vary between newborns with CMV infection who are symptomatic versus those who are asymptomatic at birth?
See Table 11-2.

38. What is the risk to the fetus if the mother is infected with parvovirus B19 during pregnancy?
The risk of fetal loss is 2–10% and is greatest when maternal infection occurs during the first half of pregnancy. Fetal loss occurs as a consequence of hydrops, which develops as a result of parvovirus-induced anemia. An elevated maternal serum alpha-fetoprotein level may be a marker for an adverse outcome. The signs of parvovirus infection in adults are not very distinctive but may include fever, a maculopapular or lace-like rash, and joint pain.

39. What are the consequences of primary varicella infection during the first trimester?
The **congenital varicella syndrome** consists of a constellation of features:

- Limb atrophy, usually associated with a cicatricial (scarring) lesion

- Neurologic and sensory defects
- Eye abnormalities (chorioretinitis, cataracts, microphthalmia, Horner syndrome)

This syndrome usually follows maternal infection during the first trimester, although it may be seen after infection up to 20 weeks into gestation. The largest prospective study reported to date found four cases of fetal varicella syndrome in 141 pregnancies, yielding an incidence of <3%.

TABLE 11-2. COMPLICATIONS IN SYMPTOMATIC VERSUS ASYMPTOMATIC NEWBORNS WITH CMV

Complication	Percentage of occurrence	
	Symptomatic	Asymptomatic
Death	5.8	0.3
Microcephaly	37.5	1.8
Sensorineural hearing loss	58	7.4
Bilateral hearing loss	37	2.7
Moderate-to-profound hearing loss (60–90 dB)	27	1.7
Chorioretinitis	20.4	2.5
Intelligence quotient of <70	55	3.7
Seizures	23.1	0.9
Paresis/paralysis	12.5	0

Adapted from Remington JS, Klein JO: Infections of the Fetus and Newborn Infant, 5th ed. Philadelphia, W.B. Saunders, 2001, p 408.

40. **When should varicella zoster immune globulin (VZIG) be given to a newborn?**
    VZIG should be given as soon as possible to a newborn whose mother developed varicella from 5 days before to 2 days after delivery. During this period of high risk, the fetus is exposed to high circulating titers of the virus without the benefit of maternal antibody synthesis. Premature neonates exposed to varicella during the neonatal period are also candidates for VZIG:
    - If the infant is ≥28 weeks' gestation and the mother has no history of chickenpox
    - If the infant is <28 weeks' gestation or weighs ≤1,000 gm, regardless of maternal history, because little maternal antibody crosses the placenta before the third trimester of pregnancy.

KEY POINTS: INDICATIONS FOR ORAL ACYCLOVIR IN VARICELLA-ZOSTER VIRUS INFECTIONS

1. Patients >12 years old

2. Patients with chronic pulmonary or cutaneous disorders

3. Patients receiving long-term salicylate therapy

4. Patients receiving corticosteroids (oral or aerosolized)

41. **Do urogenital mycoplasmas have a role in neonatal disease?**

    Ureaplasma urealyticum has been associated with low birth weight and bronchopulmonary dysplasia. This organism has been recovered from neonates with respiratory distress, pneumonia, and meningitis, but a causative role in these diseases has not been proven. Several reports of apparent *Mycoplasma hominis* meningitis and eye infection have been published.

42. **If a mother is culture positive for *Ureaplasma urealyticum* or *M. hominis*, what is the likelihood of transmission to the newborn infant?**

    Vertical transmission occurs in up to 60% of exposed newborns. Risk of transmission is higher in preterm and low-birthweight infants and correlates with the prolonged rupture of membranes and maternal fever. Infants delivered by cesarean section over intact membranes have a very low rate of colonization as compared with infants delivered vaginally.

43. **What are the features of congenital rubella syndrome?**

    The most characteristic features of congenital rubella syndrome are congenital heart disease, cataracts, microphthalmia, corneal opacities, glaucoma, and radiolucent bone lesions. The features of congenital rubella syndrome can be divided into three broad categories:
    - **Transient:** Low birthweight, hepatosplenomegaly, thrombocytopenia, hepatitis, pneumonitis, and radiolucent bone lesions
    - **Permanent:** Deafness, cataracts, and congenital heart lesions (patent ductus arteriosus > pulmonary artery stenosis > aortic stenosis > ventricular septal defects)
    - **Developmental:** Psychomotor delay, behavioral disorders, and endocrine dysfunction

44. **Should all pregnant women be screened for herpes simplex virus (HSV) infection during pregnancy?**

    Existing data indicate that antepartum cultures of the maternal genital tract fail to predict viral shedding at the time of delivery. As a consequence, routine antepartum cultures are not recommended.

45. **What are risk factors for the development of neonatal HSV disease?**

    Among infants born vaginally to mothers with primary herpes genitalis, 30–50% will develop HSV disease. Only 3–5% of infants born to mothers with active recurrent disease become infected. Distinguishing between primary and recurrent herpes infections by history and clinical examination is often difficult. Low birthweight is an independent risk factor. Fetal scalp monitoring may result in direct inoculation of the virus into the baby's scalp.

    Many experts advocate cesarean section for women who are in labor at term and have visual evidence of active genital HSV lesions, especially if membranes have been ruptured for less than 4–6 hours. If membranes have been ruptured for longer periods of time, operative delivery is less effective for reducing the risk of neonatal infection.

46. **What are the three forms of neonatal HSV disease?**

    Occurring with approximately equal frequency, the three patterns of neonatal HSV disease are as follows:
    - **Mucocutaneous disease** (localized to the skin, eye, or mouth)
    - **Encephalitis**
    - **Disseminated disease** (± central nervous system [CNS] involvement) with a picture that resembles bacterial sepsis

      It is important to note that only one third of infants with either localized encephalitis or disseminated disease will have visible skin lesions.

47. **How should the neonate with suspected HSV disease be treated?**

    Both acyclovir and vidarabine have activity against HSV. Acyclovir is the preferred drug and is administered in a dose of 20 mg/kg intravenously every 8 hours pending definitive diagnosis.

For mucocutaneous disease, treatment is continued for 14 days. For encephalitis and disseminated disease, treatment is continued for 21 days.

48. **In which groups of women is prenatal hepatitis B surface antigen (HBsAg) screening recommended?**
In the past, women were screened for HBsAg if they fell into a high-risk group based on ethnic origin, immunization status, or history of exposure to blood products, intravenous drugs, or a high-risk partner. However, historic information reveals only a portion of HBsAg carriers were captured using these screening criteria, and thus it is recommended that *all* pregnant women be screened for HBsAg.

49. **What is the relationship between age of acquisition of hepatitis B virus and the likelihood of chronic hepatitis B infection?**
Chronic hepatitis B virus infection with persistence of HBsAg occurs in as many as 90% of infants who are infected by perinatal transmission, in an average of 30% of children who are 1–5 years old when infected, and in 2–6% of older children, adolescents, and adults who become infected.

Schiff ER: Update in hepatology. Ann Intern Med 130:52–57, 1999.

50. **How should infants born to mothers with hepatitis A infection be managed?**
Neonates born to mothers with active hepatitis A infection are unlikely to contract the virus, and efficacy of postnatal prophylaxis with hepatitis A immune globulin has not been proven. With this information in mind, no prophylaxis is recommended.

51. **How should infants born to mothers with hepatitis B infection be managed?**
For infants born to women who are HBsAg-positive, hepatitis B immune globulin (0.5 mL intramuscularly) and the first dose of hepatitis B vaccine should be administered *within 12 hours of delivery* to reduce the risk of infection. Although breast milk is capable of transmitting the hepatitis B virus, the risk of transmission in HBsAg-positive mothers whose infants have received timely hepatitis B immune globulin and hepatitis B vaccine is *not* increased by breast feeding.

52. **How should infants born to mothers with hepatitis C infection be managed?**
The risk of vertical transmission of hepatitis C virus is approximately 5%, and no preventive therapy exists. Mothers with hepatitis C infection should be advised that transmission of hepatitis C by breast feeding has not been documented. Accordingly, maternal hepatitis C infection is not a contraindication to breast feeding, although mothers with cracked or bleeding nipples should consider abstaining.

53. **How do the clinical features of early and late congenital syphilis differ?**
The manifestations of congenital syphilis are protean and may be divided into early and late findings. Early manifestations occur during the first 2 years of life; late manifestations occur after 2 years of age (Table 11-3).

54. **Describe the appearance of Hutchinson's teeth.**
The permanent central incisors are typically peg-shaped or notched.

55. **How is the diagnosis of congenital syphilis made?**
- Pregnant women and infants should be screened for possible infection with a nontreponemal test for *Treponema pallidum*. Such tests include the rapid plasma reagin card test and the Venereal Disease Reference Laboratory (VDRL) slide test.
- If blood from the mother or infant yields a positive nontreponemal serologic test, a specific - treponemal test should be performed on the infant's blood. Examples include the fluorescent - treponemal antibody absorption test and the microhemagglutination test for *T. pallidum*.

- Evaluation of infants with suspected congenital syphilis should also include a complete blood count, analysis of the cerebrospinal fluid (including a CSF VDRL), and long-bone radiographs (unless the diagnosis has been otherwise established).

TABLE 11-3. EARLY AND LATE MANIFESTATIONS OF CONGENITAL SYPHILIS			
Early Congenital Syphilis (310 Patients)		**Late Congenital Syphilis (271 Patients)**	
Hepatomegaly	32%	Pseudoparalysis of Parrot	87%
Skeletal abnormalities	29%	Short maxilla	84%
Splenomegaly	18%	High palatal arch	76%
Birthweight <2,500 gm	16%	Hutchinson triad	75%
Pneumonia	16%	Saddle nose	73%
Severe anemia, hydrops, edema	16%	Mulberry molars	65%
Skin lesions	15%	Hutchinson teeth	63%
Hyperbilirubinemia	13%	Higoumenakia sign	39%
Snuffles, nasal discharge	9%	Relative protuberance of mandible	26%
Painful limbs	7%	Interstitial keratitis	9%
Cerebrospinal fluid abnormalities	7%	Rhagades	7%
Pancreatitis	5%	Saber shin	4%
Nephritis	4%	VIII nerve deafness	3%
Failure to thrive	3%	Scaphoid scapulae	0.7%
Testicular mass	0.3%	Clutton joint	0.3%
Chorioretinitis	0.3%		
Hypoglobulinemia	0.3%		

Adapted from Sanchez PJ, Gutman LT: Syphilis. In Feigin RD, Cherry JE, Demmler GJ, Kaplan SL (eds): Pediatric Infectious Diseases, 5th ed. Philadelphia, W.B. Saunders, 2004, pp 1730–1732.

56. **What are the pitfalls of rapid plasma reagin and VDRL testing?**
    - Cord blood specimens from the infant can produce false-positive results; therefore, serum from the infant is preferred.
    - A mother who has been treated adequately for syphilis during pregnancy can still passively transfer antibodies to the neonate, which results in a positive titer in the infant in the absence of infection. In this circumstance, the infant's titer is usually less than the mother's and reverts to negative over several months.

57. **If a pregnant woman is found to have *Chlamydia trachomatis* in her birth canal, what is the most appropriate course of action?**
    A pregnant woman with a known chlamydial infection should be treated with oral erythromycin, azithromycin, or amoxicillin to reduce the risk of neonatal chlamydial pneumonia and conjunctivitis. Simultaneous treatment of the male partner(s) with doxycycline (100 mg orally twice daily) or azithromycin (1 gm orally as a single dose) should also be undertaken.

58. **What is the risk to a fetus after primary maternal *Toxoplasma* infection?**
    The risk depends on the time during pregnancy that the mother becomes infected. Assuming that the mother is untreated, first-trimester infection is associated with a fetal infection rate of

approximately 25%, second-trimester infection with a rate >50%, and third-trimester infection with a rate of roughly 65%. The severity of clinical disease in congenitally infected infants is inversely related to gestational age at the time of primary maternal infection.

59. **If a mother acquires *Toxoplasma* during pregnancy, can transmission to the fetus be prevented?**
The existing literature is conflicting. Some studies suggest that treatment with spiramycin before 17 weeks' gestation or with pyrimethamine plus sulfadiazine after 17 weeks' gestation can reduce the risk of transmission of the parasite to the fetus by 50–60%, although other studies show no effect of treatment on transmission. The rationale for such treatment is based on the observation that there may be a significant lag period between the onset of maternal infection and infection of the fetus.

Gilbert R, Gras L; European Multicentre Study on Congenital Toxoplasmosis: Effect of timing and type of treatment on the risk of mother to child transmission of *Toxoplasma gondii.* Brit J Obstet Gynecol 110:112–120, 2003.
Wallon M, Liou C, Garner P, Peyron F: Congenital toxoplasmosis: Systematic review of evidence of efficacy during pregnancy. BMJ 318:1511–1514, 1999.

60. **What is the typical presentation of congenital toxoplasmosis?**
As with other congenital infections, the presentations are varied, ranging from severe disease with fever, hepatosplenomegaly, chorioretinitis, and/or neurologic features (e.g., seizures, hydrocephalus, microcephaly) in approximately 10% of infected infants to an apparent lack of signs or symptoms in roughly two thirds of cases. Among asymptomatic infants, intracranial calcifications are often present, and long-term risks include impaired vision, learning disabilities, mental retardation, and seizures.

61. **How can a woman minimize the chance of acquiring a *Toxoplasma* infection during pregnancy?**
Measures relate to personal hygiene, food preparation, and exposure to cats.
- Prepare meat by cooking to >150°F, smoking it, or curing it in brine.
- Wash fruits and vegetables before consumption.
- Wash hands and kitchen surfaces thoroughly after contact with raw meat and unwashed fruits or vegetables, and wash thoroughly after gardening.
- Avoid changing cat litter boxes, or wear gloves while changing the litter and wash hands thoroughly afterward. Changing the litter every 1–2 days will also reduce risk.

THE FEBRILE CHILD

62. **Fever in children: is it friend or foe?**
In certain situations, fever is beneficial, and in others it is detrimental. Gonococci and some treponemes are killed at temperatures of ≥40°C (104°F), and benefits from fever therapy have been reported in cases of gonococcal urethritis and neurosyphilis. In addition, fever appears to hamper the growth of some types of pneumococci and some viruses. Fever is also associated with a decrease in the amount of free serum iron, which is an essential nutrient for many pathogenic bacteria. Modest fever can accelerate a variety of immunologic responses, including phagocytosis, leukocyte chemotaxis, lymphocyte transformation, and interferon production.

On the other hand, other data indicate that high fever can impair the immune response. In addition, although the metabolic effects of fever are well tolerated by most children, in some situations these effects can be dangerous. Examples include patients at risk for cardiac or respiratory failure and those with neurologic disease or with septic shock. Fever can precipitate febrile seizures in the susceptible population, which is children between 6 months and about 5 years of age.

63. **At what temperature does a child have fever?**
This is a simple question without a simple answer. Because body temperatures vary among individuals and age groups and vary over the course of the day in a given individual (lowest around 4:00–5:00 AM and highest in late afternoon and early evening), a precise cutoff point is difficult to determine. In children between the ages of 2 and 6 years, diurnal variation can range up to 0.9°C (1.6°F). Infants tend to have a higher baseline temperature pattern, with 50% having daily rectal temperatures of >37.8°C (100.0°F); after the age of 2 years, this elevated baseline falls. In addition, activity and exercise (within 30 minutes), feeding or meals (within 1 hour), and hot foods (within 1 hour) can cause body temperature elevations. Most authorities agree that, for a child <3 months old, a rectal temperature of >38°C (100.4°F) constitutes fever. In infants between the ages of 3 and 24 months (who tend to have a higher baseline), a temperature of ≥38.3°C (101°F) likely constitutes fever. In those >2 years old, as the baseline falls, fever more commonly is defined as a rectal temperature of >38°C (100.4°F).

64. **Where did the popular notion that a normal temperature is 98.6°F originate?**
The temperature 98.6°F was established as the mean healthy temperature in 1868 after >1 million temperatures from 25,000 patients were analyzed. Ironically, these were axillary temperatures, and the waters of what constitutes normal have been muddied since.

Mackowiak PA, Wasserman SS, Levine MM: A critical appraisal of 98.6°F, the upper limit of the normal body temperature, and other legacies of Carl Reinhold August Wunderlich. JAMA 268:1578–1580, 1992.

65. **How does temperature vary among different body sites?**

Rectal	Standard
Oral	0.5–0.6°C (1°F) lower
Axillary	0.8–1.0°C (1.5–2.0°F) lower
Tympanic	0.5–0.6°C (1°F) lower

66. **How should the temperature of young infants be taken?**
In infants who are <3 months old (when fever can be more significant clinically), a rectal temperature is the preferred method. Tympanic recordings are much less sensitive in this age group, because the narrow, tortuous external canal can collapse, thereby resulting in readings obtained from the cooler canal rather than the warmer tympanic membrane. Axillary temperatures often underestimate fever. The oral route is usually not used until a child is 5–6 years old.

67. **Can excessive bundling raise an infant's temperature?**
Prospective studies have found mixed results. One study of newborns in a warm environment of 80°F found that rectal temperatures in bundled infants could be elevated to >38°C, which is the "febrile range." Another study of infants ≤3 months old found that, in room temperatures of 72–75°F, the bundling of infants for up to 65 minutes did not produce any rectal temperatures >38°C. A clinical method that may help to distinguish disease-related fevers from possible environmental overheating is the "abdomen-toe" temperature differential. A foot as warm as the abdomen suggests an overly warm environment, whereas a foot that is cooler suggests fever with peripheral vasoconstriction.

Grover C, Berkowitz CD, Lewis RJ, et al: The effects of bundling on infant temperature. Pediatrics 94:669–673, 1994.

Cheng TL, Partridge JC: Effect of bundling and high environmental temperatures on neonatal body temperature. Pediatrics 92:238–240, 1993.

68. **Does teething cause fever?**
Long a doctrine of grandmothers, the suggested association between teething and temperature elevation may have some basis in fact. In one study of 46 healthy infants with rectal temperatures recorded for 20 days before the eruption of the first tooth, nearly half had a new temperature elevation of >37.5°C on the day of the eruption. Other studies have shown some

statistical association with slight temperature increase. In any event, significantly elevated fever should not be ascribed simply to teething. Listen to the grandmothers, but verify.

Jaber L, Cohen IJ, Mor A: Fever associated with teething. Arch Dis Child 67:233–234, 1992.

Macknin ML, Piedmonte M, Jacobs J, Skibinski C: Symptoms associated with infant teething: A prospective study. Pediatrics 105:747–752, 2000.

69. **What is occult bacteremia?**
Occult bacteremia refers to the finding of bacteria in the blood of patients, usually between the ages of 3 and 36 months, who are febrile without a clinically apparent focus of infection. This term should be distinguished from *septicemia*, which refers to the growth of bacteria in the blood of a child with the clinical picture of toxicity and shock.

70. **Is there an association between the degree of fever and the incidence of bacteremia?**
In children, the relationship between fever and the likelihood of bacteremia has been examined most thoroughly in patients who are febrile yet have no localizing signs on physical examination. In general, the risk of bacteremia in this population increases with the magnitude of fever. In a classic study involving febrile children <2 years old who were seen in an ambulatory clinic, bacteremia was present only if the rectal temperature was $\geq$38.9°C (102°F). In another series of febrile children seen in a pediatric emergency room, among patients with temperatures of >41.1°C (106°F), the incidence of bacteremia was 13%.

McCarthy PL, Dolan TF: Hyperpyrexia in children: Eight-year emergency room experience. Am J Dis Child 130:849–851, 1976.

Teele DW, Pelton SI, Grant MJ, et al: Bacteremia in febrile children under 2 years of age: Results of cultures of blood of 600 consecutive febrile children in a "walk-in" clinic. J Pediatr 87:227–230, 1975.

71. **What are the Yale Observation Scales?**
This set of six items of observation and physical signs was designed at Yale to assist in detecting serious illness in febrile children who were <24 months old. Normal (1 point), moderate impairment (3 points), and severe impairment (5 points) scores are given for **quality of cry**, **reaction to parental stimulation**, **state of alertness**, **color**, **hydration**, and **response to social overtures**. Scores of $\leq$10 correlate with a low likelihood of serious illness, primarily in infants >2 months old.

McCarthy PL, Sharpe MR, Spiesel SZ, et al: Observation scales to identify serious illness in febrile children. Pediatrics 70:802–809, 1982.

72. **What is the proper way to evaluate and manage febrile illness in infants who are <60 days old?**
This is a highly contentious area. On average, about 10% of febrile infants who are <2 months old have serious bacterial infections (bacteremia, meningitis, osteomyelitis, septic arthritis, urinary tract infection, or pneumonia). One third to one half of these infections are associated with bacteremia. In the past, the approach to the evaluation and management of febrile young infants has varied. Many studies have attempted to identify criteria for a "low-risk" group of infants with a very small risk of serious bacterial infection. Clinical algorithms have ranged from routine lumbar punctures and empiric antibiotic use to neither lumbar punctures nor empiric antibiotics for well-appearing infants. One approach to the outpatient management of the febrile infant (29–60 days; temperature $\geq$38°C) is the one developed by clinicians at Children's Hospital of Philadelphia. Patients are categorized as "low risk" and followed as outpatients without antibiotic therapy if the following criteria are met:

- Well-appearing infant
- No evidence of focal infection on physical examination
- Total peripheral blood white blood cell (WBC) count 5,000–15,000/mm^3
- CSF WBC count <8/mm^3 and gram-negative

- Urinalysis: <10 WBCs per high-power field and ≤3 bacteria per high-power field on spun specimen
- No pulmonary infiltrate on chest radiograph, if performed

Of infants who meet these criteria and who were observed without antibiotics, the risk of serious infection is exceedingly low. The experiences of the Children's Hospital of Philadelphia and others suggest that infants who meet low-risk criteria may not require antibiotic therapy and/or hospitalization, provided the social setting is suitable and close outpatient follow-up is possible.

Currently, infants <28 days old are generally hospitalized for empiric therapy, but some authors advocate the outpatient management of selected "low-risk" neonates.

Avner JR, Baker MD: Management of fever in infants and children. Emerg Med Clin North Am 20:49–67, 2002.

Pantell RH, Newman TB, Bernzweig J, et al: Management and outcomes of care of fever in early infancy. JAMA 291:1203–1212, 2004.

73. **How should older infants and toddlers (2–36 months old) with fever and no apparent source be managed?**

As with infants <2 months old, this remains controversial. The basis for this controversy relates to the difficulty of distinguishing viral illness from occult bacteremia and the fear of occult bacteremia leading to more serious infection, especially meningitis. In recent years, consideration of this issue has been influenced by the remarkable success of the *Haemophilus influenzae* vaccination program. In the past, *H. influenzae* occult bacteremia was relatively common and, in approximately 10% of cases, was associated with progression to meningitis. Since the introduction of the heptavalent pneumococcal conjugate vaccine, the incidence of *Streptococcus pneumoniae* bacteremia has diminished, although this organism still accounts for the majority of episodes of occult bacteremia. Fortunately, occult bacteremia with *S. pneumoniae* seldom progresses to meningitis.

Strategies for the management of febrile young children between the ages of 2 and 36 months vary. For patients with temperatures of ≥39°C, some experts advocate use of an evaluation protocol that includes the following:

- Urine culture for males <6 months old and females <2 years old
- Stool culture if stool has blood or mucus or >5 WBCs per high-power field
- Blood culture

Empiric antibiotics (e.g., oral amoxicillin, intramuscular ceftriaxone) are then prescribed pending culture results. Other specialists consider the degree of fever and the height of the WBC count or absolute neutrophil count when assessing the likelihood of bacteremia and the need for empiric antibiotic therapy (a WBC count of ≥15,000/mm^3 and an absolute neutrophil count of ≥10,000/mm^3 are associated with a greater risk of occult bacteremia). Still others advise no testing and no empiric therapy and emphasize that parents be provided with specific information about signs and symptoms that should prompt reevaluation. This is particularly true for children who have received a heptavalent pneumococcal conjugate vaccine and who are at a much lower risk for invasive disease.

American College of Emergency Physicians: Clinical policy for children younger than three years of age presenting to the emergency department with fever. Ann Emerg Med 42:530–545, 2003.

Klein JO: Management of the febrile child without a focus of infection in the era of universal pneumococcal immunization. Pediatr Infect Dis J 21:584–588, 2002.

McCarthy PL: Fever without apparent source on clinical examination. Curr Opin Pediatr 15:112–120, 2003.

74. **How helpful is the band count for distinguishing the likelihood of viral versus bacterial infections in young infants?**

Alas, the song from the band has no lyrics. A study looking at the value of the band count in the peripheral blood smear in young febrile infants (3–24 months old) was not of value for distinguishing bacterial from viral infections. Band counts may be more helpful in infants who are <3 months old.

Kupperman N, Walton EA: Immature neutrophils in the blood smears of young febrile children. Arch Pediatr Adolesc Med 153:261–266, 1999.

75. When is a chest radiograph indicated for a febrile young infant?

Although some clinicians believe that chest x-rays should be performed for all febrile infants who are <2–3 months old, others reserve this study for infants who have respiratory symptoms or signs, including cough, tachypnea, irregular breathing, retractions, rales, wheezing, or decreased breath sounds. In a study of infants <8 weeks old who were admitted with fever, 31% of patients with respiratory manifestations had an abnormal chest x-ray, compared with only 1% of asymptomatic infants.

Crain EF, Bulas D, Bijur PE, Goldman HS: Is a chest radiograph necessary in the evaluation of every febrile infant less than 8 weeks of age? Pediatrics 88:821–824, 1991.

76. Does changing needles during the collection of blood cultures reduce contamination?

No. In one study of 303 children, replacing the needle used for venipuncture with a fresh, sterile needle before inoculating the blood into a culture medium resulted in no change in the contamination rate. As a side note, if the incubation of a blood culture is delayed by ≥2 hours, the likelihood of positivity may be significantly decreased, especially for *Streptococcus pneumoniae* and *Neisseria meningitidis*.

Roback MG, Tsai AK, Hanson KL: Delayed incubation of blood culture bottles: Effect on recovery rate of *Streptococcus pneumoniae* and *Haemophilus influenzae* type B. Pediatr Emerg Care 10:268–272, 1994.

Isaacman DJ: Lack of effect of changing needles on contamination of blood cultures. Pediatr Infect Dis J 9:274–278, 1990.

77. How long should one wait before a blood culture is designated negative?

Bacterial growth is evident in the vast majority of cultures of infected blood within 48 hours. With the use of conventional culture techniques and subculture at 4 and 14 hours, Pichichero and Todd found that 101 of 105 positive cultures yielded growth within 48 hours. Using a radiometric technique, Rowley and Wald reported that 40 of 41 cultures positive for group B streptococcus and 15 of 16 cultures growing *Escherichia coli* were identified within 24 hours. The use of continuous monitoring culture techniques at Children's Hospital of Philadelphia allowed for the detection of 95% of critical pathogens in <24 hours.

Although 48–72 hours is generally sufficient time to isolate common bacteria present in the bloodstream, fastidious organisms may take longer to grow. Therefore, when one suspects anaerobes, fungi, or other organisms with special growth requirements, a longer time should be allowed before concluding that a culture is negative.

McGowan KL, Foster JA, Coffin SE: Outpatient pediatric blood cultures: Time to positivity. Pediatrics 106:251–255, 2000.

Pichichero ME, Todd JK: Detection of neonatal bacteremia. J Pediatr 94:958–960, 1979.

Rowley AH, Wald ER: Incubation period necessary to detect bacteremia in neonates. Pediatr Infect Dis J 5:590–591, 1986.

78. How should a child with fever and petechiae be evaluated?

In these patients, the most significant concern is serious systemic bacterial infection. Fortunately, when prospectively evaluated, the incidence of bacteremia or clinical sepsis in this setting is low (<2%), and none of 357 well-appearing children had meningococcemia when evaluated.

History: Elicit information about exposures, travel, animal contacts, and immunizations.

Physical examination: Assess vital signs, general appearance, signs of toxicity, evidence of nuchal rigidity, presence of purpura, and distribution of petechiae (patients with systemic bacterial infection rarely have petechiae confined to the head and neck).

Laboratory: Obtain blood culture, complete blood count with differential, and prothrombin and partial thromboplastin times; consider the examination of cerebrospinal fluid.

Again, one should counsel parents about signs and symptoms that warrant reevaluation.

Mandl KD, Stack AM, Fleisher GR: Incidence of bacteremia in infants and children with fever and petechiae. J Pediatr 131:398–404, 1997.

79. **When is a fever considered a fever of unknown origin (FUO)?**

    FUO is defined as the presence of persistent daily fever (temperature of >38°C [>100.4°F]) in a patient in whom a careful history, a thorough physical examination, and preliminary laboratory data fail to reveal the probable cause. For study purposes, in adults the duration of fever that constitutes an FUO is ≥3 weeks, whereas in children the quoted duration varies from ≥8 days to ≥2–3 weeks.

80. **What is the eventual etiology of fever in children with FUO?**

    In a summary of 446 cases, the following causes were identified:

	No. of cases	Percentage of cases
Infection	198	44.4%
Respiratory	102	22.9%
Other	96	21.7%
Collagen disease	57	12.8%
Inflammatory bowel disease	7	1.6%
Neoplasm	25	5.6%
No diagnosis	48	10.7%
Resolved	56	12.6%
Miscellaneous	54	12.1%

    Gartner JC, Jr.: Fever of unknown origin. Adv Pediatr Infect Dis 7:1–24, 1992.

81. **How should a child with FUO be evaluated?**

    FUO is more likely to be an unusual presentation of a common disorder than a common presentation of a rare disorder. After obtaining a complete and detailed history and performing a thorough physical examination, one should avoid indiscriminately ordering a large battery of tests. Laboratory studies should be directed as much as possible toward the most likely diagnostic possibilities.

82. **In children with FUO, how helpful are computed tomography (CT) scans and nuclear medicine studies for determining the diagnosis?**

    Minimally. In a prospective study of 109 patients with FUO, scanning procedures (e.g., abdominal CT scan, gallium or indium scanning, technetium bone scanning) had very low utility in the absence of clinical findings that suggested a localized process. Similarly, bone marrow examination had little value when hematologic abnormalities were lacking in the peripheral blood.

    Steele RW, Jones SM, Lowe DA, Glasier CM. Usefulness of scanning procedures for diagnosis of fever of unknown origin in children. J Pediatr 119:526–530, 1991.

83. **What is PFAPA?**

    PFAPA is the acronym for the syndrome of **p**eriodic **f**ever, **a**phthous stomatitis, **p**haryngitis, and cervical **a**denitis, a clinical syndrome of unclear etiology that is responsive to very short courses of corticosteroids for individual episodes and is perhaps the most common cause of regular, recurrent fevers in children.

    Feder HM, Jr.: Periodic fever, aphthous stomatitis, pharyngitis, adenitis: A clinical review of a new syndrome. Curr Opin Pediatr 253–256, 2000.

    Long S: Syndrome of periodic fever, aphthous stomatitis, pharyngitis, and adenitis (PFAPA): What it isn't. What is it? J Pediatr 135:1–5, 1999.

84. **In addition to PFAPA, which syndromes are associated with periodic fevers?**
Predictable periodic fever is a cardinal feature of a small number of diseases and is uncommon in infectious diseases and malignancies. The most common periodic fever syndromes are summarized in Table 11-4.

TABLE 11-4.   CHARACTERISTICS OF PFAPA VERSUS OTHER SELECTED FEVER SYNDROMES

	PFAPA	Familial Mediterranean fever	Hyper-IgD syndrome	Systemic-onset juvenile rheumatoid arthritis	TNF-receptor-associated periodic syndrome
Age at onset	Childhood	<20 years	Childhood	Childhood	Variable
Length of fever episode	4 days	2 days	4–6 days	>30 days	1–3 weeks
Interval between fever episodes	2–8 weeks	Not periodic	Not periodic	Hectic quotidian	Variable
Associated symptoms and signs	Aphthous stomatitis, pharyngitis, adenitis	Painful pleuritis, peritonitis	Headache, cervical adenopathy, splenomegaly	Rash, generalized lymphadenopathy, hepatosplenomegaly, arthritis	Abdominal pain, myalgias, orbital edema
Ethnic	None	Mediterranean	Dutch	None	Scottish, Irish
Gene	Unknown	*MEFV*	*MVK*	Unknown	*TNFSF1A*
Protein	Unknown	Pyrin	Mevalonate kinase	Unknown	Type 1 TNF receptor
Sequelae	None	Amyloidosis	None	Symmetric polyarthritis	Amyloidosis

HUMAN IMMUNODEFICIENCY VIRUS INFECTION

85. **When did human immunodeficiency virus (HIV) testing begin on blood that is intended for transfusion?**
Spring of 1985. Patients at greatest risk for acquired immunodeficiency syndrome (AIDS) from a transfusion are those who received their transfusions from 1978 to the spring of 1985.

86. **How common is the maternal-to-infant transmission of HIV?**
Virtually all infants born to HIV-1 seropositive mothers will acquire antibody to the virus transplacentally. Approximately 25% of these infants will ultimately develop active HIV infection. In non–breast-feeding populations, approximately 30% of maternal-to-infant HIV transmission occurs in utero, and the remainder occurs intrapartum. Vertical transmission of HIV-2 is less common, occurring in 0–4% of cases.

Abrams EJ, Weedon J, Bertolli J, et al; New York City Pediatric Surveillance of Disease Consortium. Centers for Disease Control and Prevention: Aging cohort of perinatally human immunodeficiency virus-infected children in New York City. New York City Pediatric Surveillance of Disease Consortium. Pediatr Infect Dis J. 20:511–517, 2001.

87. **What drugs have been proven effective for reducing the maternal-to-infant transmission of HIV?**

In a landmark study published in 1994, treatment with zidovudine (AZT) administered antepartum and intrapartum to the mother and postnatally to the infant reduced transmission by approximately two thirds. In a more recent study conducted in Africa, treatment with nevirapine administered intrapartum to the mother (200 mg at the onset of labor) and postnatally to the infant (2 mg/kg at 72 hours of life or time of discharge) resulted in a 47% decrease in the rate of transmission. However, this regimen of nevirapine appears to result in high rates of nevirapine resistance.

Currently, HIV-infected pregnant women in the United States are treated the same as non-pregnant adults, generally with combination antiretroviral therapy. Treatment with AZT alone is reserved for the rare pregnant woman with a normal CD4 count and a low or undetectable viral load who otherwise would not require therapy. All HIV-exposed newborn infants should receive AZT at 2 mg/kg/dose every 6 hours for the first 6 weeks of life. Among infants born to mothers with high viral loads and multidrug-resistant strains, treatment with additional agents is advisable.

Committee on Pediatric AIDS: Evaluation and treatment of the human immunodeficiency virus-1-exposed infant. Pediatrics 114:497–505, 2004.

Jackson JB, Musoke P, Fleming T, et al: Intrapartum and neonatal single dose nevirapine compared with zidovudine for prevention of mother to child transmission of HIV-1 in Kampala, Uganda: 18-month follow-up of the HIVNET 012 randomised trial. Lancet 354:795–802, 1999.

88. **What are the risk factors for perinatal transmission of HIV?**

- AZT monotherapy during pregnancy (as compared with combination antiretroviral therapy)
- High maternal viral load
- Rupture of membranes >4 hours
- Fetal instrumentation with scalp electrodes and forceps
- Vaginal delivery (Currently there are no recommendations from the American College of Obstetrics and Gynecology to routinely perform elective C-sections on HIV-infected women. Instead, the decision should be made by individual obstetricians and their patients.)
- Breast feeding

Nduati R, John G, Mbori-Ngacha D, et al: Effect of breast feeding and formula feeding on transmission of HIV-1: A randomized clinical trial. JAMA 283:1167–1174, 2000.

The International Perinatal HIV Group: The mode of delivery and the risk of vertical transmission of human immunodeficiency virus type 1. N Engl J Med 340:977–987, 1999.

89. **How is a newborn infant whose mother is infected with HIV confirmed to also be infected?**

Because maternal antibody may persist in the infant well into the second year of life, enzyme-linked immunosorbent assay testing and Western blot testing are unreliable until approximately 18 months of age. The diagnosis of HIV infection in the newborn therefore usually relies on the direct detection of the virus or viral components in the infant's blood or body fluids. Three methods are currently available:

- **DNA PCR** (most common and most sensitive)
- **Antigen detection** (least sensitive)
- **Culture** (available in only a few laboratories)

Infants born to HIV-infected women should be tested by HIV DNA PCR during the first 48 hours of life, then at between 2 weeks and 2 months of age, and then at 3–6 months of age. Any time a positive result is obtained, testing should be repeated on a second blood sample as soon as possible. The diagnosis of HIV infection is established if two separate samples are found to be positive by PCR.

Committee on Pediatric AIDS: Evaluation and treatment of the human immunodeficiency virus-1-exposed infant. Pediatrics 114:497–505, 2004.

90. **How is the diagnosis of HIV infection excluded in an infant?**
The diagnosis can be excluded when results from two HIV DNA PCR assays performed at or after 1 month of age and a third performed at or after 4 months of age are negative. In addition, two blood samples that are negative for HIV antibody and that are obtained after 6 months of age and separated by at least 1 month are sufficient to exclude the diagnosis.

91. **What are the earliest and most common manifestations of congenital HIV infection?**
- The vast majority of infants with congenital HIV infection are asymptomatic at birth, although occasional patients have diffuse lymphadenopathy and hepatosplenomegaly.
- Older infants with HIV infection commonly present symptoms of failure to thrive, mucocutaneous candidiasis, hepatosplenomegaly, interstitial pneumonitis, or a combination of these features.
- Toddlers and older children with HIV infection may have generalized lymphadenopathy, recurrent bacterial infections, parotitis, or neurologic disease.

Pizzo PA, Wilfert CM: Preventing *Pneumocystis carinii* pneumonia in human immunodeficiency virus-infected children: New guidelines for prophylaxis. Pediatr Infect Dis J 15:165–168, 1996.

Center for Disease Control: 1994 Revised classification system for human immunodeficiency virus infection in children less than 13 years of age. MMWR 43(RR12):1–10, 1995.

92. **When should *Pneumocystis* prophylaxis begin and end for an HIV-exposed infant?**
Historically, the peak incidence of *Pneumocystis* pneumonia in HIV-infected infants occurred at the age of 3 months (range, 4 weeks–6 months). Given that vertical transmission of HIV cannot be excluded until the patient is ≥4 months old, *Pneumocystis* prophylaxis should be initiated at the age of 4–6 weeks and continued until the infant is ≥4 months old. If the HIV status of the child is indeterminate or confirmed positive, *Pneumocystis jiroveci* pneumonia prophylaxis should be continued until the child is 12 months old.

93. **Among infants with HIV infection, how does the CD4 count influence classification?**
According to the 1994 revised Pediatric HIV Classification System, for children ≤12 months of age, the following categories are used:
- **Category 1** (no immunosuppression): CD4 counts ≥1,500/mL and ≥25% of total lymphocytes
- **Category 2** (moderate suppression): CD4 counts 750–1,499/mL or 15–24% of total lymphocytes
- **Category 3** (severe suppression):CD4 counts <750/mL or <15% of total lymphocytes

94. **How common is the transmission of HIV from infected children to household contacts?**
Extremely rare. Only two case reports clearly implicate an infected sibling as the source of HIV infection. Nevertheless, children with HIV infection should be instructed regarding good hygiene and appropriate behavior, and their families should be counseled about HIV and its transmission.

95. **Should a classroom teacher be told that a child is HIV-positive?**
There is no absolute requirement to inform a classroom teacher, a school principal, or any other school official about a child's HIV status. It is not necessary for anyone except the child's physician to be aware of the diagnosis. Nevertheless, in certain circumstances, it may be advisable for a family to communicate with a teacher or a principal.

American Academy of Pediatrics: Human immunodeficiency virus. In Pickering, LK (ed): 2003 Red Book: Report of the Committee on Infectious Diseases, 26th ed. Elk Grove Park, IL, American Academy of Pediatrics, 2003, p 378.

96. **What are the risk factors for HIV transmission after a needlestick injury?**
- High viral inoculum (patient with advanced disease or acute retroviral syndrome)
- Large volume of blood (from a large-diameter needle)
- Deep puncture wound

Overall, the risk of transmission from needles contaminated with the blood of an HIV-infected patient is roughly 0.3%. The above risk factors were identified in a case-control study that involved 33 health care workers and 665 controls.

> Cardo DM, Culver DH, Ciesielski CA, et al: A case-control study of HIV seroconversion in health care workers after percutaneous exposure. Centers for Disease Control and Prevention Needlestick Surveillance Group. N Engl J Med 337:1485–1490, 1997.

97. **When should postexposure prophylaxis be given after a needlestick injury?**
Data from health care workers suggest that prophylaxis is most effective when given within 1–2 hours of exposure, and data from animal studies suggest that prophylaxis is not effective if it is initiated >24 hours after exposure. It is recommended that postexposure prophylaxis be continued for 4 weeks. Postexposure prophylaxis has been shown to reduce the transmission of HIV in healthcare workers by approximately 81%.

> Center for Disease Control: Public health service guidelines for the management of health-care worker exposures to HIV and recommendations for postexposure prophylaxis. MMWR 47(RR-7):1–28, 1998.

98. **What are the major classes of antiretroviral agents used to treat HIV, and what are their mechanisms of action?**
Nucleoside reverse transcriptase inhibitors (NRTIs) competitively inhibit the HIV reverse transcriptase (which converts HIV RNA into DNA) and terminate the elongation of viral DNA. They require intracellular phosphorylation for activation. NRTIs have little or no effect on chronically infected cells because their site of action is before the incorporation of viral DNA into host DNA. This class of drugs includes AZT, lamivudine, stavudine, zalcitabine, didanosine (ddI), and abacavir.

Nonnucleoside reverse transcriptase inhibitors also inhibit the HIV reverse transcriptase, although they do so at a different site than do the NRTIs. They bind directly to the active site of HIV reverse transcriptase and do not require activation. This class of drugs includes delavirdine, efavirenz, and nevirapine.

Protease inhibitors inhibit the HIV protease, which cuts HIV polyprotein precursors before viral budding. This class of drugs includes amprenavir, nelfinavir, ritonavir, indinavir, saquinavir, and lopinavir.

Fusion inhibitors are synthetic peptides that bind to the C-terminal region of gp41 and prevent it from folding into a six-helix bundle, which is a necessary step for the fusion of viral and cell membranes. Enfuvirtide is an example of a fusion inhibitor.

Immune modulators include the following:
- IL-2, which increases CD4 counts but alone has not been shown to decrease viral load;
- interferons, which may act by decreasing virion budding from the cell surface; and
- recombinant CD4, which binds the gp120 protein of HIV and prevents its attachment to host cells via the cellular CD4.

> Hanson IC and Shearer WT: Human Retroviruses. In Feigin RD, Cherry JD, Demmler GJ, et al (eds): Textbook of Pediatric Infectious Diseases, 5th ed. Philadelphia, W.B. Saunders, 2004, p 2475.
> Hussey RE, Richardson NE, Kowalski M, et al: A soluble CD4 protein selectively inhibits HIV replication and syncytium formation. Nature 331:78–81, 1998.
> Jiang S, Zhao Q, Debnath AK: Peptide and non-peptide HIV fusion inhibitors. Curr Pharm Des 8:563–580, 2002.
> Stellbrink HJ, van Lunzen J, Westby M, et al: Effects of interleukin-2 plus highly active antiretroviral therapy on HIV-1 replication and proviral DNA (COSMIC Trial). AIDS 16:1479–1487, 2002.

99. **What are the common bone marrow toxicities associated with antiretroviral therapy?**
    - **Anemia** occurs in up to 9% of children receiving AZT (as compared with 4–5% of those on other regimens). **Neutropenia** occurs in 6–27% of children receiving antiretroviral therapy, particularly those taking AZT and ddI.
    - **Thrombocytopenia** occurs in 30% of untreated children with HIV infection and is more commonly an initial presentation of HIV infection rather than a complication of antiretroviral therapy. In initial trials, severe thrombocytopenia was seen in 2% of children receiving either ddI and AZT or lamivudine and AZT.
    - **Lipodystrophy** occurs in children treated with protease inhibitors.

IMMUNIZATIONS

100. **Why are the buttocks a poor location for intramuscular injections in infants?**
    The gluteus maximus is not a good choice for injections because of the following:
    - The gluteus muscles are incompletely developed in some infants.
    - There is a potential for injury to the sciatic nerve or the superior gluteal artery if the injection is misdirected.
    - Some vaccinations may be less effective if they are injected into fat (e.g., vaccines for rabies, influenza, and hepatitis B).

    If injections into the buttocks are given to older children, the proper site is the gluteus medius in the upper outer quadrant rather than the gluteus maximus, which is more medial.

    Lawton EL, Hayden GF: Immunization, medication and tuberculin skin test administration procedures. In Lohr JA (ed): Pediatric Outpatient Procedures. Philadelphia, J.B. Lippincott, 1991, pp 25–26.
    Zuckerman JN: The importance of injecting vaccines into muscle. BMJ 321:1237–1238, 2000.

101. **Is there any risk associated with administering multiple vaccines simultaneously?**
    Most vaccines can be administered simultaneously at separate sites without concern about effectiveness because the immune response to one vaccine generally does not interfere with immune responses to others. However, some exceptions exist. For example, the simultaneous administration of cholera vaccine and yellow fever vaccine is associated with interference.

    Immunization Action Coalition: www.immunize.org.

102. **Should premature babies receive immunization on the basis of post-conception age or chronologic age?**
    In most cases, premature babies should be immunized in accordance with postnatal chronologic age. If a premature infant is still in the hospital at 2 months of age, the vaccines routinely scheduled for that age should be administered, including diphtheria, tetanus, acellular pertussis, *Haemophilus influenzae* type b, heptavalent pneumococcal, and inactivated poliovirus vaccines.

    Among premature infants who weigh <2 kg at birth, seroconversion rates to hepatitis B vaccine are relatively low when immunization is initiated shortly after birth. Accordingly, in these infants, if the mother is HBsAg negative, immunization should be delayed until just before hospital discharge or until 30 days of age.

    Saari TN; American Academy of Pediatrics Committee on Infectious Diseases: Immunization of preterm and low birth weight infants. American Academy of Pediatrics Committee on Infectious Diseases. Pediatrics 112:193–198, 2003.

103. Which vaccines are egg-embryo–based vaccines?
Of the immunizations that are commonly administered to children, **measles** and **mumps** (MMR) vaccine preparations are grown in chick embryo fibroblast culture. Recent studies indicate that children with egg allergy are at low risk for anaphylaxis to MMR and do not require skin testing before the administration of this vaccine.

Influenza vaccine contains egg protein and on rare occasions induces immediate hypersensitivity reactions, including anaphylaxis. In children who have a history of severe anaphylactic reactions to eggs and who are scheduled to receive influenza vaccine, skin testing is recommended. However, in most cases these children should not receive the influenza vaccine and should instead be prescribed chemoprophylaxis as necessary.

104. What is the difference between whole-cell and acellular pertussis vaccines?
Whole-cell pertussis vaccines consist of whole bacteria that have been inactivated and are nonviable. These vaccines contain lipo-oligosaccharide and other cell-wall components that result in a high incidence of adverse effects.

Acellular pertussis vaccines contain one or more *Bordetella pertussis* proteins that serve as immunogens. All acellular pertussis vaccines contain at least detoxified pertussis toxin, and most contain other antigens as well, including filamentous hemagglutinin, fimbrial proteins, and pertactin. The acellular vaccines are associated with a much lower incidence of side effects and thus are preferred for all doses in the United States.

105. What are the absolute contraindications to pertussis immunization?
The adverse events after pertussis immunization that represent absolute contraindications to further administration of pertussis vaccine include the following:
- Immediate anaphylactic reaction
- Encephalopathy within 7 days of vaccination
The adverse events that represent precautions for further administration of pertussis vaccine include the following:
- A seizure (with or without fever) within 3 days of immunization
- Persistent, severe, inconsolable screaming or crying for ≥3 hours within 2 days of immunization
- Collapse or shock-like state within 2 days of vaccination
- Fever of ≥40.5°C (104.9°F), unexplained by another cause, within 2 days of immunization
When a contraindication to pertussis immunization exists, diphtheria-tetanus vaccine should be administered instead.

Advisory Committee on Immunization Practices of the CDC: www.cdc.bov/nip/acip

106. How often do major neurologic complications or death occur from pertussis vaccine?
The only case-controlled study addressing this issue was the National Childhood Encephalopathy Study, which was conducted in England from 1976–1979 and examined the relationship between diphtheria-tetanus-pertussis immunization and neurologic illness. The results of this study and of a 10-year follow-up study provide no evidence for a causal relationship between whole-cell pertussis immunization and permanent neurologic injury. Limited experience with acellular pertussis vaccines does not allow conclusions about an association with rare serious neurologic effects.

Committee on Infectious Diseases: The relationship between pertussis vaccine and central nervous system sequelae: Continuing assessment. Pediatrics 97:279–281, 1996.

107. How long does protection against pertussis last after infection versus immunization?
Vaccine-induced immunity to pertussis is relatively short lived. On the basis of studies of patients who have been immunized with a whole-cell pertussis vaccine and exposed to a

sibling with pertussis, protection against infection is approximately 80% during the first 3 years after immunization, dropping to 50% at 4–7 years and to near zero at 11 years.

Protective immunity after natural infection with *B. pertussis* is long lasting, and it is superior to immunity induced by immunization, even during the first 3 years after immunization.

Wardlaw AC, Parton R (eds): Pathogenesis and Immunity in Pertussis. New York, John Wiley & Sons, 1988, p 284.

108. What are the age restrictions of pertussis vaccination?
On the basis of recommendations given as of 2004, pertussis vaccines generally should not be given to children >7 years old. With whole-cell pertussis vaccine, there is an increased incidence of localized reactions to the vaccine in older children and adults. Acellular pertussis vaccines are associated with less reactogenicity and will likely be recommended for use in adolescents in the near future.

109. What is the difference between the pediatric (DT) and adult (dT) types of diphtheria and tetanus toxoid vaccines?
The **DT vaccine** contains standard doses of diphtheria and tetanus toxoids and should be used to immunize all children who are <7 years old when pertussis immunization is not required or is contraindicated. The **dT vaccine** contains a much smaller dose of diphtheria toxoid as compared with the DT vaccine and should be used to immunize children who are >7 years old and adults. A booster dose of dT is required every 10 years to ensure continuing tetanus and diphtheria immunity in adulthood.

110. What is the relationship between the MMR vaccine, autism, and inflammatory bowel disease?
In the late 1990s, a report from Great Britain suggested that increased immunization rates with the MMR vaccine might be a cause of apparent increasing rates of autism and a risk factor for the development of Crohn's disease and ulcerative colitis. However, subsequent published studies have not supported any such association, and the original article was recently retracted.

Murch SH, Anthony A, Casson DH, et al: Retraction of an interpretation. Lancet 363:750, 2004.
Madsen KM, Hviid A, Vestergaard M, et al: A population-based study of measles, mumps, and rubella vaccination and autism. N Engl J Med 347:1477–1482, 2002.

111. Under what circumstances should hepatitis A vaccine be used?
- As preexposure prophylaxis for susceptible people traveling to countries with intermediate or high endemic rates of hepatitis A infection (In this circumstance, vaccine is preferable, but immunoglobulin is an acceptable alternative.)
- For children living in communities with consistently elevated hepatitis A rates, which are defined as twice the national average
- For people with chronic liver disease
- For homosexual and bisexual men
- For users of injection and noninjection illegal drugs
- For patients with clotting-factor disorders
- For people at risk of occupational exposure to hepatitis A (e.g., handlers of nonhuman primates and individuals working with hepatitis A virus in a laboratory setting)

Hepatitis A vaccine should also be considered for staff at day care centers, staff at custodial care institutions, hospital personnel, and food handlers.

Currently, two inactivated hepatitis A vaccines (Havrix and Vaqta) are available in the United States. Both vaccines are approved for individuals >2 years old and are administered in a two-dose schedule.

112. Who should receive the pneumococcal vaccines?
According to recommendations from the American Academy of Pediatrics Committee on Infectious Diseases, the heptavalent conjugate vaccine should be administered to all children

23 months old and younger at 2, 4, 6, and 12–15 months of age. In addition, the heptavalent vaccine is recommended for all children 24–59 months old who are at high risk for invasive pneumococcal disease, including children with sickle cell disease, other causes of functional or anatomic asplenia, HIV infection, chronic cardiac disease, chronic pulmonary disease, chronic renal insufficiency, diabetes mellitus, CSF leak, primary immunodeficiency, or a condition that is associated with immunosuppression (e.g., organ or bone marrow transplantation, drug therapy, radiation therapy). To provide protection against a broader range of serotypes, these high-risk children should also receive a dose of the 23-valent plain polysaccharide vaccine at least 6–8 weeks after the last dose of the conjugate vaccine. When elective splenectomy is performed for any reason, scheduled immunization with either the heptavalent or the 23-valent vaccine should be performed at least 2 weeks before the splenectomy. Similarly, when possible, patients anticipating cancer chemotherapy or immunosuppression should be immunized at least 2 weeks before the initiation of therapy.

113. **How effective is the pneumococcal conjugate vaccine?**

The heptavalent pneumococcal conjugate vaccine is highly effective against invasive pneumococcal disease, reducing rates by up to 90% in children during the first 2 years of life. This vaccine has a modest effect on pneumococcal otitis media, preventing approximately 35% of culture-confirmed cases in young children. The effect of the vaccine on pneumococcal pneumonia is more difficult to quantify, but episodes of pneumonia defined by an abnormal chest x-ray (without information about specific etiology) are decreased by roughly 20–30% in children younger than 1–2 years old.

Kaplan SL, Mason EO Jr, Wald ER, et al: Decrease of invasive pneumococcal infections in children among 8 children's hospitals in the United States after the introduction of the 7-valent pneumococcal conjugate vaccine. Pediatrics 113:443–449, 2004.

Whitney CG, Farley MM, Hadler J, et al; Active Bacterial Core Surveillance of the Emerging Infections Program Network: Decline in invasive pneumococcal disease after the introduction of protein-polysaccharide conjugate vaccine. N Engl J Med 348:1737–1746, 2003.

114. **What are the pediatric indications for the influenza vaccine?**

Two types of inactivated influenza vaccine are available: one that is licensed for children ≥6 months old and the other licensed for those ≥4 years old. Each year, new preparations are made that are intended to cover the expected antigenic types for the winter season. When the vaccine is given for the first time in children <9 years of age, two doses are given, 1 month apart; during subsequent years, the same patient should be given only one dose. Recently, a live attenuated intranasal vaccine was licensed for use in individuals between 5 and 49 years old. The inactivated and live attenuated vaccines are not recommended for children <6 months old. Children who should be vaccinated against influenza include the following:

1. Children between 6 and 23 months old
2. Children at high risk for severe influenza infection because of the following:
   - chronic lung disease (e.g., asthma, bronchopulmonary dysplasia, cystic fibrosis)
   - congenital heart disease causing significant hemodynamic disturbance
   - sickle cell anemia or another hemoglobinopathy
   - immunosuppressive disorder or immunosuppressive therapy
   - chronic renal dysfunction
   - chronic metabolic disease, including diabetes mellitus
3. Children requiring long-term aspirin therapy, which may increase the risk for developing Reye's syndrome after influenza
4. Children who are close contacts of high-risk patients

Cox NJ, Subbarao K: Influenza. Lancet 354:1277–1282, 1999.

Neuzil KM, Mellen BG, Wright PF, et al: The effect of influenza on hospitalizations, outpatient visits, and courses of antibiotics in children. N Engl J Med 342:225–231, 2000.

McIntosh K, Lieu T: Is it time to give the influenza vaccine to healthy infants? N Engl J Med 342: 275–276, 2000.

115. **Under what circumstances should meningococcal vaccine be given?**

Two quadrivalent meningococcal vaccines containing capsular polysaccharide from serogroups A, C, Y, and W135 are available in the United States, including a plain poly-saccharide vaccine that is approved for use in children ≥2 years old and a polysaccha-ride diphtheria toxoid conjugate vaccine that is licensed for use in individuals 11–55 years old. Of note, serogroup B isolates account for approximately one third of cases of meningococcal disease, but serogroup B polysaccharide is absent from these vaccines.

All 11–12 year olds should be vaccinated with the conjugate vaccine routinely. In addition, unvaccinated college freshmen living in dormitories should be offered either the plain polysac-charide vaccine or the conjugate vaccine. Vaccination is considered advisable for children ≥2 years old who are in high-risk groups, including those with functional or anatomic asplenia or complement deficiency.

A meningococcal vaccine is given to all military recruits in the United States and should be considered for individuals traveling to areas of epidemic or hyperendemic disease. In addition, the current vaccines may be useful as an adjunct to chemoprophylaxis for the control of out-breaks caused by a vaccine serogroup.

Bilukha 00, Rosentein N: Prevention and control of meningococcal disease: Recommendations of the Advisory Committee on Immunization Practices. MMWR 54(RR07):1–21, May 27, 2005.

116. **How effective is the varicella vaccine (Varivax) if given after exposure to the illness?**

Varivax is highly effective (95% for the prevention of any disease, 100% for the prevention of moderate to severe disease) when used within 36 hours of exposure in an environment involv-ing close contact. The reason for the high efficacy is that naturally acquired varicella zoster virus usually takes 5–7 days to propagate in the respiratory tract before primary viremia and dissemination occur, whereas vaccine virus may elicit humeral and cellular immunity in significantly less time.

Watson B, Seward J, Yang A, et al: Postexposure effectiveness of varicella vaccine. Pediatrics 105:84–88, 2000.

117. **Of the vaccines included in the routine schedule, which ones contain live viruses?**

MMR and **varicella.** Oral polio vaccine is a live attenuated virus vaccine, but it is no longer recommended for routine use. Other live virus vaccines include cold-adapted, live-attenuated influenza, adenovirus, and yellow fever virus vaccines.

118. **What are the indications for palivizumab (Synagis)?**

Palivizumab is a humanized mouse monoclonal antibody that is directed against a respiratory syncytial virus (RSV) protein and that is approved for the prevention of RSV disease in selected children. According to the American Academy of Pediatrics, recommendations for the *consideration* of palivizumab administration include the following:

- Infants and children <2 years old with chronic lung disease who have required medical therapy for their lung disease within 6 months of the expected RSV season
- Infants born at ≤32 weeks' gestation within 6 months of the expected RSV season
- Infants and children <2 years old with hemodynamically significant congenital heart disease
- Children with severe immunodeficiencies (e.g., severe combined immunodeficiency, advanced AIDS)

119. **What are the recommendations regarding the administration of live-virus vaccines to patients receiving corticosteroid therapy?**

Children receiving corticosteroid treatment can become immunosuppressed. Although some uncertainty exists, there is adequate experience to make recommendations about the administration of live-virus vaccines to previously healthy children receiving steroid treatment.

In general, live-virus vaccines should *not* be administered to children who have received prednisone or its equivalent in a dose of ≥2 mg/kg/day (or ≥20 mg per day for individuals whose weight is >10 kg) for 14 days or more. Treatment for shorter periods, with lower doses, or with topical preparations or local injections should not contraindicate the use of these vaccines.

120. **What is thimerosal?**

Thimerosal is a mercury-containing preservative that has been used as an additive to vaccines for decades because of its effectiveness for preventing contamination, especially in open, multidose containers. In an effort to reduce exposure to mercury, vaccine manufacturers, the U.S. Food and Drug Administration, the American Academy of Pediatrics, and other groups have worked to remove thimerosal from vaccines that contain this compound. By the end of 2001, all vaccines in the routine schedule for children and adolescents were free or virtually free of thimerosal.

121. **Does thimerosal cause autism?**

There is no compelling evidence that thimerosal causes autism, attention-deficit/hyperactivity disorder, or other neurodevelopmental disorders.

INFECTIONS WITH RASH

122. **What is the traditional numbering of the "original" six exanthemas of childhood, and when were they first described?**

First disease	Measles (rubeola), 1627
Second disease	Scarlet fever, 1627
Third disease	Rubella, 1881
Fourth disease	Filatov-Dukes disease (described in 1900 and felt to be a distinct scarlatiniform type of rubella, attributed more recently to exotoxin-producing *Staphylococcus aureus;* term is no longer used)
Fifth disease	Erythema infectiosum, 1905
Sixth disease	Roseola infantum (exanthem subitum), 1910

Weisse ME: The fourth disease: 1900-2000. Lancet 357:299–301, 2001.

123. **What is "atypical" about atypical measles?**

- Koplik's spots are unusual.
- Conjunctivitis and coryza are not part of the prodrome.
- The rash begins on the distal extremities and spreads toward the head (in typical measles, the exanthem spreads from the head to the feet).
- Hepatosplenomegaly is common.

Atypical measles occurs primarily in patients who have received inactivated measles vaccine.

Cherry JD: Measles. In Feigin RD, Cherry JD, Demmler GJ, Kaplan SL (eds): Textbook of Pediatric Infectious Diseases, 5th ed. Philadelphia, W.B. Saunders, 2004, pp 2292–2293.

124. **What are the circumstances associated with measles cases in the United States?**

From 1989 to 1991, the incidence of measles in the United States increased primarily as a consequence of low immunization rates among preschool-aged children. Since 1992, the incidence of measles in the United States has been low, with fewer than 1,000 reported cases per year. Cases continue to occur from importation of the virus from other countries. In addition, vaccine failure occurs in approximately 5% of vaccine recipients after a single dose of vaccine and is responsible for some cases. Waning immunity after immunization may be a factor in occasional cases. Vaccine failure after two doses of measles vaccine administered after 12 months of age is uncommon.

Center for Disease Control: Global measles control and regional elimination, 1998-1999. MMWR 48(49):1124–1130, 1999.

National Vaccine Advisory Committee: The measles epidemic: The problems, barriers, and recommendations. JAMA 266:1547–1552, 1991.

125. **Why is post-measles blindness so common in underdeveloped countries?**
As many as 1% of all patients with measles in underdeveloped regions experience the progression of keratitis to blindness. By contrast, measles keratitis in developed countries is usually self-limited and benign. There are two principal reasons for the progression to blindness among patients with measles in underdeveloped countries:
- **Vitamin A deficiency:** Vitamin A is needed for corneal stromal repair, and a deficiency allows epithelial damage to persist or worsen. Many malnourished children have accompanying vitamin A deficiency, and vitamin A supplements may be of benefit during active illness.
- **Malnutrition:** Malnutrition may predispose a patient to corneal superinfection with herpes simplex virus.

126. **How common is human herpesvirus type-6 (HHV-6) infection in children?**
Infection with HHV-6 is ubiquitous and occurs with high frequency in infants, 65% of whom have serologic evidence of primary infection by their first birthday. HHV-6 infection results in typical cases of roseola and is also associated with a number of other common pediatric problems, including "fever without localizing findings," nonspecific rash, and Epstein-Barr virus-negative mononucleosis. In a study by Hall and colleagues, up to one third of all febrile seizures in children <2 years old were to the result of HHV-6 infections. On rare occasions, the virus has been associated with fulminant hepatitis, encephalitis, and a syndrome of massive lymphadenopathy called Rosai-Dorfman disease.

Hall CB, Long CE, Schnabel KC, et al: Human herpesvirus-6 infection in children. N Engl J Med 331:432–438, 1994.

127. **What are the etiologic agents of exanthem subitum (roseola)?**
Multiple agents are likely. HHV-6 was discovered in 1986, and, in 1988, Japanese investigators isolated it from four children with exanthem subitum. In 1994, human herpesvirus type 7 was also isolated from children with the clinical features of roseola.

128. **What are the typical features of roseola?**
Most children have an abrupt onset of high fever (>39°C) with no prodrome. Fever usually lasts 3–4 days but can range from 1–8 days. Within 24 hours of defervescence, a discrete erythematous macular or maculopapular rash appears on the face, neck, and/or trunk. Erythematous papules (Nakayama spots) may be noted on the soft palate and the uvula in two thirds of patients. Other common findings on examination include mild cervical lymph node enlargement, edematous eyelids, and a bulging anterior fontanel in infants. A variety of symptoms can accompany the fever, including diarrhea, cough, coryza, and headache.

Caserta MT, Hall CB, Schnabel K, et al: Primary human herpesvirus 7 infection: A comparison of human herpesvirus 7 and human herpesvirus 6 infections in children. J Pediatr 133:386–389, 1998.

129. **What is the spectrum of disease caused by parvovirus B19?**
- Erythema infectiosum (most common; a childhood exanthem, also called fifth disease or "slapped-cheek disease" because of the classic appearance of the rash)
- Arthritis and arthralgia (most common in adults)
- Intrauterine infection with hydrops fetalis
- Transient aplastic crisis in patients with underlying hemolytic disease

- Persistent infection with chronic anemia in patients with immunodeficiencies
- No symptoms

Young NS, Brown KE: Parvovirus B19. N Engl J Med 350:586–597, 2004.

130. Describe the characteristic rash of Rocky Mountain spotted fever.
- Usually seen by day 3 of illness (5–11 days after tick bite)
- Begins as blanching red macules which evolve into petechiae
- Begins on wrists and ankles and spreads to extremities and trunk within hours
- Involves palms and soles

Razzaq S, Schutze GE: Rocky Mountain spotted fever. Pediatr Rev 26:125–130, 2005.

131. How common is rash in patients with ehrlichiosis?
In adults, approximately 25% of patients have a rash. In children, the incidence of rash is roughly 60%. In most cases, the rash is erythematous or petechial. On occasion, the rash is an erythroderma, resembling the rash that is associated with toxic shock syndrome.

132. How long after exposure to chickenpox (varicella) do symptoms develop?
Ninety-nine percent of patients develop symptoms between 11 and 20 days after exposure.

133. Should "well" children with varicella be treated with acyclovir?
Studies have shown that oral acyclovir therapy (20 mg/kg, up to 800 mg) four times daily for 5 days, initiated within 24 hours after the onset of rash, decreases the maximum number of lesions by 15–30%, shortens the duration of the development of new lesions, and shortens the duration of fever by 1 day. The American Academy of Pediatrics Committee on Infectious Diseases opted not to recommend acyclovir for routine use in uncomplicated varicella for otherwise healthy children <13 years old because of "marginal therapeutic effect, the cost of the drug, feasibility of drug delivery in the first 24 hours of illness, and the currently unknown and unforeseen possible dangers of treating as many as 4 million children each year."

American Academy of Pediatrics: Varicella-zoster infections. In Pickering LK (ed): 2003 Red Book, Report of the Committee on Infectious Diseases, 26th ed. Elk Grove Village, IL, American Academy of Pediatrics, 2003, p 674.

Committee on Infectious Diseases: Use of oral acyclovir in otherwise healthy children with varicella. Pediatrics 91:674–676, 1993.

134. What is the risk of varicella-associated complications in normal children 1–14 years old?
The most common complications of varicella zoster infection include secondary bacterial skin infections (generally due to streptococci or staphylococci), neurologic syndromes (cerebellitis, encephalitis, transverse myelitis, and Guillain-Barré syndrome), and pneumonia. Thrombocytopenia, arthritis, hepatitis, glomerulonephritis, and Reye's syndrome occur less commonly. Myocarditis, pericarditis, pancreatitis, and orchitis are described but are rare.

The frequency of these complications in normal children is not precisely known, but it is estimated to be low on the basis of hospitalization and mortality data. Before the development of varicella vaccine, approximately 4 million cases of chickenpox occurred in the United States each year, resulting in roughly 10,000 hospitalizations and 100 deaths. Since the introduction of routine immunization against varicella, rates of infection have decreased by approximately 80%.

Gershon AA, Takahashi M, Seward J: Varicella vaccine. In Plotkin SA, Orenstein WA, Offit PA (eds): Vaccines, 4th ed. Philadelphia, W.B. Saunders, 2004, pp 783–823.

Arvin AM: Varicella-zoster virus. Clin Microbiol Rev 9: 361–381, 1996.

Preblud SR: Varicella: Complications and costs. Pediatrics 78:728–735, 1986.

135. How common are second episodes of varicella?
Approximately 1 in 500 cases involve a second episode. These are more likely to occur in children who develop their first episode during infancy or whose first episode is subclinical or very mild.

Gershon A: Second episodes of varicella: Degree and duration of immunity. Pediatr Infect Dis J 9:306, 1990.

136. What are shingles?

Reactivated varicella-zoster infection. After the primary infection of chickenpox, the virus establishes a latent infection in the dorsal root ganglion. When reactivation occurs, the virus spreads to the skin via nerves, and a typical vesicular pattern along dermatomal lines occurs (Fig. 11-1). In its primary form, the infection is varicella; in its recurrent form, it is zoster.

137. In children with herpes zoster, what is the distribution of the rash?

As compared with adults, children have relatively more cervical and sacral involvement with resultant extremity and inguinal lesions:

- 50% thoracic
- 20% cervical
- 20% lumbosacral
- 10% cranial nerve

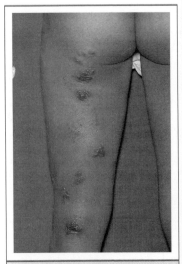

Figure 11-1. Herpes zoster with distribution along the S1 dermatome. (From Lissauer T, Clayton G: Illustrated Textbook of Pediatrics, 2nd ed. London, Mosby, 2001, p 193.)

If there are lesions on the tip of the nose, herpes zoster keratitis is more likely because of possible involvement of the nasociliary nerve. When the geniculate ganglion is involved, there is risk of developing the **Ramsay Hunt syndrome,** which consists of ear pain with auricular and periauricular vesicles and facial nerve palsy.

Feder HM Jr., Hoss DM: Herpes zoster in otherwise healthy children. Pediatr Infect Dis J 23:451–457, 2004.

138. Should children with zoster be treated with antiviral agents?

Routine antiviral therapy is not indicated. In general, the prognosis for children with herpes zoster is very good, with extremely low probabilities of postherpetic neuralgia or of associations with undiagnosed malignancy.

Petursson G, Helgason S, Gudmundsson S, Sigurdsson JA: Herpes zoster in children and adolescents. Pediatr Infect Dis J 17:905–908, 1998.

139. Who gets herpes gladiatorum?

Herpes gladiatorum is a term used to describe ocular and cutaneous infection with herpes simplex virus type 1, which occurs in wrestlers and rugby players. The infection is transmitted primarily by direct skin-to-skin contact and is endemic among high-school and college wrestlers.

140. What is the Tzanck prep?

It is a cytodiagnostic method that is used to examine blistering lesions for herpes simplex, herpes zoster, and varicella. A blister is unroofed, and scrapings of the base are placed and stained on a slide. The presence of multinucleated giant cells is diagnostic of one of those conditions (Fig. 11-2).

141. What is hand-foot-and-mouth disease?

Hand-foot-and-mouth disease is an illness that is caused most commonly by coxsackie A viruses (especially A16) or enterovirus 71. It is associated with a petechial or vesicular exanthem involving the hands, the feet, and the oral mucosa.

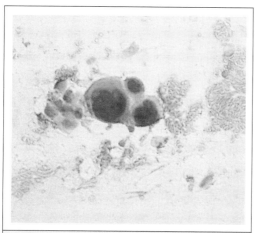

Figure 11-2. Tzanck preparation with multinucleated cells. (From Zitelli BJ, Davis HW: Atlas of Pediatric Physical Diagnosis, 4th ed. St. Louis, Mosby, 2002, p 277.)

LYMPHADENITIS/LYMPHADENOPATHY

142. **What are the most common causes of lymphadenitis in normal, otherwise healthy children, in order of frequency?**
   1. *Staphylococcus aureus*
   2. Group A *Streptococcus*
   3. *Bartonella henselae* (cat-scratch disease)
   4. *Mycobacterium tuberculosis*
   5. Nontuberculous mycobacteria
   6. Tularemia (frequency varies by geographic region)

143. **What vectors are commonly associated with tularemia?**
   Ticks, rabbits, deer, and muskrats have been associated with outbreaks of tularemia, although *Francisella tularensis* (the causative agent) has also been isolated from other mammals.

144. **An intensely erythematous but nontender submandibular or tonsillar node is most suggestive of what infectious process?**
   Nontuberculous mycobacterial infection.

145. **How is the diagnosis of nontuberculous mycobacterial disease made?**
   Definitive diagnosis of nontuberculous mycobacterial infection depends on culture of the organism from infected tissue. Histopathologic examination of the tissue cannot adequately differentiate nontuberculous mycobacterial infection from tuberculosis. Skin test antigens specific for nontuberculous mycobacteria are of limited usefulness as a result of cross-reactivity with antigens of *Mycobacterium tuberculosis*. Suggestive clinical features include adenopathy with minimal warmth and tenderness together with induration in response to PPD skin testing and a negative chest x-ray.

146. **How is nontuberculous mycobacterial disease treated?**
   Most experts recommend excision of the infected lymph node. Clarithromycin, rifampin, and ethambutol are effective against many strains of nontuberculous mycobacteria and are

generally used when excision is incomplete because of nearby nervous tissue or vascular structures or when surgery is contraindicated.

147. **Swollen, tender pectoral nodes are most suggestive of what infection?**
Cat-scratch disease.

148. **What is the etiologic agent of cat-scratch disease?**
The cause of cat-scratch disease is *Bartonella henselae*, which is detected in most cases by serologic tests and occasionally by PCR or culture. This organism was first isolated in 1991 and has also been associated with bacillary angiomatosis and peliosis hepatis, which occur primarily in adults with HIV infection.

149. **What is the typical course of the lymphadenitis in cat-scratch disease?**
Typically, an otherwise healthy child or adolescent presents symptoms of regional lymphadenopathy of several weeks' duration. The lymph nodes are usually moderately tender and are associated with overlying erythema and fluctuance. The lymph nodes most commonly involved are axillary, epitrochlear, cervical, submandibular, inguinal, and preauricular. Enlarged pectoral nodes are highly suggestive of cat-scratch disease. In most cases, fever is absent or low grade.

150. **How common is disseminated infection in cat-scratch disease?**
It is seen in 5–25% of cases. This form of the disease is characterized by severe, prolonged systemic symptoms, including fever, malaise, fatigue, myalgia, arthralgia, and abdominal pain. Granulomatous lesions may be detected by ultrasound in the liver and spleen.

151. **Describe the typical presentation of cat-scratch encephalitis.**
Approximately 46–80% of patients with cat-scratch encephalitis experience convulsions. Combative behavior is common, occurring in nearly 40% of patients. Other common signs and symptoms include headache and malaise. In one series of 76 patients with neurologic complications of cat-scratch disease, 61 had encephalopathy. CSF parameters are typically normal or reveal a mild elevation in protein. CT scans and magnetic resonance imaging (MRI) scans are usually normal. Fortunately, the prognosis for full neurologic recovery is excellent.

Bass JW, Vincent JM, Person DA: The expanding spectrum of *Bartonella* infections: II. Cat-scratch disease. Pediatr Infect Dis J 16: 163–179, 1997.

Grando D, Sullivan LJ, Flexman JP, et al: *Bartonella henselae* associated with Parinaud's oculoglandular syndrome. Clin Infect Dis 38:1156–1158, 1999.

KEY POINTS: CLINICAL FORMS OF CAT-SCRATCH DISEASE

1. Lymphadenitis

2. Parinaud's oculoglandular syndrome

3. Encephalitis

4. Retinitis

5. Osteomyelitis

6. Hepatosplenic disease

152. **Are antibiotics indicated for cat-scratch disease?**
The use of antibiotics in patients with uncomplicated cat-scratch disease is controversial because commonly used antibiotics are ineffective, and most patients recover spontaneously.

In a small randomized, placebo-controlled study of patients (n = 35) with cervical lymphadenitis, azithromycin was associated with a greater likelihood of decrease in cervical lymph node size to 20% of the original lymph node volume by 4 weeks after therapy than was placebo.

On the basis of in vitro antibiotic susceptibility testing and uncontrolled clinical studies, several antibiotics appear to offer benefit in patients with more severe forms of *Bartonella* infection. Examples include azithromycin, doxycycline, trimethoprim-sulfamethoxazole, ciprofloxacin, gentamicin, and rifampin.

Arisoy ES, Correa AG, Wagner ML, Kaplan SL: Hepatosplenic cat-scratch disease in children: Selected clinical features and treatment. Clin Infect Dis 28:778–784, 1999.

Bass JW, Freitas BC, Freitas AD, et al: Prospective randomized double-blind, placebo-controlled evaluation of azithromycin for treatment of cat-scratch disease. Pediatr Infect Dis J 17: 447–452, 1998.

153. How is the diagnosis of cat-scratch disease made?

Bartonella henselae is difficult to culture, although some experienced laboratories have reported success with chocolate or blood agar plates incubated for at least 30 days. Most cases of cat-scratch disease are diagnosed on the basis of serology. Cross reactivity exists between *B. henselae* and *Bartonella quintana,* so high positive antibody titers to *B. henselae* are sometimes associated with low positive titers to *B. quintana.*

Warthin-Starry silver staining of infected tissues is sometimes helpful for establishing a diagnosis. However, in one series, only 4 of 32 patients with serologically confirmed cat-scratch disease had a positive Warthin-Starry stain. Thus, silver staining is considered unreliable for excluding the diagnosis of cat-scratch disease.

PCR is performed at the Centers for Disease Control and Prevention and in some clinical microbiology laboratories, and it appears to be very sensitive.

154. What are the common presentations for Epstein-Barr virus (EBV) infections?

EBV infection is frequently asymptomatic in young children. In adolescents and young adults, infection typically results in infectious mononucleosis, which is characterized as follows:

- **Clinical:** Fever, pharyngitis, lymphadenopathy (75–95%), splenomegaly (50%)
- **Hematologic:** >50% mononuclear cells, > 10% atypical lymphocytes
- **Serologic:** Transient appearance of heterophil antibodies; emergence of persistent antibodies to EBV

A wide variety of symptoms (e.g., malaise, headache, anorexia, myalgias, chills, nausea) can occur. Neurologic presentations are rare but can include encephalitis, meningitis, myelitis, Guillain-Barré syndrome, and cranial or peripheral neuropathies.

155. How was the monospot test developed?

In 1932, Paul and Bunnell observed that patients with infectious mononucleosis make antibodies that agglutinate sheep red blood cells (RBCs). These antibodies are referred to as "heterophil antibodies" and serve as the basis for the monospot test, which is a rapid slide agglutination test. Today, horse or beef RBCs are usually used because they are more sensitive to agglutination than are sheep RBCs. Heterophil antibodies can also occur in serum sickness and as a normal variant. If there is clinical confusion, differential absorption can pinpoint the cause. Heterophil antibodies in infectious mononucleosis do not react with guinea pig kidney cells, whereas those of serum sickness do. Normal variant heterophil antibodies do not react with beef RBCs.

Durbin WA, Sullivan JL: Epstein-Barr virus infections. Pediatr Rev 15:63–68, 1994.

156. How common are heterophil antibodies in infectious mononucleosis?

In typical infectious mononucleosis with fever, tonsillopharyngitis, and lymphadenopathy, 75% of older children and adolescents have heterophil antibodies by the end of the first week of illness, and 85–90% have heterophil antibodies by the third week. These percentages are much lower in infants and children <4 years old, and false-negative screening with the monospot test is common in these groups and in patients without classic infectious mononucleosis.

157. **What is the natural course of serologic responses to EBV infection?**
A variety of distinct EBV antigens, including viral capsid antigen, early antigen, and nuclear antigen, can elicit antibody responses. Acute infection is best characterized by the presence of anti-viral capsid antigen immunoglobulin M.

> Junker AK: Epstein-Barr virus. Pediatr Rev 26:79–85, 2005.

158. **When are steroids indicated for children with EBV infection?**
Among patients with acute EBV infection, steroids should be considered for the relief of respiratory obstruction as a result of enlarged tonsils. Some authorities have also advocated their use for severe autoimmune hemolytic anemia, aplastic anemia, neurologic disease, and severe life-threatening infection (e.g., liver failure).

159. **Which other organisms can cause an infectious mononucleosis-like picture?**
Cytomegalovirus, *Toxoplasma gondii*, human herpesvirus-6, adenovirus, HIV, and rubella.

160. **What are the clinical presentations of acquired CMV infection?**
In normal hosts who develop symptomatic acquired CMV infection, clinical manifestations include fever, malaise, and nonspecific aches and pains. The peripheral blood smear reveals an absolute lymphocytosis and many atypical lymphocytes. By contrast with EBV-infectious mononucleosis, exudative pharyngitis is not prominent. Liver involvement is very common, and liver function tests are usually abnormal. Like EBV disease, CMV mononucleosis can persist for several weeks.

MENINGITIS

161. **What are the most common signs and symptoms of meningitis in infants <2 months old?**
In general, the findings among neonates and young infants with meningitis are minimal and often subtle. Temperature instability (fever or hypothermia) occurs in approximately 60% of infected infants; increasing irritability is present in about 60%, poor feeding or vomiting in roughly 50%, and seizures in about 40%. Lethargy, respiratory distress, and diarrhea are frequent nonspecific manifestations of meningitis in this patient group. On physical examination, approximately 25% of newborns and young infants have a bulging fontanelle, and only 13% have nuchal rigidity. The diagnosis of meningitis cannot be excluded on the basis of the absence of these physical findings in infants.

> Pong A, Bradley JS: Bacterial meningitis and the newborn infant. Infect Dis Clin North Am 13:711–733, 1999.

162. **What percentage of neonates with bacterial sepsis and positive blood cultures have meningitis?**
Up to 25% of infants <28 days old with bacterial sepsis and positive blood cultures will have culture-confirmed meningitis.

163. **What is the most common cause of aseptic meningitis?**
Aseptic meningitis is defined as clinical and laboratory evidence of inflammation of the meninges (e.g., CSF pleocytosis and increased protein) without evidence of bacterial infection on Gram stain or culture. More than 80% of cases are caused by *enteroviruses* (i.e., coxsackievirus, enterovirus, echovirus, and, rarely, poliovirus). West Nile virus is an increasingly common cause of aseptic meningitis, especially in the late summer and early fall.

164. **What is the diagnostic test of choice for enteroviral meningitis?**
PCR is highly sensitive and specific, and it is more rapid than viral cultures, which typically take 2–5 days to become positive.

165. **Is intracranial pressure elevated in patients with meningitis?**
In acute bacterial meningitis, pressure is elevated in up to 95% of cases. Elevation is also common among patients with tuberculous or fungal meningitis. The frequency of elevation in patients with viral meningitis is less well studied.

166. **Should CT scans be performed before a lumbar puncture (LP) during the evaluation of possible meningitis?**
CT scans are not routinely indicated before an LP, unless one of the following is present:
- Signs of herniation (rapid alteration of consciousness, abnormalities of pupillary size and reaction, absence of oculocephalic response, fixed oculomotor deviation of eyes)
- Papilledema
- Abnormalities in posture or respiration
- Generalized seizures (especially tonic), which are often associated with impending cerebral herniation
- Overwhelming shock or sepsis
- Concern about a condition mimicking bacterial meningitis (e.g., intracranial mass, lead intoxication, tuberculous meningitis, Reye's syndrome)

   Haslam RH: Role of CT in the early management of bacterial meningitis. J Pediatr 119:157–159, 1991.

167. **What is the range of values found in CSF of infants and children who do not have meningitis?**
- **Preterm newborn infants:** WBC count, 0–29/mm^3; protein, 65–150 mg/dL; blood glucose, 55–105 mg/dL
- **Term newborn infants:** WBC count, 0–32/mm^3; protein, 20–170 mg/dL; glucose, 44–248
- **Infants and children:** WBC count, 0–6/mm^3; protein, 15–45 mg/dL; glucose, 60–90

   McCracken GH: Current management of bacterial meningitis in infants and children. Pediatr Infect Dis J 11:169–174, 1992.

168. **If bloody CSF is collected during a lumbar puncture, how is CNS hemorrhage distinguished from a traumatic artifact?**
Most often, the blood is a result of the traumatic rupture of small venous plexes that surround the subarachnoid space, but pathologic bloody fluid can be seen in multiple settings (e.g., subarachnoid hemorrhage, herpes simplex encephalitis). Distinguishing features that suggest pathologic bleeding include the following:
- Bleeding that does not lessen during the collection of multiple tubes
- Xanthochromia of the CNS supernatant
- Crenated RBCs noted microscopically

169. **How do the CSF findings vary in bacterial, viral, fungal, and tuberculous meningitis in children beyond the neonatal period?**
Although a large overlap is possible (e.g., bacterial meningitis can be associated with a low WBC count early in the illness, or viral meningitis can often be associated with a predominance of neutrophils early or even persistently in the illness). The usual findings are summarized in Table 11-5.

170. **How is a traumatic lumbar puncture interpreted?**
To interpret the number of WBCs in the CSF after a traumatic lumbar puncture, the following correction factor can be applied. It is important to emphasize that the corrected WBC count is an estimate and should be considered in the context of other clinical information.

$$\text{"True" WBCs (CSF)} = \text{Actual WBCs (CSF)} - \frac{[\text{WBCs (blood)} \times \text{RBCs (CSF)}]}{\text{RBCs (blood)}}$$

Ashwal S, Perkin RM, Thompson JR, et al: Bacterial meningitis in children: Current concepts of neurologic management. Curr Probl Pediatr 24:267–284, 1994.

TABLE 11-5. TYPICAL FINDINGS IN BACTERIAL, VIRAL, FUNGAL, AND TUBERCULOUS MENINGITIS			
Cerebrospinal fluid findings	Bacterial	Viral	Fungal/tuberculous
White blood cells per mm³	>500	<500	<500
Polymorphonuclear neutrophils	>80%	<50%	<50%
Glucose (mg/dL)	<40	>40	<40
Cerebrospinal fluid to blood ratio	<30%	>50%	<30%
Protein (mg/dL)	>100	<100	>100

Adapted from Powell KR: Meningitis. In Hoekelman RA, Friedman SB, Nelson NM, et al (eds): Primary Pediatric Care, 3rd ed. St. Louis, Mosby, 1997, p1423.

171. **When is the best time to obtain a serum glucose level in an infant with suspected meningitis?**

Because the stress of a lumbar puncture can elevate serum glucose, the serum sample is ideally obtained just before the lumbar puncture. When the blood glucose level is elevated acutely, it can take at least 30 minutes before there is equilibration with the CSF.

172. **How often does bacterial meningitis appear in younger patients with normal findings on the initial CSF examination?**

In up to 3% of cases in children between the ages of 3 weeks and 18 months with positive bacterial cultures of the CSF, the initial CSF evaluation (i.e., cell count, protein and glucose concentrations, and Gram stain) can be normal. Of note is that, in almost all of these cases, physical examination reveals evidence of meningitis or suggests serious illness and the need for empiric antibiotics.

Polk DB, Steele RW: Bacterial meningitis presenting with normal cerebrospinal fluid. Pediatr Infect Dis J 6:1040–1042, 1987.

173. **Does antibiotic therapy before lumbar puncture affect CSF indices?**

In most cases, shortly after the initiation of antibiotics, the CSF Gram stain still demonstrates bacteria with typical staining properties, and chemistry values and cell counts are abnormal. Even when children have received appropriate antibiotic therapy for 44–68 hours, chemical and cytologic analysis of the CSF generally still reflects a bacterial process. In earlier studies of patients with *Haemophilus influenzae* meningitis who received oral antibiotic therapy before lumbar puncture, CSF cultures often grew the organism. By contrast, there is a tendency for oral therapy to sterilize the CSF of children with meningococcal disease or with meningitis as a result of sensitive *Streptococcus pneumoniae*.

174. **What are the most common organisms responsible for bacterial meningitis in the United States?**

0–1 month old
- Group B streptococci
- *Escherichia coli*

- *Listeria monocytogenes*
- *Streptococcus pneumoniae*
- Miscellaneous Enterobacteriaceae
- *Haemophilus influenzae* (especially other than type b)
- Coagulase-negative staphylococci (in hospitalized preterm infants)

1–23 months old
- *Streptococcus pneumoniae*
- *Neisseria meningitidis*
- Group B streptococci

2–18 years old
- *Neisseria meningitidis*
- *Streptococcus pneumoniae*

Schuchat A, Robinson K, Wenger JD, et al: Bacterial meningitis in the United States in 1995. Active Surveillance Team. N Engl J Med 337:970–976, 1997.

KEY POINTS: MINIMAL DURATION OF THERAPY FOR BACTERIAL MENINGITIS

1. Five days of therapy for meningococcal meningitis

2. Between 7 and 10 days for *Haemophilus influenzae* meningitis

3. Ten days for pneumococcal meningitis

4. Between 14 and 21 days for group B streptococcal or *Listeria monocytogenes* meningitis

5. Twenty-one days or more for gram-negative enteric bacilli (after the cerebrospinal fluid has become sterile)

6. Among patients with complications (e.g., brain abscess, subdural empyema, delayed cerebrospinal fluid sterilization, persistence of meningeal signs, prolonged fever), the duration of therapy should be individualized and may need to be extended

175. **Why are *Haemophilus influenzae* type B strains more virulent than nontypeable *Haemophilus* strains?**
   H. influenzae type b expresses the type b polysaccharide capsule, which is a polymer of ribose and ribitol-5 phosphate. In the absence of type-specific antibody, the type b capsule promotes intravascular survival by preventing phagocytosis and complement-mediated bactericidal activity. It is likely that other factors also contribute to the unique virulence of *H. influenzae* type b.

176. **What are the drugs of choice for the empirical treatment of bacterial meningitis in children >1 month old?**
   In cases of suspected bacterial meningitis, both vancomycin and a third-generation cephalosporin are recommended for empirical therapy because resistance to penicillin and cephalosporins is present in 10–30% of *Streptococcus pneumoniae* isolates. The exception is when the Gram stain suggests another etiology (e.g., gram-negative diplococci). Treatment failures have been reported when the dosage of vancomycin is <60 mg/kg/day. Vancomycin should not be used alone to treat *S. pneumoniae* meningitis because data from animal models indicate that bactericidal levels may be difficult to maintain. The combination of vancomycin plus cefotaxime or ceftriaxone has been shown to produce a synergistic effect in vitro, in animal models, and in the CSF of children with meningitis.

Ahmed A: A critical evaluation of vancomycin for treatment of bacterial meningitis. Pediatr Infect Dis J 16: 895–903, 1997.

American Academy of Pediatrics, Committee on Infectious Diseases: Therapy for children with invasive pneumococcal infections. Pediatrics 99:289–299, 1997.

177. **How quickly is the CSF sterilized in children with meningitis?**
In successful therapy, the CSF is usually sterile *within 36–48 hours* of the initiation of antibiotics. In patients with meningococcal meningitis, CSF is typically completely sterile in no longer than 2 hours after starting treatment. With other organisms, the time until sterilization is generally at least 4 hours.

Kanegaye JT, Soliemanzadeh P, Bradley JS: Lumbar puncture in pediatric bacterial meningitis: Defining the time interval for recovery of cerebrospinal fluid pathogens after parenteral antibiotic pretreatment. Pediatrics 108:1169–1174, 2001.

178. **How long after treatment has been initiated must individuals with meningitis remain in respiratory isolation?**
24 hours. Respiratory isolation is recommended for patients with suspected *Haemophilus influenzae* type b or meningococcal meningitis, but it can be discontinued after 24 hours of therapy.

179. **What is the accepted duration of treatment for bacterial meningitis?**
The duration of antibiotic treatment is based on the causative agent and clinical course. In general, a minimum of 5 days of therapy is required for meningococcal meningitis, 7–10 days for *Haemophilus influenzae* meningitis, and 10 days for pneumococcal meningitis. Disease as a result of group B streptococci or *Listeria monocytogenes* should be treated for 14–21 days, and meningitis caused by gram-negative enteric bacilli should be treated for a minimum of 21 days after the CSF has become sterile. Among patients with complications such as brain abscess, subdural empyema, delayed CSF sterilization, persistence of meningeal signs, or prolonged fever, the duration of therapy may need to be extended and should be individualized.

180. **What is the role of corticosteroids in the treatment of bacterial meningitis?**
The inflammatory response plays a critical role in producing the CNS pathology and resultant sequelae of bacterial meningitis. Several studies have demonstrated that treatment with dexamethasone reduces the incidence of hearing loss and other neurologic sequelae in infants and children with *Haemophilus influenzae* meningitis. For cases of meningitis caused by pathogens other than *H. influenzae*, the current recommendations by the American Academy of Pediatrics are to *consider* the use of dexamethasone. The role of steroids in meningitis caused by other bacterial pathogens (particularly *Streptococcus pneumoniae)* remains controversial.

Arditi M, Mason EO, Jr., Bradley JS, et al: Three-year multicenter surveillance of pneumococcal meningitis in children: Clinical characteristics, and outcome related to penicillin susceptibility and dexamethasone use. Pediatrics 102:1087–1097, 1998.

Feigin RD: Use of corticosteroids in bacterial meningitis. Pediatr Infect Dis J 23:355–357, 2004.

McIntyre PB, Berkey CS, King SM, et al: Dexamethasone as adjunctive therapy in bacterial meningitis. A meta-analysis of randomized clinical trials since 1988. JAMA 278:925–931, 1997.

181. **Should children receiving therapy for bacterial meningitis be retapped?**
It is widely agreed that a repeat LP is advisable for patients with meningitis caused by penicillin-resistant *Streptococcus pneumoniae* or gram-negative enteric bacilli and in children who show no clinical response to therapy within 24–36 hours. In addition, repeat LP is recommended for patients with prolonged or recurrent fever, for patients with recurrent meningitis, and for immunocompromised hosts. Some experts also recommend repeat LP in neonates with meningitis because of the greater difficulty of tracking the infant's clinical course as a measure of CSF sterilization and because of the variable response of the immature neonatal immune system. An end-of-treatment LP is sometimes considered for neonates; the purpose

of this is to provide a baseline if a subsequent febrile illness develops and reevaluation for sepsis and meningitis is performed.

Wubbel L, McCracken GH: Management of bacterial meningitis. Pediatr Rev 19:78–84, 1998.

182. **In a patient with meningitis, what are the indications for a CT scan or MRI?**
The following suggest the presence of an intracranial complication and should prompt a neuroimaging study:
- Prolonged obtundation
- Prolonged irritability
- Seizures developing after the third day of therapy
- Focal seizures
- Focal neurologic deficits
- Increasing head circumference
- Persistent elevation of CSF protein or neutrophil count
- Recurrence of disease

In cases of neonatal meningitis caused by *Citrobacter koseri* (formerly called *Citrobacter diversus*), brain abscess should be anticipated, and a CT scan or MRI should be performed early in the course. For these patients, repeat scans are useful to monitor the response to antibiotic therapy and to determine the need for surgical intervention.

Wubbel L, McCracken GH: Management of bacterial meningitis. Pediatr Rev 19:78–84, 1998.

183. **How common is persistent or recurrent fever in patients with meningitis?**
In the absence of dexamethasone treatment, fever persists for at least 4–5 days after the initiation of antibiotics in most children with meningitis. It lasts for 5–9 days in 10–15% of cases and for ≥10 days in another 10–15% of patients. Fever that returns after a minimum of 24 hours of normal temperatures is considered recurrent fever and occurs in approximately 15% of patients.

Arditi M, Mason EO, Jr., Bradley JS, et al: Three-year multicenter surveillance of pneumococcal meningitis in children: Clinical characteristics, and outcome related to penicillin susceptibility and dexamethasone use. Pediatrics 102:1087–1997, 1998.

Lin TY, Nelson JD, McCracken GH, Jr.: Fever during treatment for bacterial meningitis. Pediatr Infect Dis J 3:319–32, 1984.

184. **What are the most common causes of prolonged fever in patients with meningitis?**
- Disease at other foci (e.g., arthritis)
- Nosocomial infection
- Thrombophlebitis (related to intravenous catheters and infusates)
- Sterile or infected abscesses from intramuscular injections
- Drug fever

Subdural effusions have also been associated with prolonged fever, but these occur commonly among children with meningitis and are probably not a cause of fever.

185. **How should prolonged fever during treatment for meningitis be managed?**
Patients who remain febrile for >5 days and who are irritable or have persistent neck stiffness should undergo a repeat lumbar puncture. Similarly, children who appear well yet have fever for ≥10 days should also undergo repeat lumbar puncture. If the CSF examination reveals a protein concentration of >100 mg/dL, a glucose concentration of <30 mg/dL, or >25% neutrophils, persistent infection is a possibility. Studies should be obtained to exclude an abscess or resistant isolate. If the CSF values are approaching normal, antibiotic therapy can usually be discontinued at the usual time. In this situation, nosocomial viral infection or drug fever would be likely.

Nelson JD: Management problems in bacterial meningitis. Pediatr Infect Dis J 4:S41–S44, 1985.

186. **How commonly are subdural effusions noted in patients with bacterial meningitis?**

Subdural effusions are common in bacterial meningitis and should be considered part of the disease rather than a complication. Estimates of their incidence vary from 10–50%. The incidence is highest in young infants and in patients with *Haemophilus influenzae* meningitis. Approximately 1% of patients with meningitis will have a subdural *empyema*; the typical presentation is fever, irritability, and meningeal signs. Subdural empyema can be diagnosed by CT and requires drainage and prolonged antibiotic therapy.

187. **If a child develops bacterial meningitis, what should the parents be told about long-term outcomes?**

Disease resulting from *Streptococcus pneumoniae* is associated with considerably more mortality and morbidity than is infection caused by *Neisseria meningitidis* or *Haemophilus influenzae*. Mortality ranges from 8–15%. A recent 3-year multicenter surveillance study of invasive pneumococcal infections examined outcomes of meningitis caused by *S. pneumoniae* in 180 children. Twenty-five percent of children had evidence of neurologic sequelae at the time of hospital discharge, and 32% had unilateral or bilateral deafness. Predictors of mortality included coma on admission, requirement for mechanical ventilation, and shock.

Arditi M, Mason EO, Jr., Bradley JS, et al: Three-year multicenter surveillance of pneumococcal meningitis in children: Clinical characteristics and outcome related to penicillin susceptibility and dexamethasone use. Pediatrics 102:1087–1097, 1998.

Baraff LJ, Lee SI, Schriger DL: Outcomes of bacterial meningitis in children: A meta-analysis. Pediatr Infect Dis J 12:389–394, 1993.

188. **How should contacts of children with *Neisseria meningitidis* disease be managed?**

Antibiotic prophylaxis is indicated for household and day care or nursery school contacts of patients with invasive meningococcal disease. Only those medical personnel who have had intimate contact with the patient (e.g., through intubation or mouth-to-mouth resuscitation) require antibiotic prophylaxis. In most instances, options for chemoprophylaxis include rifampin, ceftriaxone, and ciprofloxacin (for those ≥18 years of age).

American Academy of Pediatrics: Meningococcal infections. In Pickering LK (ed): 2003 Red Book: Report of the Committee on Infectious Diseases, 26th ed. Elk Grove Village, IL, American Academy of Pediatrics, 2003, p 432–434.

Committee on Infectious Diseases: Meningococcal disease prevention and control strategies for practice-based physicians. Pediatrics 97:404–412, 1996.

OCULAR INFECTIONS

189. **Among neonates with conjunctivitis, what is the timing for the various etiologies?**

Cause	Time of Onset
Chemical	<2 days
Neisseria gonorrhoeae	2–7 days
Chlamydia trachomatis	5–14 days
Herpes simplex virus	6–14 days

190. **In children with conjunctivitis and otitis media, what is the most likely etiologic agent?**

Nontypeable *Haemophilus influenzae* is the most common cause of the so-called conjunctivitis-otitis syndrome, which is characterized by concurrent conjunctivitis and otitis media.

KEY POINTS: DURATION OF MIDDLE-EAR EFFUSION PERSISTENCE AFTER OTITIS MEDIA

1. Two weeks: 70%

2. One month: 40%

3. Two months: 20%

4. Three months: 5–10%

191. **Can bacterial conjunctivitis be distinguished from viral conjunctivitis on clinical grounds alone?**

Classically, bacterial conjunctivitis is more common in infants and young children, with the discharge being purulent or mucopurulent. Viral conjunctivitis is accompanied by a serous exudate in children of all ages. Bacterial infections are commonly associated with otitis media, and otoscopy should be performed on all patients. However, clinical findings can overlap. Both bacteria and viruses can cause unilateral or bilateral symptoms.

Aside from culture, the best way to distinguish the culprit is by Giemsa stain of a conjunctival scraping. Neutrophils predominate in bacterial infections, lymphocytes in viral infections, and eosinophils in allergic conjunctivitis.

Weiss A: Acute conjunctivitis in childhood. Curr Probl Pediatr 24:4–11, 1994.

192. **What is keratoconjunctivitis?**

Keratoconjunctivitis is an inflammatory process that involves both the conjunctiva and the cornea. Superficial inflammation of the cornea occurs commonly in association with viral and bacterial conjunctivitis, particularly in adults. Hence, many cases of conjunctivitis are more correctly called *keratoconjunctivitis*.

Epidemic keratoconjunctivitis is caused by adenovirus serotypes 8, 19, and 37. Some organisms, including *Pseudomonas aeruginosa*, *Neisseria gonorrhoeae*, and herpes simplex virus, have a propensity to cause more severe infection of the cornea. Infection as a result of these pathogens must be recognized early to prevent corneal scarring with subsequent vision loss.

193. **When are topical antibiotics not sufficient for treating acute conjunctivitis?**

Topical therapy for neonatal chlamydial conjunctivitis should never be used as sole therapy because of the high likelihood of concomitant respiratory tract colonization (which can eventually progress to pneumonia). Infections resulting from *Neisseria gonorrhoeae*, *Pseudomonas aeruginosa*, *Haemophilus influenzae* type b, and *Neisseria meningitidis* require systemic therapy to prevent the serious complications seen with these organisms. Of course, viral conjunctivitis does not respond to topical antibiotics.

194. **What is the best method of prophylaxis for ophthalmia neonatorum?**

Chlamydia is now the predominant etiology of neonatal conjunctivitis. As a consequence, erythromycin 0.5% ophthalmic ointment and tetracycline 1.0% ophthalmic ointment are now used routinely in nurseries the United States, although their efficacy for preventing chlamydial disease remains unclear. Worldwide, other methods are used. In one large study of >3000 infants in Kenya, 2.5% povidone-iodine ophthalmic solution was more effective than silver nitrate drops or erythromycin ointment as prophylaxis against neonatal conjunctivitis.

Isenberg SJ: A controlled trial of povidone-iodine as prophylaxis against ophthalmia neonatorum. N Engl J Med 332:562–566, 1995.

195. **Can newborns with chlamydial conjunctivitis be treated with topical therapy alone?**
Newborns diagnosed with chlamydial conjunctivitis should receive systemic therapy with oral erythromycin (50 mg/kg/day in four divided doses) for 14 days. Topical therapy will not eradicate the organism from the upper respiratory tract, and it fails to prevent the development of chlamydial pneumonia. Close follow-up evaluation is indicated to ensure the absence of relapse.

196. **Are ophthalmic solutions better than ophthalmic ointments for eradicating conjunctivitis?**
Ophthalmic ointments are usually preferred for infants and young children because they can be instilled more reliably and remain in the eye for a longer time. In older children, ophthalmic solutions may be preferred to prevent the blurring of vision that occurs with ointments. In general, the efficacy of ophthalmic ointments is presumed to be superior to that of solutions. However, several antibiotics are available in high-concentration solutions. These "fortified" formulations have not been compared prospectively with other preparations, but they are widely used because of their presumed enhanced efficacy.

197. **What is the most common cause of Parinaud's oculoglandular syndrome?**
Parinaud's syndrome is characterized by granulomatous or ulcerating conjunctivitis and prominent preauricular or submandibular adenopathy. The most common cause is **cat-scratch disease**, but other causes include tularemia, sporotrichosis, tuberculosis, syphilis, and infectious mononucleosis.

198. **How is orbital cellulitis distinguished from periorbital (or preseptal) cellulitis?**
Periorbital cellulitis involves the tissues anterior to the eyelid septum (Fig. 11-3), whereas **orbital cellulitis** involves the orbit and is sometimes associated with abscess formation and cavernous sinus thrombosis. Distinction between these processes requires assessment of ocular mobility, pupillary reflex, visual acuity, and globe position, which are normal in periorbital cellulitis but may be abnormal in orbital cellulitis. An abnormality in any of these four areas mandates radiologic evaluation (usually CT scan of the orbit) and possible surgical drainage.

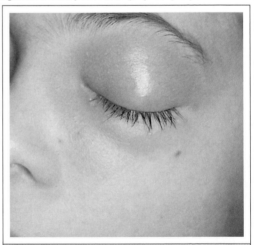

Figure 11-3. Periorbital cellulitis. (From Zitelli BJ, Davis HW: Atlas of Pediatric Physical Diagnosis, 4th ed. St. Louis, Mosby, 2002, p 848.)

199. **What is the difference between a hordeolum, a stye, and a chalazion?**
  - A **hordeolum** is a purulent infection of any one of the sebaceous or apocrine sweat glands of the eyelid, including the glands of Moll and Zeis, which drain near the eyelash follicle, and the meibomian glands, which drain nearer the conjunctiva. Clinically, a hordeolum is recognized as a red, tender swelling. It is usually caused by *Staphylococcus aureus*.

- A **stye** is an external hordeolum, on the skin side of the eyelid.
- A **chalazion** is an internal hordeolum, on the conjunctival side of the eyelid.

In all cases, these lesions are treated with warm compresses and topical antibiotic drops and usually resolve within 7 days. A chalazion is more likely to become chronic and require surgical excision.

200. **What are the most common etiologies of endophthalmitis?**
- Postoperative cases: *Staphylococcus epidermidis*
- Penetrating trauma: *Bacillus cereus* and *Streptococcus* species
- Patient with a central venous catheter or prolonged antibiotic therapy: *Candida albicans*

Alfaro DV, Roth D, Liggett PE: Posttraumatic endophthalmitis. Causative organisms, treatment, and prevention. Retina 14:206–211, 1994.

OTITIS MEDIA

201. **How commonly does cerumen obscure the diagnosis of otitis media?**
As many as 30% of cases of otitis media are obscured by this waxy roadblock.

Schwartz RH, Rodriguez WJ, McAveney W, Grundfast KM: Cerumen removal. How necessary is it to diagnose acute otitis media? Am J Dis Child 137:1065–1068, 1983.

202. **What is the best way to remove cerumen?**
Removal by curettage via direct visualization (preferably through an otoscope) is commonly used, but this approach can be uncomfortable and difficult if immobilization of the child is incomplete. When time permits, ceruminolytic agents can be instilled to soften the wax, with subsequent gentle irrigation. A recent study compared docusate sodium (Colace) with triethanolamine polypeptide (Cerumenex) and found the former to be more effective. Water jet irrigation devices are used but can result in perforation, especially at higher pressures.

Singer AJ, Sauris E, Viccellio AW: Ceruminolytic effects of docusate sodium: A randomized, controlled trial. Ann Emerg Med 36:228–232, 2000.

203. **Is ear pulling a reliable sign of infection?**
In the absence of other signs or symptoms (e.g., fever, upper respiratory infection symptoms), ear pulling alone is a very poor indicator of acute otitis media.

Baker RB: Is ear pulling associated with ear infection? [letter] Pediatrics 90:1006–1007, 1992.

204. **What are the landmarks of the tympanic membrane?**
See Fig. 11-4.

205. **What are the most reliable ways, on physical examination, to accurately diagnosis acute otitis media?**
Good visualization of the tympanic membrane (TM) with use of a pneumatic otoscope is key.
- **Visualization of position:** Bulging of the TM implies fluid under pressure, whereas retraction is more commonly seen with effusion rather than suppuration
- **Color/translucence:** Normal TM color is pearly gray and translucent; cloudiness implies suppuration; distinct redness (especially if unilateral) can indicate infection but can be seen in other settings, particularly with fever
- **Mobility:** Immobility of the TM to positive pressure by pneumatic otoscopy implies a fluid-filled space

Rothman R, Owens T, Simel DL: Does this child have acute otitis media? JAMA 290:1633–1640, 2003.

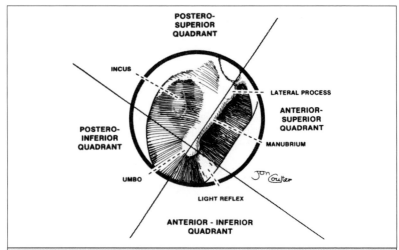

Figure 11-4. Right tympanic membrane. (From Bluestone CD, Klein JO: Otitis Media in Infants and Children. Philadelphia, W.B. Saunders, 1988, p 76.)

206. **How often will acute otitis media resolve spontaneously without antibiotics?**
In 60% of cases or more. The likelihood of spontaneous resolution depends on the microbiologic etiology and is estimated at 20% with *Streptococcus pneumoniae*, 50% with *Haemophilus influenzae*, 80% with *Moraxella catarrhalis*, and 100% with respiratory viruses.

207. **Should all children with acute otitis media be treated with antibiotics?**
Because of the high rate of spontaneous improvement, some suggest that children may not require antibiotic therapy for uncomplicated otitis media. However, placebo-controlled trials have demonstrated that treatment with an antimicrobial agent shortens the duration of symptoms and reduces the likelihood of persistent infection, especially in children <2 years old. According to new recommendations from the American Academy of Pediatrics and the American Academy of Family Practitioners, decisions about antibiotic treatment should be based on diagnostic certainty, age, illness severity, and assurance of follow-up. In particular, antibiotic treatment should be seriously considered for all infants <6 months old, for children between 6 months and 2 years old with a certain diagnosis of otitis media *or* severe illness, and for children >2 years old with a certain diagnosis of otitis media *and* severe illness.

American Academy of Pediatrics: Diagnosis and management of acute otitis media. Pediatrics 113:1451–1465, 2004.

208. **How should young infants with otitis media be managed?**
With infants 0–8 weeks old, the main concern is whether a localized infection (i.e., otitis media) has disseminated and become systemic. Controversial issues include the extent of work-up (e.g., lumbar puncture) and the need for hospitalization. Serious bacterial infection is infrequently associated with isolated otitis media in nontoxic-appearing infants between the ages of 2 and 8 weeks. Some experts argue that outpatient management is appropriate. Febrile infants should have a more extensive laboratory evaluation. Clinical practice varies with regard

to inpatient versus outpatient management of those infants with essentially normal blood, urine, and CSF tests. This variation is in large part the result of the decreased reliability of clinical observation in infants <2 months old.

Nozicka CA, Hanly JG, Beste DJ, et al: Otitis media in infants aged 0-8 weeks: Frequency of associated serious bacterial disease. Pediatr Emerg Care 15:252–254, 1999.

209. **After an acute episode of otitis media, how long does the middle ear effusion persist?**
Approximately 70% of patients will continue to have an effusion at 2 weeks, 40% at 1 month, 20% at 2 months, and 5–10% at 3 months.

210. **What are the most common viral and bacterial agents that cause otitis media?**
Tympanocentesis yields positive bacterial cultures in 65–90% of cases of acute otitis media. Virus or viral antigen is detected from middle ear fluid in 10–25% of cases (Table 11-6). The significance of virus in middle ear fluid is debated, although it seems clear that antecedent viral infection is an important factor in the pathogenesis of otitis media and that concomitant viral infection may prolong the course of bacterial otitis media and lead to treatment failures.

Heikkinen T, Chonmaitree T: Increasing importance of viruses in acute otitis media. Ann Med 32:157–163, 2000.

TABLE 11-6. COMMON BACTERIA AND VIRUSES IDENTIFIED IN MIDDLE EAR FLUID			
Bacterial isolates		**Viral isolates***	
Streptococcus pneumoniae	43%	Respiratory syncytial virus	7%
Moraxella catarrhalis	21%	Rhinovirus	3%
Haemophilus influenzae	18%	Influenza virus	2%
Streptococcus pyogenes	4%	Adenovirus	2%
Other	4%	Parainfluenza virus	2%

*Viruses are given as the percentage of total aspirates.
Adapted from Ruuskanen O, Arola M, Heikkinen T, et al: Viruses in acute otitis media: Increasing evidence for clinical significance. Pediatr Infect Dis J 10:425–427, 1991.

211. **What percentage of otitis media is caused by penicillin-resistant organisms?**
In some areas, up to 40% of *Streptococcus pneumoniae* has some degree of ampicillin resistance because of alterations in penicillin-binding proteins. In addition, approximately 30% of *Haemophilus influenzae* isolates and more than 80% of *Moraxella catarrhalis* isolates produce beta-lactamase. Given the prevalence of *H. influenzae* and *M. catarrhalis* as additional causes of otitis media, roughly 20–30% of all cases will have relative resistance to amoxicillin. Many authorities have recommended that amoxicillin be given at higher doses (70–90 mg/kg/day), particularly in children who have received antibiotic therapy during the previous 3 months.

Bradley JS: Oral versus intramuscular antibiotic therapy for acute otitis media: Which is best? Pediatr Infect Dis J 18:1147–1151, 1999.
McCracken GH: Prescribing antimicrobial agents for treatment of otitis media. Pediatr Infect Dis J 18:1141–1146, 1999.

212. Among patients with otitis media, what are the indications for tympanocentesis?

- A "toxic"-appearing child
- An unsatisfactory response to antibiotics
- A suppurative complication
- Underlying immunosuppression

Some experts would also consider tympanocentesis in newborn infants with otitis media, because the spectrum of potential pathogens may be broader than that seen in an older child.

213. When should prophylactic antibiotics be considered for children with recurrent otitis media?

Several studies have demonstrated that chronic use of an oral antimicrobial agent can marginally decrease the incidence of recurrent otitis media. Amoxicillin (20 mg/kg once daily) and sulfisoxazole have been studied most thoroughly, although trimethoprim-sulfamethoxazole and erythromycin have also been found to be effective.

In an effort to control the use of antibiotics and to minimize selection for resistant organisms, antibiotic prophylaxis should be reserved for patients with three or more distinct and well-documented episodes per 6 months or four or more episodes per 12 months. When initiated, the duration of prophylactic therapy should be no more than 6 months.

Dowell SF, Schwartz B, Phillips WR: Appropriate use of antibiotics for URIs in children: Part I. Otis media and acute sinusitis. Am Fam Physician 58:113–118, 1998.

214. What are the indications for tympanostomy tubes?

Tympanostomy tubes are most commonly inserted for the treatment of otitis media with effusion or for prophylaxis against recurrent otitis media.

A child with otitis media with effusion that lasts ≥3 months or that is associated with suspected hearing loss, language delay, or learning problems should undergo hearing evaluation. If significant hearing impairment is detected, placement of tympanostomy tubes should be considered, although prompt placement does not appear to improve developmental outcome at the age of 3 years. Tympanostomy tubes have been shown to improve hearing during the initial 6 months after the procedure. On the other hand, benefits are less marked beyond 6 months, partially as a result of extrusion of the tubes.

For patients with recurrent otitis media, the benefit of tube placement is modest and must be weighed against the risk of complications, which include sclerosis, retraction, and atrophy of the eardrum.

American Academy of Pediatrics: Otitis media with effusion. Pediatrics 113:1412–1429, 2004.
Otitis Media Guideline Panel: Managing otitis media with effusion in young children. Pediatrics 94:766–772, 1994.
Paradise JL, Feldman HM, Campbell TF, et al: Effect of early or delayed insertion of tympanostomy tubes for persistent otitis media on developmental outcomes at the age of three years. N Engl J Med 344:1179–1187, 2001.

215. Should a child with tympanostomy tubes be allowed to swim?

Otolaryngologists differ widely in their guidance to parents about issues of swimming and bathing. Controlled studies have shown that the rate of otorrhea is similar between nonswimmers (15%) and surface swimmers without earplugs (20%). If diving or underwater swimming is planned, fitted earplugs are recommended. Bath water with shampooing can cause inflammatory changes in the middle ear, and thus earplugs should be used if head dunking is anticipated during bathing. An in vitro study (using a head model) found water entry greatest with submersion in soapy water and with deeper swimming.

Hebert RL, II, King GE, Bent JP, III: Tympanostomy tubes and water exposure: A practical model. Arch Otolaryngol Head Neck Surg 124:1118–1121, 1998.
Isaacson G, Rosenfeld RM: Care of the child with tympanostomy tubes: A visual guide for the pediatrician. Pediatrics 93:924–929, 1994.

216. **A child with the acute onset of ear pain and double vision likely has what condition?**

   Gradenigo's syndrome is an acquired paralysis of the abducens muscle with pain in the area that is served by the ipsilateral trigeminal nerve. It is caused by inflammation of the sixth cranial nerve in the petrous portion, with involvement of the gasserian ganglion. The inflammation is usually the result of infection from otitis media or mastoiditis. Symptoms may include weakness of lateral gaze on the affected side, double vision, pain, photophobia, tearing, and hyperesthesia.

PHARYNGEAL/LARYNGEAL INFECTIONS

217. **Can group A streptococcal pharyngitis be diagnosed clinically?**

   Streptococcal pharyngitis is a disease with variable clinical manifestations. Clues that suggest streptococcal disease include the abrupt onset of headache, fever, and sore throat with the subsequent development of tender cervical lymphadenopathy, tonsillar exudate, and palatal petechiae. The presence of concurrent conjunctivitis, rhinitis, or cough suggests a viral process. The physical findings are by no means diagnostic. Even the most skilled clinician cannot exceed an accuracy rate of about 75%. A throat culture or a rapid antigen test is essential for confirming streptococcal infection.

218. **What is the rationale for the treatment of group A streptococcal pharyngitis?**
   - To prevent acute rheumatic fever (even with the low incidence of acute rheumatic fever in the United States, it is still prevalent in much of the world)
   - To shorten the course of the illness, including headache, sore throat, and lymph node tenderness
   - To reduce the spread of infection and prevent suppurative complications
   - To prevent some cases of acute glomerulonephritis

219. **Should patients with group A streptococcal pharyngitis have a post-treatment throat culture?**

   In general, repeated courses of antibiotics are not indicated for patients who become asymptomatic but whose throat cultures remain positive for group A streptococci after appropriate antibiotic therapy. Accordingly, post-treatment throat cultures are of little value. Exceptions include individuals with a history of rheumatic fever and patients who have family members with rheumatic heart disease.

   Dajani A, Taubert K, Ferrieri P, et al: Treatment of acute streptococcal pharyngitis and prevention of rheumatic fever: A statement for health professionals. Committee on Rheumatic Fever, Endocarditis, and Kawasaki Disease of the Council on Cardiovascular Disease in the Young, the American Heart Association. Pediatrics 96:758–764, 1995.

220. **How does one differentiate a patient with a sore throat who is a streptococcal carrier with an intercurrent viral pharyngitis from one who is having repeated episodes of group A streptococcal pharyngitis?**

   Streptococcal carrier
   - Signs and symptoms of viral infection (rhinorrhea, cough, conjunctivitis, diarrhea)
   - Little clinical response to antibiotics (sometimes difficult to assess because of the self-resolving nature of viral infections)
   - Group A streptococcus present on cultures between episodes
   - No serologic response to infection (i.e., anti-streptolysin O, anti-DNase B)
   - Same serotype of group A streptococcus in sequential cultures

   Recurrent group A streptococcal pharyngitis
   - Signs and symptoms consistent with group A streptococcal infection

- Marked clinical response to antibiotics
- No group A streptococcus on cultures between episodes
- Positive serologic response to infection
- Different serotypes of group A streptococcus on sequential cultures

Gerber MA: Treatment failures and carriers: Perception or problems? Pediatr Infect Dis J 13:576–579, 1994.

Pichichero ME, Marsocci SM, Murphy ML, et al: Incidence of streptococcal carriers in private practice medicine. Arch Pediatr Adolesc Med 153:624–628, 1999.

221. What are the acceptable alternative therapies for group A streptococcal pharyngitis?

Penicillin V is the drug of choice for group A streptococcal pharyngitis, except in penicillin-allergic individuals. There are no documented reports of group A streptococci that are resistant to penicillin. The dose is 250 mg two to three times per day for 10 days for children and 500 mg two to three times per day for 10 days for adolescents and adults. Intramuscular benzathine penicillin or Bicillin (a mixture of benzathine penicillin and procaine penicillin) is an alternative and has the advantage of guaranteed compliance but the disadvantage of associated pain. A single daily dose of amoxicillin for 10 days is also effective. For patients with allergy to penicillin, erythromycin has been used most widely, but clarithromycin for 10 days and azithromycin for 5 days are appropriate as well. Narrow-spectrum cephalosporins and clindamycin represent additional options. Tetracyclines, sulfisoxazole, and trimethoprim-sulfamethoxazole should not be used because many strains of group A streptococcus are resistant to tetracyclines, and sulfonamides fail to eradicate group A streptococci from the pharynx.

222. When can children treated for positive streptococcal throat cultures return to school or day care?

Although clinical improvement often occurs promptly, most patients remain culture positive at 14 hours after the initiation of antibiotics. However, by 24 hours, nearly all patients are culture negative. To minimize contagion, children should receive a full 24 hours of antibiotic therapy before returning to school or child care.

Snellman LW, Stang HJ, Stang JM, et al: Duration of positive throat cultures for group A streptococci after initiation of antibiotic therapy. Pediatrics 91:1166–1170, 1993.

223. Do toddlers <2 years old get strep pharyngitis?

Traditional teaching has been that toddlers rarely develop strep pharyngitis. Recent studies indicate that the incidence of infection and the prevalence of carriage is greater than previously thought. In studies of patients <2 years old with fever and clinical pharyngitis, the range of group A beta-hemolytic streptococcus positivity was 4–6%; among well children, the carrier rate is about 6%. The rate of rheumatic fever is exceedingly low in children <3 years old.

Berkovitch M, Vaida A, Zhovtis D, et al: Group A streptococcal pharyngotonsillitis in children less than 2 years of age—more common than is thought. Clin Pediatr 38:365–366, 1999.

Nussinovitch M, Finkelstein Y, Amir J, Varsano I: Group A beta-hemolytic streptococcal pharyngitis in preschool children aged 3 months to 5 years. Clin Pediatr 38:357–360, 1999.

224. How long after the development of streptococcal pharyngitis can treatment be initiated and still effectively prevent rheumatic fever?

Treatment should be started as soon as possible, but little is lost in waiting for throat culture results to establish the diagnosis. Antibiotic treatment prevents acute rheumatic fever even when therapy is initiated as long as 9 days after the onset of the acute illness.

225. What are other bacterial causes of pharyngitis?

Arcanobacterium haemolyticum is an important cause of pharyngitis in adolescents. Lancefield group C and G beta-hemolytic streptococci have been associated with pharyngitis and a variety of other suppurative infections. Tularemia and *Neisseria gonorrhoeae* are additional bacterial etiologies of pharyngitis.

226. **What diagnosis should be suspected in a teenager with pharyngitis followed by multifocal pneumonia and sepsis?**
Lemierre syndrome. The syndrome of "postanginal septicemia" was first reported by Schottmuller in 1918 and was recorded in more detail by Lemierre in 1936. It represents septic thrombophlebitis of the internal jugular vein as a result of pharyngeal infection and is typically caused by the anaerobic gram-negative rod *Fusobacterium necrophorum*. Bacteremia ensues, and multifocal embolic pneumonia leads to respiratory failure in untreated cases. Anaerobic blood cultures, ultrasonography of the jugular vessels, and CT scan of the chest are helpful for establishing the diagnosis. In addition to supportive care, patients should receive appropriate systemic antibiotics, which can include penicillin, metronidazole, and ampicillin-sulbactam.

> Lemierre A: On certain cepticemias. Lancet 1:70–73, 1936.
> Schottmuller H: Uber die Pathogenität anaëro ber Bazillen. Dtsch Med Wochenschr 44:1440, 1918.

227. **What is the difference between herpangina and Ludwig's angina?**
- **Herpangina** is a common viral infection during the summer and fall and is characterized by posterior pharyngeal, buccal, and palatal vesicles and ulcers. Coxsackieviruses A and B and echoviruses are the most common causative agents. In young children, it is often accompanied by a high fever (103–104°F). Herpangina is distinguished from herpes simplex infections of the mouth, which are more anterior and involve the lips, tongue, and gingiva.
- **Ludwig's angina** is an acute diffuse infection (usually bacterial) of the submandibular and sublingual spaces with brawny induration of the floor of the mouth and tongue. Airway obstruction can occur. The infections usually follow oral cavity injuries or dental complications (e.g., extractions, impactions).

228. **What is quinsy?**
Peritonsillar abscess (from the Lower Latin for "an inflammation of the throat").

229. **How is a peritonsillar abscess distinguished from peritonsillar cellulitis?**
A peritonsillar abscess is diagnosed when a discrete mass is palpated, usually in school-aged children and adolescents. The bulging abscess causes lateral displacement of the uvula. Trismus occurs more commonly in the setting of abscess than does simple *cellulitis*, which is characterized by signs of diffuse inflammation only.

230. **What x-ray features suggest the diagnosis of a retropharyngeal abscess?**
When a patient's neck is extended, a measurement of the prevertebral space that exceeds two times the diameter of the C2 vertebra suggests an abscess. Pockets of air in the prevertebral space also suggest abscess. The retropharynx extends to T1 in the superior mediastinum, so empyema or mediastinitis is also possible whenever a retropharyngeal abscess is identified. CT scanning can delineate the extent of these deep neck infections.

231. **Which age group is most susceptible to retropharyngeal abscess?**
This disease is most common in children between the ages of 1 and 6 years. There are several small lymph nodes in the retropharynx that usually disappear by the age of 4 or 5. These lymph nodes drain the posterior nasal passages and nasopharynx, and they may become involved if those sites are infected.

232. **What are the indications for removing adenoids?**
Infectious
- Persistent symptoms of adenoiditis despite two courses of antibiotic therapy
- Otitis media with effusion of >3 months that is refractory to antibiotic therapy and when a second set of tympanostomy tubes is required for treatment of same effusion
- >4 episodes of purulent nasopharyngitis during the previous 12 months in a patient <12 years old

Obstructive

- Nasopharyngeal obstruction with sleep disturbances, hypopnea, and apnea
- Association with pulmonary hypertension, cor pulmonale, and failure to thrive
- Abnormalities in craniofacial growth and dental occlusion as a result of adenoidal hypertrophy
- Significant hyponasal speech

Kazahaya K, Potsic WP: Tonsillectomy and adenoidectomy. In Burg FD, Ingelfinger JR, Polin RA, et al (eds): Current Pediatric Therapy, 17th ed. Philadelphia, W.B. Saunders, 2002, pp 929–932.

233. **What are the indications for removing the tonsils?**

Infectious

- Recurrent acute tonsillitis (>6 episodes in a year or >3 per year for 2 years)
- Recurrent acute streptococcal tonsillitis with complicating medical conditions (e.g., cardiac valvular disease, recurrent febrile seizures)
- Chronic tonsillitis that is unresponsive to medical management
- Chronic or recurrent tonsillitis that is associated with group A beta-hemolytic streptococcus carrier state
- Chronic or recurrent peritonsillar abscesses
- Chronic halitosis associated with recurrent tonsillar disease
- Infectious mononucleosis with tonsillomegaly that is unresponsive to medical management

Obstructive

- Similar to adenoids
- Asymmetric hypertrophy with suspicion of malignancy

Kazahaya K, Potsic WP: Tonsillectomy and adenoidectomy. In Burg FD, Ingelfinger JR, Polin RA, et al (eds): Current Pediatric Therapy, 17th ed. Philadelphia, W.B. Saunders, 2002, pp 929–932.

234. **How should children with epiglottitis be managed?**

Acute epiglottitis is a medical emergency, and all children should be assumed to have a critical airway (i.e., of the potential for imminent occlusion exists). Because of the risk of airway obstruction upon agitation, the patient should be allowed to remain with parents, free from restraint. Examination should be performed as cautiously as possible. Continuous observation regardless of the setting (e.g., radiology suite), avoidance of supine positioning, and arrangements for admission to an intensive care unit are mandatory. Ideally, the epiglottis is visualized directly in an operating room, and the child is intubated immediately afterward.

Previously, >90% of cases were caused by *Haemophilus influenzae* type b. However, because of the routine use of *H. influenzae* type b vaccines in infants, the incidence of epiglottitis has decreased dramatically, and pneumococci, staphylococci, and streptococci now account for a relatively large percentage of cases.

235. **How is epiglottitis distinguished clinically from croup?**

See Table 11-7.

236. **What are the criteria for the admission of a child with viral croup?**

- **Clinical signs of impending respiratory failure:** Marked retractions, depressed level of consciousness, cyanosis, hypotonicity, and diminished or absent inspiratory breath sounds
- **Laboratory signs of impending respiratory failure:** PCO_2 >45 mmHg, PaO_2 <70 mmHg in room air
- **Clinical signs of dehydration**
- **Social considerations:** Unreliable parents, excessive distance from hospital
- **Historic considerations:** High-risk infant with history of subglottic stenosis or prior intubations

TABLE 11-7. CLINICAL DISTINCTIONS BETWEEN CROUP AND EPIGLOTTITIS

	Croup	Epiglottitis
Age	Younger (6 months–3 years)	Older (3–7 years)
Onset of stridor	Gradual (24–72 hours)	Rapid (8–12 hours)
Symptoms	Prodromal upper respiratory Infection	Minimal rhinitis Little coughing
	Harsh, brassy cough	Muffled voice
	Hoarseness	Pain in throat
	Slightly sore throat	
Signs	Mild fever	High fever (>39° C)
	Not toxic	Toxic appearance
	Variable distress	Severe distress; sits upright; may drool
	Harsh inspiratory stridor	Low-pitched inspiratory stridor
	Expiratory sounds uncommon	May have a low-pitched expiratory sound
Radiology	Subglottic narrowing	Edema of epiglottis and aryepi- glottic folds (positive "thumb" sign)

237. Are steroids efficacious for the treatment of croup?

The use of corticosteroids (including oral and intramuscular dexamethasone and nebulized budesonide) has been shown to be beneficial for patients hospitalized for croup. In particular, corticosteroid treatment reduces the incidence of intubation and results in more rapid respiratory improvement. In addition, among patients with mild or moderate croup, corticosteroids appear to reduce the use of nebulized racemic epinephrine and the need for hospitalization. At present, the most common dose of dexamethasone is 0.6 mg/kg, but lower doses are under study. The dose of budesonide is 2–4 mg.

Ausejo M, Saenz A, Pham B, et al: The effectiveness of glucocorticoids in treating croup: Meta-analysis. BMJ 319:595–600, 1999.

Johnson DW, Jacobson S, Edney PC, et al: A comparison of nebulized budesonide, intramuscular dexamethasone, and placebo for moderately severe croup. N Engl J Med 339:498–503, 1998.

238. If a child has received racemic epinephrine as a treatment for croup, is hospitalization required?

In earlier days, children treated with racemic epinephrine were routinely hospitalized to observe for potential rebound mucosal edema and airway obstruction, regardless of how they appeared clinically. However, a number of recent studies have shown that children who are free of significant stridor or retractions at rest 2–3 hours after the administration of racemic epinephrine can be safely discharged, provided that adequate follow up is assured. In most of these studies, oral or intramuscular dexamethasone (0.6 mg/kg) was also administered.

Ledwith CA, Shea LM, Mauro RD: Safety and efficacy of nebulized racemic epinephrine in conjunction with oral dexamethasone and mist in the outpatient treatment of croup. Ann Emerg Med 25:331–337, 1995.

Rizos JD, DiGravio BE, Sehl MJ, Tallon JM: The disposition of children with croup treated with racemic epinephrine and dexamethasone in the emergency department. J Emerg Med 16:535–539, 1998.

239. Is a cool-mist vaporizer truly of benefit for patients with croup?

The usual advice for the home management of croup includes the use of a cool-mist vaporizer. The theory is that the coolness serves as a vasoconstrictor and that the mist serves to thin respiratory secretions. Interestingly, this therapy remains time honored but is largely unproven. One small study found no differences between control and mist-treated infants. The calming effects of being held by a parent during the mist treatment may have greater impact.

Bourchier D, Dawson KP, Fergusson DM: Humidification in viral croup: A controlled trial. Aust Paediatr J 20:289, 1984.

240. What are membranous and pseudomembranous croup?

Membranous croup is the historic term for diphtheria, and **pseudomembranous croup** is the historic term for bacterial tracheitis.

Bacterial tracheitis is usually caused by *Staphylococcus aureus* and occurs after trauma to the neck or trachea or after a viral respiratory tract infection such as croup. The presentation of bacterial tracheitis is similar to that of severe croup or epiglottitis, and consequently a lateral neck radiograph is frequently obtained. In bacterial tracheitis, this study often reveals narrowing of the tracheal lumen as the result of a thick, purulent exudate that can extend into both mainstem bronchi.

241. What is spasmodic croup?

Spasmodic croup is a poorly understood cause of recurrent stridor in young children (usually 1–3 years old) and resembles acute infectious laryngotracheobronchitis in many respects. However, unlike infectious croup, a prodrome of upper respiratory symptoms is usually absent, and the patient is usually afebrile. The onset is sudden, typically at night, with inspiratory stridor and a brassy cough that responds to therapies used for infectious croup (e.g., cool mist, racemic epinephrine, corticosteroids). Recurrence is common. The pathogenesis is unclear, but allergic and hypersensitivity components are suspected. In the rare patient who requires intubation, the typical finding is the pale and boggy mucosa of allergy and not the inflamed swelling of a primary infection.

SINUSITIS

242. When do the sinuses develop during childhood?

The maxillary and ethmoid sinuses are present at birth. Pneumatization of the sphenoid sinuses begins at approximately 2–3 years of age and is usually complete by about age 6. Frontal sinus pneumatization varies considerably, beginning around 3–7 years of age and finishing by age 12.

243. What percentage of teenagers do not have frontal sinuses when x-rays are obtained?

Frontal sinus pneumatization is absent in approximately 10% of the normal population.

244. List the predisposing factors for the development of chronic sinusitis.

- Allergic rhinitis
- Anatomic abnormalities (e.g., polyps, enlarged adenoids)
- Impairment of mucociliary clearance (e.g., cystic fibrosis, primary ciliary dyskinesia)
- Foreign bodies (e.g., nasogastric tube)
- Abnormalities in immune defense

245. Does a thick, green nasal discharge on day two of a respiratory illness indicate a bacterial sinus infection?

Absolutely not. The character of nasal secretions (e.g., purulent, discolored, tenacious) does not distinguish viral from bacterial. Early treatment (<7–10 days) of purulent nasal discharge is a common cause of antibiotic overuse.

246. **Is transillumination helpful for diagnosing sinusitis in children?**
In general, transillumination of the sinuses is of very limited value in the diagnosis of acute sinusitis in young children.

247. **What is the role of plain radiographs in the diagnosis of sinusitis?**
Acute sinusitis usually appears in one of two ways, either with the acute onset of fever of >39°C and purulent nasal discharge or with prolonged nasal discharge and cough continuing without improvement for >10 days. Most clinicians treat suspected acute sinusitis empirically, without performing imaging studies. Although plain radiographs are easy to obtain and are relatively inexpensive, they lack sensitivity for diagnosing sinusitis. In addition, they lack specificity, especially in children without clinical symptoms of sinusitis.

248. **Which radiographic views are potentially useful for evaluating sinusitis?**
In children <6 years old, only the maxillary and ethmoid sinuses are clinically important, and 80% of children in this age group with acute sinusitis will have both sets of sinuses involved. Caldwell (anteroposterior) and Waters (occipitomental) views are necessary to assess these sinuses. To evaluate the frontal and sphenoid sinuses of older children, a lateral view is most informative.

249. **What constitutes an abnormal sinus x-ray?**
- Complete opacification of a sinus cavity
- Mucosal thickening of at least 4 mm
- Presence of an air-fluid level

  Although these findings are not specific for sinusitis, they are helpful for confirming a diagnosis of acute sinusitis in patients with suggestive signs and symptoms (i.e., nasal discharge and cough persisting for >10 days without improvement or high fever and purulent nasal discharge for >3 days).

250. **When should CT scans be considered for the diagnosis of sinusitis?**
In most cases, a sinus CT scan is unnecessary. CT scans are more sensitive than sinus x-rays but also suffer from a lack of specificity. Scenarios that might warrant the use of CT scanning include the following:
- Complicated sinus disease with either orbital or CNS abnormalities
- Multiple recurrences
- Prolonged symptoms that are unresponsive to treatment and that suggest possible anatomic abnormalities, thereby raising sinus surgery as a consideration

  Nash D, Wald ER: Sinusitis. Pediatr Ann 22:111–117, 2001.

251. **Which organisms are responsible for acute and chronic sinusitis in the pediatric age group?**
In acute, uncomplicated sinusitis, the etiologic organisms closely parallel those associated with acute otitis media: *Streptococcus pneumoniae*, *Haemophilus influenzae*, and *Moraxella catarrhalis*. In patients with chronic sinusitis, the most common pathogens remain *S. pneumoniae*, *H. influenzae*, and *M. catarrhalis*, along with *Staphylococcus aureus* and anaerobes. Fungal infection with zygomycosis (mucormycosis) is an important concern in immunosuppressed patients, and *Pseudomonas aeruginosa* must always be considered in patients with cystic fibrosis.

252. **For how long should sinus infections be treated?**
The duration of therapy for acute sinusitis in children has not been studied systematically. However, for patients whose symptoms improve dramatically within 3–4 days of initiating treatment, a 10-day course of therapy is usually effective. For patients who respond more slowly to antibiotics, treatment until symptoms resolve plus another 7 days is reasonable. Often 3 weeks of treatment are required.

KEY POINTS: PNEUMATIZATION OF THE PARANASAL SINUSES

1. Maxillary and ethmoid: Present at birth

2. Sphenoid: Begins at 2–3 years of age, complete by age 6

3. Frontal: Begins at 3–7 years of age, complete by age 12

TUBERCULOSIS

253. Who should be screened for tuberculosis (TB)?
Previously, routine periodic screening with multiple puncture tests (tine tests) was a norm for the entire population of children. However, routine screening of low-risk children in low-prevalence areas is no longer advised. Current recommendations are as follows:
Children who should be tested immediately
- Contacts of persons with confirmed or suspected infectious TB
- Children with radiographic or clinical findings that are suggestive of TB
- Children emigrating from endemic countries
- Children with a history of travel to endemic countries

Children who should be tested annually
- Children with HIV or living in a household with an HIV-infected person
- Incarcerated adolescents

Children who should be tested every 2–3 years
- Children exposed to the following groups: HIV-infected persons, homeless persons, nursing home residents, institutionalized adolescents or adults, illicit drug users, and migrant farm workers

Children who should be considered for testing at 4–6 and 11–16 years of age
- Children whose parents immigrated from endemic regions of the world
- Children residing in high-prevalence areas

American Academy of Pediatrics. Tuberculosis. In Pickering LK (ed): 2003 Red Book: Report of the Committee on Infectious Diseases, 26th ed. Elk Grove Village, IL: American Academy of Pediatrics, 2003, p 646.

254. When are the various strengths of PPD used?
The standard-strength PPD (Mantoux test) contains 5 tuberculin units (TU) of purified protein derivative and is designated intermediate strength. This preparation is used for routine skin test screening. PPD is also available in 1-TU and 250-TU strengths, but these preparations are not generally recommended.

255. How is the Mantoux test interpreted in children?
The Mantoux test is interpreted in the context of clinical signs and symptoms and epidemiologic risk factors (e.g., known exposure). Positive tests are defined as follows:
Reaction of ≥5 mm
- Children in close contact with confirmed or suspected cases of TB
- Children with radiographic or clinical evidence of TB disease

- Children receiving immunosuppressive therapy
- Children with immunodeficiency disorders, including HIV infection

Reaction of ≥10 mm

- Children <4 years old
- Children with diabetes mellitus, chronic renal failure, malnutrition, or other chronic conditions
- Children born in high-prevalence regions of the world, whose parents were born in such areas, or who have traveled to such areas
- Children frequently exposed to adults who are infected with HIV, homeless, incarcerated, illicit drug users, or migrant farm workers

Reaction of ≥15 mm

- Children >4 years old with no risk factors

American Academy of Pediatrics. Tuberculosis. In Pickering LK (ed): 2003 Red Book, Report of the Committee on Infectious Diseases, 26th ed. Elk Grove Village, IL, American Academy of Pediatrics, 2003, p 643.

256. **What are the reasons for false-negative skin testing with PPD?**
- Testing during the incubation period (2–10 weeks)
- Problems with the administration technique
- Severe systemic TB infection (miliary or meningitis)
- Immunosuppression, malnutrition, or immunodeficiency
- Concurrent infection: Measles, varicella, HIV, Epstein-Barr virus, *Mycoplasma*, mumps, rubella
- Recent measles immunization

Callahan CW: Tuberculosis. In Schidlow DV, Smith DS (eds): A Practical Guide to Pediatric Respiratory Diseases. Philadelphia, Hanley & Belfus, 1994, p 107.

257. **Why is a multiple puncture test (tine test) not considered an ideal test for TB?**
- The exact dose of antigen (either PPD or old tuberculin) cannot be standardized, and thus interpretation is difficult. As a result, any positive test must be confirmed with a Mantoux test.
- In a patient with a positive tine test, the need for a follow-up Mantoux test can lead to a booster phenomenon if the patient has had a previous bacille Calmette-Guérin (BCG) vaccine or infection with nontuberculous mycobacteria, again making interpretation difficult.
- Significant variability exists among false-negative rates and especially among false-positive rates.
- The use of tine tests has a tendency to result in parental reporting, which can be very unreliable.

Starke JR, Correa AG: Management of mycobacterial infection and disease. Pediatr Infect Dis J 14:455–470, 1995.

258. **How should patients with a positive tuberculin test be evaluated?**
History should search for clues that are suggestive of active infection, such as recurrent fevers, weight loss, adenopathy, or cough. A history of recurrent infections in the patient or a family member may be suggestive of HIV infection, which is a risk factor for infection with *Mycobacterium tuberculosis*. Information from previous tuberculin skin testing is invaluable. Epidemiologic information includes an evaluation of possible exposure to TB. A family history is obtained, including questions pertaining to chronic cough or weight loss in a family member or other contact. Travel history and current living arrangements should be elucidated. If the patient has immigrated to North America, a history of BCG vaccination should be ascertained.

Physical examination should focus on pulmonary, lymphatic, and abdominal systems. Examination should corroborate a history of BCG vaccination.

Laboratory evaluation, including a chest x-ray with a lateral film, is the next stage. Family members and close contacts should undergo skin testing. In certain circumstances, chest x-rays should be performed on the child's contacts.

If any of the preceding evaluation suggests active infection, sputum, gastric aspirates, and other appropriate specimens (e.g., lymph-node tissue) should be obtained for mycobacterial culture and Ziehl-Neelsen or auramine-rhodamine staining.

259. **In a younger child that is suspected of having TB, how should gastric aspirates be obtained?**

Because children <10 years old rarely produce sputum, gastric aspirates are a better source for the culture of mycobacteria in these patients, yielding the organism in up to 40% of cases. The aspirate should be obtained early in the morning as the child awakens to sample the overnight accumulation of respiratory secretions. The sample should be collected in a saline-free fluid, and the pH should be neutralized if any delay in processing is anticipated.

260. **How are children with active pulmonary TB treated?**

Recommendations for the treatment of active TB in children have evolved over the past several years. Previously, at least 9 months of therapy were suggested for uncomplicated pulmonary disease. Studies in adults and children have demonstrated that 6 months of combined antituberculous therapy (short-course therapy) is as effective as 9-month therapy. To date, the combined results of multiple studies in pediatric patients have demonstrated the efficacy of 6-month therapy to be >95%.

The current standard regimen for active pulmonary TB in children consists of 2 months of daily isoniazid, rifampin, and pyrazinamide followed by 4 months of isoniazid and rifampin (daily or twice weekly). If drug resistance is a concern, either ethambutol or streptomycin is added to the initial three-drug regimen until drug susceptibilities are determined.

261. **Why are multiple antibiotics used for the treatment of TB?**

Two features of *Mycobacterium tuberculosis* make the organism difficult to eradicate after infection has been established. First, mycobacteria replicate slowly and may remain dormant for prolonged periods, but they are susceptible to drugs only during active replication. Second, drug-resistant organisms exist naturally within a large population, even before the initiation of therapy. These features render the organism—when it is present in significant numbers—extremely difficult to eradicate with a single agent. Indeed, the ability to cure patients with asymptomatic infection with a single agent is based on the presence of a small number of organisms that are exposed to a bactericidal antibiotic for an extended period of time.

262. **Why is pyridoxine supplementation given to patients who are receiving isoniazid?**

Isoniazid interferes with pyridoxine metabolism and may result in peripheral neuritis or convulsions. The administration of pyridoxine is generally not necessary for children who have a normal diet because they have adequate stores of this vitamin. Children and adolescents with diets deficient in milk or meat, breast-fed infants, and pregnant women should receive pyridoxine supplementation during isoniazid therapy.

263. **How effective is BCG vaccination?**

The BCG vaccines are among the most widely used in the world at present and are also perhaps the most controversial. The difficulties stem from the marked variation in reported efficacy of BCG against *Mycobacterium tuberculosis* and *Mycobacterium leprae* infections. Depending on the population studied, efficacy against TB has ranged from 0–80%. Similarly, the efficacy against leprosy has ranged from 20–60% in prospective trials.

The vaccines were derived from a strain of *Mycobacterium bovis* in 1906 and were subsequently dispersed to several laboratories around the world, where they were propagated under nonstandardized conditions. Hence, the vaccines in use today cannot be considered homogeneous. This may explain the observed variation in efficacy.

264. How does BCG immunization influence TB skin testing?

Generally, the interpretation of PPD tests is the same in BCG recipients as it is in nonvaccinated children. If positive, consideration should be given to several factors when deciding who should receive antituberculous therapy. These factors include time since BCG immunization, number of doses received, prevalence of TB in the country of origin, contacts in the United States, and radiographic findings.

265. Why do children with TB rarely infect other children?

TB is transmitted via infected droplets of mucus that become airborne when an individual coughs or sneezes. As compared with adults, children with TB have several factors that minimize their contagiousness:

- Low density of organisms in sputum
- Lack of cavitations or extensive infiltrates on chest x-ray
- Lower frequency of cough
- Lower volume and higher viscosity of sputum
- Shorter duration of respiratory symptoms

Starke JR: Childhood tuberculosis during the 1990s. Pediatr Rev 13:343–353, 1992.

266. In addition to TB, what other airborne microbes can cause respiratory disease?

See Table 11-8.

TABLE 11-8. AIRBORNE MICROBIAL DISEASES	
Disease	**Airborne source**
Aspergillosis	Conidia spores from decaying vegetation and soil
Brucellosis	Aerosolized from carcasses of domestic and wild animals
Chickenpox	Aerosolized from respiratory secretions
Coccidioidomycosis	Arthroconidia from soil and dust
Cryptococcosis	Aerosolized from bird droppings
Histoplasmosis	Conidia spores from bat or bird droppings
Legionnaires' disease	Aerosolized contaminated water, especially from air-conditioning cooling towers
Measles	Aerosolized respiratory secretions
Mucormycosis	Spores from soil
Psittacosis	*Chlamydia psittaci* from birds
Q fever	*Coxiella burnetii* from a variety of farm and other animals
Tularemia	Aerosolized from multiple wild animals, especially rabbits
Viral nasopharyngitis, bronchiolitis, and pneumonia	Aerosolized respiratory secretions

ZOONOSES AND EMERGING INFECTIONS

267. How long should domestic animals be observed in confinement when rabies is a concern?

Animals with rabies almost always become ill within 4–5 days after the onset of shedding of rabies virus. In some experimental settings, this asymptomatic period can last for up to 14 days. The standard in the United States is to confine dogs, cats, or ferrets for *10 days* following a suspicious human contact. There has not been a report of a case of rabies transmission by an animal that remained healthy during that time period.

268. Which wild animals are capable of transmitting rabies?

The wild animals that are most often infected with rabies include *bats, raccoons, foxes,* and *skunks.* Bites and scratches by these animals pose a significant risk for the transmission of infection. If the animal can be captured, it should be put to sleep promptly for examination of the brain by local health authorities. If the animal escapes, rabies immunization should be commenced immediately. Bites of livestock, squirrels, hamsters, gerbils, rabbits, mice, and other rodents almost never require antirabies treatment.

269. What advice should be given to a patient who finds a bat in the bedroom upon waking up?

There are reports of human rabies cases in which a bat encounter with no known direct contact has occurred. Most experts recommend that individuals who may have had contact with a bat during sleep should be given rabies prophylaxis. If the bat is captured and examination of the brain is negative for rabies virus, the vaccination series can be discontinued.

270. What are the features of West Nile virus infection?

West Nile virus is acquired through the bite of an infected mosquito; birds such as crows and jays act as intermediate hosts, and humans are incidental (dead-end) hosts. The majority of infections are asymptomatic. Between 10% and 15% of infected individuals will develop a nonspecific febrile illness, whereas <1% will develop infection of the central nervous system. Altered mental status, focal neurologic deficits, and seizures can occur. Most patients survive. Severe disease and mortality are more likely in the elderly.

271. What virus was most recently identified as a cause of lower respiratory tract infection in children?

Various studies have established that *human metapneumovirus,* a paramyxovirus related to RSV and to avian pneumovirus, is responsible for 5–20% of pediatric lower respiratory tract infections that previously lacked a specific etiologic diagnosis. The pathogen can be detected by PCR of respiratory samples such as nasopharyngeal swabs and nasal washes.

272. What was the source of the 2003 U.S. outbreak of monkeypox?

Monkeypox infection in the U.S. Midwest resulted from the distribution of prairie dogs to a variety of pet stores from a single center in Illinois. The prairie dogs had been housed with Gambian giant rats en route from Africa.

273. What pathogen was responsible for the contamination of the mail in 2001?

Twenty-two patients were infected with *Bacillus anthracis* delivered in the form of a powder that contaminated mail sorting systems in Washington, D.C., and other locations. Eleven individuals contracted the inhalational form of anthrax; five of these patients died. The other 11 patients developed cutaneous anthrax, and all were treated successfully. Numerous people received 60-day courses of ciprofloxacin for prophylaxis.

274. **What is the difference between classic and variant Creutzfeldt-Jakob disease (CJD)?**

CJD is a fatal neurodegenerative disorder and is thought to be caused by prions, which are infectious proteins that are acquired from food or environmental sources. Classic CJD occurs rarely and sporadically and can be transmitted iatrogenically through contaminated neurosurgical instruments. Variant CJD is acquired from the ingestion of meat (especially beef) that is contaminated with infected neural tissue. The variant form of CJD has a comparatively lower age of onset (and death), with the earlier manifestation of psychiatric symptoms. In an effort to prevent variant CJD, a ban on ruminant tissues as cattle feed was enacted by the U.S. Food and Drug Administration in 1997.

275. **What disease is classically associated with attending livestock births?**

Q fever is acquired by the inhalation of aerosols that contain *Coxiella burnetii*, which can be created during parturition in domesticated mammals, including sheep, goats, and cows. Acute infection can cause fever, cough, chills, headache, and hepatitis, but the infected individual may also be asymptomatic.

CHAPTER 12

NEONATOLOGY

Philip Roth, MD, PhD

CLINICAL ISSUES

1. **Should an asymptomatic infant with a single umbilical artery have a screening ultrasound done for renal anomalies?**

   This point has been argued for years. A single umbilical artery is a rare phenomenon. In one study of nearly 35,000 infants, examination of the placenta showed that only 112 (0.32%) had a single umbilical artery. All 112 underwent renal ultrasonography, and 17% had abnormalities (45% of which persisted). In a recent study, a single umbilical artery was detected in 2% of fetuses. Fetuses with a single umbilical artery had significantly more chromosomal (10.3%) and congenital anomalies (27%) than those with two umbilical arteries. Because of the rarity of the condition and the increased association of abnormalities, patients with single umbilical arteries should probably receive a screening renal ultrasound.

   > Bourke WG, Clarke TA, Mathews TG, et al: Isolated single umbilical artery: The case for routine renal screening. Arch Dis Child 68:600–601, 1993.
   > Prucka S, Clemens M, Craven C, McPherson E: Single umbilical artery: What does it mean for the fetus? A case-control analysis of pathologically ascertained cases. Genet Med 6:54–57, 2004.

2. **How does the handling of the umbilical cord at birth affect neonatal hemoglobin concentrations?**

   At the time of birth, the placental vessels may contain up to 33% of the fetal-placental blood volume. Constriction of the umbilical arteries limits blood flow from the infant, but the umbilical vein remains dilated. The extent of drainage from the placenta to the infant via the umbilical vein is very dependent on gravity. The recommendation is to keep the baby at least 20–40 cm below the placenta for approximately 30 seconds before clamping the cord. More elevated positioning or rapid clamping can minimize the placental transfusion and decrease red-cell volume.

   > Brugnara C, Platt OS: The neonatal erythrocyte and its disorders. In Nathan DG, Orkin SH, Ginsburg D, Look AT (eds): Nathan and Oski's Hematology of Infancy and Childhood, 6th ed. Philadelphia, W.B. Saunders, 2003, pp 30–31.

3. **What is the best method of umbilical cord care during the immediate neonatal period?**

   No single method of cord care has been determined to be superior for preventing colonization and infections. Antimicrobial agents, such as bacitracin or triple dye, are commonly used, but there are no efficacy data (other than reduced colonization). Alcohol accelerates the drying of the cord, but it has not been shown to reduce the rates of colonization or omphalitis. The use of topical antibiotics has been shown to delay cord separation. Therefore, simply keeping the cord dry and clean appears to be as safe and effective as using antibiotics.

   > Mullany LC, Darmstadt GL, Tielsch J: Role of antimicrobial applications to the umbilical cord in neonates to prevent bacterial colonization and infection: A review of the evidence. Pediatr Infect Dis J 11:996–1002, 2003.
   > Zupan J, Garner P, Omari AA: Topical umbical cord care at birth. Cochrane Database Syst Rev 3:CD001057, 2004.

4. **Which way does the umbilical cord twist?**
    Usually *counterclockwise*. Coiling of the umbilical cord occurs in approximately 95% of new-borns, and most are twisted in a sinistral manner. Because this helical arrangement is absent in species in which fetuses are arranged longitudinally in a bicornuate uterus, spiraling may result from the mobility of the primate fetus. Noncoiled cords may be associated with an increased likelihood of anomalies. In a recent study, placenta previa was more common in patients with a right umbilical cord twist as compared with a left umbilical cord twist (6.0% versus 1.5%; $p < .05$). There was a trend toward an increased incidence of single umbilical artery in patients with a right umbilical cord twist (2.5% versus 0%; $p = .06$).

    Kalish RB, Hunter T, Sharma G, Baergen RN: Clinical significance of the umbilical cord twist. Am J Obstet Gynecol 189:736–739, 2003.
    Strong TH Jr, Finberg HJ, Mattox JH: Antepartum diagnosis of noncoiled umbilical cords. Am J Obstet Gynecol 170:1729–1733, 1994.

5. **When should a parent begin to worry if an umbilical cord has not fallen off?**
    The umbilical cord generally dries up and sloughs by 2 weeks of life. Delayed separation can be normal up to 45 days. However, because neutrophilic and/or monocytic infiltration appears to play a major role in autodigestion, persistence of the cord beyond 30 days should prompt consideration of an underlying functional abnormality of neutrophils (leukocyte adhesion deficiency) or neutropenia.

    Kemp AS, Lubitz L: Delayed cord separation in alloimmune neutropenia. Arch Dis Child 68:52–53, 1993.
    Roos D, Laws SK: Hematologically important mutations: Leukocyte adhesion deficiency. Blood Cell Mol Dis 6:1000–1004, 2001.

6. **How do you estimate the insertion distance necessary for umbilical catheters?**
    Measuring the distance from the umbilicus to the shoulder (lateral end of clavicle) allows for an estimation of desired length (Table 12-1). Alternatively, insertion distance in centimeters for the following situations is given below:
    - "High" umbilical artery catheter = $[3 \times \text{weight (kg)}] + 9$
    - Umbilical venous catheter = $[\frac{1}{2} \times \text{UAC insertion distance}] + 1$

TABLE 12-1. INSERTION DISTANCE FOR UMBILICAL CATHETERS (CM)

Shoulder to umbilicus	Aortic catheter to diaphragm	Aortic catheter to aortic bifurcation	Venous catheter to right atrium
9	11	5	6
10	12	5	6–7
11	13	6	7
12	14	7	8
13	15	8	8–9
14	16	9	9
15	17	10	10
16	18	10–11	11
17	20	11–12	11–12

Data from Dunn PM: Localization of umbilical catheters by post mortem measurement. Arch Dis Child 41:69–75, 1966.

7. **What are the increased risks of twin pregnancies?**
   - Premature delivery
   - Intrauterine growth retardation, including discordant growth (which may occur in up to one third of twin pregnancies)
   - Increased perinatal mortality, especially for premature, monozygotic, and discordant twins
   - Spontaneous abortion
   - Birth asphyxia
   - Fetal malposition
   - Placental abnormalities (abruptio placentae, placenta previa)
   - Polyhydramnios

8. **Why are monozygotic twins considered higher risk than dizygotic twins?**
   Monozygotic twins (identical twins) arise from the division of a single fertilized egg. Depending on the timing of the division of the single ovum into separate embryos, the amnionic and chorionic membranes can either be shared (if division occurs >8 days after fertilization), separate (if division occurs <72 hours after fertilization), or mixed (separate amnion, shared chorion if division occurs 4–8 days after fertilization). Sharing of the chorion and/or amnion is associated with potential problems of vascular anastomoses (and possible twin-twin transfusions), cord entanglements, and congenital anomalies. These problems increase the risk of intrauterine growth retardation and perinatal death. **Dizygotic twins**, however, result from two separately fertilized ova and, as such, usually have a separate amnion and chorion.

9. **Who is at higher risk, the first- or second-born twin?**
   The *second-born twin* has a twofold to fourfold increased risk of developing respiratory distress syndrome and is more likely to be asphyxiated. However, the risks for sepsis and necrotizing enterocolitis may be increased in first-born twins.

10. **How extensive is insensible water loss in preterm infants?**
    Insensible water loss is the loss of water through the lungs during respiration and from the skin by evaporation. A rough guide to the amount of insensible loss in mL/kg/day for infants in humidified isolettes is given in Table 12-2.

TABLE 12-2.	INSENSIBLE LOSS (ML/KG/DAY) FOR INFANTS IN HUMIDIFIED ISOLETTES					
	Body Weight (gm)					
Age (days)	500–750	751–1,000	1,001–1,250	1,251–1,500	1,501–1,750	1,751–2,000
0–7	100	65	55	40	20	15
7–14	80	60	50	40	30	20

Data from Avery GB, Fletcher MA, MacDonald MG: Neonatology: Pathophysiology and Management of the Newborn. Lippincott Williams & Wilkins, Philadelphia, 1999, p 348.

11. **What factors affect insensible water loss?**
    - **Increase:** Prematurity, activity, fever, radiant warmer, phototherapy, and skin breakdown/defect
    - **Decrease:** High humidity and mechanical ventilation (with humidified air)

12. **Do infants receiving phototherapy require additional fluids?**

Unless there is evidence of dehydration, routine intravenous fluid or other supplementation of term and near-term infants is not necessary. Preterm infants weighing <1,500 gm should receive a 25% increment while receiving phototherapy.

Subcommittee on Hyperbilirubinemia: Management of hyperbilirubinemia in the newborn infant 35 or more weeks of gestation. Pediatrics 114:297–316, 2004.

13. **You are informed during sign-out rounds that a newborn is suspected of having funisitis. Where should you look for that infection?**

Funisitis is inflammation of the umbilical cord vessels and Wharton's jelly, and it has been described as either an acute exudative or subacute necrotizing process that accompanies chorioamnionitis. The predominant organisms that have been identified as etiologic agents are gram-negative bacteria, including *Escherichia coli*, *Klebsiella*, and *Pseudomonas*. Gram-positive organisms (e.g., streptococci, staphylococci) and candidal species are less-commonly responsible.

14. **Which infants require ophthalmologic evaluation for retinopathy of prematurity (ROP)?**

The American Academy of Pediatrics recommends that an individual experienced in neonatal ophthalmology and indirect ophthalmoscopy examine the retinas of all neonates with a birth weight of <1,500 gm or a gestational age of <28 weeks and of those selected infants weighing between 1,500 and 2,000 gm who have had unstable clinical courses, placing them at increased risk. Unless full retinal vascularization is noted on examination, all infants should undergo two examinations, with the first performed at 4–6 weeks postnatal age or 31–32 weeks postconceptional age, whichever is later.

American Academy of Pediatrics, American Association for Pediatric Ophthalmology and Strabismus: Screening examination of premature infants for retinopathy of prematurity. Pediatrics 108:809–811, 2001.

15. **What are the stages of ROP?**

Stage I: Line of demarcation separates vascular and avascular retina
Stage II: Ridging of line of demarcation as a result of scar formation
Stage III: Extraretinal fibrovascular proliferation present (In addition, in stages II and III, the term *plus disease* refers to active inflammation as manifested by tortuosity of retinal vessels, which increases the risk of progression of ROP.)
Stage IV: Subtotal retinal detachment
Stage V: Complete retinal detachment

16. **What are the indications for cryotherapy or laser therapy among patients with ROP?**

In a multicenter trial by the Cryotherapy for ROP Cooperative Group, "threshold" disease, which was defined as a level of severity at which the risk of blindness approaches 50%, was chosen for treatment. This diagnosis required the presence of at least five contiguous or eight cumulative 30° sectors (clock hours) of stage III ROP (in zone 1 or 2) and the presence of plus disease. In a recent multicenter trial, study results indicated that earlier intervention in certain high-risk prethreshold eyes resulted in improved vision.

Hardy RJ, Good WV, Dobson V, et al; Early Treatment for Retinopathy of Prematurity Cooperative Group: Multicenter trial of early treatment for retinopathy of prematurity: Study design. Control Clin Trials 3:311–325, 2004.

17. **If maternal drug abuse is suspected, which specimen from the infant is most accurate for detecting exposure?**

Although urine has traditionally been tested when maternal drug abuse is a possibility, **meconium** has a greater sensitivity than urine and positive findings that persist longer. It may contain metabolites gathered over multiple weeks as compared with urine, which represents more recent exposure. It is important to remember that maternal self-reporting is notoriously inaccurate as an indicator of drug use. In addition, in some states, informed maternal consent must be given before drug screening of the neonate, which can hinder diagnosis and surveillance.

Ostrea EM, Jr. Brady M, Gause S, et al: Drug screening of newborns by meconium analysis: A large-scale, prospective, epidemiologic study. Pediatrics 89:107–113, 1992.

18. **What are the manifestations of drug withdrawal in the neonate?**
The signs and symptoms of drug withdrawal in the neonate can be remembered by using the acronym **WITHDRAWAL:**
    - **W** = **W**akefulness
    - **I** = **I**rritability
    - **T** = **T**remulousness, temperature variation, tachypnea
    - **H** = **H**yperactivity, high-pitched persistent cry, hyperacusis, hyperreflexia, hypertonus
    - **D** = **D**iarrhea, diaphoresis, disorganized suck
    - **R** = **R**ub marks, respiratory distress, rhinorrhea
    - **A** = **A**pneic attacks, autonomic dysfunction
    - **W** = **W**eight loss or failure to gain weight
    - **A** = **A**lkalosis (respiratory)
    - **L** = **L**acrimation

Committee on Drugs: Neonatal drug withdrawal. Pediatrics 72:896, 1983.

19. **What bone is the most frequently fractured in the newborn?**
The **clavicle**. This injury, which stems from excessive traction during delivery, generally results in a greenstick fracture (Fig. 12-1).

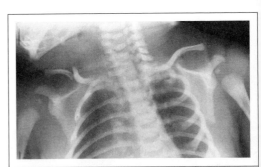

Figure 12-1. X-ray of right clavicular fracture. (From Clark DA: Atlas of Neonatology. Philadelphia, W.B. Saunders, 2000, p 8.)

20. **Should palpable lymph nodes in a newborn be considered pathologic?**
No. Up to 25% of newborns have palpable nodes, particularly in the inguinal and cervical regions. By 1 month of age, the prevalence is nearly 40%.

Bamji M, Stone RK, Kaul A, et al: Palpable lymph nodes in healthy newborns and infants. Pediatrics 78:573–575, 1986.

21. **How valuable is the footprinting of newborns for the permanent medical record?**
This is a time-honored tradition that is, alas, of minimal benefit. Although the American Academy of Pediatrics recommended discontinuing the practice in 1983 as a result of the fact that, in nearly 80% of cases, the quality was so poor as to render the print useless, up to 80% of U.S. hospitals continue footprinting as a means of identification. Footprinting is legally mandated only in New York State. Recently, DNA "fingerprinting" has been introduced, but it is primarily available through private commercial ventures.

22. **What are the two most common causes of fetal death?**
Chromosomal abnormalities (especially during early pregnancy) and **congenital malformations**.

23. **How long should a healthy term newborn remain hospitalized?**
This is a controversial issue. Although some neonatal problems do not appear until several days of age, most are apparent by 6 hours of life. Nevertheless, there is an increased frequency of hospital readmissions, most commonly for hyperbilirubinemia, in patients discharged at <48 hours (some studies even suggest 72 hours) and especially in those discharged at <24 hours.

> Maisels MJ, Kring E: Length of stay, jaundice, and hospital readmission. Pediatrics 101:995–998, 1998.
> Braveman P, Kessel W, Egerter S, Richmond J: Early discharge and evidence-based practice. Good science and good judgment. JAMA 278:334–336, 1997.

24. **What are Spitzer's laws of neonatology?**
    1. The more stable a baby appears to be, the more likely he will "crump" that day.
    2. The nicer the parents, the sicker the baby.
    3. The likelihood of bronchopulmonary dysplasia (BPD) is directly proportional to the number of physicians involved in the care of that baby.
    4. The longer a patient is discussed during rounds, the more certain it is that no one has the faintest idea of what is going on or what to do.
    5. The sickest infant in the nursery can always be discerned by the fact that he or she is being cared for by the newest, most inexperienced nursing orienteer.
    6. The surest way to have an infant linger interminably is to inform the parents that death is imminent.
    7. The more miraculous the "save," the more likely that you will be sued for something totally inconsequential.
    8. If they are not breathin', they may be seizin'.
    9. Antibiotics should always be continued for ____ days. (Fill in the blank with any number 1–21.)
    10. If you cannot figure out what is going on with a baby, call the surgeons. They won't figure it out either, but they will sure as hell do something about it.

> From Spitzer A: Spitzer's laws of neonatology. Clin Pediatr 20:733, 1981.

25. **What is Throckmorton's sign?**
Throckmorton's sign is the extension of the suspensory ligament of the penis before micturition in newborn infants. However, thousands of house officers have come to believe that this sign relates to the radiographic finding in a male in which the penis points to the side of pathology.

THE DELIVERY ROOM

26. **What is the clinical significance of fetal decelerations?**
The character or pattern of decelerations often seen during fetal heart rate monitoring can be a valuable indicator of fetal well-being or need for intervention.
- **Early decelerations:** Associated with head compression; usually of no consequence
- **Variable decelerations:** Observed with cord compression; may indicate fetal distress when prolonged and associated with bradycardia
- **Late decelerations:** Indicate uteroplacental insufficiency and hypoxemia; both variable and late decelerations may be associated with acidosis and fetal compromise

27. **How sensitive is fetal heart rate monitoring for detecting fetal asphyxia?**
Abnormal decelerations have a poor positive-predictive value, with only 15–25% being associated with a significantly compromised fetus. However, normal studies have a much higher predictive value with regard to ongoing fetal well-being.

28. **What is an acceptable scalp pH for the fetus?**

    Fetal scalp sampling to measure blood pH is used in conjunction with electronic fetal heart rate monitoring to assess fetal well-being during labor (Table 12-3). The range of acceptable values for fetal pH is broad. Clinically significant acidemia is defined as a scalp pH of <7.2. A scalp pH of >7.25 is considered normal. Values between 7.0 and 7.25 are considered borderline and warrant further sampling. A low pH does not predict subsequent cerebral palsy.

TABLE 12-3. NORMAL FETAL SCALP BLOOD VALUES IN LABOR			
	Early First Stage	**Late First Stage**	**Second Stage**
pH	7.33 ± 0.03	7.32 ± 0.02	7.29 ± 0.04
PCO_2 (mmHg)	44 ± 4.05	42 ± 5.1	46.3 ± 4.2
PO_2 (mmHg)	21.8 ± 2	21.3 ± 2.1	16.5 ± 1.4
Bicarbonate (mmol/L)	20.1 ± 1	19.1 ± 2.1	17 ± 2
Base excess (mmol/L)	3.9 ± 1.9	4.1 ± 2.5	6.4 ± 1.8

Data from Gilstrap LC: Fetal acid-base balance. In Creasy RK, Resnik R (eds): Maternal-Fetal Medicine, 4th ed. Philadelphia, W.B. Saunders, 2004, p 431.

29. **Is length of labor the same for male and female babies?**

    No. Labor length for boys is about 1 hour longer than that of girls.

30. **How long has meconium been present in the amniotic fluid if an infant has evidence of meconium staining?**

    Gross staining of the infant is a surface phenomenon that is proportional to the length of exposure and meconium concentration. With heavy meconium, staining of the umbilical cord begins in as little as 15 minutes; with light meconium, it occurs after 1 hour. Yellow staining of the newborn's toenails requires 4–6 hours. Yellow staining of the vernix caseosa takes about 12–14 hours.

    Miller PW, Coen RW, Benirschke K: Dating the time interval from meconium passage to birth. Obstet Gynecol 66:459–462, 1985.

31. **Is meconium staining a good marker for neonatal asphyxia?**

    No. Because 10–20% of all deliveries have in utero passage of meconium, meconium staining alone is not a good marker for neonatal asphyxia.

32. **If meconium is noted before or during the time of delivery, what is the recommended course of action?**

    Regardless of the nature of the fluid, the obstetrician should suction the infant's oro- and nasopharynx before delivery of the shoulders. An 8- or 10-Fr flexible catheter is much more effective than simple bulb syringing. The next course of action depends on the clinical appearance of the baby. If the infant is crying and vigorous, visualization of the larynx and intubation is not necessary. In a depressed infant, the infant's pharynx should be suctioned, and this should be followed by endotracheal intubation with suctioning below the vocal cords.

    Gelfand SL, Fanaroff JM, Walsh MC: Meconium stained fluid: Approach to the mother and the baby. Pediatr Clin North Am 51:655–667, 2004.

33. **During asphyxia, how is primary apnea distinguished from secondary apnea?**
A regular sequence of events occurs when an infant is asphyxiated. Initially, gasping respiratory efforts increase in depth and frequency for up to 3 minutes, and this is followed by approximately 1 minute of primary apnea. If oxygen (along with stimulation) is provided during the apneic period, respiratory function spontaneously returns. If asphyxia continues, gasping then resumes for a variable period of time, terminating with the "last gasp" and followed by secondary apnea. During secondary apnea, the only way to restore respiratory function is with positive-pressure ventilation (PPV) and high concentrations of oxygen.
    Thus, a linear relationship exists between the duration of asphyxia and the recovery of respiratory function after resuscitation. The longer the artificial ventilation is delayed after the "last gasp," the longer it will take to resuscitate the infant. However, clinically, the two conditions are indistinguishable.

34. **How does one estimate the size of the endotracheal tube required for resuscitation?**
See Table 12-4.

TABLE 12-4. ENDOTRACHEAL TUBES NEEDED FOR RESUSCITATION		
Tube size (internal diameter in mm)	Weight (gm)	Gestational age (weeks)
2.5	<1,000	<28
3.0	1,001–2,000	28–34
3.5	2,001–3,000	34–38
3.5–4.0	>3,000	>38

Adapted from Hertz D: Principles of neonatal resuscitation. In Polin RA, Yoder MC, Burg FD (eds): Workbook in Practical Neonatology, 3rd ed. Philadelphia, W.B. Saunders, 2001, p 13.

35. **What is the "7-8-9" rule?**
The "7-8-9" rule is an estimate of the length (in cm) that an oral endotracheal tube should be inserted into a 1-, 2-, or 3-kg infant, respectively. A variation of this rule is the tip-to-lip rule of adding 6 to the weight in kilograms of the infant to determine the insertion distance. With good visualization, the tube should be inserted 1.0–1.5 cm below the vocal cords. Tube placement should always be verified radiographically.

36. **When should epinephrine be given during a resuscitation in the delivery room?**
In a depressed infant with gasping or absent respirations, 100% oxygen should be given via PPV. Depending on the extent of asphyxia (and depression of heart rate to <60 bpm), cardiac compressions are usually initiated within 30 seconds. If there is no response (i.e., increased heart rate to >60 bpm) after at least 30 seconds of PPV with 100% oxygen and chest compressions, epinephrine is indicated. Epinephrine (1:10,000) can be given intravenously or via the umbilical vein or an endotracheal tube at a dose of 0.1–0.3 mL/kg.

37. **When is sodium bicarbonate administered in resuscitation?**
If there is no response to epinephrine in a severely asphyxiated infant (with continued apnea and a heart rate of <60 bpm), sodium bicarbonate (and/or a volume expander) should be considered. If an infant is being adequately ventilated, the partial correction of metabolic acidosis may improve pulmonary blood flow and improve oxygenation. Half-strength (4.2% solution or 0.5 mEq/L) bicarbonate is preferable, given in a dose of 2 mEq/kg slowly over 2–5 minutes.

38. **Are there complications of sodium bicarbonate therapy in infants?**
The relative risks of sodium bicarbonate therapy in infants are related to dosage (higher > lower), rapidity of administration (faster > slower), and osmolality (higher > lower). Physiologic complications include a transient increase in $PaCO_2$ and fall in PaO_2. The sudden expansion of blood volume and an increase in cerebral blood flow may increase the risk of periventricular-intraventricular hemorrhage (IVH) in preterm infants (unproven).

39. **If the newborn is stabilized and the extent of acidosis determined by an arterial blood gas, how is the therapeutic correction calculated?**

$$HCO_3 \text{ (mEq)} = \text{Base deficit (mEq/L)} \times 0.3 \text{ L/kg} \times \text{body weight (kg)}$$

Generally, it is safest to correct half of the base deficit initially and then reassess acid-base status to determine if further correction is necessary. Under optimal circumstances, sodium bicarbonate should be infused in small doses over 20–30 minutes as a dilute solution (0.5 mEq/mL).

40. **Should umbilical arterial catheters be kept in a "low" or "high" position?**
Umbilical catheters kept in a low position (L3–L5) are associated with a somewhat higher incidence of lower-limb blanching and cyanosis as compared with high lines (T6–T10). In addition, high lines are associated with a lower incidence of clinical vascular complications (e.g., ischemic events, aortic thrombosis) without an increase in any adverse sequelae. Periventricular-intraventricular hemorrhage, death, and necrotizing enterocolitis did not occur with greater frequency in low versus high catheters. Therefore, high catheters should be used whenever possible.

> Barrington KJ: Umbilical artery catheters in the newborn: Effects of catheter materials. Cochrane Database Syst Rev 2:CD000949, 2000.

41. **After a "traumatic" delivery, what are the commonly injured systems?**
   - **Cranial injuries:** Caput succedaneum, subconjunctival hemorrhage, cephalohematoma, subgaleal hematoma, skull fractures, intracranial hemorrhage, cerebral edema
   - **Spinal injuries:** Spinal cord transection
   - **Peripheral nerve injuries:** Brachial palsy (Erb-Duchenne paralysis, Klumpke's paralysis), phrenic nerve and facial nerve paralysis
   - **Visceral injuries:** Liver rupture or hematoma, splenic rupture, adrenal hemorrhage
   - **Skeletal injuries:** Fractures of the clavicle, femur, and humerus

42. **Who was Virginia Apgar?**
Virginia Apgar, an anesthesiologist at Columbia Presbyterian Medical Center in New York City, introduced the Apgar scoring system in 1953 to assess the newborn infant's response to the stress of labor and delivery.

43. **How does one remember the Apgar score?**
   A = **A**ppearance (pink, mottled, or blue)
   P = **P**ulse (>100, <100, or 0 bpm)
   G = **G**rimace (response to suctioning of the nose and mouth)
   A = **A**ctivity (flexed arms and legs, extended limbs, or limp)
   R = **R**espiratory effort (crying, gasping, or no respiratory activity)
   Each category is assigned a rating of 0, 1, or 2 points, with a total score of 10 indicating the best possible condition.

44. **Is a low Apgar score alone sufficient to diagnose a neonate as asphyxiated?**
No. It is not acceptable to label an infant as asphyxiated simply because of a low Apgar score. Typically, a sentinel hypoxic event before or during labor is followed by fetal bradycardia or

absent variability in the presence of variable and/or late decelerations If asphyxiated, neonates typically have a profound metabolic acidosis and demonstrate abnormalities within 72 hours of birth in multiple organ systems. Signs referable to the central nervous system (CNS) are often most prominent. The cardinal features of hypoxic-ischemic encephalopathy include seizures, alterations of consciousness, and abnormalities of tone. Disorders of reflexes, respiratory pattern, oculovestibular responses, and autonomic function are less-significant components of this entity. Early imaging studies may also show evidence of acute nonfocal cerebral abnormality.

Committee on Fetus and Newborn: Use and abuse of the Apgar score. Pediatrics 98:141–142, 1996.

Hankins GDV, Speer M: Neonatal encephalopathy and cerebral palsy: Defining the pathogenesis and pathophysiology. Obstet Gynecol 102:628–636, 2003.

Leuthner SR, Das U: Low Apgar scores and the definition of birth asphyxia. Pediatr Clin North Am 51: 737–745, 2004.

45. **When should neonatal resuscitation be stopped?**
Although each case should be considered individually, the discontinuation of efforts is generally appropriate after 15 minutes of absent heart rate despite adequate resuscitative measures. Current data suggest that asystole for >10 minutes is highly unlikely to result in survival or survival without severe disability.

American Heart Association: Neonatal Resuscitation Textbook. Dallas, American Heart Association, 2000, pp 7–20.

KEY POINTS: DELIVERY ROOM AND RESUSCITATION ✓

1. Infants born of multiple gestations contribute a disproportionate share of neonatal complications and neonatal intensive care unit admissions.

2. Apgar scores at 1 and 5 minutes do not predict long-term outcome.

3. Sodium bicarbonate should never be administered without first ensuring adequate ventilation, whether spontaneous or artificial.

4. Every delivery room resuscitation should follow the same algorithm and proceed systematically on the basis of clinical assessment at each step.

DEVELOPMENT AND GROWTH

46. **What is the best way to assess gestational age in the fetus?**
Nägele's rule, which dates pregnancy from the first day of the last menstrual period, has historically been the most reliable way to assess gestational age. However, **ultrasound** measurements done between 5 and 20 weeks of gestation can predict gestational age quite accurately. Before 12 weeks of gestation, crown-rump length is the measurement of choice; beyond 12 weeks, biparietal diameter is the preferred study. During later gestation, the accuracy of fetal age determination is improved by the assessment of multiple variables (e.g., femur length, abdominal circumference, biparietal diameter) and by serial determinations. Maternal dates should always be used as the "gold standard" unless ultrasound studies are highly discrepant. Estimates of **uterine size**, which approximate gestational age from 16–38 weeks, may also be clinically useful.

47. **What features constitute the biophysical profile?**
The biophysical profile is a scoring system that assesses fetal well-being before birth. Five variables are assessed:
1. Fetal breathing movements
2. Gross body movements

3. Fetal tone
4. Reactive fetal heart rate
5. Qualitative amniotic fluid volume
   Normal results equate to 2 points per variable, for a possible total of 10 points.

48. **What factors influence biophysical profile performance?**
    - Drugs (sedatives, theophylline, cocaine, and indomethacin)
    - Cigarette smoking, hyperglycemia, and hypoglycemia
    - Spontaneous premature rupture of membranes
    - Fetal arrhythmia
    - Periodic decelerations
    - Acute disasters (e.g., abruptio placentae)

49. **What is the first bone in the human fetus to ossify?**
    The **clavicle.** In the long bones, the process of ossification occurs in the primary centers of ossification in the diaphysis during the embryonic period of fetal development. Although the femora are the first long bones to show traces of ossification, the clavicles, which develop initially by intramembranous ossification, begin to ossify before any other bones in the body.

50. **What external characteristics are useful for estimating gestational age?**
    See Table 12-5.

TABLE 12-5. EXTERNAL GESTATIONAL AGE CHARACTERISTICS				
External characteristics	**Gestational age**			
	28 weeks	**32 weeks**	**36 weeks**	**40 weeks**
Ear cartilage	Pinna soft, remains folded	Pinna slightly harder but remains folded	Pinna harder, springs back	Pinna firm, stands erect from head
Breast tissue	None	None	1–2 mm nodule	6–7 mm nodule
External genitalia				
Male	Testes undescended, smooth scrotum	Testes in inguinal canal, few scrotal rugae	Testes high in scrotum, more scrotal rugae	Testes descended, pendulous scrotum covered with rugae
Female	Prominent clitoris, small, widely separated labia	Prominent clitoris, larger separated labia	Clitoris less prominent, labia majora covers labia minora	Clitoris covered by labia majora
Plantar surface	Smooth	1–2 anterior creases	2–3 anterior creases	Creases cover sole

From Volpe JJ: Neurology of the Newborn, 4th ed. Philadelphia, W.B. Saunders, 2001, p 104.

51. **At what gestational age does pupillary reaction to light develop?**
Pupillary reaction to light may appear as early as 29 weeks into gestation but is not consistently present until approximately 32 weeks.

52. **At what gestational age does a sense of smell develop?**
By 32 weeks of gestation, normal premature infants respond to concentrated odor.

53. **When does the fetal heart begin to contract in utero?**
Contractions begin by the 22nd day of gestation. These contractions resemble peristaltic waves and begin in the sinus venosus. By the end of the fourth week, they result in the unidirectional flow of blood.

54. **How does fetal circulation differ from neonatal circulation?**
   - Intra- and extracardiac shunts are present (i.e., placenta, ductus venosus, foramen ovale, and ductus arteriosus).
   - The two ventricles work in parallel rather than in series.
   - The right ventricle pumps against a higher resistance than the left ventricle.
   - Blood flow to the lung is only a fraction of the right ventricular output.
   - The lung extracts oxygen from the blood instead of providing oxygen for it.
   - The lung continually secretes a fluid into the respiratory passages.
   - The liver is the first organ to receive maternal substances (e.g., oxygen, glucose, amino acids).
   - The placenta is the major route of gas exchange, excretion, and acquisition of essential fetal chemicals.
   - The placenta provides a low resistance circuit.

   Allen HD, Gutgesell HP, Clark EB, Driscoll DJ (eds): Moss and Adams' Heart Disease in Infants, Children, and Adolescents, 6th ed. Baltimore, Williams & Wilkins, 2001, pp 41–63.

55. **How does postmaturity differ from dysmaturity?**
   - **Postmature:** An infant born of a postterm pregnancy (>42 weeks of gestation)
   - **Dysmature:** Features of placental insufficiency are present (e.g., loss of subcutaneous fat and muscle mass; meconium staining of the amniotic fluid, skin, and nails)

56. **What is the normal rate of head growth in the preterm infant?**
The rate is approximately 0.5–1 cm/wk during the first 2–4 months of life. An increase in the circumference of the head of approximately 2 cm in 1 week should raise a suspicion of CNS pathology, such as hydrocephalus. However, some premature infants may experience rapid "catch-up" head growth after significant early stress or illness. The ratio of body length to head circumference may be used to distinguish normal from abnormal head growth. A ratio of 1.42–1.48 is reportedly normal, whereas a low ratio of 1.12–1.32 indicates relative or absolute macrocephaly.

57. **How is the ponderal index used to classify growth-retarded infants?**

$$\text{Ponderal index} = \frac{\text{weight (gm)}}{(\text{length [cm]})^3} \times 100$$

This index has been used to estimate the adequacy of intrauterine fetal nutrition. Values of <2.0 between 29 and 37 weeks of gestation and of 2.2 beyond 37 weeks of gestation have been associated with fetal malnutrition. Growth-retarded infants with low ponderal indices also appear to be at increased risk for the development of neonatal hypoglycemia. Maternal conditions associated with a low ponderal index (fetal malnutrition) include poor maternal weight gain, lack of prenatal care, preeclampsia, and chronic maternal illness.

58. **What morbidities (short- and long-term) are known to occur more frequently in growth-retarded babies?**
    - **Short-term morbidities:** Perinatal asphyxia, meconium aspiration, fasting hypoglycemia, alimented hyperglycemia, polycythemia-hyperviscosity, and immunodeficiency
    - **Long-term morbidities:** Poor developmental outcome and altered postnatal growth.
      Most studies demonstrate normal intelligence and developmental quotients in small for gestational age (SGA) infants, although there seems to be a higher incidence of behavioral and learning problems. The presence or absence of severe perinatal asphyxia is extremely important for predicting later intellectual and neurologic function. Recent population studies suggest an increased likelihood of hypertension, hypercholesterolemia, and diabetes mellitus in adulthood.

      Strauss RS: Adult functional outcome of those born small for gestational age: Twenty-six year follow-up of the 1970 British Birth Cohort. JAMA 283:625–632, 2000.

59. **When do premature infants "catch up" on growth charts?**
    Most catch-up growth takes place during the first 2 years of life, with maximal growth rates occurring between 36 and 40 weeks after conception. Little catch-up growth occurs after the chronologic age of 3 years. Approximately 15% of infants born prematurely remain below normal weight at 3 years of age.

60. **What is the outcome for extremely premature babies?**
    Although outcomes differ by centers, summaries of data indicate that severe disability occurs in about 33% of infants born at 23 weeks of gestation, 25% of infants born at 24 weeks of gestation, and 20% of infants born at 25 weeks of gestation. However, in infants who do not suffer early IVH with subsequent CNS injury, cognitive function improves between 3 and 8 years of age. Nonetheless, infants born before the 29 weeks of gestation represent <1% of all births but 30% of all cases of cerebral palsy.

      March of Dimes Birth Defects Foundation: www.modimes.org.
      Ment LR, Vohr B, Allan W, et al: Change in cognitive function over time in very low birth weight infants. JAMA 289:705–711, 2003.

GASTROINTESTINAL ISSUES

61. **When does the newborn infant's stomach begin to secrete acid?**
    The pH of gastric fluid in newborns is usually neutral or slightly acidic and decreases shortly after birth. pH values are <3 by 6–8 hours of age and then increase again during the second week of life. Preterm infants frequently demonstrate gastric pH values of >7.

62. **When is meconium usually passed after birth?**
    Most infants pass some meconium during the first 12 hours of life. Overall, 99% of term infants and 95% of premature infants pass meconium by 48 hours of life. However, the smallest of premature infants may have a delayed passage of meconium as a result of the relative immaturity of rectal sphincteric reflexes.

63. **What differentiates meconium ileus from meconium plug syndrome?**
    - **Meconium ileus:** Obstruction of the distal ileum occurs as a result of thick, tenacious concretions of inspissated meconium. A barium enema may reveal a microcolon, and 25% of cases have associated intestinal atresia as a result of intrauterine obstruction. Meconium ileus is a common presentation of cystic fibrosis during the newborn period.
    - **Meconium plug syndrome:** This condition presents symptoms of either the delayed passage of meconium or intestinal obstruction. Barium enema usually demonstrates a normal-caliber colon with multiple filling defects. Small preterm infants, infants of diabetic mothers, and infants

born to mothers who received magnesium sulfate are especially likely to develop meconium plug syndrome. There is also an increased frequency of cystic fibrosis among infants with meconium plug syndrome, although this is much less than that seen among infants with meconium ileus.

64. **After an asphyxial event, how long should feeding be delayed?**
During an asphyxial event, vasoconstriction of the mesenteric vessels can result in intestinal ischemia. Because of the relationship between ischemia and the incidence of necrotizing enterocolitis, feedings should be delayed for 2–3 days to allow for repair of the intestinal mucosa.

65. **How is gastroschisis differentiated from omphalocele in the newborn infant?**
Both are ventral wall defects, yet their pathogenesis and prognosis differ markedly (Table 12-6).

TABLE 12-6. GASTROSCHISIS VERSUS OMPHALOCELE IN NEWBORN INFANTS		
	Gastroschisis	Omphalocele
Incidence	1 in 50,000 births	1 in 5,000 births
Location of defect	Right paraumbilical	Central umbilical
Umbilical cord insertion	Normal	Apex of sac
Herniation of liver	Rare	Common
Extraintestinal anomalies	Rare	Common
Chromosomal abnormalities	Rare	Common

66. **Which conditions are associated with intra-abdominal calcifications?**
Meconium peritonitis and **intra-abdominal tumors** are the most common disorders associated with intra-abdominal calcifications in the neonate. The calcifications of meconium peritonitis are streaky or plaque-like and occur over the abdominal surface of the diaphragm or along the flanks. Intraintestinal calcifications appear as small round densities that follow the course of the intestine and occur in association with intestinal stenoses, atresias, and aganglionosis. Intra abdominal calcifications have also been observed in infants with adrenal hemorrhages and congenital infections.

67. **What is necrotizing enterocolitis (NEC)?**
NEC is a necrotizing inflammatory intestinal disorder that is the most common acquired gastrointestinal emergency in newborns. Signs and symptoms include abdominal distention, increasing gastric residuals, stool with blood, erythema of the abdominal wall, and lethargy.

68. **Are positive blood cultures common in babies with NEC?**
Approximately 25% will have a positive blood culture at the time of diagnosis.

69. **What are the most important risk factors for NEC in preterm infants?**
In an analysis of 15,072 neonates born at 98 centers over a 2-year period, the most important variables associated with NEC were **gestational age** and **birth weight**. Apgar score was not related. Other variables associated with an increased risk of NEC included the use of a ventilator on the first day of life and exposure to both glucocorticoids and indomethacin during the first week of life. Delivery by cesarean section and the use of breast milk were associated with a lower risk of surgical NEC.

Guthrie SO, Gordon PV, Thomas V, et al: Necrotizing enterocolitis among neonates in the United States. J Perinatology 23:278–285, 2003

70. **Is pneumatosis intestinalis pathognomonic for NEC?**
No. Pneumatosis intestinalis can be seen in various other conditions, including Hirschsprung's disease, pseudomembranous enterocolitis, neonatal ulcerative colitis, and ischemic bowel disease. However, it is a characteristic finding in 85% of patients with NEC. Dark, concentric rings within the bowel wall represent hydrogen as a byproduct of bacterial metabolism (Fig. 12-2).

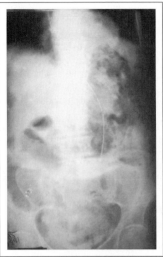

71. **Is it safe to feed infants with umbilical, arterial, or venous catheters?**
The association of umbilical arterial catheters with NEC is weak. In a recent survey of 549 neonatal intensive care units, 92% of medical directors believed that it was safe to provide trophic feedings with an umbilical venous catheter in place, and 88% practiced this most of the time. Seventy-nine percent of medical directors used trophic feedings with an umbilical arterial catheter in place most or some of the time.

Tiffany KF, Burke BL, Collins-Odoms C, Oelberg DG: Current practice regarding the enteral feeding of high-risk newborns with umbilical catheters in situ. Pediatrics 112:20–23, 2003.

Figure 12-2. Pneumatosis intestinalis. X-ray of the abdomen shows extensive changes of linear and bubbly forms. (From Katz DS, Math KR, Groskin SA: Radiology Secrets. Philadelphia, Hanley & Belfus, 1998, p 114.)

72. **How long should infants with NEC receive nothing by mouth?**
Infants with true NEC (radiographic or surgical evidence) should continue to receive nothing by mouth for a minimum of 2–3 weeks. Infants in whom the diagnosis is suspected but not proved should be treated conservatively; many of these infants may be fed after 3–7 days.

73. **Does the feeding of immunoglobulin to infants or the use of prophylaxis prevent NEC?**
The evidence does not support the administration of oral immunoglobulin for the prevention of NEC. There are no randomized controlled trials of oral immunoglobulin A alone for the prevention of NEC.

Foster J, Cole M: Oral immunoglobulin for preventing necrotizing enterocolitis in preterm and low birth-weight neonates. Cochrane Database Syst Rev 1:CD001816, 2004.

74. **Does the prophylactic administration of antibiotics prevent NEC?**
In a meta-analysis of five relevant trials, the administration of enteral antibiotics resulted in a statistically significant reduction in the incidences of NEC and NEC deaths. One study found an increased incidence of colonization with resistant bacteria. Because of the concerns about the development of resistant flora, enteral antibiotics should not be used at this time.

Bury RG, Tudehope D: Enteral antibiotics for preventing necrotizing enterocolitis in low birthweight or preterm infants. Cochrane Database Syst Rev 1:CD000405, 2001.

75. **What are the proven ways to decrease the incidence of NEC?**
There are no proven ways to prevent NEC. However, data support the following interventions: cohorting of infants during epidemics, breast-milk feedings, cautious advancement of feedings, antenatal steroids, and restriction of fluid intake.

76. **How is NEC classified?**
    - **Stage 1 (suspected NEC):** Signs of sepsis, feeding intolerance, ± bright red blood per rectum
    - **Stage 2 (proven NEC):** All of the above, pneumatosis, ± portal vein gas, ± metabolic acidosis, ± ascites
    - **Stage 3 (advanced NEC):** All of the above, clinical instability, definite ascites, ± pneumoperitoneum

    Walsh MC, Kleigman RM: Necrotizing enterocolitis: treatment based on staging criteria. Pediatr Clin North Am 33:179–201, 1986.

77. **Does the rapid advancement of feedings cause NEC?**
    Retrospective studies suggest an association. A prospective trial by Rayyis and colleagues comparing 15 cc/kg/day with 35 cc/kg/day did not demonstrate increased risk. In a recent prospective trial, Berseth and colleagues compared infants maintained on trophic feeds (20 mL/kg for 10 days) with those advanced on feeds (20 mL/kg/day), and they demonstrated a higher risk of NEC in infants who were advanced on feeds. However, infants fed advancing volumes reached full oral feedings sooner, required fewer central lines, and were discharged sooner.

    Berseth CL, Bisquera JA, Paje VU: Prolonging small feeding volumes early in life decreases the incidence of necrotizing enterocolitis in very low birth weight infants. Pediatrics 111:529–534, 2003.
    Rayyis SF, Ambalavanan N, Wright L, Carlo WA: Randomized trial of "slow" versus "fast" feed advancements on the incidence of necrotizing enterocolitis in very low birth weight infants. J Pediatr 134:293–297, 1999.

78. **How is the volume of gastric aspirate helpful for the diagnosis of intestinal obstruction in a newborn?**
    A large aspirate during the first 15 minutes after birth suggests obstruction. In normal-term newborns, the mean gastric aspirate is about 5 mL. In newborns with obstruction (e.g., duodenal atresia, jejunal atresia, annular pancreas), the mean aspirate is approximately 60 mL. Any gastric aspirate of >20 mL should be viewed as suspicious.

    Britton JR, Britton HL: Gastric aspirate volume at birth as an indication of congenital intestinal obstruction. Acta Pediatr 84:945–946, 1995.

HEMATOLOGIC ISSUES

79. **When does the switch from fetal to adult hemoglobin synthesis occur in the neonate?**
    The switch from the production of hemoglobin F to hemoglobin A begins in a very programmed fashion in the fetus and neonate at approximately 32 weeks of gestation. At birth, approximately 50–65% of hemoglobin is type F.

80. **Does the definition of anemia vary by gestational age?**
    For the term infant, most authorities consider a venous blood hemoglobin of <13 gm/dL or a capillary hemoglobin of <14.5 gm/dL as consistent with anemia. In preterm infants beyond 32 weeks of gestation, hematologic values differ only minimally from those of full-term infants, and therefore the same values may be used.

81. **Describe the changes in hemoglobin concentration seen during the first few days of life.**
    In all newborn infants, hemoglobin levels rise slightly during the first few hours of life (because of hemoconcentration) and then fall somewhat during the remainder of the first day. In healthy full-term infants, the hemoglobin concentration then stays relatively constant for the rest of the

first week of life. However, appropriate-for-gestational-age infants of <1,500-gm birth weight may show a decline of 1.0–1.5 gm/day during this same period.

82. **What are the indications for red blood cell transfusions in premature infants?**
In recent years, the criteria for red blood cell transfusions have become far more stringent. The following guidelines are derived from the U.S. Multicenter Trial of Erythropoietin in Treating Anemia of Prematurity.
Transfuse infants with hematocrit levels of ≤20%:
- If asymptomatic with reticulocytes <100,000/μL

Transfuse infants with hematocrit levels of ≤30%:
- If receiving <35% supplemental hood oxygen
- If receiving continuous positive airway pressure or mechanical ventilation with mean airway pressure (MAP) <6 cm H_2O
- If significant apnea and bradycardia are noted (>9 episodes in 12 hours or >2 episodes requiring bag-and-mask ventilation) while receiving therapeutic doses of methylxanthines
- If heart rate is >180 bpm or respiratory rate is >80 breaths per minute persistently for 24 hours (and no other etiology is evident)
- If weight gain is <10 gm/day over 4 days while receiving 100 kcal/kg/d
- If undergoing surgery

Transfuse infants with hematocrit levels of ≤35%:
- If receiving >35% supplemental hood oxygen
- If receiving continuous positive airway pressure or mechanical ventilation with MAP = 6–8 cm H_2O

Do not transfuse:
- To replace blood removed for laboratory tests alone
- For low hematocrit alone

Shannon KM, Keith JF, III, Mentzer WC, et al: Recombinant human erythropoietin stimulates erythropoiesis and reduces erythrocyte transfusions in very low birth weight preterm infants. Pediatrics 95:1–8, 1995.

83. **Is there a practical way to assess the need for transfusion in the preterm infant?**
No. Because there is no easy way to determine tissue oxygenation, red-cell transfusions in preterm infants are generally given at preset levels, depending on the age and level of respiratory support. Although a variety of clinical signs (apnea, poor weight gain) have been attributed to anemia, they are often unaffected by red-cell transfusion.

Murray NA, Roberts IAG: Neonatal transfusion practice. Arch Dis Child Fetal Neonatal Ed 89:101–107, 2004.

84. **Should erythropoietin be used in preterm infants?**
The largest reduction in transfusion requirements has been observed when erythropoietin is given soon after birth and at a high dose (750–1500 IU/kg/wk). Unfortunately, it takes 1–2 weeks to produce a rise in the hematocrit with erythropoietin. Because two thirds of red blood cell transfusions are given during the first few weeks of life, erythropoietin has had a limited impact on transfusion requirements. Erythropoietin has been shown to significantly increase the number of preterm infants who never require a transfusion. However, the treatment of every infant weighing <1,000 gm is expensive and means giving unnecessary treatment to the a third of infants who would never have required a transfusion.

Murray NA, Roberts IAG: Neonatal transfusion practice. Arch Dis Child Fetal Neonatal Ed 89:F101–F107, 2004.

85. **How can Rh disease be prevented?**
Unsensitized pregnant women who are Rh-negative should have a repeat antibody screen at approximately 28 weeks of gestation and receive 300 mg of Rh-immune globulin (RhoGAM) prophylactically. After delivery, if the infant is Rh-positive, the mother should receive an additional dose of RhoGAM. At the time of delivery, the dose of RhoGAM may be increased if the fetomaternal hemorrhage is excessively large.

86. **Why is the direct Coombs' test frequently negative or weakly positive in infants with ABO incompatibility?**
There are fewer A or B antigenic sites on the newborn red cell, and there is also a greater distance between antigenic sites as compared with adult red cells. There is also absorption of serum antibody by ABO antigens located on tissues throughout the body.

87. **If fetomaternal hemorrhage is suspected as a cause of neonatal anemia, how is this diagnosed?**
The **Kleihauer-Betke test** detects the presence of fetal cells in the maternal circulation. Because fetal hemoglobin is resistant to elution with acid, the treatment of a maternal blood smear with acid will result in darkly stained fetal cells among the maternal "ghost" cells. From the percentage of fetal red cells and the estimated maternal blood volume, the size of the hemorrhage can be determined. One percent fetal cells in the maternal circulation indicates a bleed of approximately 50 mL.

88. **If a gastric aspirate contains blood shortly after birth, what test can determine if the blood is swallowed maternal blood or fetal hemorrhage?**
The **Apt test.** This test relies on the increased sensitivity of adult hemoglobin to alkali as compared with fetal hemoglobin.
Method: Mix the specimen with an equal quantity of tap water. Centrifuge or filter. Supernatant must have pink color to proceed. To five parts of supernatant, add one part of 0.25 N (1%) NaOH.
Interpretation: A pink color persisting for >2 minutes indicates fetal hemoglobin. Adult hemoglobin gives a pink color that becomes yellow in ≤2 minutes, thereby indicating the denaturation of hemoglobin.

89. **How is polycythemia defined?**
Polycythemia is defined by a venous hematocrit of 65% because this exceeds the mean hematocrit found in normal newborns by two standard deviations. As the central venous hematocrit rises above 65%, there is a dramatic increase in viscosity. Because direct measurements of blood viscosity are not readily available in most laboratories, a high hematocrit level is felt to be the best indirect indicator of hyperviscosity.

90. **What are the clinical manifestations of polycythemia?**
In symptomatic infants, the most common presentations relate to CNS abnormalities, including lethargy, hypotonia, tremulousness, and irritability. With severe CNS involvement, seizures can result. Hypoglycemia is common. Other organ systems can be involved, including the gastrointestinal tract (vomiting, distension, NEC), the kidneys (renal vein thrombosis, acute renal failure), and the cardiopulmonary system (respiratory distress, congestive heart failure). However, infants with polycythemia are often asymptomatic.

91. **Which infants with polycythemia should be treated?**
Because polycythemia results from a diverse array of etiologies, it is difficult to determine whether outcome depends more on etiology or the chronic elevation of viscosity. There is controversy regarding guidelines for treatment. Many authorities recommend a partial exchange transfusion, regardless of symptoms, in infants with a central venous hematocrit level of ≥70%

(because of the correlation with laboratory-measured hyperviscosity) or in those with a central hematocrit level of ≥65% if there are signs and symptoms attributable to polycythemia.

92. **Describe the preferred method for partial exchange transfusions in polycythemic neonates.**

    Partial exchange transfusions can be performed through an umbilical venous catheter, an umbilical arterial catheter, or a peripheral venous catheter. Aliquots equal to 5% of the estimated blood volume are withdrawn and historically have been replaced either with fresh frozen plasma, Plasmanate, 5% albumin, or normal saline. Adult plasma poses the risk of transfusion-acquired infections and may actually raise neonatal blood viscosity, whereas albumin offers no proven benefit. Therefore, the amount of blood volume to be exchanged with readily available crystalloid may be calculated using the following formula:

    $$\frac{\text{Blood volume}}{\text{to be exchanged}} = \frac{\text{Observed hematocrit} - \text{desired hematocrit}}{\text{Observed hematocrit}} \times \text{blood volume} \times \text{weight (kg)}$$

93. **What is the definition of thrombocytopenia in the neonate?**

    Platelet counts of <100,000/mm^3 should be considered abnormal in term or preterm neonates, whereas counts in the 100,000–150,000/mm^3 range may be seen in some healthy newborns. Consequently, patients with counts in this latter category should have repeat counts as well as further studies if illness is suspected.

94. **At what platelet count should platelet transfusion be considered?**

    Platelet counts should be maintained at >50,000/mm^3 in preterm infants (weighing <1,000 gm) who are at high risk for intracranial hemorrhage. The greatest risk for these infants is during the first week of life. In the nonbleeding neonate, platelets should not be given unless the count is <25,000/mm^3. In the bleeding infant, the platelet count should be kept at ≥100,000/mm^3.

95. **What features on physical examination suggest a specific cause of thrombocytopenia?**

    - "Blueberry muffin rash" (**T**oxoplasmosis **R**ubella **C**ytomegalovirus **H**erpes [TORCH] or viral infection)
    - Absence of radii (**T**hrombocytopenia **A**bsent **R**adii [TAR] syndrome)
    - Palpable flank mass and hematuria (renal vein thrombosis)
    - Hemangioma, large, often with bruit (Kasabach-Merritt syndrome)
    - Abnormal thumbs (Fanconi syndrome, albeit thrombocytopenia is less likely in newborns)
    - Markedly dysmorphic features (chromosomal abnormalities, particularly trisomy 13 or 18)

96. **What are the two main types of neonatal thrombocytopenia caused by maternal antibody?**

    Transplacental passage of antibody from the mother to infant can be due to maternal idiopathic thrombocytopenic purpura (with the newborn a secondary target) and isoimmune thrombocytopenia (with the newborn a primary target). The diseases can have a similar clinical appearance. Babies generally appear well, do not have hepatosplenomegaly, and have thrombocytopenia that persists for 3–12 weeks postnatally.

97. **In the mother with new-onset thrombocytopenia during pregnancy, how can one determine the risk to the fetus?**

    The maternal platelet count is a poor predictor of the risk of thrombocytopenia in the fetus. However, an elevated maternal titer of circulating antiplatelet immunoglobulin G (IgG) places the infant at high risk for thrombocytopenia. When maternal thrombocytopenia is limited to late pregnancy, however, the risk for developing severe neonatal thrombocytopenia is low. In mothers who have circulating antiplatelet antibody (IgG), the infant should be delivered via cesarean section, or a cordocentesis should be performed to demonstrate a normal platelet count before a vaginal delivery.

98. **How long do transfused platelets survive?**
If thrombocytopenia is not the result of increased platelet destruction, the platelet count will fall approximately 10% each day and reach pretransfusion levels in approximately 1 week.

99. **When do the prothrombin time and partial thromboplastin time "normalize" to adult values?**
The prothrombin time reaches adult values at approximately 1 week of age, whereas the partial thromboplastin time does not attain adult values until 2–9 months.

100. **How is disseminated intravascular coagulation (DIC) diagnosed in the neonate?**
The laboratory findings of DIC include evidence of red-cell fragmentation on peripheral smear; elevation of prothrombin time, partial thromboplastin time, and thrombin time; thrombocytopenia; decreased levels of factors V, VIII, and fibrinogen; and, in some cases, the presence of fibrin split products.

101. **How should newborn infants with DIC be managed?**
Treatment should be directed primarily at the underlying disease rather than just at the coagulation defects. In many cases, treatment of the former makes specific treatment of the latter unnecessary. However, in cases in which the stabilization of coagulopathy is not imminent, treatment with fresh frozen plasma and platelets is recommended. In cases in which fluid overload is a major concern, exchange transfusion with fresh whole blood may be used. However, this second approach is not superior to the first with respect to the resolution of DIC. The use of heparin in patients with DIC is currently reserved for cases of thrombosis of major vessels or purpura fulminans.

102. **What causes hemorrhagic disease of the newborn?**
For evolutionary reasons that are unclear, a newborn has only about 50% of the normal vitamin K–dependent cofactors. Unless vitamin K is given, these levels steadily decline during the first 3 days of life. In addition, breast milk is low in vitamin K. Early hemorrhagic disease can be observed during the first few days of life in infants who are exclusively breast fed and who do not receive vitamin K prophylaxis at birth; they may bleed from various sites (e.g., umbilical cord, circumcision). Infants born to mothers who have received medications that affect the metabolism of vitamin K (e.g., warfarin, antiepileptic medications, antituberculous drugs) are at risk to develop severe life-threatening intracranial hemorrhages at or shortly after delivery.

HYPERBILIRUBINEMIA

103. **What are the normal changes in bilirubin levels in full-term healthy newborns?**
All newborn infants exhibit a progressive rise in serum bilirubin concentrations following birth. Beginning with an average bilirubin in cord blood of 2 mg/dL, serum levels rise and peak at 5–6 mg/dL between 60 and 72 hours of life. The 97th percentile for bilirubin in healthy full-term infants is 12.4 mg/dL for bottle-fed infants and 14.8 mg/dL for breast-fed infants.

104. **How common is extreme hyperbilirubinemia in newborns?**
If untreated, at least 1–2% of newborns will develop bilirubin levels of 20 mg/dL.

Newman TB, Xiong B, Gonzalez VM, Escobar GJ: Prediction and prevention of extreme neonatal hyperbilirubinemia in a mature HMO. Arch Pediatr Adolesc Med 154:1140–1147, 2000.

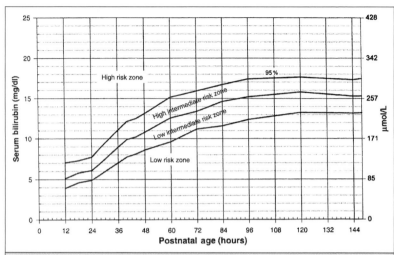

Figure 12-3. Assessment of jaundice. (From Subcommittee on Hyperbilirubinemia: Management of hyperbilirubinemia in the newborn infant 35 or more weeks of gestation. Pediatrics 114:297–316, 2004.)

105. How should infants be assessed for jaundice before discharge?

The American Academy of Pediatrics recommends two clinical options individually or in combination: a predischarge total serum bilirubin (or transcutaneous bilirubin) and/or assessment of clinical risk factors. Predischarge bilirubins should be plotted on the chart in Fig. 12-3 to assess risk.

106. How soon should infants be evaluated for jaundice after discharge?

All infants discharged before the age of 24 hours should be seen by 72 hours of age by a qualified health care professional. Infants discharged between 24 and 47.9 hours should be evaluated by 96 hours of age, and those discharged after 48 hours should be seen by 120 hours of age.

Subcommittee on Hyperbilirubinemia: Management of hyperbilirubinemia in the newborn infant 35 or more weeks of gestation. Pediatrics 114:297–316, 2004.

107. What factors suggest hemolytic disease as a cause of jaundice in the newborn?

- Family history of hemolytic disease
- Bilirubin rise of >0.5 mg/dL/h
- Failure of phototherapy to lower serum bilirubin levels
- Ethnicity suggestive of inherited disease (e.g., glucose 6-phosphate dehydrogenase deficiency)
- Onset of jaundice before 24 hours of age
- Reticulocytosis (>8% at birth, >5% during first 2–3 days, >2% after first week)
- Changes in peripheral smear (microspherocytosis, anisocytosis, target cells)
- Significant decrease in hemoglobin
- Pallor and hepatosplenomegaly

Provisional Committee for Quality Improvement and Subcommittee on Hyperbilirubinemia: Practice parameter: Management of hyperbilirubinemia in the healthy term newborn. Pediatrics 94:558–565, 1994.

108. Which infants are "set ups" for ABO incompatibility?

Infants who are type A or B and whose mothers are type O. In individuals with type A or B blood, naturally occurring anti-A and anti-B isoantibodies are primarily immunoglobulin M and do not cross the placenta. However, in type O individuals, isoantibodies are frequently IgG. These antibodies can cross the placenta and cause hemolysis. Although approximately 12% of maternal/infant pairs qualify as "set ups" for ABO incompatibility, < 1% of infants have significant hemolysis.

109. **What screening tests should pregnant women have to identify infants at risk for hyperbilirubinemia?**
All pregnant women should be tested for ABO and RH (D) blood types and have a serum screen for unusual isoimmune antibodies.

Subcommittee on Hyperbilirubinemia: Management of hyperbilirubinemia in the newborn infant 35 or more weeks of gestation. Pediatrics 114:297–316, 2004.

110. **When calculating bilirubin levels (and thus potential toxicity), should the direct component be subtracted from the total?**
In general, the direct-reacting component should not be subtracted from the total serum bilirubin concentration. In rare circumstances in which the direct component is 50% or more of the total, consultation with a neonatologist is recommended.

111. **What is "vigintiphobia"?**
Vigintiphobia, translated from the Latin, is the "fear of 20." Traditionally, it has been common to do exchange transfusions in term infants without evidence of isoimmunization or hemolysis at bilirubin levels of 20 mg/dL to prevent kernicterus. Critics argue that this practice is without scientific evidence, and there is support for tolerating higher levels of bilirubin (in infants without ABO incompatibility or other causes of hemolysis) before intervention has grown.

Watchko JF, Oski FA: Bilirubin 20 mg/dL = vigintiphobia. Pediatrics 71:660–663, 1983.

112. **What are the clinical features of bilirubin toxicity?**
The early clinical manifestations of bilirubin toxicity can be subtle. In addition, they can progress rapidly to severe and life-threatening manifestations. Acutely, toxicity is called **bilirubin-induced neurological dysfunction** (BIND). For chronic cases, the term **kernicterus** is generally used. Using the BIND score, infants with subtle signs of bilirubin toxicity can be identified (Table 12-7).

TABLE 12-7. CLINICAL FEATURES OF BILIRUBIN–INDUCED NEUROLOGIC DYSFUNCTION (BIND)

Signs	Mild	Moderate	Severe

Behavior	Too sleepy
	Decreased feeding
	Decreased vigor
		Lethargy and/or irritable
		  (depending on
		  arousal state)
		Very poor feeding
			Semicoma
			Apnea
			Extreme irritability
			Seizures
			Fever

Muscle tone	Slight but persistent
	  decrease in tone
		Mild to moderate
		  hypertonicity
		Mild nuchal or
		  truncal arching
			Severe hypo- or hypertonia
			Atonic
			Opisthotonus
			Posturing, bicycling

Cry pattern	High-pitched	Shrill and piercing
		  (especially when
		  stimulated)
			Inconsolable, very weak,
			  and cries only with
			  stimulation

113. When should phototherapy be instituted in infants of ≥35 weeks of gestation?
The American Academy of Pediatrics guidelines for instituting phototherapy in term and near-term infants are shown in Figure 12-4.

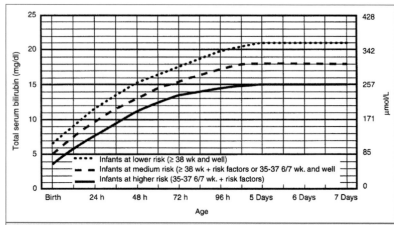

Figure 12-4. American Academy of Pediatrics guidelines for instituting phototherapy. (From Subcommittee on Hyperbilirubinemia: Management of hyperbilirubinemia in the newborn infant 35 or more weeks of gestation. Pediatrics 114:297–316, 2004.)

114. What distinguishes "breast-feeding jaundice" from "breast-milk jaundice"?
Hyperbilirubinemia in breast-fed infants during the first week of life is called *breast-feeding jaundice* and is thought to be the result of poor caloric intake and/or dehydration. Hyperbilirubinemia in breast-fed infants after the first week of life is known as *breast-milk jaundice*. The cause of breast-milk jaundice is uncertain; however, possible etiologies include an increased enterohepatic circulation of bilirubin as a result of the presence of beta-glucuronidase in human milk and/or to the inhibition of the hepatic glucuronosyl transferase by a factor such as free fatty acids in some human milk samples. The incidence and duration as compared with physiologic jaundice are noted in Table 12-8.

TABLE 12-8. COMPARISON OF PHYSIOLOGIC, BREAST–FEEDING, AND BREAST–MILK JAUNDICE

	Physiologic jaundice	Breast-feeding jaundice	Breast-milk jaundice
Time of onset (TSB >7 mg/dL)	After 36 hours	2–4 days	4–7 days
Usual time of peak bilirubin	3–4 days	3–6 days	5–15 days
Peak TSB	5–12 mg/dL	>12 mg/dL	>10 mg/dL
Age when total bilirubin <3 mg/dL	1–2 weeks	>3 weeks	9 weeks
Incidence in full-term neonates	56%	12–13%	2–4%

TSB = total serum bilirubin.
From Gourley G: Pathophysiology of breast milk jaundice. In Polin RA, Fox W (eds): Fetal and Neonatal Physiology. Philadelphia, W.B. Saunders, 1992, p 1174.

115. **Why should infants at risk for breast-feeding jaundice be fed more frequently?**
Breast-fed infants exhibit their maximum weight loss by day 3 of life and lose on average 6.1% ± 2.5% of their birth weight. Infants breast fed an average of >8 times per day during the first 3 days of life have significantly lower serum bilirubin concentrations than those who are less-frequently breast fed. This practice accelerates and enhances the acquisition of milk supply. With increased milk available, dehydration is less likely to occur, and the excretion of bilirubin via the gastrointestinal tract is more rapid. Infants with adequate intake should have 4–6 wet diapers per day.

116. **Should breast feeding be discontinued in an infant with hyperbilirubinemia?**
Only in rare metabolic disorders (e.g., galactosemia) should breast feeding be permanently discontinued. Breast-feeding infants do respond more slowly to phototherapy as compared with formula-fed infants. Martinez and colleagues compared three interventions (cessation of breast feeding and formula substitution, phototherapy, and cessation of breast feeding and phototherapy) with no intervention in breast-fed newborns with a serum bilirubin concentration of ≥17 mg/day (Table 12-9). The authors concluded that most infants (86%) do not require any intervention because they will never reach a serum bilirubin of 20 mg/dL. If phototherapy is used, there is no need to discontinue breast feeding.

TABLE 12-9.	SUMMARY OF MARTINEZ STUDY	
	Intervention	Treatment failure*
Group I	Continued breast feeding until TSB rose to 20 mg/dL, then breast feeding stopped and phototherapy begun	24%
Group II	Breast feeding stopped and formula substituted; phototherapy begun at TSB of 20 mg/dL	19%
Group III	Breast feeding stopped, formula substituted, and phototherapy begun immediately	3%
Group IV	Breast feeding continued and phototherapy begun	14%

*TSB rose to 20 mg/dL.
TSB = total serum bilirubin.
Data from Martinez JC, Maisels MJ, Otheguy L, et al: Hyperbilirubinemia in the breast-fed newborn: A controlled trial of four interventions. Pediatrics 91:470–473, 1993.

117. **Where does bilirubin go when you turn on the lights?**
It becomes *lumirubin* (through a cyclization reaction) and is rapidly excreted in bile, with a half-life of about 2 hours. In addition to the aforementioned principal pathway of bilirubin elimination, photoisomers are also formed, and, because of their water solubility, they can be excreted in the urine.

118. **What are the factors that affect the efficacy of phototherapy?**
- Spectrum of light emitted (blue-green is most effective)
- Spectral irradiance (intensive phototherapy = 30 uwatts/cm^2/nm)
- Spectral power (expose maximal surface area)
- Cause of jaundice (phototherapy is less effective with hemolysis/cholestasis)
- Total bilirubin at start (the higher the bilirubin, the greater the decline)

  Subcommittee on Hyperbilirubinemia: Management of hyperbilirubinemia in the newborn infant 35 or more weeks of gestation. Pediatrics 114:297–316, 2004.

119. **Does phototherapy need to be administered continuously?**
No. Phototherapy may be interrupted for procedures and parental visits.

120. **What are the contraindications to phototherapy?**
Infants with a family history of **light-sensitive porphyria** should not receive phototherapy. The presence of direct hyperbilirubinemia is not considered a contraindication, but it will decrease the effectiveness of phototherapy.

121. **What are the common adverse effects of phototherapy?**
Diarrhea, increased insensible water loss, skin rashes, overheating, and the potential for burns if the lights are placed too close to the infant's skin. If direct hyperbilirubinemia is present, the bronze baby syndrome can result.

122. **A newborn develops dark skin discoloration and dark urine after beginning phototherapy. What is the diagnosis?**
Bronze baby syndrome. Infants who develop the syndrome typically have an elevated direct serum bilirubin concentration. The bronze baby syndrome results from the retention of photoproducts (e.g., lumirubin) that cannot be excreted in the bile. Most infants appear to recover without complications. Direct hyperbilirubinemia is not a contraindication to phototherapy.

123. **How quickly does the bilirubin rebound after an exchange transfusion?**
Although 87% of the infant's circulating bilirubin is removed in a two-volume exchange, the serum bilirubin concentration is only reduced to 45% of the pre-exchange level. Equilibration with bilirubin in tissues is complete by 30 minutes, at which time the bilirubin rises to 60% of the pre-exchange value.

KEY POINTS: HEMATOLOGY/HYPERBILIRUBINEMIA

1. The switch from fetal to adult hemoglobin occurs in a preprogrammed manner.

2. Near-term infants are at higher risk than term infants for bilirubin encephalopathy.

3. Although ABO incompatibility is common, sensitization and hemolysis are not.

4. Exchange transfusion for hyperbilirubinemia in healthy full-term infants without evidence of hemolysis is almost never required.

124. **What are the complications of exchange transfusions in the newborn?**
Acute
- Hypocalcemia (as a result of the binding of calcium by citrate)
- Thrombocytopenia (as a result of the removal of platelets and the use of stored blood that may be low in platelets)
- Hyperkalemia (as a result of the higher potassium levels of stored blood)
- Hypovolemia (if blood replacement is inadequate)
- Diminished oxygen delivery (if blood stored for >5–7 days is used, the resultant loss of 2,3-DPG may have deleterious effects on oxygen delivery)

Late
- Anemia (for unknown reasons)
- Graft-versus-host disease (as a result of the introduction of donor lymphocytes into a relatively immunocompromised neonatal host)

125. **How often does prolonged unconjugated hyperbilirubinemia occur?**
About one third of healthy breast-fed infants will have persistent jaundice for 14 days. Among formula-fed infants, this prolonged jaundice occurs in <1% of neonates.

126. **What is the relationship between delayed neonatal jaundice and urinary tract infection (UTI)?**
Unexplained jaundice developing between 10 and 60 days of age can be associated with a UTI in infants. The typical patient is usually afebrile (in two thirds of cases) with hepatomegaly and minimal systemic symptoms. Hyperbilirubinemia is usually conjugated, and liver transaminases may be normal or mildly elevated. Treatment of the UTI (usually caused by *Escherichia coli*) results in reversal of the liver dysfunction, which is believed to be the result of endotoxins.

127. **Who was Sister Ward?**
In the early 1950s, Sister Ward was the nurse in charge of the unit for premature infants at Rochford General Hospital in Essex, England. On warm summer days, Sister Ward would take her infants to the courtyard to give them a little fresh air and sunshine. It was after such an afternoon of sunshine that Sister Ward observed that sunlight was able to "bleach" the skin of jaundiced neonates. The account of her discovery, as recorded by R.H. Dobbs, follows:

> One particularly fine summer's day in 1956, during a ward routine, Sister Ward diffidently showed us a premature baby, carefully undressed and with fully exposed abdomen. The infant was pale yellow except for a strongly demarcated triangle of skin very much yellower than the rest of the body. I asked her, "Sister, what did you paint it with—iodine or flavine—and why?" But she replied that she thought it must have been the sun. "What do you mean Sister? Suntan takes days to develop after the erythema has faded." Sister Ward looked increasingly uncomfortable, and explained that she thought it was a jaundiced baby, much darker where a corner of the sheet had covered the area. "It's the rest of the body that seems to have faded." We left it at that, and as the infant did well and went home, fresh air treatment of prematurity continued.

METABOLIC ISSUES

128. **How frequently are the various metabolic disorders detected by newborn screening?**

Disorder	Frequency
Tay-Sachs disease (U.S. Jews)	1 in 3,000
Phenylketonuria	1 in 10,000–25,000
Galactosemia	1 in 40,000–60,000
Biotinidase deficiency	1 in 70,000
Homocystinuria	1 in 50,000–150,000
Maple syrup urine disease	1 in 250,000–300,000

129. **Which common sugar does the Clinitest screen not detect?**
Sucrose. Reducing sugars (e.g., glucose, fructose, galactose, pentoses, lactose) are detected, but sucrose is not a reducing sugar. The test method is straightforward. Five drops of urine and 10 drops of water are mixed, and a Clinitest tablet is added. Color changes are then compared with a standard chart to determine the percentage of reducing substances. Testing for sucrose can be done by substituting hydrochloric acid for the water and boiling for a few seconds. This hydrolyzes the sucrose, and a negative test will become positive.

130. **In what settings should inborn errors of metabolism be suspected?**
- Onset of symptoms that correlates with dietary changes
- Loss or leveling of developmental milestones

- Patient with strong food preferences or aversions
- Parental consanguinity
- Unexplained sibling death, mental retardation, or seizures
- Unexplained failure to thrive
- Unusual odor
- Hair abnormalities, especially alopecia
- Microcephaly or macrocephaly
- Abnormalities of muscle tone
- Organomegaly
- Coarsened facial features, thick skin, limited joint mobility, and hirsutism

131. **What key urine odors are associated with inborn errors of metabolism?**

Cabbage	Tyrosinemia, type I
Cat urine	3-methylcrotonyl-CoA carboxylase deficiency
Fish	Trimethylaminuria
Hops	Oasthouse urine disease
Maple syrup	Maple syrup urine disease
"Mousy" or musty	Phenylketonuria
Sweaty feet or cheesy	Isovaleric acidemia; glutaric aciduria, type II

132. **What is the definition of neonatal hypoglycemia?**
The definition is controversial, but most investigators would treat a plasma glucose level of <40 mg/dL.

133. **When is hypoglycemia most likely to occur in a neonate?**
During gestation, glucose is freely transferred across the placenta by the process of facilitated diffusion. However, after birth, the infant must adjust to the sudden withdrawal of this transplacental supply. In all infants, there is a nadir in blood sugar between 1 and 3 hours of life. During the first 12–24 hours of life, newborns are at increased risk for hypoglycemia because gluconeogenesis and especially ketogenesis are incompletely developed. These factors are accentuated in preterm infants, infants of diabetic mothers, infants with erythroblastosis fetalis, asphyxiated infants, and infants who are small or large for gestational age.

Sperling MA, Menon RK: Differential diagnosis and management of neonatal hypoglycemia. 51:703–723, 2004.

134. **How should hypoglycemia be treated?**
Both symptomatic and asymptomatic hypoglycemia should be treated. If an asymptomatic infant can take oral feedings, these may suffice initially. Otherwise, the infant should receive therapy based on his or her response:

- If an intravenous line is in place and the infant is asymptomatic, the glucose infusion rate should be increased to 6–8 mg/kg/min. Glucose should be rechecked within 15 minutes.
- If an infant is symptomatic (or asymptomatic and unresponsive to a glucose infusion rate of 6–8 mg/kg/min), a bolus of intravenous glucose (200 mg/kg or 2 mL/kg of 10% dextrose water [D10W]) should be given and followed by a glucose infusion of 6–8 mg/kg/min (3.6–4.8 mL/kg/h of D10W), with rechecking of glucose within 15 minutes, frequent glucose monitoring, and increases in infusion rates and concentrations as needed.
- Glucagon (1 mg intramuscularly) can be given as an anti-insulin measure until an intravenous line is established, but glucagon is not as helpful in the low-birth-weight infant.
- If 15–20 mg/kg/min of glucose is required, glucocorticoids (hydrocortisone, 5 mg/kg/day, or prednisone, 2 mg/kg/day) can enhance gluconeogenesis. Diazoxide (10–15 mg/kg/day) can suppress insulin secretion. For these therapies and others (e.g., somatostatin), an endocrinologist should be consulted

135. **What features on physical examination suggest the etiology of hypoglycemia?**
- **Macrosomia:** This occurs in infants of diabetic mothers, infants with severe congenital hyperinsulinism, and infants with Beckwith-Wiedemann syndrome; recall that insulin is a growth factor and that hyperinsulinism leads to macrosomia.
- **Midline defects:** Congenital pituitary deficiency can be associated with midline defects such as cleft lip, cleft palate, single central incisor, and micro-ophthalmia.
- **Micropenis:** Congenital gonadotropin deficiency and possible pituitary abnormalities cause this condition.
- **Hepatomegaly:** This is associated with glycogen storage diseases and fatty acid oxidation disorders.

136. **What are manifestations of hypocalcemia in the neonate?**
The major manifestations are jitteriness and seizures. Additional signs such as high-pitched cry, laryngospasm, Chvostek's sign (facial muscle twitching on tapping), and Trousseau's sign (carpopedal spasm) may be present, but more commonly these are absent during the neonatal period.

137. **What is the differential diagnosis of hypocalcemia in the neonate?**
Early neonatal hypocalcemia (first 3 days of life)
- Premature infants
- Infants with birth asphyxia
- Infants of diabetic mothers

Late neonatal hypocalcemia (after the end of the first week of life)
- High-phosphate cow's milk formula
- Intestinal malabsorption
- Postdiarrheal acidosis
- Hypomagnesemia
- Neonatal hypoparathyroidism
- Rickets
- Decreased ionized fraction of calcium (with either normal or decreased total calcium)
- Citrate (exchange transfusion)
- Increased free fatty acid (Intralipid)
- Alkalosis

138. **When should hypocalcemia be treated in the neonate?**
Hypocalcemia should be treated when it is associated with signs or symptoms or when the serum calcium level is <7.0 mg/dL or the ionized calcium level is <4 mg/dL. The first line of therapy generally consists of increasing the amount of calcium in the intravenous infusion to achieve 20–75 mg of elemental Ca/kg/day and evaluating serum levels every 6–8 hours. After normal calcium levels are achieved, the intravenous dose can be weaned over 2–3 days. The infusion of a bolus of intravenous calcium (10% calcium gluconate, 2 mL/kg) over 10 minutes should be reserved for the infant with seizures. In the asymptomatic infant, hypocalcemia most frequently resolves spontaneously without the need for further therapy.

139. **In which neonates should the serum magnesium concentration be measured?**
- Any hypocalcemic infant who is not responding to calcium therapy
- Hypotonic infants born to mothers who received magnesium sulfate therapy before delivery
- Infants with seizures of unknown etiology

140. How is hypomagnesemia treated?

Hypomagnesemic infants should be treated with 0.25 mL/kg of a 50% solution (100 mg of elemental magnesium per milliliter) given intramuscularly. Magnesium levels are followed and the dosage repeated, if necessary.

NEONATAL SEPSIS

141. Can sepsis be distinguished from other causes of respiratory distress in the neonate?

Not reliably. Diagnosis is confirmed only by a positive blood, urine, or CSF culture.

142. What laboratory tests can rule out sepsis on admission?

None. Total WBC counts, immature-to-total (I:T) ratios of neutrophils, and C-reactive protein are of limited value as single tests for the diagnosis of bacterial sepsis in the newborn. In one third of infants with proven bacterial disease, total WBC counts are normal, particularly early during the course of infection. The most sensitive neutrophil index for identifying septic infants is the I:T neutrophil ratio. An I:T ratio of >0.2 has been considered abnormal, although some studies have suggested that a ratio as high as 0.27 may be seen in healthy term newborns. Neutropenia (total WBC <5,000/mm^3 or absolute neutrophil count <1,750/mm^3) is the most specific indicator. The least sensitive neutrophil index is the absolute band count (normal, <2,000/mm^3). Generally, abnormal neutrophil indices have low positive-predictive values and therefore are not helpful as sole tests for clearly identifying which infants are infected. However, they have a much higher negative-predictive value, particularly if repeated 12 hours after birth, and thus they can be very helpful for determining which infants do not have infection.

143. How should asymptomatic infants born to mothers with risk factors for infection be evaluated?

The major risk factors for infection are prolonged rupture of membranes, signs or symptoms of chorioamnionitis, and colonization with group B streptococci. The algorithms in Figures 12-5 and 12-6 use a "sepsis screen" to identify asymptomatic infants who do not require antibiotics or in whom antibiotics can be used. A positive sepsis screen is defined as two abnormal values (C-reactive protein >1 mg/dL; I:T ratio >0.2; absolute neutrophil count <1,750/mm^3; absolute band count >2,000/mm^3).

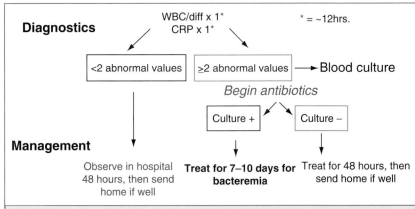

Figure 12-5. Evaluation of asymptomatic infants ≥35 weeks of gestation with one or more risk factors for neonatal sepsis. (From Gerdes JS, Polin RA: Neonatal septicemia. In Burg FD, Ingelfinger JR, Polin RA, Gerschon AA (eds): Current Pediatric Therapy, 17th ed. Philadelphia, W. B. Saunders, 2002, pp 347–351.)

144. **How should symptomatic infants be evaluated?**
The algorithm in Fig. 12-7 use a "sepsis screen" to identify symptomatic infants who do not require antibiotics or in whom antibiotics can be used.

145. **How helpful is a gastric aspirate for the evaluation of infection?**
The examination of gastric aspirates for leukocytes and bacteria was previously thought to be useful for identifying infants at risk for sepsis. However, the leukocytes are of maternal origin, and the bacteria represent organisms colonizing or infecting the amniotic cavity. They do not necessarily indicate fetal or neonatal infection.

146. **Should a lumbar puncture (LP) be performed on all newborns as part of the sepsis evaluation?**
The need for LP as part of the sepsis evaluation of a newborn is controversial, with some authors suggesting its omission in asymptomatic infants. However, in symptomatic infants,

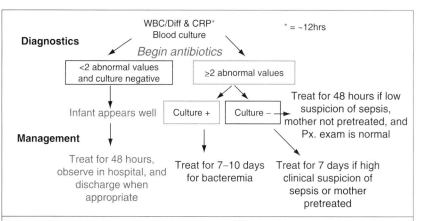

Figure 12-6. Evaluation of asymptomatic infants <35 weeks of gestation with one or more risk factors for neonatal sepsis. (From Gerdes JS, Polin RA: Neonatal septicemia. In Burg FD, Ingelfinger JR, Polin RA, Gerschon AA (eds): Current Pediatric Therapy, 17th ed. Philadelphia, W. B. Saunders, 2002, pp 347–351.)

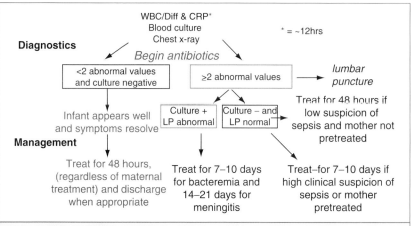

Figure 12-7. Evaluation of symptomatic infants for neonatal sepsis. (From Gerdes JS, Polin RA: Neonatal septicemia. In Burg FD, Ingelfinger JR, Polin RA, Gerschon AA (eds): Current Pediatric Therapy, 17th ed. Philadelphia, W. B. Saunders, 2002, pp 347–351.)

an LP should be strongly considered because of the following: (1) bacterial meningitis can be present in newborns without CNS symptoms; (2) a significant number of infants (15–30%) can have meningitis without bacteremia; and (3) meningitis can coexist in premature infants with suspected respiratory distress syndrome. The procedure should be postponed in an infant with cardiorespiratory instability or significant thrombocytopenia.

Wiswell TE, Baumgart S, Gannon CM, Spitzer AR: No lumbar puncture in the evaluation for early neonatal sepsis: Will meningitis be missed? Pediatrics 95:803–806, 1995.

147. **What is the ideal position to use for an infant undergoing LP?**
Infants who undergo LP in an upright position (with head support and spinal flexion) exhibit less hypoxia and hypercarbia. If a lateral recumbent position is used, partial neck extension helps to minimize the respiratory stresses.

148. **Are skin surface cultures helpful for the evaluation of suspected neonatal sepsis?**
The theoretic value of these cultures is that they might help to identify the possible etiologic agents and thus guide therapy. However, an analysis of nearly 25,000 cultures in >3,300 patients revealed that surface cultures correlated with urine, blood, or CSF cultures in only about 50% of cases. Most agree that surface cultures in this setting have little clinical value.

Evans ME, Schaffner W, Federspiel CF, et al: Sensitivity, specificity, and predictive value of body surface cultures in a neonatal intensive care unit. JAMA 259:248–252, 1988.

Fulginiti VA, Ray CG: Body surface cultures in the newborn infant: An exercise in futility, wastefulness, and inappropriate practice. Am J Dis Child 142:19–20, 1988.

149. **What are the two strategies to determine which maternal carriers of group B streptococci (GBS) warrant prophylactic antibiotics?**
Antepartum screening based and **risk factor based.** The American Academy of Pediatrics guidelines for the prevention of early onset GBS infection proposes two strategies: one uses prenatal cultures at 35–37 weeks of gestation, and the other uses risk factors without prenatal culture screening. If the culture-based strategy is employed, all women identified as GBS carriers should be offered intrapartum prophylaxis even if no risk factors are present. If the results of culture are not available at the onset of labor or the rupture of membranes, prophylaxis should be administered on the basis of risk factors: gestational age of <37 weeks, membranes ruptured for >18 hours, maternal temperature during labor of >38°C, and history of a previous baby with invasive GBS disease or a urine culture positive for GBS during the current pregnancy.

Schrag SJ, Gorwitz R, Fultz–Butts K, Schuchat A: Prevention of perinatal Group B streptococcal disease: Revised guidelines from CDC. MMWR 51:1–22, 2002.

150. **How successful are these screening strategies?**
The incidence of early-onset GBS disease in the United States has fallen by 70% from 1.7 per 1,000 live births (1993) to 0.5 per 1,000 live births (1999) since the introduction of these strategies in the mid-1990s. Despite this impressive decline, however, risk-factor–based strategy identifies only about 75% of affected infants' mothers, and screening-based strategy identifies about 85–90%. Twenty-five percent of infants with blood-culture–positive GBS disease are born to mothers who have received intrapartum antibiotics.

Schrag SJ, Gorwitz R, Futtz–Butts K, Schuchat A: Prevention of perinatal Group B streptococcal disease: Revised guidelines from CDC. MMWR 51:1–22, 2002.

151. **Do intrapartum antibiotics change the clinical presentation of early-onset GBS sepsis?**
No. In a study of 319 infants with early-onset GBS disease, the administration of intrapartum antibiotics to the mother did not affect the constellation and timing of clinical signs of disease.

All infants born to pretreated mothers became ill during the first 24 hours of life (80% within the first 6 hours of life).

Bromberger P, Lawrence JM, Braun D, et al: The influence of intrapartum antibiotics on the clinical spectrum of early-onset group B streptococcal infection in term infants. Pediatrics 106:244–250, 2000.

KEY POINTS: SEPSIS

1. Because there are no reliable screening tests for sepsis, clinical judgment is paramount.

2. Screening cultures for group B *Streptococcus* should be performed for all pregnant women at 35–37 weeks of gestation.

3. Coagulase-negative staphylococci are the most common bacterial pathogens that are responsible for nosocomial infections.

4. Neonatal meningitis can occur in the absence of a positive blood culture.

5. Fungal infection must be considered in sick preterm infants who are evaluated for sepsis.

152. **In cultures that are positive for coagulase-negative staphylococci, what distinguishes contamination from "true" infection?**
To help with the differentiation of a true coagulase-negative staphylococcal infection from blood-culture contamination (especially in infants with central catheters), blood cultures should be obtained from two different sites. In infants with infections, both cultures should grow coagulase-negative staphylococci with identical sensitivity patterns. If only a single blood culture is obtained, some authors have suggested that a colony count of >50 CFU/mL is sug-gestive evidence of true bacteremia. In clinical practice, however, that number of CFUs has a relatively poor predictive accuracy.

153. **What are the most common pathogens that are responsible for late-onset sepsis in the newborn infant?**
- Coagulase-negative *staphylococci* (48%)
- *Staphylococcus aureus* (8%)
- Enterococcus (3%)
- Gram-negative enterics (18%)
- Candida (9%)

Stoll BJ, Hansen N, Fanaroff AA, et al: Late-onset sepsis in very low birth weight neonates: The experience of the NICHD Neonatal Research Network. Pediatrics 110:285–291, 2002.

154. **What are the major risk factors for nosocomial sepsis?**
- Prematurity
- Use of parenteral alimentation and central lines
- Intravenous fat emulsions
- H_2 blockers
- Steroids for BPD
- Prolonged duration of mechanical ventilation
- Overcrowding
- Heavy staff workloads

155. **How is systemic candidiasis diagnosed in the neonate?**
By cultures of blood, urine, and CSF or other body fluids that are generally sterile. Because cultures are only intermittently positive, multiple systemic cultures should be obtained.

A urinalysis demonstrating budding yeasts or hyphae should raise suspicion of systemic infection. Gram stains of buffy coat smears may also demonstrate organisms. An ophthalmologic examination may indicate the presence of candidal endophthalmitis. Renal and brain ultrasounds should be performed to look for characteristic lesions. In addition, echocardiography should be performed in infants with central catheters to rule out cardiac vegetations.

NEUROLOGIC ISSUES

156. What are normal CSF values for healthy neonates?
More than 15 cells in a CSF specimen should be considered suspicious, and >20 cells is suggestive of meningitis. Protein concentration in the CSF of term infants should be <100 mg/dL. There is an inverse relationship between protein concentrations in CSF and gestational age. Glucose values should be one half to two thirds of serum levels.

Ahmed A, Hickey SM, Ehrett S, et al: Cerebrospinal fluid values in the term neonate. Pediatr Infect Dis J 15:298–303, 1996.
Rodriguez AF, Kaplan SL, Mason EO, Jr. Cerebrospinal fluid values in the very low birth weight infant. J Pediatr 116:971–974, 1990.

157. After a difficult delivery, what three major forms of extracranial hemorrhage can occur?
1. Caput succedaneum
2. Cephalhematoma
3. Subgaleal hemorrhage

Fig. 12-8 and Table 12-10 characterize the major forms of extracranial hemorrhages.

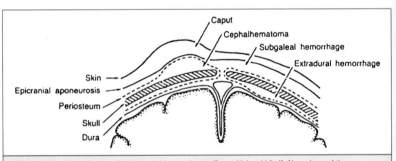

Figure 12-8. Major forms of extracranial hemorrhage. (From Volpe JJ [ed]: Neurology of the Newborn, 4th ed. Philadelphia W.B. Saunders, 2001, p 814.)

TABLE 12-10. MAJOR VARIATIONS OF TRAUMATIC EXTRACRANIAL HEMORRHAGE

Lesion	Features of external swelling	Increases after birth	Crosses suture lines	Marked acute blood loss
Caput succedaneum	Soft pitting	No	Yes	No
Subgaleal hemorrhage	Firm, fluctuant	Yes	Yes	Yes
Cephalhematoma	Firm, tense	Yes	No	No

From Volpe JJ (ed): Neurology of the Newborn, 3rd ed. Philadelphia, W.B. Saunders, 1995, p 770.

158. **If a cephalhematoma is suspected, should a skull x-ray be performed to evaluate for fracture?**
Cephalhematomas occur in up to 2.5% of live births. In studies, the incidence of associated fractures ranges from 5–25%. These fractures are almost always linear and nondepressed and do not require treatment. Thus, in an asymptomatic infant with a cephalhematoma over the convexity of the skull and without suspicion of a depressed fracture, x-ray is not necessary. If the examination suggests cranial depression or neurologic signs are present, radiographic imaging is warranted.

159. **Should all preterm infants be examined by cranial ultrasound?**
Because of the relative noninvasiveness of ultrasound, most neonatologists recommend that a single cranial ultrasonogram be obtained during the first week of life in infants born at a gestational age <35 weeks.

160. **When screening for IVH, when is the best time to perform an ultrasound?**
In a series of infants studied by ultrasonography, approximately 50% had the onset of hemorrhage on the first day of life, 25% on the second day, and 15% on the third day. Thus, a single scan on the fourth day of life would be expected to detect >90% of IVHs. However, approximately 20–40% of hemorrhages show evidence of extension within 3–5 days after initial diagnosis, and thus a second scan is indicated to take place about 5 days after the first to determine the maximal extent of hemorrhage.

161. **How are IVHs classified?**
Most traditional systems of classification include a grading system that is in accordance with increasing severity:
- **Grade I:** Germinal matrix hemorrhage only
- **Grade II:** IVH without ventricular dilatation
- **Grade III:** IVH with ventricular dilatation
- **Grade IV:** Grade III hemorrhage plus intraparenchymal involvement
   Some authorities have abandoned the grade IV classification in favor of "periventricular hemorrhagic infarction" to emphasize that these lesions have a different pathophysiology and are not simply extensions of matrix or IVH into parenchymal tissue. As such, the extent of parenchymal involvement rather than the grade of hemorrhage is more important for determining prognosis.

162. **What is the cause of hydrocephalus after an intracranial hemorrhage?**
The acute hydrocephalus is believed to be a result of impairment of CSF absorption by the arachnoid membrane caused by the particulate blood clot. In subacute/chronic hydrocephalus, ventricular enlargement is the result of an obliterative arachnoiditis (likely a chemical inflammatory response from the continued presence of blood), which usually causes a communicating hydrocephalus. Less commonly, obstruction of the aqueduct of Sylvius can lead to a noncommunicating hydrocephalus.

163. **How common is progressive posthemorrhagic ventricular enlargement?**
The likelihood of this phenomenon depends on the extent of the initial hemorrhage, ranging from only about a 5% likelihood in patients with grade I IVH to 80% in those with grade IV IVH.

164. **Can serial LPs prevent posthemorrhagic hydrocephalus?**
No. Although LPs are useful for lowering increased intracranial pressure and for treating hydrocephalus after it has developed, they are of no benefit for preventing the onset. Infants with slowly progressive ventricular dilation and increasing head circumference who do not show signs of spontaneous arrest and improvement within 4 weeks should undergo a trial of

serial LPs. Their effectiveness should be assessed with ultrasound. If there is no benefit, the placement of a ventriculoperitoneal shunt is necessary.

165. **How much fluid should be removed by LP in an infant with ventriculomegaly?**
Because the volume of CSF in the dilated ventricles of infants with posthemorrhagic hydrocephalus is large, the removal of a significant amount of fluid (10–15 mL/kg) is usually required.

166. **What is the most common brachial plexus palsy?**
Erb's palsy. Neonatal brachial plexus injuries occur in <0.5% of deliveries and are often associated with shoulder dystocia and breech or forceps delivery.
- Involves upper plexus (C5, C6)
- In 50% of cases, C7 affected
- Arm held limply adducted, internally rotated, and pronated with wrist flexed and fingers flexed ("waiter's tip" position)
- Biceps reflex absent, Moro reflex with hand movement but no shoulder abduction, palmar grasp present
- Ipsilateral diaphragmatic involvement in 5%

167. **What is Klumpke's paralysis?**
A brachial plexus palsy involving injury to the *lower* plexus (C8, T1). It is associated with weakness of the flexor muscles of the wrist and the small muscles of the hand ("claw hand"). Up to one third of these patients have an associated Horner syndrome.

168. **How is brachial plexus injury treated?**
Therapy must be aimed at preventing contractures. For the first 7–10 days, the arm is gently immobilized against the abdomen to minimize further hemorrhage and/or swelling. After this initial period, passive range of motion exercises at the shoulder, elbow, wrist, and hand are performed. In addition, wrist splints to stabilize the fingers and avoid contractures should be used. Improvements in microsurgical techniques have increased interest in this modality if recovery is delayed beyond 3 months, particularly in cases of nerve root avulsion. Surgical options include sural nerve graft or local root grafts. Other therapies include the use of botulinum toxin with physical therapy if severe contractures have evolved.

Noetzel MJ, Wolpaw JR: Emerging concepts in the pathophysiology of recovery from neonatal brachial plexus injury. Neurology 55:5–6, 2000.

169. **What is the outcome of neonatal brachial plexus palsy?**
Approximately 90% of patients have normal examinations by 12 months of age. Onset of recovery within 2 weeks and involvement of only the proximal upper extremity are both favorable prognostic signs.

Strombeck C, Krumlinde-Sundholm L, Forssberg H: Functional outcome at 5 years in children with obstetrical brachial plexus palsy with and without microsurgical reconstruction. Dev Med Child Neurol 42:148–157, 2000.

170. **In newborns with facial paralysis, how is peripheral nerve involvement distinguished from central nerve involvement?**
- **Peripheral:** This usually results from compression of the peripheral portion of the nerve by prolonged pressure from the maternal sacral promontory. The use of forceps alone is not thought to be an important causative factor. Peripheral paralysis is unilateral. The forehead is smooth on the affected side, and the eye is persistently open.
- **Central:** This type often results from contralateral CNS injury (temporal bone fracture and/or posterior fossa hemorrhage or tissue destruction). It involves only the lower half or two thirds of the face; the forehead and eyelids are not affected.

In both forms of paralysis, the mouth is drawn to the normal side when crying, and the nasolabial fold is obliterated on the affected side.

171. Is ankle clonus normal in the newborn infant?
Bilateral ankle clonus of 5–10 beats may be a normal finding, especially in infants who are crying, hungry, or jittery. This is particularly true if the clonus is unaccompanied by other signs of upper motor neuron dysfunction.

172. Do newborns prefer to turn their heads to the right or to the left?
Healthy neonates prefer to turn their heads to the **right**, which may reflect the normal asymmetry of cerebral function at this age. This preference has been observed as early as 28 weeks of gestation. By 39 weeks of gestation, 90% of newborn infants spend 80% of the time with their heads turned to the right side.

NUTRITION

173. How many calories are required daily for growth in a healthy, growing preterm infant?
Preterm infants need *approximately 120 cal/kg/day*. About 45% of the caloric intake should be carbohydrate, 45% should be fat, and 10% should be protein. Infants who expend increased calories (e.g., those with chronic lung disease, fever, or cold stress) may need up to 150 cal/kg/ day.

KEY POINTS: NEUROLOGY

1. The major forms of neonatal extracranial hemorrhages can be distinguished clinically.

2. In >90% of cases, intraventricular hemorrhages in preterm infants occur during the first 3 days of life.

3. Posthemorrhagic hydrocephalus is most likely to occur after the most severe intraventricular hemorrhages.

4. Recovery occurs in approximately 90% of patients with brachial plexus injuries.

5. Signs of neuromuscular maturation along with physical characteristics can be used to estimate gestational age at birth with an accuracy of ±1 week.

174. How should enteral feedings be started in the preterm infant?
All preterm infants should receive parenteral nutrition until feedings can be established. Minimal enteral feedings (trophic feedings) are usually begun on day 2 of life if there is no cardiovascular instability. Trophic feedings are provided as breast milk or as a formula designed for preterm infants at a volume equal to 15–20 mL/kg/day. Feedings are usually given every 3 hours by gavage. The number of days that an infant is maintained on trophic feedings (before feeding advancement) is variable, but it usually ranges from 4–7 days. If tolerated, enteral feedings are advanced about 20 mL/kg/day until the infant receives 110–120 cal/kg/day. The preterm infant is often started on formula feeds that are one-quarter or one-half strength.

Berseth CL: Feeding methods for the preterm infant. Semin Neonatol 6:417–24, 2001.

175. What are the documented medical benefits of breast feeding?
Proven benefits
- Fewer episodes of otitis media and respiratory and gastrointestinal illness occur in breast-fed infants.

- Human milk facilitates the growth of beneficial, nonpathogenic flora as compared with the pathogenic anaerobes and coliforms that predominate in infants who are fed formula.
- Formula-fed infants have reduced quantities of host-defense proteins in the gastrointestinal tract (e.g., lactoferrin, secretory immunoglobulin A).

Suggested but unproven benefits
- Decreased incidence of neonatal sepsis and necrotizing enterocolitis in preterm infants
- Enhancement of subsequent intelligence
- Reduction in incidence of atherosclerosis
- Reduction in incidence of diabetes mellitus

176. **How does maternal breast milk differ for a full-term versus a premature baby?**
The composition of human milk for preterm infants differs from that for term infants in a number of ways. For every 100 mL, it is higher in calories (67–72 kcal versus 62–68 kcal), higher in protein (1.7–2.1 gm versus 1.2–1.7 gm), higher in lipids (3.4–4.4 gm versus 3.0–4.0 gm), lower in carbohydrates, higher in multiple minerals and trace elements (especially sodium [Na], chloride [Cl], iron[Fe], Zinc [Zn], and copper [Cu]), and higher in vitamins (especially vitamins A and E). However, as breast milk becomes mature, many of these nutritional advantages are lost.

177. **How does colostrum differ from mature human breast milk?**
Colostrum is the thick, yellowish mammary secretion that is characteristic of the first postpartum week. It is higher in phospholipids, cholesterol, and protein concentration and lower in lactose and total fat composition than mature breast milk. Colostrum is particularly rich in immunoglobulins, especially secretory immunoglobulin A.

178. **With regard to breast feeding, how do fore milk and hind milk differ?**
The caloric density of human milk increases in a nonlinear fashion while the infant is breast feeding. **Hind milk** (produced at the end of the feeding) can have a fat content that is 50% higher than **fore milk**. In preterm infants with poor weight gain, hind milk may offer a nutritional advantage.

179. **What are contraindications to breast feeding?**
- **Inborn errors of metabolism:** Galactosemia, phenylketonuria, and urea-cycle defects
- **Infections:** Human immunodeficiency virus, tuberculosis (before treatment), human T-cell lymphotropic virus (HTLV) types I and II, cytomegalovirus (in preterm infants), and herpes simplex (when lesions are present on the breast)
- **Substance abuse/use:** Cocaine, narcotics, stimulants, and marijuana
- **Medications:** Sulfonamides (for ill, stressed, or preterm infants or infants with hyperbilirubinemia and glucose-6-phosphate-dehydrogenase deficiency), radioactive medicines, chemotherapeutic agents (alkylating agents), bromocriptine (suppresses lactation), and lithium (In general, psychotropic drugs should be used with caution.)

   American Academy of Pediatrics Committee on Drugs: The transfer of drugs and other chemicals in human milk. Pediatrics 108:776–789, 2001.

180. **Should babies who are breast fed receive water supplements?**
Although a common practice, there is no basis for the supplementation of breast feeding with water. Babies with water supplementation do not have any lesser degree of physiologic jaundice. They may have more weight loss than babies who do not receive water, and they are less likely to be breast fed at 3 months than those who do not receive supplements.

181. **How long should infants be breast fed per feeding?**
Infants nurse between 4 and 20 minutes per breast. Although the majority of milk volume is consumed during the first 4 minutes of nursing, the caloric density is greater during the later phase of breast feeding. If >25 minutes is needed by an infant to empty a breast, one should suspect poor milk production, an abnormal "let-down" response, or ineffective "latch-on."

182. **What advice should be given to a mother who plans to express and save breast milk for later feedings?**
Ideally, she should collect the milk as cleanly as possible and then store it rapidly at ≤3°–4°C; the milk should then be used within 5 days. Alternatively, breast milk can be stored in the freezer compartment of a refrigerator for approximately 6 months. If more prolonged storage is necessary (12 months), the milk should be kept frozen at a temperature of ≤−20°C (usually in a separate freezer). After the milk has thawed, it should not be refrozen.

183. **What are the advantages of a 60/40 whey-to-casein ratio in infant formulas?**
The term 60/40 refers to the percentage of whey (lactalbumin) and casein in human milk or cow's milk formulas. This ratio makes for small curds and therefore easy digestibility by the infant. The 60/40 ratio is of particular advantage for the preterm infant because it is associated with lower levels of serum ammonia and a decreased incidence of metabolic acidosis. Only human milk or formulas that supply protein in this ratio provide adequate amounts of the amino acids cystine and taurine, which may be essential for the preterm infant.

184. **How much formula should an average infant drink per day?**
A healthy term newborn in the first 1–2 days of life may drink only 0.5–1 oz every 3–4 hours. After feedings are well established, infants may ingest 200 mL/kg/day or more.

185. **Must infant formulas be sterilized?**
As a rule, no. The terminal sterilization of prepared formula by boiling the bottle for 25 minutes offers no advantage over the simple cleansing of the bottles and nipples in hot, soapy water and the subsequent use of unsterilized tap water in formula preparation. If bacteriologically safe tap water is used, no differences in rates of gastroenteritis occur.

Gerber MA, Berliner BC, Karolus JJ: Sterilization of infant formula. Clin Pediatr 22:344–349, 1983.

186. **"Low-iron" or "regular iron-fortified" formulas: which are preferred for infants?**
Generally, low-iron formula has 1.5 mg/L of elemental iron, whereas regular iron-fortified formula has 12 mg/L. Infants who are not breast fed should be placed on regular iron-fortified formula. Although a greater percentage of iron is absorbed from the ingested low-iron formula, the quantity may not be sufficient to protect against the development of iron-deficiency anemia. In addition, despite anecdotal experiences, the incidence of colic, constipation, vomiting, and fussiness does not vary between infants fed the two formulas.

187. **May milk be heated in a microwave oven?**
No. Microwave heating produces uneven temperatures, and human milk is easily damaged by high temperatures.

188. **Is vitamin supplementation necessary for exclusively breast-fed term infants?**
As a result of the growing concerns about the relationship of sunlight exposure and skin cancer, the low concentration of vitamin D in breast milk, and the inability to predict adequate exposure as a result of diverse lifestyle and cultural practices, cases of rickets in breast-fed infants have been reported.

- All breast-fed infants should be supplemented with 200 IU/day of vitamin D to prevent the occurrence of rickets, per American Academy of Pediatrics recommendations.
- Malnourished mothers may need to supplement their breast-fed babies with multivitamins.
- Mothers who are strict vegetarians may have low concentrations of B vitamins in their breast milk, and infants may need supplementation.

American Academy of Pediatrics: Prevention of rickets and vitamin D deficiency: New guidelines for vitamin D intake. Pediatrics 111:908–910, 2003.

189. **If alimentation is being administered through a peripheral vein, is heparinization necessary?**

The administration of heparin to premature infants in a concentration of 0.5–1.0 U/mL has been shown to improve the clearance of lipids. Therefore, heparin should be used whenever fats are being administered intravenously.

190. **What is nonnutritive sucking?**

Nonnutritive sucking is a mode of sucking that is unique to humans and that is characterized by a highly regular, burst-pause pattern. Nonnutritive sucking occurs in all sleep and awake states, although it is seen less often during quiet sleep and crying. It assumes a recognizable rhythmic pattern after 33 weeks of gestation.

191. **How do protein requirements vary with the mode of nutrient delivery (intravenous versus enteral)?**

Whether delivered intravenously or enterally, the protein requirements needed to achieve in utero accretion rates are similar. Preterm infants have slightly higher protein requirements (3.0–3.5 gm/kg/day) than term infants (2.0–2.5 gm/kg/day).

192. **Which fatty acids are essential for the neonate?**

Linoleic acid and **linolenic acid.** In infants weighing <1,750 gm who experience delay in or difficulty with maintaining full enteral feedings, arachidonic and docosahexaenoic fatty acids may also be essential. These fatty acids are vital for normal brain development, myelination, cell proliferation, and retinal function. Fatty acids in human milk are composed of 12–15% linoleic acid.

193. **What are the proven advantages of supplementing formulas with long-chain polyunsaturated fatty acids?**

- Docosahexaenoic acid–supplemented infants demonstrate improved behaviorally based and electrophysiologically based measurements of visual acuity.
- The beneficial effects on visual function may be transient.
- The effects on cognitive development are controversial.

SanGiovanni JP, Parra-Cabrera S, Colditz GA, et al: Meta-analysis of dietary essential fatty acids and long-chain polyunsaturated fatty acids as they relate to visual resolution acuity in healthy preterm infants. Pediatrics 105:1292–1298, 2000.

194. **What are the manifestations of essential fatty-acid deficiency?**

Scaly dermatitis, alopecia, thrombocytopenia (and platelet dysfunction), failure to thrive, and increased susceptibility to recurrent infection. To prevent and treat fatty-acid deficiency, 4–5% of caloric intake should be provided as linoleic acid and 1% as linolenic acid. This requirement can be met by 0.5–1.0 gm/kg/day of intravenous lipids.

195. **Why are nucleotides being added to a number of infant formulas?**

Dietary nucleotides may play a role during early neonatal life in the desaturation and elongation of essential fatty acids, which are necessary for brain and retinal development. The addition of nucleotides to formula (simulating the composition of breast milk) may be especially important during early development. Nucleotides are present in relatively large amounts in human milk, and several studies have suggested an important role for nucleotides in immune function, gastrointestinal function, and lipoprotein metabolism.

196. **What are the manifestations of vitamin E deficiency in the neonate?**
    Hemolytic anemia (with reticulocytosis), **peripheral edema**, and **thrombocytosis**. Vitamin E is important for stabilizing the red-cell membrane, and a deficiency can result in a mild hemolytic anemia. The American Academy of Pediatrics recommends that 0.7 IU of vitamin E per 100 kcal be present in feedings for preterm infants. There is current consensus that infants weighing <1,000 gm require 6–12 IU of vitamin E per kilogram per day and that this can generally be met by preterm formulas that provide 4–6 IU per 100 kcal.

KEY POINTS: GROWTH AND NUTRITION

1. Infants with late-onset in utero growth retardation have a low ponderal index.

2. Breast milk is protective against infection and may reduce the incidence of adult chronic diseases.

3. The presence of an umbilical artery catheter is not a contraindication to breast feeding.

4. Breast-milk feedings for preterm infants should be fortified.

5. Premature infant feeding regimens attempt to mimic the growth achieved in utero.

RESPIRATORY ISSUES

197. **What causes infants to grunt?**
    Infants with respiratory disease tend to expire through closed or partially closed vocal cords to elevate transpulmonary pressure and to therefore increase lung volume. The latter effect results in an improved ventilation/perfusion ratio with better gas exchange. It is during the last part of expiration, when gas is expelled through the partially closed vocal cords, that the audible grunt is produced.

198. **What do hyperpnea and tachypnea signify in the neonate?**
    - **Hyperpnea** refers to deep, relatively unlabored respirations at mildly increased rates. It is typical of situations in which there is reduced pulmonary blood flow (e.g., pulmonary atresia), and it results from the ventilation of underperfused alveoli.
    - **Tachypnea** refers to shallow, rapid, and somewhat labored respirations, and it is seen in the setting of low lung compliance (e.g., primary lung disease, pulmonary edema).

199. **Until what age are infants obligate nose breathers?**
    Although 30% of newborn infants breathe through their mouth or nose and mouth, the remaining 70% are obligate nose breathers until the third to sixth week of life.

200. **What are the effects of severe hypercarbia (PCO_2 = 100 mmHg) if there is no associated hypoxia?**
    There are few data about human newborns regarding the effects of isolated severe hypercarbia in the absence of hypoxia. However, results from animal studies and limited clinical observations in humans suggest that this condition can lead to a pressure-passive cerebral circulation and a possible increased risk of IVH. In addition, the high $PaCO_2$ may disrupt the blood-brain

barrier and enhance the deposition of molecules such as bilirubin in the CNS, thereby leading to kernicterus. Finally, on a more cellular level, data in animal model systems demonstrate alterations in brain-cell membrane lipid peroxidation as well as Na+-K+ ATPase activity. The significance of these latter findings remains undetermined. Moderate degrees of hypercarbia may be neuroprotective, and it may decrease lung injury in ventilated neonates.

201. **In an infant who is receiving mechanical ventilation, what is an acceptable range for pH, PCO_2, and PO_2?**
   - **PaO_2:** 50–70 mmHg (in term infants with primary pulmonary hypertension [PPHN]): 80–120 mmHg
   - **$PaCO_2$:** 50–70 mmHg (in term infants with PPHN: 35–45)
   - **pH:** ≥7.2 (in term infants with PPHN: 7.3–7.4)

202. **What mechanical ventilator settings are likely to affect PO_2 and PCO_2?**
   - **PaO_2 is increased** by raising the positive end expiratory pressure (PEEP), the peak inspiratory pressure, the inspiratory-to-expiratory ratio, or the inspired oxygen concentration.
   - **PCO_2 is decreased** by increasing the rate or peak inspiratory pressure. An increase in PEEP may increase the $PaCO_2$ by decreasing the tidal volume.

203. **What are the physiologic effects of PEEP?**
   PEEP can prevent alveolar collapse, maintain lung volume at end expiration, and improve ventilation-perfusion mismatch. However, an increase in PEEP may decrease tidal volume and impede CO_2 elimination. Elevations in PEEP to nonphysiologic values may decrease lung compliance, impair venous return, decrease cardiac output, and reduce tissue oxygen delivery.

204. **Is there a role for nasal ventilation?**
   Although providing positive-pressure breaths in a noninvasive manner would potentially avoid the complications of intubation, there are no data to support the use of nasal ventilation as a primary treatment for pulmonary disorders. However, this type of ventilation has been successfully employed to prevent extubation failures, especially those that result from severe apnea.

   Barrington KJ, Bull D, Finer NN: Randomized trial of nasal synchronized intermittent mandatory ventilation compared with continuous positive airway pressure after extubation of very low birth weight infants. Pediatrics 107:638–641, 2001.

   Lin CH, Wang ST, Lin YJ, Yeh TF: Efficacy of nasal intermittent positive pressure ventilation in treating apnea of prematurity. Pediatr Pulmonol 26:349–353, 1998.

205. **Should newborn infants receiving mechanical ventilation be pharmacologically paralyzed?**
   Neuromuscular paralysis is not recommended as routine treatment for mechanically ventilated infants. However, in specific instances (e.g., persistence of fetal circulation), neuromuscular paralysis may benefit infants whose activity/agitation may increase right-to-left shunting and decrease oxygenation. Paralysis may also reduce the incidence of pneumothorax and IVH in infants with respiratory distress.

206. **How do high-frequency oscillatory ventilation and high-frequency jet ventilation differ?**
   In general, high-frequency jet ventilation has been used more commonly to treat infants with severe air leak syndromes, whereas high-frequency oscillatory ventilation has been of greater value for infants with difficulties achieving adequate oxygenation and requiring "high" settings. Neither ventilator has been proven to be superior to conventional ventilation for the management of infants with uncomplicated respiratory distress syndrome (RDS). Furthermore, there

is controversy surrounding whether either form of high-frequency ventilation lessens the incidence of BPD (*see* Table 12-11).

Stark AR: High-frequency oscillatory ventilation to prevent bronchopulmonary dysplasia—Are we there yet? N Engl J Med 347:682–683, 2002.

207. **Has nasal prong continuous positive airway pressure (CPAP) been proven to decease the risk of BPD?**
   No. The beneficial effects of CPAP are unproven, although there is considerable anecdotal data supporting its efficacy. Multicenter randomized clinical trials are in progress.

   Polin RA, Sahni R: Newer experience with CPAP. Semin Neonatol 7:379–389, 2002.

TABLE 12-11. HIGH-FREQUENCY OSCILLATORY VENTILATION VERSUS HIGH-FREQUENCY JET VENTILATION

	High-frequency oscillatory ventilation	High-frequency jet ventilation
Frequency	10–30 Hz	10–40 Hz
Total volume	Determined by oscillator	Increased by gas entrainment
I:E ratio	Constant	Variable
Expiratory phase	Active, less risk of gas trapping	Passive, more risk of gas trapping
Airway damage	Similar to IPPV	Necrotizing tracheobronchitis
May be used in combination with IPPV	Yes	Yes

I:E = inspiratory-to-expiratory, IPPV = intermittent positive pressure ventilation.

208. **Have antenatal steroids or surfactant been proven to decrease the risk of chronic lung disease?**
   No. Although both treatments offer benefits with regard to preventing and treating RDS, neither one has been shown to lower the incidence of BPD.

   Van Marter LJ, Allred EN, Leviton A, et al; Neonatology Committee for the Developmental Epidemiology Network: Antenatal glucocorticoid treatment does not reduce chronic lung disease among surviving preterm infants. J Pediatr 138:198–204, 2001.

209. **What is the function of surfactant?**
   Surfactant is a surface-active material that is made up of a mixture that is rich in phosphatidyl-choline (64%), phosphatidylglycerol (8%), and lesser amounts of proteins and other lipids. Surfactant acts as an anti-atelectasis factor in the alveolar lining by lowering surface tension at diminished lung volumes and increasing it at high volumes. This allows for the maintenance of functional residual capacity, which acts as a reservoir to prevent wide fluctuation in arterial PO_2 and PCO_2 during respiration. In patients with RDS, surfactants have been shown to decrease the need for supplemental oxygen therapy, to lower mortality rates, and to decrease the incidence of air-leak syndromes. The incidence of BPD has also been reduced in some studies.

210. **Do the kinds of surfactant used to treat infants with RDS differ in effectiveness?**
   Two general classes of surfactant are available for replacement therapy: *natural surfactants* prepared from mammalian lungs (e.g., Survanta, Infasurf, Curosurf) and *synthetic surfactants*

(e.g., Exosurf, ALEC). Although natural surfactant extracts seem to have a better immediate effect (i.e., less supplemental oxygen required, fewer pneumothoraces), long-term clinical outcomes (e.g., chronic lung disease, death) with synthetic surfactants were not significantly different. Natural surfactants may be associated with a higher risk of intracranial hemorrhage, but they are still considered to be preferable.

Soll RF, Blanco F: Natural surfactant extract versus synthetic surfactant for neonatal respiratory distress syndrome. Cochrane Database Syst Rev 2:CD000144, 2001.

211. **In surfactant therapy, is "prophylaxis" or "rescue" treatment better?**
Although some institutions administer surfactant as soon as possible after birth (preventilatory or within minutes of ventilation) as **prophylaxis** and others wait for the development of RDS to administer **rescue** therapy, earlier administration is advantageous, even with the latter approach. Recent data suggest that, for the most immature babies (<28 weeks or possibly <26 weeks), prophylaxis improves survival and lessens the severity of RDS, but it appears to not reduce the incidence of chronic lung disease.

Soll RF, Morley CJ: Prophylactic versus selective use of surfactant in preventing morbidity and mortality in preterm infants. Cochrane Database Syst Rev 2:CD000510, 2001.

212. **What are the adverse effects of prophylactically administering surfactant in the delivery room?**
- Approximately 20–60% of healthy infants whose gestational age is ≥30 weeks will be treated unnecessarily.
- It imposes extra risks and unwarranted expenses.
- The use of surfactant may lead to a transient decrease in oxygen saturation.
- It delays resuscitation efforts and stabilization if administered before ventilation.

213. **Which infants benefit most from extracorporeal membrane oxygenation (ECMO)?**
ECMO is prolonged cardiopulmonary bypass that is used to treat newborn infants (<1 week old) with reversible pulmonary disease that has been complicated by persistent pulmonary hypertension. Although overall survival is approximately 70–80%, it varies by diagnosis, with rates of >90% for meconium aspiration syndrome, 75% for sepsis, and approximately 50% for congenital diaphragmatic hernia.

214. **What are the risks of and contraindications to ECMO?**
The risk of thrombosis is an ever-present threat during ECMO therapy. Therefore, all infants receiving ECMO are heparinized. However, heparinization creates an increased risk for systemic bleeding and/or intracranial hemorrhage. Long-term morbidities are generally referable to the CNS.

Contraindications to ECMO include uncontrolled bleeding, grade II or greater IVH, pulmonary hemorrhage, irreversible pulmonary disease, history of severe asphyxia, prolonged mechanical ventilation (>7–14 days), lethal genetic condition, and significant prematurity (birthweight <2,000 gm; gestational age <35 weeks).

215. **What characterizes the diagnosis of BPD?**
Since BPD was first reported in 1967, the clinical definition and diagnosis have evolved to include all patients who, after mechanical ventilation, remain oxygen-dependent at 36 weeks postconceptional age and who have persistent changes on chest radiographs. The pathologic diagnosis remains unchanged and is characterized by areas of emphysema and collapse with interstitial edema and fibrosis. The airway epithelium demonstrates hyperplasia and squamous metaplasia, and the smooth muscle in the airways and vasculature frequently demonstrates hyperplasia.

216. **What are the advantages and disadvantages of long-term diuretic therapy for BPD?**

Long-term diuretic therapy in infants with BPD improves pulmonary function, decreases airway resistance, increases pulmonary compliance, and allows for the weaning of supplemental oxygen. However, the duration of supplemental oxygen may not be shortened. Furthermore, the long-term effect on infant mortality is not entirely clear. Diuretic therapy is not without side effects, including electrolyte imbalance, nephrocalcinosis, bone demineralization, and ototoxicity.

Brion LP, Primhak RA: Intravenous or enteral loop diuretics for preterm infants with (or developing) chronic lung disease. Cochrane Database Syst Rev 1:CD001453, 2002.

KEY POINTS: RESPIRATORY SYSTEM

1. Hypercarbia is tolerated to avoid barotrauma and to minimize the occurrence of chronic lung disease.

2. Whether surfactant is administered as "prophylaxis" or "rescue," the earlier the time of administration, the more potent the effects.

3. Outside of clinical trials and clinical respiratory disease unresponsive to maximal support, postnatal steroids should not be administered to prevent chronic lung disease or to facilitate extubation.

4. Apnea of prematurity may be central, obstructive, or mixed.

5. Continuous positive airway pressure is used to prevent extubation failure and apnea and may avert the need for mechanical ventilation in patients with primary lung disease.

217. **Are diuretics of any benefit for infants with RDS?**

No. There are no convincing data that diuretics improve the outcomes of infants with RDS.

Brion LP, Soll RF: Diuretics for respiratory distress syndrome in preterm infants. Cochrane Database Syst Rev 2:CD001454, 2001.

218. **What is the role of vitamin A supplementation for preventing or reducing the severity of BPD?**

Because vitamin A is involved in the proliferation and differentiation of epithelial cells, it is thought to play an important role in the repair process in the lung after barotrauma and oxygen exposure. Although vitamin A deficiency has been associated with the development of BPD, studies examining the effects of vitamin A supplementation on the incidence of BPD have shown conflicting results. However, the most recent large multicenter trial has demonstrated a modest reduction in the incidence of chronic lung disease in extremely low–birth-weight infants while reducing the biochemical evidence of vitamin A deficiency.

Tyson JE, Wright LL, Oh W, et al: Vitamin A supplementation for extremely-low-birth-weight infants. National Institute of Child Health and Human Development Neonatal Research Network. N Engl J Med 340:1962–1968, 1999.

219. **When should steroids be initiated in neonates with BPD?**

Studies of long-term follow up have demonstrated an increased incidence of cerebral palsy and adverse neurodevelopmental sequelae in premature infants who have been treated with postnatal steroids. Consequently, this treatment should be limited to patients who are participating in controlled clinical trials or to those receiving maximal ventilatory and oxygen support who are showing no signs of progress and at significant risk of death.

American Academy of Pediatrics and Canadian Pediatric Society: Postnatal corticosteroids to treat or prevent chronic lung disease in preterm infants. Pediatrics 109:330–338, 2002.

220. **Why are infants with BPD at increased risk for poor neurodevelopmental outcome?**
   - Recurrent episodes of hypoxia occurs as a result of chronic lung disease and BPD spells.
   - BPD is associated with IVH and periventricular leukomalacia.
   - Poor nutrition is an issue during periods of critical brain growth.
   - Prolonged illness and hospitalization preclude normal stimulation and parent-infant interaction.

   Gerdes JS: Bronchopulmonary dysplasia. In Polin RA, Yoder MC, Burg FD (eds): Workbook in Practical Neonatology, 3rd ed. Philadelphia, W.B. Saunders, 2001, p 198.

221. **What is the difference between apnea and periodic breathing?**
   Apnea is the cessation of respiration for >20 seconds or for a shorter duration if it is associated with cyanosis and/or bradycardia. **Periodic breathing** is commonly seen in preterm infants, and it is defined as a pattern of three or more respiratory pauses of >3 seconds' duration with <20 seconds of respirations between pauses. Periodic breathing is not associated with bradycardia. Both apnea and periodic breathing reflect a lack of maturation of respiratory control centers in the preterm infant.

222. **When should apnea be treated?**
   In all cases of apnea, an underlying cause should be sought and treated if found. In idiopathic apnea, therapy should be initiated when episodes do not resolve with gentle tactile stimulation and require vigorous stimulation or when patients have a frequency of more than four episodes in eight hours.

223. **What methods are effective for treating apnea of prematurity?**
   - Use of oscillating waterbeds
   - Administration of CPAP (this is especially helpful in apnea with an obstructive component)
   - Provision of supplemental oxygen (with or without CPAP) (If supplemental oxygen is used, the PaO_2 must be carefully monitored either directly by arterial blood gases or indirectly by noninvasive oxygen monitoring devices [e.g., pulse oximetry].)
   - Administration of respiratory stimulants (primarily methylxanthines)

224. **Is caffeine or theophylline more effective for lessening apnea of prematurity?**
   There is no evidence to date that one methylxanthine is more effective than another for reducing the frequency of apnea in premature infants. Caffeine, however, has become the preferred medication for several reasons: it is excreted more slowly, it can be given once daily, it achieves a more stable plasma level, and it has fewer gastrointestinal and CNS side effects.

   Steer PA, Henderson-Smart DJ: Caffeine versus theophylline for apnea in preterm infants. Cochrane Database Syst Rev 2:CD000273, 2000.

225. **What are the criteria for discontinuing the use of an apnea monitor or methylxanthines?**
   Methylxanthines are usually discontinued after an apnea-free period of 4–8 weeks. Alternatively, 44 weeks postconceptional age can be used as a "milestone" for the maturation of respiratory control in virtually all babies. The apnea monitor is then discontinued 4–8 weeks later if there is no recurrence of symptomatic apnea. A home pneumogram or a downloading of the data stored in the home "smart monitor" should be recorded before monitor discontinuance.

226. **Do home apnea monitors help prevent sudden infant death syndrome (SIDS)?**
    Epidemiologic studies have not been able to demonstrate any impact of home monitoring on
    the incidence of SIDS. On that basis, the American Academy of Pediatrics recommends that
    home monitors not be prescribed to prevent SIDS. Indications for monitoring include the
    following:
    - Premature infants with persistent apnea and bradycardia
    - Technology-dependent infants
    - Infants with neurologic or metabolic disorders that affect respiratory control
    - Infants with chronic lung disease, especially those requiring O_2, CPAP and/or mechanical
      ventilation

    American Academy of Pediatrics: Apnea, SIDS and home monitoring. Pediatrics 111:914–917, 2003.

ACKNOWLEDGMENT

The editors gratefully acknowledge contributions by Drs. Mary Catherine Harris, Carlos Vega-Rich, and Peter Marro that were retained from the first three editions of *Pediatric Secrets*.

CHAPTER 13

NEPHROLOGY

Michael E. Norman, MD

ACID-BASE, FLUIDS, AND ELECTROLYTES

1. **In what situations can a child be hyponatremic but not hypotonic?**
   - **Increased extracellular osmotically active solutes:** When excessive glucose, mannitol, glycerol, or another osmotically active substances are added to or increased in the extracellular space, the osmotic gradient pulls water from the cells and dilutes the serum sodium concentration.
   - **Elevated plasma lipids and plasma proteins:** A measurement of 100 mL of *serum* actually contains approximately 93 mL of water and 7 mL (gm) of *plasma* lipids and proteins. Increases in plasma lipids and protein decrease the amount of water (and sodium) in a fixed volume, and so the serum sodium concentration as measured per volume is artifactually decreased.

2. **How is the cause of hyponatremia established?**
   Artifactual causes of hyponatremia should be ruled out. If the urine specific gravity is <1.003, causes of water intoxication (e.g., administration of inappropriate intravenous fluids, use of low-solute formulas or plain water in infants, excessive use of tap-water enemas, pathologic drinking behavior in psychiatric patients) should be sought by history. If none of these causes are likely, clinical evaluation on the basis of the patient's volume status and urinary sodium concentration will help categorize the disorder:
   1. If the patient is **hypovolemic**, evaluate urinary sodium concentration.
      i. If the urinary sodium concentration is <20 mEq/L, consider extrarenal losses:
         - Gastrointestinal problems (vomiting, diarrhea, drainage tubes, fistulas, gastrocystoplasty)
         - Skin problems (cystic fibrosis, heat stroke)
         - Third spacing (burns, pancreatitis, muscle trauma, effusions, ascites, peritonitis)
      ii. If the urinary sodium concentration is >20 mEq/L, consider renal losses:
         - Diuretic induced
         - Osmotic diuresis
         - Salt-losing nephritis
         - Bicarbonaturia (renal tubular acidosis, metabolic alkalosis)
         - Mineralocorticoid deficiency
         - Pseudohypoaldosteronism
   2. If the patient is **euvolemic**, urine sodium concentration is usually >20 mEq/L, and the following should be considered:
         - Glucocorticoid or thyroid problem
         - Reset osmostat
         - Excessive antidiuretic hormone
   3. If the patient is **hypervolemic**, evaluate urinary sodium concentration:
      i. If the urinary sodium concentration is <20 mEq/L, consider edema-forming states:
         - Nephrosis
         - Congestive heart failure
         - Cirrhosis

ii. If the urinary sodium concentration is >20 mEq/L, consider acute or chronic renal failure.

Avner ED: Clinical disorders of water metabolism: Hyponatremia and hypernatremia. Pediatr Ann 24:23–30, 1995.

3. **What symptoms are associated with hyponatremia?**
Symptoms can range from gastrointestinal complaints (anorexia, nausea, vomiting) to mental status changes (headaches, irritability, disorientation, clouded sensorium), and these may lead to seizures, coma, and death. Symptoms of hyponatremia usually do not occur until the plasma Na+ is <120 mEq/L, but they may occur at higher concentrations if the change has been sudden.

4. **Describe the emergency treatment of symptomatic hyponatremia.**
Patients with central nervous system symptoms should receive urgent treatment with **hypertonic saline (3%)**; 1 mL/kg (which is equal to 0.513 mEq of sodium/mL) raises the serum Na by almost 1 mEq/L. Infusions of hypertonic saline at a rate of 3 mL/kg every 10–20 minutes are generally safe. Increasing the serum sodium by only 5–10 mEq/L is usually sufficient to stop hyponatremic seizures.

5. **How is the cause of hypernatremia established?**
A combination of history, clinical assessment of the patient's volume status, and urinary sodium concentration measurement is helpful for establishing the diagnostic categories:
1. If the patient is **hypovolemic**, evaluate urinary sodium concentration:
    i. If the urinary sodium concentration is <20 mEq/L, consider extrarenal losses:
        - Diarrhea
        - Excessive perspiration
    ii. If the urinary sodium concentration is >20 mEq/L, consider renal losses:
        - Renal dysplasia
        - Obstructive uropathy
        - Osmotic diuresis
2. If the patient is **euvolemic**, urinary sodium concentration is variable, and the following should be considered:
    - Extrarenal losses (insensible: dermal, respiratory)
    - Renal losses (central diabetes insipidus, nephrogenic diabetes insipidus)
3. If the patient is **hypervolemic**, urinary serum concentration is usually >20 mEq/L, and the following should be considered:
    - Improperly mixed formula in tube feeding
    - $NaCHO_3$ administration
    - NaCl administration, poisoning
    - Primary hyperaldosteronism (rare in children)

Avner ED: Clinical disorders of water metabolism: Hyponatremia and hypernatremia. Pediatr Ann 24:23–30, 1995.

6. **Why can correcting hypernatremia too rapidly cause seizures?**
Children with severe hyponatremia usually seize before treatment is started, whereas those with hypernatremia may develop seizures in response to therapy. In patients with hypernatremic dehydration, the increased extracellular tonicity draws fluid from the intracellular compartment, and cells shrink in size, including those in the brain. However, the brain can generate "idiogenic osmoles" to minimize the loss of fluids. These idiogenic osmoles are principally amino acids and other organic solutes that cause the brain to reabsorb some that water. In fact, in chronic hypernatremia, brain size is back to almost normal. It takes approximately 24 hours to begin to generate or dissipate these idiogenic osmoles. If the correction of chronic

(>24 hours duration) hypernatremia is too rapid, water flows from the extracellular compartment back into the cerebral intracellular compartment, thereby causing cerebral edema. This can lead to seizures, cerebral hemorrhage, and even death. To prevent this situation, in patients with chronic hypernatremia, the serum Na should not be allowed to fall faster than 0.5 mEq/L/h and ideally not more than 15 mEq/L in 24 hours.

7. **How does serum potassium concentration change with alterations in serum pH?**
In patients with **alkalosis**, potassium moves into cells as hydrogen moves out of cells in an effort to diminish the alkalinity. The opposite occurs in conditions of **acidosis**. For every 0.1 unit rise or fall in pH, there is a change in the opposite direction in the potassium concentration of between 0.4 and 0.6 mEq/L (i.e., lower pH leads to a higher potassium concentration). This is true in individuals and laboratory animals with acidosis as a result of mineral acids (e.g., HCl or NH_4Cl). The effects of organic acids on serum potassium are much less predictable.

8. **What are the clinical and physiologic consequences of progressive hypokalemia?**
   - Muscle weakness and paralysis, which can lead to hypoventilation and apnea
   - Constipation, ileus
   - Increases susceptibility for ventricular ectopic rhythms and fibrillation, especially in children receiving digitalis
   - Interference with the ability of the kidney to concentrate urine, leading to polyuria

9. **What should be the maximum rate and concentration of potassium infusions?**
Ideally, if potassium supplementation or replacement is needed, the concentration of potassium in the intravenous fluids should *not exceed* 40 mEq/L if given via a *peripheral vein* or 80 mEq/L if given via a *central vein*. Infusion rates should not be >0.3 mEq K^+/kg/h. Faster delivery can lead to local irritation of the veins, paresthesias and/or weakness, and cardiac arrest because of changes in transmembrane potentials. For life-threatening conditions that result from hypokalemia (e.g., cardiac dysrhythmias, respiratory paralysis in a patient without alkalosis or acidosis), the rate may be increased up to 1 mEq K^+/kg/h given centrally by an infusion pump. A continuous electrocardiogram monitor should be in place.

Cronan KM, Norman ME: Renal and electrolyte emergencies. In Fleisher GR, Ludwig S (eds): Textbook of Pediatric Emergency Medicine, 4th ed. Baltimore, Lippincott Williams &Wilkins, 2001, pp 819–820.

10. **List the common causes of hypokalemia.**
    - Diuretics, occasionally laxatives
    - Metabolic alkalosis, especially in patients with pyloric stenosis
    - Severe diabetic ketoacidosis with dehydration
    - Diarrhea
    - Renal tubular acidosis, types I and II
    - Fanconi syndrome
    - Bartter syndrome, Gitelman's syndrome
    - Hypermineralocorticoid states: Primary hyperaldosteronism, Cushing's syndrome, adrenal tumors, rare forms of congenital adrenal hyperplasia, dexamethasone-suppressible hypertension
    - Pituitary tumors producing adrenocorticotropic hormone
    - Hyperreninemic states

11. **Which foods are high in potassium?**
See Table 13-1.

TABLE 13-1. FOODS HIGH IN POTASSIUM		
Food	Portion	Potassium (mg)
Raisins	⅔ cup	751
Baked potato	1 medium	503
Cocoa	1 cup	480
Orange juice	8 oz	474
Banana	1 medium	451
French fries	⅜ cup	364
Carrot	1 raw	341

12. **List the causes of hyperkalemia in children.**
Increased intake
- Oral including salt substitutes
- Intravenous
- Exchange transfusion, use of aged, unwashed, packed red blood cells (RBCs)
- Hypovolemia

Decreased renal excretion
- Acute oliguric renal failure: Acute glomerulonephritis or acute tubular necrosis
- Oliguric end-stage renal failure
- Hypoaldosteronism

Transcellular outward movement
- Metabolic and acute respiratory acidosis
- Insulin deficiency and hyperglycemia in uncontrolled diabetes mellitus
- Increased tissue catabolism: Trauma, chemotherapy, hemolysis, rhabdomyolysis
- Exercise
- Medication related: Digoxin, beta-blockers, succinylcholine, arginine
- Familial hyperkalemic periodic paralysis
- Medications: Potassium-sparing diuretics, angiotensin-converting enzyme inhibitors
- Distal renal tubular acidosis, type IV
- Renal defect in potassium excretion (familial or obstructive)

Pseudohyperkalemia (laboratory artifact)
- Thrombocytosis, leukocytosis, hemolysis
- Abnormal leaky RBC membrane

   McDonald RA: Disorders of potassium balance. Pediatr Ann 24:31–37, 1995.

13. **When are calcium infusions indicated in a patient with elevated serum potassium?**
If the patient's **serum potassium level is >8 mEq/L** or **cardiac arrhythmia** is present. Calcium is the quickest way to treat an arrhythmia that is associated with hyperkalemia, but it has no effect on serum potassium concentrations. Hyperkalemia leads to an increase in the cell's membrane potential, thereby making cells more arrhythmogenic. Hypercalcemia raises the cell's threshold potential, restores the voltage difference between these two potentials, and decreases the likelihood of an arrhythmia. The effect of calcium infusion is transient, whereas potassium concentrations remain unchanged.

14. **What therapies are used for the emergency treatment of hyperkalemia?**
    - **Reversal of membrane effects** with 10% calcium gluconate, 0.5 mL/kg, administered intravenously over 2–5 minutes; onset of action within minutes; duration of action: 30–60 minutes. ECG should be monitored, and treatment should be discontinued if the pulse rate rises above 100 bpm.
    - **Movement of potassium into cells** with sodium bicarbonate, 7.5% (1 mEq = 1 mL), 2–3 mL/kg, or glucose 50% plus insulin (regular), 1 unit for every 5–6 gm of glucose, administered over 30–60 minutes; onset of action within 30 minutes; duration of action: 1–4 hours. Sodium bicarbonate may be used in the absence of acidosis; monitoring of blood glucose level is required with use of glucose plus insulin.
    - **Enhanced excretion of potassium** with Kayexalate, 1 gm/kg; can be given in 10% glucose (1 gm in 4 mL) every 4–6 hours; onset of action within hours; variable duration of action; route of administration: oral or rectal.

      Cronan K, Norman ME: Renal and electrolyte emergencies. In Fleisher GR, Ludwig S (eds): Textbook of Pediatric Emergency Medicine, 4th ed. Baltimore, Lippincott Williams & Wilkins, 2001, p 822.

15. **What is the normal serum anion gap from infancy to adulthood?**
    The anion gap or *delta* is the difference between the serum Na and the sum of the serum Cl^- plus serum bicarbonate, usually measured as total CO_2. This difference represents the unmeasured anions, such as organic acids, sulfate, and phosphate. The mean anion gap in children from age 9 months to 19 years is 8 ± 2 mEq/L if the blood is assayed immediately; however, if the blood is analyzed 4 hours later, the mean is closer to 11 mEq/L, which is similar to that of adults (12 ± 2 mEq/L). An elevated anion gap, in practice, occurs when this difference is >15–16 mEq/L.

16. **What are the causes of an elevated anion-gap acidosis?**
    The mnemonic **MUDPILES** is commonly used to recall these acidoses, which occur in a variety of clinical scenarios, including certain ingestions:
    M = **M**ethanol
    U = **U**remia (renal failure)
    D = **D**iabetic ketoacidosis, diarrhea of infancy
    P = **P**araldehyde, phenformin
    I = **I**ron, isoniazid, inborn errors of metabolism
    L = **L**actic acidosis (seen in clinical situations associated with hypoxia, severe cardiorespiratory depression, shock, and prolonged seizures)
    E = **E**thanol, ethylene glycol
    S = **S**alicylates

17. **How limited is the respiratory response to metabolic alkalosis?**
    Metabolic alkalosis occurs when a net gain of alkali or loss of acid leads to a rise in the serum bicarbonate concentration and pH. In metabolic alkalosis (as in metabolic acidosis), there is a measure of respiratory compensation in response to the change in pH. This response, which is accomplished by alveolar hypoventilation, is limited by the overriding need to maintain an adequate blood oxygen concentration. Usually the PCO_2 will not rise above *50–55 mmHg,* despite severe alkalosis.

18. **What is the differential diagnosis for a child presenting symptoms of primary metabolic alkalosis?**
    Metabolic alkalosis can be divided into two major categories on the basis of the urinary Cl^- concentration and the response to volume expansion with a saline infusion. The **saline-responsive** metabolic alkaloses usually involve a urine Cl^- concentration that is <10 mEq/L and significant volume depletion. Treatment with intravenously administered normal saline usually corrects the metabolic alkalosis; the classic example is pyloric stenosis.

The **saline-resistant** alkaloses are associated with a high urine Cl^- and often hypertension. The administration of normal saline tends to aggravate rather than correct the metabolic alkalosis. In most cases, mineralocorticoid excess plays the central role in the generation of the acid-base disturbance.

Causes of saline-responsive metabolic alkalosis	Causes of saline-resistant metabolic alkalosis
Pyloric stenosis	Primary hyperaldosteronism
Vomiting	(extremely rare in children)
Excessive upper gastrointestinal suctioning	Hyperreninemic hypertension
Congenital chloride diarrhea	Renal artery stenosis
Laxative abuse synthesis	Heritable block in steroid hormone
Diuretic abuse	17a-OH deficiency
Cystic fibrosis	11b-OH deficiency
Chloride-deficient formulas in infants	Licorice
Posthypercapnia syndrome	Liddle syndrome
Poorly reabsorbable anion administration	Bartter syndrome or Gitelman's syndrome
Posttreatment of organic acidemias	Severe potassium deficiency

19. **What is the pathophysiologic basis for "contraction alkalosis"?**

Alkalosis occurs as a result of an actual increase in bicarbonate recovery whenever dehydration is accompanied by the loss of chloride. Common settings include the *loss of gastric contents* (e.g., nasogastric suction, pyloric stenosis) or *intravascular dehydration* (e.g., diarrhea, diuretic abuse). In chloride-deficient states, sodium reabsorption is increased; however, as a result of a deficiency of chloride, all of the filtered bicarbonate is reabsorbed so that none can be excreted in the urine. Furthermore, because the individual is salt (and water) depleted, aldosterone levels are increased, and distal tubular sodium is reabsorbed (along with bicarbonate) in an exchange of potassium and hydrogen ion secretion. Thus, paradoxic aciduria can be seen in the setting of systemic alkalosis.

The treatment is to provide the patient with water and chloride ion. When potassium losses are not significant, NaCl alone will correct the alkalosis. Otherwise, KCl must be added to the infusion because severe hypokalemia is an independent cause of alkalosis.

CLINICAL ISSUES

20. **How is enuresis categorized?**

The terminology can be confusing. In an effort to standardize definitions, the 1998 International Children's Continence Society recommended the following:

- **Enuresis:** A normal void occurring at a socially unacceptable time or place
- **Nocturnal enuresis:** Voiding in bed during sleep that is socially unacceptable
- **Primary nocturnal enuresis:** Monosymptomatic (no other urinary symptoms) bedwetting in an individual who has never been dry at night for an uninterrupted period of 6 months
- **Dysfunctional voiding:** Functional disturbances of voiding owing to overactivity of the pelvic floor during micturition (Dysfunctional voiding is characterized by variable urinary stream, prolonged voiding, and incomplete bladder emptying, and it may be accompanied by daytime incontinence.)
- **Diurnal enuresis:** Daytime enuresis characterized by normal voiding but at a socially unacceptable time or place; voiding is complete

Norgaard JP, van Gool JD, Hjalmas K, et al: Standardization and definitions in lower urinary tract dysfunction in children. International Children's Continence Society. Br J Urol 81 Suppl 3:1–16, 1998.

21. **How common is primary nocturnal enuresis in older children?**

At the age of 5 years, approximately 20% of children (boys > girls) wet the bed at least once monthly. Nightly wetting is not as common (<5%). By the age of 7 years, the overall rate is down to 10%, and by the age of 10 years, it is down to 5%. About 1–2% of teenagers and adults persist with primary nocturnal enuresis.

22. **Why does bedwetting persist in some children?**

Ninety-seven percent or more of the causes are nonpathologic, and a number of explanations have been theorized: maturational delay of neurodevelopmental processes, small bladder capacity, genetic influence, difficulties with waking, and decreased nighttime secretion of antidiuretic hormone. Genetic influences are quite strong. If both parents were enuretic, a child's likelihood is about 75%; if one parent was involved, the likelihood is about 50%; only 3% of cases are the result of disease states. Psychological problems are an unlikely cause of nocturnal enuresis, but they are more common if daytime symptoms are present.

Thiedke CC: Nocturnal enuresis. Am Fam Physician 67:1499–1410, 2003.

23. **In what settings should a medical or surgical cause of enuresis be considered?**

Medical conditions include urinary tract infection (UTI), diabetes mellitus, diabetes insipidus, fecal impaction, and constipation. Suspicious symptoms include intermittent daytime wetness, polydipsia, polyuria, history of central nervous system trauma, and encopresis. **Surgical conditions** include ectopic ureter, neurogenic bladder, bladder calculus, and foreign body and debatably adenoidal enlargement. These should be suspected if there is constant dampness, a dribbling urinary stream with abnormalities in gait, or obstructive sleep apnea. A thorough history and physical examination along with urinalysis and urine culture (if indicated) is usually sufficient to eliminate the likelihood of any of these etiologies.

24. **What treatments are available for nocturnal enuresis?**

The therapeutic approach depends in large part on the age of the patient, the effect of the problem on the patient, and the parents' attitude. It is important to realize that 15% of patients per year will spontaneously improve.

- **Dry bed training:** Self-awakening routines, cleanliness training, bladder training, and rewards for dry nights; generally not effective as a sole intervention
- **Enuresis alarms:** Portable alarms (audio or vibratory) worn by the child at night and designed to awaken the child to the sensation of a full bladder; positive benefits in 70% of cases; safe, but requires parental and child motivation
- **Desmopressin:** Synthetic analog of vasopressin that, at a renal level, increases distal tubular retention of filtrate, thus diminishing nighttime bladder volume; available in oral and nasal forms; improvement noted in 12–65%; high relapse rate after discontinuation (similar to placebo); possible adverse effects, including nasal irritation; expensive
- **Imipramine:** Bladder effects include increasing capacity and decreasing detrusor excitability; improvement in 10–60% of cases, but high relapse rate; important central nervous system side effects in 10% (e.g., drowsiness, agitation, sleep disturbances)
- **Oxybutynin:** Provides an anticholinergic, antispasmodic effect that reduces uninhibited detrusor muscle contractions; limited studies available on effectiveness; ≤17% experience adverse reactions (e.g., dry mouth, flushing, drowsiness, constipation)

Silverstein DM: Enuresis in children: Diagnosis and management. Clin Pediatr 43:317–221, 2004.
Nield LS, Kamat D: Enuresis: How to evaluate and treat. Clin Pediatr 43:409–415, 2004.

KEY POINTS: ENURESIS

1. This is a very familial condition; 70% of enuretic children have a parent with the condition.

2. Nocturnal enuresis prevalence rates show a natural history of spontaneous resolution: 20% at 5 years, 10% at 7 years, and 5% at 10 years, with only a 1% persistence rate.

3. Isolated primary nocturnal enuresis rarely has identifiable organic pathology.

4. There is a high relapse rate when medications are stopped.

5. Enuresis alarms are the most therapeutically (especially in younger patients) and cost effective, but they require weeks of consistent use for full benefits.

25. **What are the causes of diurnal enuresis?**

Organic causes account for <5% of cases. Of these, urinary tract infections are probably the most common. An ectopic ureter should be suspected if dampness is constantly present; most children with diurnal enuresis have intermittent wetness. Rarely, a neurogenic bladder can cause this problem. Severe lower urinary tract obstruction can lead to bladder distention with overflow incontinence. Finally, pelvic masses (e.g., presacral teratoma, hydrocolpos, fecal impaction) that press on the bladder can lead to stress incontinence with running, coughing, or lifting.

Physiologic types of daytime wetting include the vaginal reflux of urine, giggle incontinence, and urgency incontinence. Reflux of urine into the vagina during micturition occurs frequently; after normal voiding, when the girl stands up and walks, the urine seeps out of the vagina and wets the underpants. Giggle incontinence is a sudden, involuntary, uncontrollable, and complete emptying of the bladder when giggling or laughing. Tickling or excitement may also lead to this problem. Urgency incontinence can be defined as an attack of intense bladder spasms that leads to abrupt voiding and wetting.

Psychogenic causes may be related to stress. Wetting can occur in any child who is significantly frightened. Chronic stress (e.g., the loss of a close relative, parental marital discord, hospitalization) can also lead to this kind of daytime wetting. The resistant child is one who is about 2½ years old and who refuses to be toilet trained. Seventy percent are males who are predominantly or totally wet. Often, this situation has occurred because of high-pressured attempts at toilet training. Most children with daytime wetness and nighttime dryness have a behavioral basis for the problem.

26. **What simple exercises may help a child with daytime incontinence?**

Kegel exercises are exercises of the pelvic muscles. The pelvic muscles can be stimulated in children by instructing them to void, then starting and stopping the urinary stream two or three times by means of pelvic contractions. These maneuvers can then be done at other times without voiding. Voluntary contracture of the pelvic floor muscles is reflexively accompanied by relaxation of the detrusor muscle. These exercises may be helpful for children with daytime incontinence.

Schneider MS, King LR, Surwit RS: Kegel exercises and childhood incontinence: A new role for an old treatment? J Pediatr 124:91–92, 1994.

27. **How do you treat labial adhesions?**

Labial adhesions are a relatively common gynecologic finding in girls between 4 months and 6 years of age. They may be complete or partial and are felt to be a result of local inflammation in a low-estrogen setting with resulting skin agglutination. Treatment consists of eliminating the underlying inflammation (if it is caused by an infection), sitz baths twice daily, maintenance of good perineal hygiene, and topical application of a 1% conjugated estrogen cream over the entire adhesion at bedtime for 3 weeks. The use of estrogen has an 80–90% cure rate and may be followed by the application of a petroleum jelly for 1–2 months nightly. It should be noted that the natural history of untreated asymptomatic labial adhesions is self-resolution: 50% resolve within 6 months, and nearly 100% resolve by 18 months. Surgical correction is almost never required.

Leung AKC, Robson WLM, Kao CP, et al: Treatment of labial fusion with topical estrogen therapy. Clin Pediatr 44:245-247, 2005.

HEMATURIA

28. **What distinguishes lower from upper tract bleeding?**
As a general rule, brown, tea- or cola-colored urine suggests *upper tract bleeding,* whereas bright red blood suggests *lower tract bleeding.* The darker urine has had more time to become oxidized within the urinary tract. However, exceptions occur. Rapid upper tract bleeding may be red, and a dissolving clot within the bladder may produce brown urine. Establishing the source of microscopic hematuria can be difficult. *Glomerular bleeding* is said to produce red cells that are small and dysmorphic with blebs or burr cells as opposed to the normal-sized red cells seen in lower tract bleeding. Unfortunately, this change is best observed with phase contrast microscopy, which is not readily available in most clinical settings. The presence of significant *proteinuria* also suggests upper tract (i.e., kidney) disease. The presence of even a single red blood cell or hemoglobin *cast* indicates a glomerular (or, rarely, tubular) etiology.

Patel HP, Bissler JJ: Hematuria in children. Ped Clin North Am 48:1519–1537, 2001.

29. **If a healthy 5-year-old child has bright red blood at the end of a previously clear urine stream, what is the likely diagnosis?**
The finding of bright red blood suggests that this is lower tract bleeding. The history of the early part of the urination producing clear urine suggests that this child has a problem with his *bladder neck* or *trigone.* In the absence of pain or other symptoms, it is most likely that this child has *benign hemorrhagic cystitis,* which is most often caused by adenovirus. In an otherwise healthy child, the family should be reassured that hematuria will resolve within several days. Bacterial urinary tract infections almost never cause gross hematuria (certainly not bright red). The absence of pain argues against a stone or bladder calculus, and the vast majority of pediatric nephrologists are still waiting to diagnose their first bladder hemangioma.

30. **How common is asymptomatic hematuria?**
Up to *3%* of all girls (and *1.5%* of boys) will have two out of three urines positive for >5 RBC per high-power field at some time between the ages of 6–12 years. This drops to only about 0.8% (0.5% for boys) if the clinician's definition of hematuria requires the presence of blood in three consecutively collected urine specimens.

31. **Which children with hematuria should be evaluated?**
Children with microscopic hematuria without proteinuria should be evaluated if the hematuria is present in essentially all tested urines over several months' time. Red flags in the history and physical examination that suggest other than a benign etiology include the following:
History
- Recent illnesses (particularly if you can associate episodes of gross hematuria with the illnesses)
- Trauma (particularly if there is gross bleeding after relatively minor trauma)
- Pain: Abdominal, suprapubic, flank, or dysuria
- Medication usage: Anticoagulants, aspirin, sulfonamide, chronic antibiotic administration, and others

- Family history of renal disease, bilateral hearing loss, hemoglobinopathies, bleeding disorders, or stone disease

Physical Examination
- Short stature
- Hypertension
- Pallor
- Significant (nonfunctional) cardiac murmurs
- Abdominal mass
- Evidence of multisystem disease

32. **What evaluations should be considered during the evaluation of isolated hematuria?**
- Blood urea nitrogen (BUN)/creatinine
- Electrolytes
- Urine calcium/creatinine ratio
- Serologic evidence of recent streptococcal infection (unless hematuria has been present for several months)
- Renal ultrasound: Evaluation for structural abnormalities (e.g., hydronephrosis, autosomal dominant or recessive polycystic kidney disease) and for Wilms' tumor in any patient <5 years old
- Hemoglobin electrophoresis: If sickle cell trait or disease is suspected
- C3, C4, antinuclear antibody (ANA), or antinuclear cytotoxic antibody (ANCA): In the absence of proteinuria or evidence of systemic involvement, *unlikely* to be positive
- Urine culture: Unnecessary for recurrent gross hematuria or in an asymptomatic child with a 6-month history because there is a *low likelihood* of positivity

KEY POINTS: HEMATURIA

1. This is a very common condition; asymptomatic, microscopic hematuria is found in 1–4% of school children.

2. In the vast majority, the condition is benign, and evaluation yields no renal or urologic disease.

3. Hypercalciuria (>4 mg/kg/day) is found in significant numbers of these patients.

4. Patients with significant proteinuria along with hematuria are much more likely to have underlying pathology.

5. If the dipstick assessment is positive for blood but microscopic urinalysis is negative for red blood cells, suspect hemolysis (positivity as a result of hemoglobin) or rhabdomyolysis (muscle breakdown with positivity as a result of myoglobin).

33. **How common is hypercalciuria as a cause of hematuria?**
This depends on where you live. In areas of the southeastern United States—often called "the stone belt"—this is a common cause of isolated hematuria, with nearly *one third* of children with microscopic hematuria having hypercalciuria as the cause. In other parts of the United States, it is significantly less common.

34. **How does hypercalciuria cause hematuria?**
The mechanism is unknown, but it has been hypothesized to involve *irritation* of the renal tubules by calcium-containing *microcrystals*. Because the amount of blood lost in this way is

minimal and never causes anemia and because only a limited number of these patients develop renal calculi, it is important to be conservative before initiating chronic therapy. If there is a history of nephrolithiasis or nephrocalcinosis, hypercalciuria can be treated by increasing fluid intake, decreasing sodium intake, and, if necessary, adding of a small dose of a thiazide diuretic.

GLOMERULONEPHRITIS

35. **During the evaluation of a patient with hematuria, what features suggest glomerulonephritis?**
Three presentations of glomerular involvement can occur:
1. **Acute glomerulonephritis:** Edema, proteinuria of 1+ or greater, hypertension, oliguria, dysmorphic RBCs (small, misshapen RBC with blebs), or red-cell casts on urinalysis
2. **Chronic glomerulonephritis:** Minimal acute symptoms; may have chronic fatigue, failure to thrive, or unexplained anemia with features of chronic renal failure, hypertension, abnormal urinalysis, and azotemia
3. **Nephrotic syndrome:** Proteinuria >40 mg/m^2/h, edema, hypoproteinemia, and hyperlipidemia

36. **If glomerulonephritis is suspected, what laboratory tests should be considered?**
   - Urinalysis
   - BUN/creatinine
   - Serum C3 (possibly C4)
   - Streptococcal serology
   - Throat culture; skin culture if lesions present
   - Serum albumin
   - ANA, anti-DNA antibodies (if systemic lupus erythematosus is suspected)
   - Hepatitis B and C serology (for patients living in endemic areas, those who have received transfusions, or those who engage in high-risk behavior)
   - ANCA (if rapidly progressive glomerulonephritis or vasculitis is suspected)

37. **Which glomerulonephritides are associated with hypocomplementemia?**
   - Poststreptococcal
   - Other postinfectious causes (may have normal complement)
   - Subacute bacterial endocarditis
   - Shunt nephritis
   - Systemic lupus erythematosus
   - Membranoproliferative

38. **Does the treatment of streptococcal skin or pharyngeal infections prevent poststreptococcal glomerulonephritis?**
No study has ever demonstrated that the treatment of impetigo or pharyngitis prevents renal complications in the index case. Clearly, acute rheumatic fever does not occur after the skin infections, and glomerulonephritis is limited to infections with a few serotypes, especially 49, 55, 57, and 60, which appear to be less prevalent in recent years. However, treatment lessens the likelihood of contagious spread to hosts who may be susceptible to renal complications. Serum antistreptolysin (ASO) titers, which are elevated in patients with pharyngeal infections, are usually not elevated after skin infections. Therefore, to confirm the diagnosis of an antecedent skin infection, antihyaluronidase and anti-DNase B titers should be obtained.

39. **What is the usual time course for poststreptococcal glomerulonephritis?**
Approximately 7–14 days after a pharyngitis and as long as 6 weeks after a pyoderma with group A beta-hemolytic streptococci, children typically have tea-colored urine and edema.

The acute phase (e.g., hypertension, gross hematuria) can as long as 3 weeks. Serum complement levels may remain depressed for up to 8 weeks, and persistence beyond this point suggests another diagnosis. Chronic microscopic hematuria can persist for up to 18 months. In pediatric patients, full recovery is expected and progression to chronic renal insufficiency is extremely rare.

40. **What percentage of children with poststreptococcal glomerulonephritis have elevated levels of serum ASO titers?**

    Approximately *80–85%* of children with documented pharyngeal streptococcal infections develop elevated ASO titers. Streptolysin O is bound to lipids in the skin so that the percentage of individuals with streptococcal impetigo who develop positive ASO titers is much lower. For this reason, a normal ASO titer does not rule out recent ASO infection. Screening for other streptococcal-associated antigens, antihyaluronidase, and antiDNAase B titers or the use of the Streptozyme test, which measures a variety of streptococcal antigens, will be positive in >95% of children with documented streptococcal infection.

41. **A 9-year-old boy with intermittent episodes of gross hematuria associated with febrile upper respiratory infections likely has what type of glomerular disease?**

    Immunoglobulin A (IgA) nephropathy (Berger's disease). This is the most common cause of chronic glomerulonephritis in persons of European or Asian descent. In children, IgA nephropathy typically causes asymptomatic microscopic hematuria with periods of gross hematuria during febrile infections. Most children are normotensive and, other than the gross hematuria, have no other kidney-related findings. Previously considered a benign condition, recent studies indicate that, after 30 years of follow up, approximately 30% of individuals will develop evidence of chronic renal insufficiency. Renal biopsy followed by specific treatment is generally reserved for those who develop evidence of progressive disease, (i.e., hypertension, persistent proteinuria, or an elevated serum creatinine concentration). The etiology of IgA nephropathy is unclear, and diagnosis is established by renal biopsy with the demonstration of IgA in the mesangium of the glomerulus.

42. **What are the most common causes of chronic glomerulonephritis in children and adolescents?**

    - IgA nephropathy (Berger's disease)
    - Diffuse proliferative glomerulonephritis
    - Membranoproliferative glomerulonephritis
    - Familial nephritis (primarily the sex-linked recessive form [Alport's syndrome])
    - Henoch-Schönlein purpura
    - Crescentic glomerulonephritis (rapidly progressive glomerulonephritis)
    - Systemic lupus erythematosus

HYPERTENSION

43. **How is hypertension defined in children?**

    The diagnosis of hypertension is made on the basis of comparison with the normative distribution blood pressure of healthy children of similar age, gender, and height. (This information is available in the article cited below.)

    - **Hypertension:** Average systolic and or diastolic blood pressure is ≥95th percentile on ≥3 occasions
    - **Prehypertension:** ≥90th percentile, but <95th percentile; as with adults, adolescents with blood pressure of ≥120/80 mmHg should be considered prehypertensive

    National High Blood Pressure Education Program Working Group on High Blood Pressure in Children and Adolescents: The fourth report on the diagnosis, evaluation, and treatment of high blood pressure in children and adolescents. Pediatrics 114:555–576, 2004.

KEY POINTS: HYPERTENSION

1. Common cause of artifactual elevation: Blood pressure cuff is too small

2. Essential (no detectable cause): Often a strong family history

3. Secondary (detectable lesion) hypertension: More likely with higher blood pressures and in younger children

4. Majority of secondary hypertension in children caused by renal disease (renal anomalies, renal parenchymal disease, renal vascular abnormalities)

44. **How do you determine the optimum cuff size for obtaining a blood pressure?**
The length of the inflatable bladder inside the cuff (easily palpated) should almost completely encircle the arm and will overestimate the blood pressure if it is too short. Additionally, the height of the cuff should be the largest that comfortably fits from the axilla to the elbow. A cuff that is too small can produce falsely elevated blood pressure readings, and one that is too large can produce falsely low blood pressure readings.

45. **Which Korotkoff sound best represents diastolic blood pressure?**
The Korotkoff sounds are produced by the flow of blood as the constricting blood pressure cuff is gradually released. There are five phases of Korotkoff sounds. The first appearance of a clear, tapping sound is called *phase I* and represents the systolic pressure. As the cuff continues to be released, soft murmurs can be auscultated; this is *phase II*. These are followed by louder murmurs during *phase III*, as the volume of blood passing through the constricted artery increases. The sounds become abruptly muffled in *phase IV* and disappear in *phase V*, which is usually within 10 mmHg of phase IV.
    In studies that compare intravascular blood pressure determinations with auscultatory readings, true diastolic pressure is most closely related to phase V (the disappearance of sound). However, in many young children, muffled sounds can be heard to zero and thus clearly do not always correlate with diastolic pressure. In these instances, it is best to record both the phase IV (the point at which sounds become muffled) and the phase V readings (e.g., 80/45/0).

46. **When should hypertension be treated in the neonate?**
Hypertension is defined as a blood pressure of >90/60 mmHg in term neonates and of >80/45 in preterm infants. A sustained systolic blood pressure of >100 mmHg in the neonate should be investigated and treated.

KEY POINTS: CONSISTENT AND STRUCTURED WAYS TO AVOID MISDIAGNOSING HYPERTENSION

1. Properly sized cuff (age-dependent)

2. Quiet room, quiet patient

3. Repeated measurements over time and the use of averaged values

4. Get rid of the white coat

5. Sit at child level when taking the measurement

47. **What are the indications for the pharmacologic treatment of hypertension in older children?**
    - Symptomatic hypertension
    - Secondary hypertension
    - Hypertensive target-organ damage (e.g., left ventricular hypertrophy on echocardiogram)
    - Diabetes (types 1 and 2)
    - Persistence despite nonpharmacologic measures

    National High Blood Pressure Education Program Working Group on High Blood Pressure in Children and Adolescents: The fourth report on the diagnosis, evaluation, and treatment of high blood pressure in children and adolescents. Pediatrics 114:555–576, 2004.

48. **During the evaluation of a child with elevated blood pressure, what risk factors should be considered for identification and/or reduction?**
    Important risk factors for hypertension in children include **family history** (if one parent has hypertension, the risk is about 25%; if both parents have hypertension, the risk is 45%), other genetic factors including **race** (African Americans have twice the incidence of hypertension as compared with Caucasians, beginning in adolescence), **obesity**, history of **renal disease**, and **dietary factors** (mainly salt intake). More recently, a history of **prematurity** has been recognized as a risk factor.

    Remembering that hypertension is a critical risk factor for cardiovascular disease, the important risk factors for this largest cause of mortality should also be addressed. These include diet and its effect on serum lipids; tobacco use; and lack of exercise.

49. **What are the most common causes of hypertension in pediatric patients?**
    - **Newborn period: Renal artery occlusion.** This is usually caused by a thromboembolism from an umbilical catheter; additionally, coarctation of the aorta must always be considered.
    - **Older infants and children: Renal** or **renovascular disease.** Included in the broad category of renal disease are virtually all categories of renal dysfunction, such as obstructive nephropathy, scarring from UTI and reflux, glomerulonephritis, polycystic kidney disease, and renal dysplasia.
    - **Adolescence:** Renal disease is also very common, but **primary** or **essential hypertension** is the most frequent cause of high blood pressure.

50. **List other causes of secondary hypertension in children and adolescents.**
    See Table 13-2.

51. **What historic information suggests a secondary cause of hypertension?**
    See Table 13-3.

52. **List the features on physical examination that suggest a secondary cause of hypertension.**
    See Table 13-4.

53. **Why should patients with hypertension and/or those using diuretics avoid licorice?**
    True licorice contains glycyrrhizic acid, which has mineralocorticoid (i.e., sodium-retaining) properties. However, most American licorice contains only licorice flavoring and thus has no mineralocorticoid properties. Some chewing tobacco also contains licorice and has been associated with an excessive mineralocorticoid syndrome. Think of this if you are called to evaluate an edematous New York Yankees batboy.

TABLE 13-2.	CAUSES OF SECONDARY HYPERTENSION IN CHILDREN AND ADOLESCENTS		
Cause	Acute hypertension	Chronic hypertension	Etiology
Renal	Acute glomerulonephritis	Congenital defects	Tumors of the kidney
	Acute renal failure	Chronic pyelonephritis	Hypoplastic kidney
	Hemolytic-uremic syndrome	Hydronephrosis	Collagen vascular disease
Endocrine	—	Pheochromocytoma	Primary aldosteronism
		Hyperthyroidism	Neuroblastoma
Vascular	Renovascular trauma	Coarctation of the aorta	Renal arteriovenous fistula
		Renal artery stenosis	Neurofibromatosis
		Takayasu arteritis	Tuberous sclerosis
Neurogenic	Increased intracranial pressure	Dysautonomia	—
	Guillain-Barré syndrome		
Metabolic	Hypercalcemia	—	—
	Hypernatremia		
Drugs	Cocaine	Nonsteroidal anti-inflammatory drugs	Anabolic steroids
	Phencyclidine		Corticosteroids
	Amphetamines	Oral contraceptives	Alcohol
Miscella-neous	Burns	Heavy metal poisons	—
	Leg traction		

Adapted from Daniels SR, Loggie JM: Essential hypertension. Adolesc Med State Art Rev 2:555, 1991.

PROTEINURIA/NEPHROTIC SYNDROME

54. **How do the bedside methods for testing protein in random urine samples compare?**
    - **Dipstick assessment:** This relies on the reaction of protein (primarily albumin) with tetrabromophenol blue in a citrate buffer impregnated on the dipstick patch. Mild false-positive reactions can occur (1–2+) when the patient's urine is alkaline or when the dipstick is allowed to sit in the urine for too long and the buffer strength is overcome. The results are reported qualitatively as trace to 4+, which corresponds to a range of 30–2,000 mg/dL.
    - **Sulfosalicylic acid:** This test precipitates protein in the urine and allows for a comparison with a group of previously prepared aqueous standards; it is reported in the same way as those standards. In contrast with the dipstick assessment, all proteins—not just albumin—are precipitated. The finding of heavy proteinuria by sulfosalicylic acid testing with minimal proteinuria using the dipstick suggests the presence of large amounts of nonalbumin protein, most often as the result of multiple myeloma and the excretion of Bence Jones proteins. Look for this during a geriatrics—not a pediatrics—rotation.

TABLE 13-3. SECONDARY CAUSE OF HYPERTENSION AS SUGGESTED BY HISTORY

History	Suggests
Known urinary tract infection; recurrent abdominal or flank pain with frequency, urgency, dysuria; secondary enuresis	Renal disease
Joint pains, rash, fever, edema	Renal disease, vasculitis
Complicated neonatal course, umbilical artery catheter	Renal artery stenosis
Renal trauma	Renal artery stenosis
Drug use (e.g., sympathomimetics, anabolic steroids, oral contraceptives, illicit drugs)	Drug-induced hypertension
Aberrant course or timing of secondary sexual characteristics; virilization	Adrenal disorder
Muscle cramping, constipation, weakness	Hyperaldosteronism (primary or secondary)
Excessive sweating, episodes of pallor and flushing	Pheochromocytoma

Adapted from Hiner LB, Falkner B: Renovascular hypertension in children. Pediatr Clin North Am 40:128–129, 1993.

TABLE 13-4. PHYSICAL FINDINGS THAT SUGGEST A POSSIBLE SECONDARY CAUSE OF HYPERTENSION

Physical finding	Possible secondary cause
Blood pressure	
>140/100 at any age	Multiple secondary causes
Leg < arm blood pressure	Coarctation of the aorta
Poor growth	**Chronic renal disease**
Short stature, features of Turner syndrome	Coarctation of the aorta
Multiple café-au-lait spots or neurofibromas	Renal artery stenosis, pheochromocytoma
Decreased or delayed pulse in leg	Coarctation of the aorta
Vascular bruits	
Over large vessels	Arteritis
Over upper abdomen, flank	Renal artery stenosis
Flank or upper quadrant mass	**Renal malformation, renal or adrenal tumor**
Excessive virilization or secondary sex characteristics inappropriate for age	Adrenal disorder
Extremities	
Edema	Renal disease
Excessive sweating	Pheochromocytoma

Adapted from Hiner LB, Falkner B: Renovascular hypertension in children. Pediatr Clin North Am 40:128–129, 1993.

55. **On a routine urinalysis, an asymptomatic 7-year-old boy has 1+ protein noted on dipstick assessment. How should this child be evaluated?**

Assuming that the child is otherwise healthy and without any of the subtle signs of renal disease (e.g., short stature, pallor, hypertension) and assuming that this is isolated proteinuria, it is important to determine whether the proteinuria is intermittent or persistent. Intermittent (transient) proteinuria is entirely benign and does not require any work-up. Persistent proteinuria may or may not be benign. The presence of persistent proteinuria can be determined by rechecking the urine at least three times over 2–3 weeks. If one of these tests is performed on a first morning urine specimen, the patient can be evaluated for orthostatic proteinuria at the same time. Causes of transient proteinuria include fever, vigorous exercise, dehydration, stress, cold exposure, and seizures.

56. **Other than a timed urine collection, what is the best "spot" method for determining the degree of proteinuria?**

Urinary protein/creatinine excretion ratio. Particularly in children, a 24-hour urine collection for protein is very difficult to obtain. Although both the dipstick and the sulfosalicylic testing methods estimate the concentration of protein in the urine, small amounts of protein in very concentrated urine will show up as more positive than the same amount of protein present in dilute urine. A number of studies have demonstrated that the urinary protein/creatinine ratio more closely approximates total 24-hour urinary protein excretion. Thus, on a random sample of urine, a urine protein/creatinine ratio of *<0.2–0.25* reflects a normal daily protein excretion, whereas values of *>1* strongly suggest the presence of the nephrotic syndrome. This test has proven very effective both for the diagnosis of the nephrotic syndrome and for follow-up evaluations in children with prolonged and difficult-to-manage proteinuria. However, the test may overestimate protein excretion in individuals with abnormally low muscle mass (and hence lower creatinine excretion rates).

57. **How is the diagnosis of orthostatic proteinuria established?**

By definition, individuals with orthostatic proteinuria have normal rates of protein excretion when lying recumbent but increased excretion rates when upright. Although all individuals excrete more protein when standing, some have an exaggerated response and may excrete as much as 1 gm of urinary protein per day. Protein excretion when recumbent can be assessed semiquantitatively with a first morning urine specimen immediately upon arising using either a urine dipstick or a sulfosalicylic acid precipitation of the urine. More accurate assessment can be obtained using the urine protein/creatinine excretion ratio or as milligrams excreted per hour. In a reasonably concentrated first morning urine specimen (urine specific gravity ≥ 1.018), a trace or negative value by dipstick assessment or sulfosalicylic acid precipitation is adequate to rule out proteinuria. At any urine specific gravity, a urine protein/creatinine ratio (mg/dL/mg/dL) of <0.25 is also considered normal. Remember, even individuals with renal disease may have increased protein excretion when standing and lower protein excretion rates when recumbent. The key to orthostatic proteinuria is that protein excretion is truly normal when recumbent and the individual is otherwise entirely healthy.

58. **What additional evaluation should be done for a patient with persistent proteinuria?**

If the child's proteinuria is persistent and not orthostatic, protein excretion needs to be determined. Although the gold standard is the timed (24-hour) urine collection, this is often difficult to obtain from children. Because substantial amounts of urine are often lost, a 24-hour urinary creatinine excretion should be determined at the same time to assess for completeness. A standard definition of proteinuria was developed by the International Study for Kidney Disease in Children. Those researchers defined proteinuria as the excretion of >4 mg/m^2 of protein per hour (or 100 mg every 24 hours for a 30-kg child). More commonly, the urine protein/creatinine ratio is used.

The evaluation of a child with persistent proteinuria includes many of the same tests required to evaluate glomerulonephritis, such as BUN/creatinine; electrolytes; serum albumin; and often tests to document evidence of immunologic activation, such as C3, C4, ANA, and anti-DNA antibodies. Rarely, ANCA may be required. Finally, renal imaging studies and renal biopsy may be necessary for diagnosis.

59. **What is the natural history of orthostatic proteinuria?**
Few prospective data exist about the long-term outcome of children and adolescents, but follow-up data for young adults for up to 50 years after diagnosis demonstrate a *benign* clinical course. Most agree that the prognosis is excellent, although the etiology remains unclear.

60. **What level constitutes "significant" proteinuria?**
Protein excretion of >4 mg/m^2/h on a timed urine collection is considered abnormal. Children with nephrosis excrete >40 mg/m^2/h. The upper limit of protein excretion in adults is 150 mg/day, but, for some reason, adolescents may excrete as much as 250 mg/day. A urine protein/urine creatinine ratio of >0.5 in children <2 years old and of >0.2 in older children is considered excessive.

61. **In the presence of gross hematuria, what amount of protein excretion is considered abnormal?**
500 mg/m^2/day.

62. **What constellation of clinical findings defines nephrotic syndrome?**
The nephrotic syndrome consists of **proteinuria**, **hypoalbuminemia**, **edema**, and **hyperlipidemia.** Of these, the proteinuria is primary, with the development of hypoalbuminemia, edema, and hyperlipidemia as secondary findings. It is not at all uncommon to find individuals with clear evidence of nephrotic-range proteinuria and mild to moderate hypoalbuminemia in whom evidence of hypolipidemia and peripheral edema are minimal.

63. **What distinguishes nephrosis from nephritis?**
The suffix "-itis" implies *evidence of inflammation*, which is seen on renal biopsy as the proliferation of the cellular elements within the glomerulus and often the presence of white blood cells. Clinically, these abnormalities produce a disruption of glomerular basement structure and function that leads to hematuria and proteinuria. The proteinuria may be minimal to massive, depending on the type and severity of the **nephritis**. The finding of RBC casts in the urine is, with rare exceptions, diagnostic of glomerulonephritis.

Nephrosis is another term for the nephrotic syndrome. "Syndrome" implies a characteristic group of findings that may have diverse causes. As noted in the answer to the previous question, the nephrotic syndrome is caused by the renal loss of protein and the development of hypoalbuminuria, edema, and hyperlipidemia. This can be caused by a number of renal conditions, some of which demonstrate proliferative and inflammatory changes and some that do not demonstrate any evidence of nephritis (e.g., minimal change nephrotic syndrome). Thus, some but not all patients with (glomerulo)nephritis may have nephrosis, and some patients with the clinical syndrome called nephrosis may have evidence of nephritis on urinalysis (e.g., RBC casts) (Fig. 13-1) or on biopsy.

64. **Which childhood diseases appear primarily as glomerulonephritis or the nephrotic syndrome?**
Most of conditions in Table 13-5 present symptoms of either a nephritic or a nephrotic picture; occasionally a mixed picture will be noted.

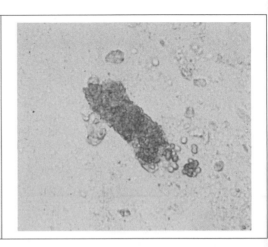

Figure 13-1. Red blood cell cast from a patient with streptococcal glomerulonephritis. These casts are almost always associated with glomerulonephritis or vasculitis and virtually exclude extrarenal disease. (From Zitelli BJ, Davis HW: Atlas of Pediatric Physical Diagnosis, 4th ed. St. Louis, Mosby, 2002, p 458.)

TABLE 13-5. CHILDHOOD DISEASES PRESENTING WITH SYMPTOMS OF GLOMERULONEPHRITIS OR NEPHROTIC SYNDROME

Glomerulonephritis	Nephrotic syndrome
Postinfectious (both streptococcal as well as other bacteria, viruses, and parasites)	Minimal change nephrosis
Henoch-Schönlein nephritis	Focal segmental glomerulosclerosis
Immunoglobulin A nephropathy glomerulonephritis	Membranoproliferative
Membranoproliferative glomerulonephritis	Membranous nephropathy
Familial nephritis	Congenital nephrotic syndrome
Systemic lupus erythematosus	Systemic lupus erythematosus
Immune complex nephritis (infective endocarditis or "shunt nephritis")	Henoch-Schönlein nephritis
Rapidly progressive glomerulonephritis (Wegener's granulomatosis or polyarteritis nodosa)	Immunoglobulin A nephropathy
Familial nephritis	

65. **At what level of albumin do children usually start to develop edema?**
When the serum albumin falls *below 2.5 gm/dL,* edema usually *begins* to develop. When it falls *below 1.8 gm/dL,* edema is almost always *present,* unless the child is receiving a diuretic.

66. **Why doesn't eating more protein restore the serum albumin concentration to normal in individuals with the nephrotic syndrome?**
The loss of urinary albumin is only part of the story. Under normal circumstances, very small amounts of albumin are filtered at the glomerulus. A very high percentage of what is filtered is then catabolized by the proximal tubular cells. Amino acids are reabsorbed from the tubular lumen back into the body and resynthesized into albumin within the liver. In patients with the

nephrotic syndrome, significantly more albumin is filtered. Even with increased catabolism and amino acids reabsorption at the renal tubular level, the rate of liver albumin synthesis is limited, and serum albumin levels fall. Feeding more protein would lead to increased protein absorption through the gastrointestinal tract, but the rate-limiting feature of insufficient liver synthesis cannot be overcome.

67. **What is the most common form of nephrotic syndrome seen in childhood?**
Minimal-change nephrotic syndrome (MCNS). Earlier names for this condition included "lipoid nephrosis" and "nil disease." MCNS is a form of primary nephrotic syndrome and has a more favorable therapeutic response and prognosis. The etiology of MCNS is unknown, but it appears to be a condition of abnormal T lymphocyte function. Other forms of *primary* nephrotic syndrome include conditions such as focal segmental glomerulosclerosis, membranous nephropathy, and membranoproliferative glomerulonephritis. *Secondary* forms of nephrotic syndrome may also occur as a consequence of infection, as a response to some medications, and as an autoimmune phenomenon.

68. **What is the most important historic factor to consider when assessing a patient for possible MCNS?**
Although the only definitive way to document the presence of MCNS is with a renal biopsy, most patients with MCNS show a constellation of signs and a response to treatment that is characteristic. The most important characteristic for a child with this condition is *age on presentation*. Between 75% and 80% of all children with nephrotic syndrome have MCNS, and approximately 80% of those present symptoms within the first 8 years of life. Appearance before the age of 1 year is unusual and should make one suspect various forms of congenital nephrotic syndrome or a secondary etiology such as congenital syphilis.

69. **What are the typical clinical features and therapeutic responses seen in patients with MCNS?**
Edema is generally present, blood pressure is normal, and gross hematuria is absent, but up to one third of these patients may have microscopic hematuria; however, RBC casts are not seen. In the absence of significant intravascular volume depletion, BUN, creatinine, and electrolytes are all within normal limits. Children who present symptoms in this manner should be started on daily prednisone; this is often called a "medical biopsy."

The standard dose recommended for the initial episode is 2 mg/kg/day with a maximum dose of 80 mg/day. A single daily dose given in the morning is as effective as split doses and may lead to fewer steroid side effects. For the initial episode, daily steroids are continued for 1 month, regardless of how soon the patient responds. If the patient responds, then the daily prednisone is changed to alternate-day dosing at the same 2 mg/kg every other day for an additional month. Thereafter, the dose is tapered over the next 2 months. Relapses are treated similarly, except the switch to alternate-day steroid is done when the urine dipstick assessment shows a negative or trace protein reaction for 3–4 days.

After the initiation of prednisone for an initial episode, <93% of patients will respond during the first month, with the mean time being 10–13 days. Response is indicated by the normalization of urinary protein excretion and diuresis. If therapy is prolonged for an additional month, another 4% will respond. Approximately 3% of children with biopsy-proven MCNS will be steroid resistant despite 2 months of therapy.

70. **When should secondary therapies be considered for MCNS?**
- For patients who do not respond to the initial course of prednisone
- For patients who become subsequent nonresponders to prednisone during relapses
- For patients who have frequent relapses
- For patients who develop significant side effects from steroids

71. **When are furosemide and albumin therapy indicated for patients with nephrotic syndrome?**

Infusion of a 25% albumin solution in a dose of 0.5–1 gm/kg of albumin over 1–2 hours and followed by a potent diuretic such as furosemide (1–4 mg/kg) can be used to induce diuresis in a child with nephrotic syndrome that is unresponsive to furosemide alone. This measure is only *temporary* because the rise in albumin will lead to increased protein excretion, thereby returning the serum level to the previous steady-state value. However, it is useful in a child with severe edema leading to incapacitating anasarca, cellulitis, skin breakdown, or respiratory embarrassment from pleural effusions. Albumin alone is useful for the child with a rising BUN caused by decreased renal perfusion; this situation is most often seen after vigorous diuretic therapy.

72. **What are the risks of the "albumin–Lasix sandwich"?**

The administration of 25% albumin and furosemide is a serious therapy with important potential risks to the patient. The unspoken assumption in this treatment is that the fluid drawn back into the intravascular space by the albumin infusion will be excreted by the kidneys after the administration of furosemide. This may not be true when the nephrotic syndrome is associated with decreased renal function as a result of coexisting glomerulonephritis. In that situation, the interstitial fluid drawn from the periphery may lead to *intravascular volume overload* and *pulmonary edema.*

73. **What is the mechanism of hypercoagulability associated with nephrotic syndrome?**

Multiple factors contribute to the hypercoagulable state. *Blood viscosity* (in part as a result of hyperlipidemia) is increased. *Platelet adhesiveness* is increased. Nearly all *coagulation factors* and *clotting inhibitors* are altered. Fibrinogen levels are increased, and antithrombin III levels are decreased as a result of urinary losses. The overall tendency favors increased coagulation and decreased fibrinolysis.

74. **Which organisms are responsible for peritonitis in children with nephrotic syndrome?**

Pneumococcus remains the most important cause, although gram-negative organisms, especially *Escherichia coli*, account for 25–50% of cases.

75. **Which causes of nephrotic syndrome are likely to progress to renal impairment?**

See Table 13-6.

76. **Discuss the prognostic factors in children with nephrotic syndrome.**

The best prognosis is associated with the presence of MCNS. For individuals with other etiologies, the two features in all categories that portend a worse prognosis are the presence of *large amounts of urinary protein* and the development of *hypertension.* Thus, the maintenance of normal blood pressures, including the liberal use of angiotensin-converting enzyme inhibitors, is widely stressed in the treatment of patients with persistent nephrotic syndrome.

77. **In which children with nephrotic syndrome should renal biopsy be considered?**

Because older children are more likely to have other forms of nephrotic syndrome (e.g., focal segmental glomerulosclerosis, membranoproliferative glomerulonephritis), most pediatric nephrologists would biopsy those who present symptoms at the age of >8 years before beginning therapy. Certainly the presence of significant hypertension, renal insufficiency, RBC casts, multiple organ involvement, partial lipodystrophy, or a low serum C3 level all speak against the finding of MCNS and require a renal biopsy for definitive diagnosis. Children of any age who do not go into remission during their initial course of prednisone or who fail to respond to prednisone after relapses will also require a renal biopsy.

TABLE 13-6. PROGRESSION OF NEPHROTIC SYNDROME TO RENAL IMPAIRMENT

Type of nephrotic syndrome failure	Percentage progressing to renal without treatment
Minimal change nephrotic syndrome	0%*
Focal segmental glomerulosclerosis	30–50%
Membranoproliferative glumerulonephritis	90%†
Membranous	30%
Systemic lupus erythematosus	30–40%
Henoch-Schönlein nephritis	1–5%
Diabetes mellitus	100%‡
AIDS nephropathy	100%

*It is generally believed that patients with minimal change nephrotic syndrome do not progress. Clinical deterioration (or developed—this is still the subject of much debate) is attributed to underlying undiagnosed focal segmental glomerulosclerosis.
†Treatment of membranoproliferative glomerulonephritis has been shown to be effective for decreasing the rate of progression to chronic renal failure over several years, but the long-term outcome is still unclear.
‡Even in the absence of intensive therapy, only 40% of individuals with diabetes mellitus will develop significant proteinuria and the nephrotic syndrome. However, those that due invariably progress to chronic renal failure. Intensive treatment of the diabetes has been shown to decrease this complication by 50–70%.

RENAL FAILURE

78. **What clinical tools, including laboratory studies, are useful for distinguishing prerenal oliguria (e.g., volume depletion) from the oliguria of intrinsic acute renal failure (ARF)?**
Clinical assessment of hydration, volume, and perfusion status are critical and are more likely to be impaired in a prerenal state. In patients with ARF, these parameters are more likely to show normal or excess volume status, including possible evidence of edema or vascular congestion. If volume status assessment suggests a volume deficit, a fluid bolus with normal saline can be both diagnostic and therapeutic. Laboratory studies of some assistance are summarized in Table 13-7.

79. **What is the most common cause of ARF in young children in the United States?**
The answer traditionally has been the **hemolytic-uremic syndrome**, which in most cases is associated with gastrointestinal infection with verotoxin-producing *Escherichia coli,* especially the O157:H7 serotype. However, when one considers *all* of the cases of **acute tubular necrosis** in childhood that most commonly result from hypoxic, hypotensive, and/or hypovolemic

insults or drug-induced injury, it is difficult to place this broad category of ARF in second place. If you are asked on rounds and are in an argumentative mood, answer "acute tubular necrosis." (No one knows the true answer because statistics are not available for large populations.)

TABLE 13-7.	LABORATORY STUDIES OF VALUE IN PRERENAL OLIGURIA AND ACUTE RENAL FAILURE	
Parameter	Prerenal	Renal
U Na-random meq/L	<20	<40–60
FE_{Na}^{*}	<1%	>3%
Urine osmolality (mOsm/L)	>500	<300

*$FE_{Na} = ([U_{Na} \times P_{Creat}]/[P_{Na} \times U_{Creat}]) \times 100\%$ (on a randomly collected, "spot" urine).

80. **Does the use of antibiotic therapy in children with diarrhea caused by *E. coli* 0157:H7 prevent hemolytic-uremic syndrome?**
   This is controversial. A 2000 study showed that children who received antibiotics (usually sulfa-containing or beta-lactam antibiotics) during outbreaks have had a much higher rate (50% versus 7%) of hemolytic-uremic syndrome, but other larger studies have reported a protective or no association.

   Safdar N, Said A, Gangnon RE, Maki DG.: Risk of hemolytic-uremic syndrome after antibiotic treatment of *Escherichia coli* 0157:H7 enteritis: A meta-analysis. JAMA 288:996–1001, 2002.

   Wong CS, Jelacic S, Habeeb RL, et al: The risk of hemolytic-uremic syndrome after antibiotic treatment of *Eshcerichia coli* 0157:H7 infections. N Engl J Med 342:1930–1936, 2000.

81. **What constitutes the triad of clinical findings of the hemolytic-uremic syndrome?**
   1. **Acute renal failure** that is usually—but not always—oligoanuric.
   2. **Microangiopathic hemolytic anemia:** Examination of the smear is essential to identify RBC fragments, burr cells, and schistocytes.
   3. **Thrombocytopenia** that may vary from mild to severe.

82. **What is the pathogenesis of renal osteodystrophy?**
   Renal osteodystrophy, which is also known as "renal metabolic bone disease" or "renal rickets," is a condition that affects bone growth and development and that occurs in patients with chronic renal insufficiency. The pathogenesis is a combination of factors that lead to hypocalcemia. These include *phosphate retention* and *hyperphosphatemia* as a result of a decreased glomerular filtration rate and decreased production of 1,25 dihydroxyvitamin D by the kidney. This leads to the decreased absorption of calcium from the gastrointestinal tract and the decreased responsiveness of bone to parathyroid hormone. The hypocalcemia leads to an increased release of parathyroid hormone, which then increases bone resorption. Chronic disease leads to secondary hyperparathyroidism and bone marrow fibrosis, which is known as *osteitis fibrosis cystica*. Recognition of osteodystrophy, which often has its origins when the glomerular filtration rate is still approximately half of the normal rate, is important, because early intervention with vitamin D and phosphate binders can prevent and/or heal the bone disease (although not necessarily enhance growth). Also, in states of chronic acidosis, the

skeleton acts as a buffer for the net acid retained. This results in the release of calcium, which contributes to osteopenia and bone disease.

83. **What are indications for dialysis?**
 Elevated BUN and creatinine: There are no established critical levels above which dialysis needs to be instituted. However, when the creatinine reaches 10 mg/dL or the BUN 100 mg/dL, the glomerular filtration rate is usually markedly reduced, which results in one or more of the following abnormalities:
 - **Hyperkalemia**, either rapidly rising or stable at a dangerously high level that is not controlled by Kayexalate-binding resin or other measures
 - **Volume-dependent hypertension** or signs of **congestive heart failure** not responsive to diuretics
 - **Severe metabolic acidosis** that cannot be treated with sodium bicarbonate
 - Signs or symptoms of **uremia** (e.g., fatigue, encephalopathy, anorexia, pruritus, cramps, bleeding, pericarditis)
 - **Other severe electrolyte disturbances**, including symptomatic hyponatremia, hypocalcemia, and hyperphosphatemia
 - Need for a **blood transfusion** in the presence of oligoanuria

84. **What are the main causes of chronic renal disease in children that result in renal transplantation?**
 - Obstructive uropathy
 - Aplastic/hypoplastic/dysplastic kidneys
 - Focal segmental glomerulosclerosis

 Chan JC, Williams DM, Roth KS: Kidney failure in infants and children. Pediatr Rev 23:47–60, 2002.

RENAL FUNCTION ASSESSMENT AND URINALYSIS

85. **What is the simplest way to estimate the glomerular filtration rate in the absence of a timed urine collection?**
 Use of the *Schwartz formula* requires only a serum creatinine level and the height of the child. No urine collection, timed or untimed, is necessary. The formula is as follows:
 Creatinine clearance (mL/min/1.73m^2) = K × Height (cm)/Serum creatinine (mg/dL)
 K is 0.45 in infants <1 year old, 0.55 in infants >1 year old, 0.33 in low birthweight infants, and 0.7 in adolescent males.

86. **How can you be confident that a 24-hour urine collection (for anything) is complete?**
 Because creatinine is produced in a continuous fashion and eliminated only via the kidneys, there is an expectation that a given amount, determined largely by muscle mass, will be excreted daily, independent of the level of renal function. Thus, the determination of total urine creatinine in a timed sample can give a reasonable estimate of whether the collection approximates that of 24 hours. The guidelines for expected creatinine excretion applicable to children and adolescents are as follows: for males, 15–25 mg/kg/day; for females, 10–20 mg/kg/day.

87. **When should routine urinalyses (UA) be performed in the pediatric age group?**
 There is some controversy regarding the use of the UA as a routine screening tool. It is a simple, inexpensive, and noninvasive study that is quite sensitive and specific, but the likelihood of this test for uncovering significant, previously undiagnosed renal dysfunction is very low. However, the landscape is strewn with nephrologists who can cite from personal experience cases of significant renal disease that were first discovered on a routine UA. The American

Academy of Pediatrics Guidelines for Health Supervision recommends a UA at the age of 5 years and another sometime between the ages of 11 and 21 years (or annual dipstick urinalysis for leukocytes for sexually active male and female adolescents).

American Academy of Pediatrics, Committee on Practice and Ambulatory Medicine: Recommendations for preventive pediatric health care. Pediatrics 105:645–646, 2000.

88. **How does Clinitest differ from typical urine dipstick testing for the evaluation of glucosuria?**
The **Clinitest tablet** detects reducing substances in the urine. These include reducing sugars (e.g., glucose, galactose, lactose, pentoses, fructose) and other compounds, including high amounts of amino acids, oxalate, ketones, and uric acid. It is also positive in the presence of many drugs, including high concentrations of ascorbic acid, penicillin, cephalosporins, nitrofurantoin, sulfonamides, and tetracycline. The **glucose oxidase square** on the dipstick is specific for glucose. The Clinitest may be helpful as an initial screening tool for a child who is suspected of having galactosemia, or it may be useful when testing the stool of a child who is suspected of having carbohydrate malabsorption/intolerance.

Liao JC, Churchill BM: Pediatric urine testing. Pediatr Clin North Am 48:1425–1440, 2001.

89. **What are the maximum and minimum urinary dilutional and concentrating capabilities of the renal system?**
Maximally dilute urine has a specific gravity of 1.001 and an osmolality of 50. Maximally concentrated urine has a specific gravity of about 1.032 and an osmolality of about 1,200. Urine that is neither concentrated nor dilute (i.e., isosthenuric) has a specific gravity of approximately 1.010 and a corresponding osmolality of 300.

90. **What is the difference between urine specific gravity and urine osmolality?**
Both tests measure the concentration or dilution of the urine, and the relationship between the two is linear and direct, although osmolality is more physiologically correct. **Specific gravity** is determined by the *density* (and thus the weight and size) of solute in solution. **Osmolality**, on the other hand, depends on the *numbers* of solute (independent of their size) in solution and their effect on changing its freezing point. Therefore, when there are solutes with a relatively large molecular weight (e.g., albumin, glucose, contrast material) in the urine, specific gravity will disproportionately increase, and osmolality will be a better indicator of true urine concentration. A urine specific gravity of 1.040 is not achievable by the human kidney; in a child with nephrotic syndrome, levels that high do not represent supernormal concentrating capacity but rather artifactual effects of heavy proteinuria.

91. **What crystal, when seen in the urinary sediment, is always pathologic?**
The presence of a **cystine crystal**, which appears as a flat, simple, hexagon-shaped crystal, is never normal and is strong evidence for the amino acid transport disorder cystinuria. In classic cystinuria, the dibasic amino acids (cystine, ornithine, arginine, and lysine) are affected. The condition would be of little clinical significance except for the fact that cystine is very insoluble and results in nephrolithiasis.

SURGICAL ISSUES

92. **What are the risks of circumcision?**
The most common complications are bleeding and infection. With poor technique, injury or amputation of the glans can occur. Meatal stenosis as a consequence of meatal ulceration is another complication.

93. **Is circumcision now medically indicated?**

The debate continues. Data support that newborn circumcision protects males against UTIs in infancy and adulthood. Circumcision may decrease the transmission of certain sexually trans-mitted diseases (e.g., syphilis, chancroid, herpes simplex, human papillomavirus, human immunodeficiency virus), but these data are not as substantial. Other benefits can include improved lifetime genital hygiene, elimination of phimosis and local foreskin infections, and a lower incidence of penile cancer. There are many proponents both for and against circumci-sion. The decision at present, however, still rests primarily on nonmedical issues.

Alanis MC, Lucidi RS: Neonatal circumcision: A review of the world's oldest and most controversial operation. Obstet Gynecol Surv 59:379–395, 2004.

94. **What is the proper method of anesthesia for neonatal circumcision?**

Up to 85% of infant males in the United States undergo circumcision, and worldwide it remains the most commonly performed operation. Until recently, it was usually performed by most without anesthesia or analgesia. Although pacifiers, topical agents (3.0% lidocaine, EMLA cream), oral sucrose, and parenteral analgesics (e.g., acetaminophen) help alleviate some dis-comfort, the most effective means of minimizing pain are a ring block or a dorsal penile nerve block. The latter consists of injecting 0.3–0.4 mL of 1% lidocaine *without* epinephrine in both sides of the dorsal penile base.

Litman RS: Anesthesia and analgesia for newborn circumcision. Obstet Gynecol Surv 56:114–117, 2001.

95. **What is hypospadias?**

Hypospadias occurs in 1–2 out of every 1,000 live births and results from the failure or delay of the midline fusion of the urethral folds. It is often associated with a ventral band of fibrous tissue (chordee) that causes ventral curvature of the penis, especially with an erection, thereby making intercourse difficult or impossible. When assessing hypospadias, it is useful to describe where the urethral meatus appears (i.e., glandular, distal shaft, proximal shaft, or perineal) and also the degree and location of chordee. The treatment of hypospadias is surgical repair, usually as a one-step procedure. With the advent of microsurgical techniques, the optimal time for repair appears to be 6–12 months of age.

96. **How are the degrees of hypospadias classified?**

The mildest and most common form of hypospadias is distal hypospadias (Fig. 13-2, *A*), which occurs in the subcoronal or glandular area in about 80–85% of cases. About 10–15% of cases occur in the penile shaft. Only 5–10% occur in the severe penoscrotal or perineal location (Fig. 13-2, *B*).

97. **What abnormalities are associated with hypospadias?**

A number of associated genitourinary abnormalities have been described with hypospadias, including meatal stenosis, inguinal hernias, undescended testes, and enlarged utricle masculi-nus (vestigial vagina). The incidence of these abnormalities rises sharply with the more severe degrees of hypospadias. In the mild forms, which account for most cases, radiography or endoscopy of the urinary tract is unnecessary.

98. **What distinguishes phimosis and paraphimosis?**

Phimosis is a narrowing of the distal foreskin, which prevents its retraction over the glans of the penis. In newborns, retraction is difficult because of normal adhesions that gradually self-resolve. Chronic inflammation or scarring can cause true phimosis with persistent narrowing and may require circumcision. **Paraphimosis** is incarceration of a retracted foreskin behind the glans. It occurs when the retracted foreskin is not repositioned. Progressive edema results, which, if uncorrected, can lead to ischemic breakdown. Local anesthesia, ice, and manual reduction usually correct the problem, but if these are unsuccessful, surgical reduction is necessary.

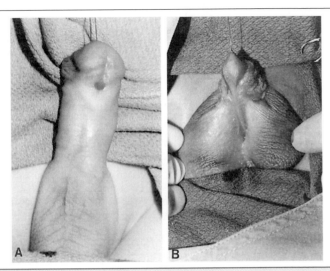

Figure 13-2. *A,* Distal hypospadias. *B,* Severe proximal hypospadias in the midscrotal area. (From Kay R: Hypospadias. In Resnick MI, Novick AC (eds): Urology Secrets, 3rd ed. Philadelphia, Hanley & Belfus, 2003, p 188.)

99. **What is the most common cause of urinary tract obstruction in the newborn?**
    Posterior urethral valves, which are more commonly seen in male infants. The obstruction is frequently associated with high intravesicular pressures, which may damage the renal parenchyma if undetected. However, the adverse obstructive effects of the valves during intrauterine life may be associated with renal dysplasia. Thus, even with prompt recognition and treatment, renal insufficiency may progress.

100. **What is the natural history of hydroceles?**
    Small hydroceles in infancy are benign and spontaneously resolve by 9–12 months of age. Large hydroceles rarely resolve and may cause vascular compromise and testicular atrophy; these should be resected. A communicating hydrocele (which changes in size) indicates a completely patent processus vaginalis and has the potential for hernia formation. This variety should also be repaired.

101. **When should undescended testicles be repaired?**
    The optimal time for surgery on an undescended testicle is *12 months of age* or shortly there-after. Traditional teaching is that cryptorchidism usually resolves without intervention. Seventy-five percent of full-term infants and 90% of premature cryptorchid newborns will have full testicular descent by the age of 9 months, although recent data suggest that the rate of spontaneous descent is much lower. Spontaneous testis descent after 9 months is unlikely. During the second year of life, ultrastructural changes in the seminiferous tubules of the undescended testes begin to appear, but these may be halted by orchiopexy.

    American Academy of Pediatrics: Timing of elective surgery on the genitalia of male children with particular reference to the risks, benefits, and psychological effects of surgery and anesthesia. Pediatrics 97:590–594, 1996.
    Wenzler DL, Bloom DA, Park JM: What is the rate of spontaneous testicular descent in infants with cryptorchidism? J Urol 171:849–851, 2004.

102. **What is the most common genitourinary abnormality found on prenatal ultrasound?**

Hydronephrosis. This descriptive term indicates distention of the renal pelvis and calyces, which is often due to obstruction. However, it can also be seen with nonobstructing entities such as vesicoureteral reflux (VUR).

103. **What are the possible causes of prenatal hydronephrosis?**
   - Ureteropelvic junction obstruction (most common)
   - Posterior urethral valves
   - VUR
   - Prune belly syndrome
   - Multicystic kidney
   - Ectopic ureter or ureterocele
   - Megaureter (obstructive and nonobstructive)
   - Urethral atresia

   Gonzalez R, Schimke CM: Ureteropelvic junction obstruction in infants and children. Pediatr Clin North Am 48:1505–1518, 2001.

104. **What is a reasonable approach to the management of prenatally detected hydronephrosis?**
   See Fig. 13-3.

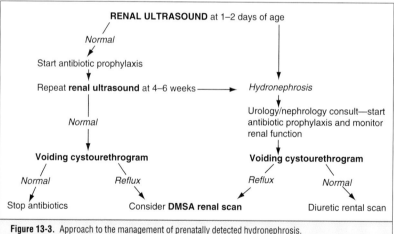

Figure 13-3. Approach to the management of prenatally detected hydronephrosis.

105. **What physical findings should prompt a search for an underlying renal abnormality?**
   - Abdominal mass
   - Neonatal ascites
   - High imperforate anus
   - Oligohydramnios
   - Perineal hypospadias
   - Anuria-oliguria (especially in neonate)
   - Exstrophy of the bladder
   - Aniridia, hemihypertrophy (Wilms' tumor)
   - Ambiguous genitalia
   - Poor urinary stream

- Prune belly syndrome
- Persistent wetness

106. **What is the differential diagnosis of abdominal masses in newborns, infants, and children?**

During the newborn period, two thirds of abdominal masses are of renal origin, particularly hydronephrosis and dysplastic and polycystic kidneys. Below is the differential diagnosis of masses based on their location on physical examination.

Liver mass
Choledochal cyst
Benign tumors
Malignant tumors
Right lower quadrant mass
Appendiceal abscess
Lymphoma
Ectopic kidney
Ovarian or testicular mass
Lower midline mass
Hydrometrocolpos
Ovarian cyst or tumor
Sacrococcygeal teratoma
Left lower quadrant mass
Fecal impaction
Ovarian or testicular mass

Flank mass
Multicystic-dysplastic kidney (MCD) kidney
Hydronephrosis
Renal vein thrombosis
Neuroblastoma
Wilms' tumor
Adrenal hemorrhage
Midline mass
Gastrointestinal duplication
Mesenteric cyst
Omental cyst
Urachal cyst
Meconium pseudocyst
Pancreatic pseudocyst

Rudolph CD: Gastroenterology and nutrition. In Rudolph CD, Rudolph AM (eds): Rudolph's Pediatrics, 21st ed. New York, McGraw-Hill, 2003, p1375.

TUBULAR DISORDERS

107. **Name the four main types of renal tubular acidosis (RTA).**

Type 1: Impairment in *distal* acidification
Type 2: Impairment in *proximal* tubule bicarbonate reclamation
Type 3: A combination of types 1 and 2
Type 4: Occurs as a result of a lack of—or insensitivity to—aldosterone
All four types are associated with a hyperchloremic normal anion gap acidosis.

108. **Describe the clinical and laboratory manifestations of the various RTAs.**

RTAs of types 1, 2, and 3 are associated with *hypokalemia*, whereas type 4 is characterized by *hyperkalemia* in addition to hyperchloremic acidosis. Hypercalciuria is typical of type 1 RTA and, in conjunction with hypocitraturia, often leads to nephrocalcinosis and renal calculi. Type 2 is often part of a more global defect of proximal tubule function, the **Fanconi syndrome**, which, in addition to bicarbonaturia, is characterized by aminoaciduria, glycosuria, phosphaturia (hypophosphatemia), and rickets. Type 4 RTA is most commonly observed in pediatric patients with obstructive uropathy, tubular unresponsiveness to aldosterone (pseudoaldosteronism) that is often transient during infancy, or decreased aldosterone secretion (hypoaldosteronism). Other signs and symptoms that are common with all forms of RTA are growth failure, polyuria, polydipsia, recurrent dehydration, and vomiting (*see* Table 13-8).

109. **How is determining the urinary anion gap helpful for the evaluation of metabolic acidosis?**

Investigation of any child with a persistent metabolic acidosis must consider some form of RTA in the differential diagnosis. The urinary anion gap is a convenient and accurate screening test for RTA. It is an indirect estimate of urinary ammonium excretion (and thus urinary acid excretion) and is calculated by the following formula after determining urinary electrolyte concentrations:

$$\text{Anion gap} = Na^+ + K^+ - Cl^-$$

If the anion gap is *negative*, it suggests a large chloride excretion and thus adequate ammonium excretion. The urinary anion gap is negative in hyperchloremic metabolic acidosis as a result of diarrhea, untreated proximal RTA, or prior administration of an acid load. If the anion gap is *positive*, it suggests an acidification defect, as is seen in patients with distal RTA. Results are not reliable if there are large amounts of unmeasured anions such as ketoacids, penicillin, or salicylates.

TABLE 13–8. CLINICAL AND LABORATORY MANIFESTATIONS OF VARIOUS RENAL TUBULAR ACIDOSES

	Type 1 (classic, distal)	Type 2 (proximal)	Type 3 (hybrid)	Type 4 (aldosterone deficiency)
Growth failure	+++	++	++	+++
Hypokalemic muscle weakness	++	+	+	Hyperkalemia
Nephrocalcinosis	Frequent	Rare	±	Rare
Low citrate excretion	+++	±	±	±
Fractional excretion of filtered HCO_3 at normal serum HCO_3 levels	<5%	>15%	5–15%	<15%
Daily alkali treatment (mEq/kg)	1–10	5–20	1–10	1–5
Daily potassium requirement	Decreases with correction	Increases with correction	±	
Urine pH	>5.5	<5.5	>5.5	<5.5
Presence of other tubular defects	Rare	Common	Rare	Rare
Metabolic bone disease	Rare	Common	Rare	Rare
Urine anion gap	Positive	Negative	Positive	Positive

+ = present, ++ = common, +++ = very common, ± = variable.
From Chan JC: Renal tubular acidosis. J Pediatr 102:327–340, 1983.
From Zelikovic I: Renal tubular acidosis. Pediatr Ann 24:48–54, 1995.

110. **What is the primary defect in type 1 RTA?**
An inability of the distal tubule to secrete hydrogen. Thus, in the presence of significant systemic acidosis, urine is not maximally acidified (pH <5.5). This defect in hydrogen secretion is associated with low rates of ammonium and titratable acid excretion.

111. **How is the diagnosis of type 1 RTA established?**
The key to this diagnosis is the demonstration of an impaired ability of the distal tubule to secrete hydrogen NH_4^+ in the setting of a persistent metabolic acidosis. If a patient is *acidotic*, the following urine studies are diagnostic of distal RTA: (1) urine pH >5.5 (measured by meter)

or (2) diminished or absent NH_4^+ excretion (i.e., positive urinary anion gap). Another test of hydrogen ion secretion involves loading the patient with bicarbonate. Normally, distally secreted hydrogen ions combine with bicarbonate to form carbonic acid, which is catalyzed to water and CO_2. In patients with distal RTA, less carbonic acid (and thus CO_2) is produced. When the difference between the urine and blood CO_2 concentration is <20 mmHg, this indicates decreased hydrogen secretion, and distal RTA is likely.

112. **What is the main renal defect in type 2 RTA?**
The primary defect is a **decreased ability of the proximal tubule to reabsorb filtered HCO_3** at normal plasma HCO_3 concentrations—a "lowered tubular reabsorptive threshold." These patients typically have a chronic hyperchloremic metabolic acidosis, acid urine (pH <5.5), and a low fractional excretion of HCO_3 (FE <5%). When plasma HCO_3 levels are increased toward normal (and thus above the lowered tubular reabsorptive threshold), patients will lose HCO_3 in the urine (FE >15%), and the urine will be alkaline (pH >6.0).

113. **What are the recommended therapies for the treatment of various forms of RTA?**
Goals of RTA therapy: Improve growth, correct metabolic bone disease, prevent nephrolithiasis/nephrocalcinosis, and control any underlying disease process. Principle therapies include the following:
- **Alkali therapy** (sodium citrate or sodium bicarbonate): This is required for all forms of RTA, with the goal of a normal plasma HCO_3 level. Patients with *distal* RTA generally require only 2–3 mEq/kg/day of alkali. However, infants may also experience some increased urinary bicarbonate wasting and require up to 10 mEq/kg/day. Patients with *proximal* RTA require large quantities of alkali (5–20 mEq/kg/day). For *type 4* RTA, patients usually need low-dose alkali therapy (1–3 mEq/kg/day) *plus* a potassium-restricted diet and mineralocorticoid therapy if there is hypoaldosteronism.
- **Potassium supplementation** (potassium citrate): This is required in distal and especially in proximal RTA.

114. **How do you diagnose RTA in a patient with a hyperchloremic metabolic acidosis and a normal serum anion gap?**
See Fig. 13-4.

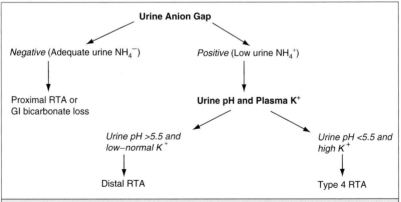

Figure 13-4. Diagnosis of renal tubular acidosis in patients with hyperchloremic metabolic acidosis and normal serum anion gap. (Adapted from Lash JP, Arruda JA: Laboratory evaluation of renal tubular acidosis. Clin Lab Med 13:117–129, 1993.)

115. **What is the clinical presentation of acute interstitial nephritis (AIN)?**
AIN is caused by an immune-mediated inflammatory response that initially involves the renal interstitium and tubules, usually sparing the glomeruli and vasculature. AIN has a wide array of clinical presentations that range from isolated tubular disorders (e.g., Fanconi syndrome) to acute renal failure. Additional findings may suggest a hypersensitivity reaction (e.g., fever, rash, arthralgias).

116. **What drugs are known to be causes of AIN?**
   - **Antibiotics** (especially penicillin analogs, cephalosporins, sulfonamides, and rifampin)
   - **Nonsteroidal anti-inflammatory drugs**
   - **Diuretics** (especially thiazides and furosemide)

117. **What laboratory abnormalities are seen in patients with AIN?**
   - **Urinary sediment:** RBCs, leukocytes (eosinophils), leukocyte casts
   - **Urinary protein excretion:** <1 gm/day; with NSAID use, may be >1 gm/day
   - **Fractional excretion of sodium:** Usually >1
   - **Proximal tubular defects:** Glucosuria, bicarbonaturia, phosphaturia, aminoaciduria, proximal RTA
   - **Distal tubular defects:** Hyperkalemia, sodium wasting, distal RTA
   - **Medullary defects:** Sodium wasting, urinary concentrating defects

   Meyers CM: Acute interstitial nephritis. In Greenberg A (ed): Primer on Kidney Diseases. National Kidney Foundation, Academic Press, San Diego, 1998, p 278.

URINARY TRACT INFECTIONS

118. **How helpful are dipstick testing and microscopic analysis of urine as screening tests for UTIs?**
Recalling that *sensitivity* is the probability that test results will be positive among patients who have UTIs and *specificity* is the probability that test results will be negative among patients who do not have UTIs, the value of the components of the urinalysis individually and in combination as screening tools for the diagnosis of a UTI are summarized in Table 13-9.

119. **What is the "enhanced urinalysis"?**
The enhanced urinalysis is a technique devised at the University of Pittsburgh as an alternative method of screening for UTIs. Traditional urinalysis has consisted of dipstick (particularly

TABLE 13-9.   EFFECTIVENESS OF SCREENING TESTS FOR URINARY TRACT INFECTIONS

Test	Sensitivity (range)	Specificity (range)
Leukocyte esterase	83% (67–94%)	78% (64–92%)
Nitrite	53% (15–82%)	98% (90–100%)
Leukocyte esterase *or* nitrite positive	93% (90–100%)	72% (58–91%)
Microscopy: White blood cells	73% (32–100%)	81% (45–98%)
Microscopy: Bacteria	81% (16–99%)	83% (11–100%)
Leukocyte esterase *or* nitrite *or* microscopy positive	99.8% (99–100%)	70% (60–92%)

From the American Academy of Pediatrics, Committee on Quality Improvement, Subcommittee on Urinary Tract Infection: Practice parameter: The diagnosis, treatment, and evaluation of the initial urinary tract infection in febrile infants and young children. Pediatrics 103:847, 1999.

leukocyte esterase and nitrite testing) and microscopic evaluation. A positive microscopic result has been ≥5 white blood cells per high-power field in a centrifuged specimen and any bacteria seen on an unstained specimen. The enhanced urinalysis modifies the approach as follows:

- **Pyuria:** Redefined as ≥10 white blood cells per mm^3 in uncentrifuged urine when viewed via a Neubauer hemocytometer
- **Bacteriuria:** Any seen on 10 oil immersion views after 2 drops of uncentrifuged urine are gram stained

The advantages of this method include the following: (1) decreased variability in results caused by centrifugation and resuspension; (2) fixed volume for examination; and (3) concise visual field with uniform illumination. This technique may have a higher sensitivity and positive-predictive value than traditional urinalysis.

Wald E: Urinary tract infections in infants and children: A comprehensive overview. Curr Opin Pediatr 16:85–88, 2004.

120. Can the diagnosis of UTI be made on the basis of urinalysis alone?

No. A urine culture is the only accurate means of diagnosing a UTI. Urinalysis can be valuable for selecting individuals for the prompt initiation of treatment while awaiting results of the urine culture. In older children (in whom UTI symptoms are more reliable indicators of infection), a negative nitrite test, a negative leukocyte esterase test, and the absence of UTI symptoms are highly correlated with the absence of infection. However, babies require a culture to exclude UTI.

121. In an infant or toddler who is not toilet-trained, how should urine for culture be obtained?

Suprapubic aspiration (SPA) is the gold standard (and, unfortunately, the most invasive). However, the batting average of house officers for obtaining urine by this method is only about 60% or less (increasing to >90% with ultrasonic guidance). **Catheter specimens** have a >90% correlation with SPA (which can be increased if the first 3 mL are discarded, as that part of the specimen is more likely to contain contaminants) and a higher collection rate. **Sterile bag collection** has very limited accuracy, with wide variations in false-positive and false-negative rates. Invasive specimen collection remains the procedure of choice in a sick febrile infant for whom the rapid initiation of therapy is warranted. When time permits, allowing parents to obtain clean-catch specimens from infants and toddlers (by holding a bowl under a child's genitalia) has shown a remarkably good correlation with SPA and can be an alternative to invasive techniques.

Dayan PS, Chamberlain JM, Boenning D, et al: A comparison of the initial to the later stream in children catheterized to evaluate for urinary tract infection. Pediatr Emerg Care 16:88–90, 2000.

Ramage IJ, Chapman JP, Hollman AS, et al: Accuracy of clean-catch urine collection in infancy. J Pediatr 135:765–767, 1999.

122. How is a suprapubic aspiration done?

1. The patient should not have voided within 1 hour of the procedure.
2. Restrain the infant in a supine, frog-leg position.
3. Clean the suprapubic area with povidone-iodine and alcohol.
4. Identify the site of puncture at 1–2 cm above the symphysis pubis in the midline.
5. Use a 22-gauge, 1.5-inch needle (with a 3-mL syringe attached to it), and puncture at a 10–20° angle of the true vertical, aiming cephalad (Fig. 13-5). A second attempt can be performed at a similar angle, aiming caudad.
6. Exert suction gently as the needle is advanced until urine enters the syringe. Aspirate the urine with gentle suction. If urine is not obtained, further trials are unlikely to be successful.

123. **What bacterial counts constitute a positive urine culture?**
    - **Suprapubic aspiration:** ≥100 colony-forming units (CFU)/mL
    - **Catheterization:** ≥10,000 CFU/mL
    - **Midstream clean catch:** ≥100, 000 CFU/mL of a single organism; 10,000–100,000 CFU/mL: suspicious and requires reculturing; <10,000: usually indicates contamination
    - **Urine bag:** May be helpful if negative, but even ≥100,000 CFU/mL has an 85% false-positive result

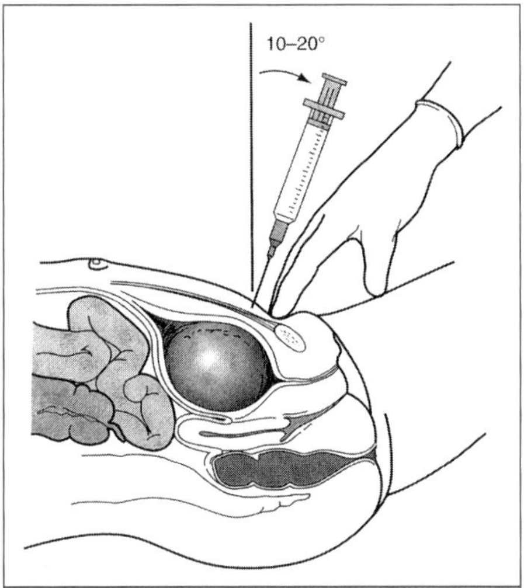

Figure 13-5. Suprapubic aspiration. (From Wald E: Cystitis and pyelonephritis. In Feigin RD, Cherry JD, Demmler GJ, Kaplan S (eds): Textbook of Pediatric Infectious Disease, 5th ed. Philadelphia, W.B. Saunders, 2004, p 546.)

124. **What factors can cause low colony counts despite significant urinary infection?**
    - High-volume urine flow
    - Recent antimicrobial therapy
    - Fastidious and slow-growing organisms (e.g., enterococci, *Staphylococcus saprophyticus*)
    - Low urine pH (<5.0) and specific gravity (<1.003)
    - Bacteriostatic agents in the urine
    - Complete obstruction of a ureter
    - Chronic or indolent infection
    - Use of inappropriate culture techniques

Bock GH: Urinary tract infections. In Hoekelman RA, Adam HM, Nelson HM, et al (eds): Primary Pediatric Care, 4th ed. St. Louis, Mosby, 2001, p 1896.

125. **Why should urine specimens be refrigerated if they cannot be immediately processed?**
    The storage of urine specimens at room temperature is one of the most common causes of false-positive results. When left at room temperature, enteric organisms in specimens have a growth-doubling time of 12.5 minutes, and thus colony counts become an unreliable guide. If a urine specimen cannot be processed within 15 minutes, it should be refrigerated at <4°C to stop in vitro replication.

126. **Which children are at increased risk for bacteriuria or a symptomatic UTI?**
    1. **Premature infants** discharged from neonatal intensive care units
    2. **Children** with the following conditions:
        - Immunodeficiencies or underlying systemic disease
        - Urinary tract abnormalities
        - Renal calculi
        - Neurogenic bladder or voiding dysfunction
        - Chronic severe constipation
        - Family history of UTI, renal anomalies, or reflux
    3. **Girls** <5 years old with a history of UTI

127. **What are the common presenting signs and symptoms of a UTI in an infant?**
The presenting findings are nonspecific and can include fever, vomiting, diarrhea, irritability, and poor feeding. These same findings are often seen in infants *without* UTIs—thus the potential importance of cultures in febrile infants.

128. **How common are UTIs in young febrile infants?**
Quite common. In infants and toddlers *between 2 and 24 months* with unexplained fever (>38.3°C), the prevalence is about 5%, with girls having twice as many infections (or more) as boys. The rate in circumcised boys is low (0.2–0.4%). In infants *<2 months old,* 7.5% had UTIs, with boys having more than girls.

Schlager TA: Urinary tract infections in infants and children. Infect Dis Clin North Am 17:353–365, 2003.

129. **What pathogens are associated with UTIs in children?**
Between 80% and 90% of initial UTIs are caused by *Escherichia coli.* Other organisms include *Proteus mirabilis, Klebsiella pneumoniae, Pseudomonas, Enterobacter,* and some *Staphylococcus* species.

130. **What are the characteristics of complicated UTIs?**
Complicated UTIs imply the presence of either an anatomic abnormality (e.g., obstruction, VUR) or a functional abnormality (e.g., neurogenic bladder, voiding dysfunction). Patients with complicated UTIs are more likely to have symptoms that are consistent with pyelonephritis and to have infections with more virulent organisms (e.g., *Proteus, Pseudomonas* species).

131. **How is cystitis distinguished clinically from pyelonephritis?**
Often with difficulty. **Pyelonephritis** tends to have more constitutional symptoms, such as fever, rigors, flank pain, and back pain, whereas **cystitis** has more bladder symptoms, such as enuresis, dysuria, frequency, and urgency. The presence of white-cell casts or impaired urinary-concentrating ability is more indicative of pyelonephritis. Patients with pyelonephritis tend to have higher sedimentation rates and C-reactive proteins, but these results can also be seen in some patients with cystitis. Renal dimercaptosuccinic acid (DMSA) scintigraphy is the most accurate study for identifying acute pyelonephritis. For most children, the treatment of cystitis and of pyelonephritis are essentially the same.

132. **Which patients with UTIs require hospitalization and parenteral antibiotics?**
- Any infant <2 months old because of an increased risk for urosepsis or other serious concomitant infections
- Any patient who is toxic, dehydrated, or unable to tolerate oral antibiotics

133. **Should all pediatric patients with clinical pyelonephritis be hospitalized?**
Traditionally, older patients with clinical evidence of pyelonephritis have been hospitalized for 24–48 hours for parenteral antibiotics and, if a good clinical response has occurred, discharged to home for additional oral antibiotic therapy. Data are emerging that the short- and long-term outcome of patients (even as young as 2 months old) with uncomplicated pyelonephritis is the same for initial therapy either intravenously or with oral, third-generation cephalosporins. Outpatient therapy clearly mandates the ability to tolerate oral antibiotics and that there be no concerns regarding compliance and careful and reliable follow-up.

Hoberman A, Wald ER, Hickey RW, et al: Oral versus initial intravenous therapy for urinary tract infection in young febrile children. Pediatrics 104:79–86, 1999.

134. **What is the duration of antibiotic therapy for a UTI?**
Standard duration of therapy is 10 days (combined oral plus parenteral) for cystitis or pyelonephritis, although shorter courses are under study; however, some experts lean toward

14 days of treatment for pyelonephritis. If the patient is not clinically improved within 2–3 days of starting therapy, the urine culture should be repeated and antibiotics adjusted, if indicated.

135. **In what cases are prophylactic antibiotics indicated for patients with UTIs?**
   - Infants or children with their **first UTI**, who have finished their 10-day course of therapy and who are awaiting the completion of studies (e.g., voiding cystourethrogram [VCUG], renal ultrasound).
   - Patients with **known urologic abnormalities** that place them at high risk for recurrent UTIs (e.g., VUR, hydronephrosis, posterior urethral valves).
   - Children and adolescents with **recurrent UTIs** and normal urinary tract anatomy: A 6- to 12-month course is indicated; if infections recur after stopping prophylaxis, antibiotics should be resumed.

136. **Which antibiotics are commonly used for prophylaxis?**
   - Trimethoprim (TMP)/sulfamethoxazole (SMX): 2 mg/kg of TMP and 10 mg/kg of SMX as a single bedtime dose *or* 5 mg/kg of TMP and 25 mg/kg of SMX twice per week
   - Nitrofurantoin: 1–2 mg/kg as single daily dose
   - Sulfisoxazole: 10–20 mg/kg divided, every 12 hours
   - Nalidixic acid: 30 mg/kg divided, every 12 hours
   - Methenamine mandelate: 75 mg/kg divided, every 12 hours

   American Academy of Pediatrics, Committee on Quality Improvement, Subcommittee on Urinary Tract Infection: Practice parameter: The diagnosis, treatment, and evaluation of the initial urinary tract infection in febrile infants and young children. Pediatrics 103:843–852, 1999.

137. **Is cranberry juice helpful for the management of UTIs in children?**
   The use of cranberry juice as a urine-acidifying agent and treatment for UTI has been popular for adults since the 1920s, and studies of adults have shown it to be helpful for diminishing the frequency of bacteriuria, possibly because of its antiadhesive properties against *Escherichia coli*. Limited studies in children that have primarily looking at the juice's role as a possible prophylactic treatment for chronic bacteriuria in children who require frequent catheterization have not shown positive benefits.

   Schlager TA, Anderson S, Trudell J, Hendley JO: Effect of cranberry juice on bacteriuria in children with neurogenic bladder receiving intermittent catheterization. J Pediatr 135:698–702, 1999.

138. **What is the role of DMSA scanning in the evaluation of UTIs?**
   Injected 99mTc DMSA is taken up by renal tubular cells. Subsequent scanning provides information about renal morphology and functioning parenchyma. When carried out at the time of an acute infection, it has been touted as a reasonably rapidly available study to help in the differentiation of renal parenchymal infections from lower-tract UTIs. When performed after the infection has been treated, the study provides an assessment of renal scars. Both local inflammation and renal scars appear as "cold" spots on the scan. Some published studies question the usefulness of the test because of a relatively high rate of false-positive and equivocal scans.

139. **Which patients with UTIs warrant imaging studies of the urinary tract?**
   - Any patient with an episode of acute pyelonephritis
   - Boys with their first UTI
   - Girls <3 years old with their first UTI
   - Girls ≥3 years old with their second UTI
   - Girls ≥3 years old with their first UTI if they have positive family history, abnormal voiding patterns, poor growth, hypertension, urinary tract abnormalities, or failure to respond promptly to treatment

   Wald E: Cystitis and pyelonephritis. In Feigin RD, Cherry JD, Demmler GJ, Kaplan S (eds): Textbook of Pediatric Infectious Disease, 5th ed. Philadelphia, Saunders, 2004, p 547.

140. What imaging studies are used for patients with UTIs who warrant evaluation?
- **VCUG or radionuclide cystogram,** to evaluate for VUR (the most common abnormality found in children with UTIs)
- **Renal ultrasound,** to screen for urinary tract obstruction or other structural genitourinary abnormalities
- **Renal cortical DMSA scanning,** recommended by some authorities to determine if there is evidence of acute pyelonephritis or permanent renal scarring

141. How soon after a UTI is diagnosed can imaging studies of the urinary tract be obtained?
- The **VCUG** or radionuclide cystogram can be performed as soon as the urine culture is sterile. A tradition recommendation has been to wait 3–6 weeks after a UTI for a VCUG to minimize the possibility of false-positive testing as a result of transient reflux from inflammatory-mediated changes at the ureterovesical junction. However, most studies indicate that reflux does not diminish during this interval and, in some settings, patients may be lost to follow-up, so the earlier evaluation is more appropriate.
- The **renal ultrasound** can be done with the above studies or at the time of hospital admission if the patient appears toxic or is hypertensive or if there is evidence of reduced renal function.
- A **DMSA scan** (if ordered to evaluate for renal scarring) should be done at least 6 months after the last acute UTI.

  McDonald A, Scranton M, Gillespie R, et al: Voiding cystourethrograms and urinary tract infections: How long to wait? Pediatrics 105:E50, 2000.

142. Is renal scarring a common occurrence in children with UTIs?
Renal scars are relatively uncommon (<10% in children <2 years old) when DMSA scanning is done 6 months after a UTI if a patient has a normal urinary tract and no bladder dysfunction. Children with recurrent UTIs and concomitant VUR are at a higher risk for renal scarring. Approximately 40%–70% of children with grades II–IV reflux will have renal scarring at the time of their initial renal scan. Much recent emphasis has focused on the importance of congenital abnormalities (e.g., hypoplasia, dysplasia) rather than ongoing VUR as contributors to chronic scarring observed after UTIs in children. The potential for the delayed appearance of renal scarring after normal initial studies remains controversial.

  Hellerstein S: Long-term consequences of urinary tract infections. Curr Opin Pediatr 12:125–128, 2000.
  Wennerstrom M, Hansson S, Jodal U, Stokland E: Primary and acquired renal scarring in boys and girls with urinary tract infections. J Pediatr 136:30–34, 2000.
  Wennerstrom M, Hansson S, Jodal U, et al: Renal function 16 to 26 years after the first urinary tract infection in children. Arch Pediatr Adolesc Med 154:339–345, 2000.

KEY POINTS: URINARY TRACT INFECTION

1. *Escherichia coli* causes 90% of cases.

2. Antibiotic sensitivity testing is important because of the increasing incidence of ampicillin-resistant *E. coli.*

3. Infections may be caused by ascending bacteria from the urethral area.

4. Clean-bagged specimens are unreliable for diagnosis because of their high contamination rate.

5. Uncircumcised males have a 10-fold greater risk of infection as compared with circumcised males.

143. **What factors increase the risk for permanent renal damage in children with UTIs?**
- Younger age
- Obstruction
- VUR
- Recurrent infections
- Pyelonephritis
- Nephrolithiasis
- Delay in diagnosis and initiation of therapy

144. **Should children be screened for asymptomatic bacteriuria?**
Although 1–2% of girls >5 old have persistent bacteriuria, mass screening at present is not recommended for the following reasons:
- In girls with radiologically demonstrable anatomic abnormalities (0.2–0.5%), most renal injury appears to occur before the age of 5 years and may not progress.
- Older girls with asymptomatic bacteriuria and normal anatomy are unlikely to have sequelae if untreated.

The screening of infants and toddlers is technically more difficult, and the merits of screening are unclear. Infants and children at high risk should be considered for screening.

UROLITHIASIS

145. **What is the composition of kidney stones in children?**
See Table 13-10.

TABLE 13-10.	COMPOSITION OF KIDNEY STONES IN CHILDREN	
Stone composition	North America (n = 340)	Europe (n = 315)
Calcium	58%	37%
Struvite	25%	54%
Cystine	6%	3%
Uric acid/urate	9%	2%
Others	2%	4%

Polinsky MS, Kaiser BA, Baluarte HJ: Urolithiasis in childhood. Pediatr Clin North Am 34:683–710, 1987.

146. **What is the most common metabolic cause of pediatric urinary calculi?**
Hypercalciuria. The most common cause of this condition is *familial idiopathic hypercalciuria*. Multiple other causes include the following:
- Increased intestinal calcium absorption (vitamin D excess)
- Renal tubular dysfunction
- Endocrine abnormalities (hypothyroidism, adrenocorticoid excess, hyperparathyroidism)
- Bone metabolism disorders (immobilization, rickets, malignancies, juvenile rheumatoid arthritis)
- Drugs (certain diuretics, corticosteroids)
- Other (hypercalcemia, UTI, Williams syndrome)

Gillespie RS, Stapleton FB: Nephrolithiasis in children. Pediatr Rev 25:131–138, 2004.

147. **How is hypercalciuria defined in the infant and child?**
The strict definition of hypercalciuria in a child is >4 mg of urinary calcium per kilogram per 24 hours on an unrestricted diet that is normal for the child's age. Twenty-four hour urine collections can be difficult in young children. Therefore, random urine collections have been used to *screen* for hypercalciuria. The urine **calcium/creatinine ratio** will vary with age. Morning nonfasting urine ratios that exceed the following correlate with quantitative hypercalciuria:

Patient age	Calcium/creatinine ratio
>7 years	>0.24
5–7 years	>0.30
3–5 years	>0.41
1–2 years	>0.56
<1 year	>0.81

148. **What laboratory studies are appropriate during the initial evaluation of children with renal stones?**
- Serum electrolytes, calcium, and creatinine
- 24-hour urine collection for calcium, creatinine, magnesium, citrate, uric acid, oxalate, and cystine
- Urine pH (by meter), urinalysis, and urine culture (if indicated)

   Minevich E: Pediatric urolithiasis. Pediatr Clin North Am 48:1571–1586, 2001.

149. **How does the manipulation of urine pH affect renal calculi?**
Calcium oxalate stones, which are the most common type of renal calculi, are *unaffected* by the urine pH. These stones can be treated with thiazides diuretics, which increase renal calcium reabsorption and thereby decrease the urinary calcium excretion. Potassium citrate can be added if the urinary citrate excretion is low. Do not restrict calcium intake unless it is excessively high. **Calcium phosphate** stones, which occur in cases of distal renal tubular acidosis, respond to treatment with *alkali*. **Uric acid** stones form in acidic urine and also respond to *alkalinization* to a pH of >6.5. Additional therapy includes a reduction in purine intake and occasionally the use of allopurinol to block the formation of uric acid. High fluid intake plus urine alkalinization (pH >7) helps to block the formation of **cystine** stones. Penicillamine may also be required in some of these patients. **Struvite** or infection stones form in extremely alkaline urine. Urine *acidification* and antibiotics are the cornerstones of treatment for these stones.

150. **When is lithotripsy or surgery indicated for children with kidney stones?**
Most children with stones will spontaneously pass them. **Lithotripsy** is useful for children with large pelvic or bladder stones that are radiopaque in whom fluoroscopy can be used to focus the shock waves. **Surgery** is generally reserved for children with stones that are causing urinary tract obstruction and for staghorn calculi that cannot be dissolved medically or fragmented by lithotripsy. Cystine stones are difficult to fragment by lithotripsy.

   Cohen TD, Ehreth J, King LR, Preminger GM: Pediatric urolithiasis: Medical and surgical management. Urology 47:292–303, 1996.

VESICOURETERAL REFLUX

151. **How is VUR graded?**
Figure 13-6 demonstrates the five grades of VUR:
1. **Grade I:** Ureter only
2. **Grade II:** Ureter, pelvis, and calices; no dilation, normal caliceal fornices

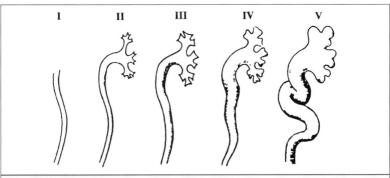

Figure 13-6. The five grades of vesicoureteral reflux.

3. **Grade III:** Mild dilation and/or tortuosity of the ureter and mild dilation of the renal pelvis; minor blunting of the fornices
4. **Grade IV:** Moderate dilation and/or tortuosity of the ureter and moderate dilation of the renal
5. **Grade V:** Significant blunting of most fornices; papillary impressions are no longer visible in most of the calices; gross dilation and tortuosity of the ureter; gross dilation of the renal pelvis and calices

   Duckett JW, Bellinger MF: A plea for standardized grading of vesicoureteral reflux. Eur Urol 8:74–77, 1982.

152. **In addition to reflux, what other pathologic bladder findings may be noted on a VCUG?**
Diverticula may be seen, especially in the presence of outflow obstruction. A posterior urethral valve or urethral stricture can be detected during the voiding phase of the study. A ureterocele may be seen and appears as a filling defect in the bladder. Other features to note are the bladder capacity, residual volume after voiding, and thickening or trabeculation of the bladder from muscular hypertrophy.

153. **What is the normal bladder capacity in children?**
Volume (in ounces) = Patient's age (in years) + 2. The normal adult bladder capacity is 12–16 oz.

154. **Discuss the comparative features of a VCUG and a radionuclide cystogram (RNC) for the evaluation of reflux.**
   - Both studies require the catheterization of the bladder and the filling of the bladder with an imaging solution.
   - The RNC allows for continuous monitoring of the filling and emptying of the bladder as compared with the intermittent fluoroscopy that occurs with the VCUG.
   - There is less radiation exposure with the RNC.
   - The VCUG provides greater anatomic detail of the urethra and bladder and can aid in the evaluation of bladder dysfunction better than the RNC.
   - The VCUG is more accurate for assessing and grading the degrees (I–V) of reflux.
   - In general, the majority of authorities prefer the VCUG for the evaluation of a child with an initial UTI.

155. **How does the radiation exposure differ between RNC and VCUG?**
RNC has approximately *100 times less* the absorbed radiation dose as compared with a single x-ray VCUG. Many authorities do recommend its use for the screening of siblings with reflux,

for evaluating the child with myelomeningocele, and for the ongoing evaluation of significant reflux.

Conway JJ, Cohn RA: Evolving role of nuclear medicine for the diagnosis and management of urinary tract infection. J Pediatr 124:87–90, 1994.

KEY POINTS: VESICOURETERAL REFLUX

1. Spontaneous resolution more likely with grades I–III.

2. Thirty percent of these patients will have siblings with vesicoureteral reflux, but sequelae are rare.

3. Between 30% and 50% of children with urinary tract infections will have vesicoureteral reflux.

4. Prophylactic antibiotics are intended to prevent pyelonephritis and to limit renal scarring and hypertension.

156. **What is the natural history of VUR?**
The likelihood that reflux will resolve spontaneously is influenced by the severity of the reflux at the time of initial diagnosis. About 80–90% of patients with grade I–II reflux, 45% with grade III reflux, and 25% with grade IV reflux will experience spontaneous resolution *within 5 years*. Grade V reflux always requires surgical intervention. The chances for resolution are better in children with unilateral—rather than bilateral—reflux.

157. **How is VUR managed: medically or surgically?**
   - **Grades I–II:** These grades are usually managed medically if the family is reliable and will comply with outpatient regimens and follow-up studies.
   - **Grades III–IV:** If followed expectantly, these types of reflux will resolve slowly, at a rate of approximately 10% per year. Surgical intervention results in the elimination of this degree of reflux at least 95% of the time. Randomized studies have not shown any significant difference in long-term renal outcome (e.g., renal scarring, hypertension, reduced function) when comparing medical versus surgical treatment.
   - **Grade V:** Surgical intervention is indicated.

   Wheeler D, Vimalachandra D, Hodson EM, et al: Antibiotics and surgery for vesicoureteric reflux: A meta-analysis of randomized controlled trials. Arch Dis Child 88:688–694, 2003.

158. **What constitutes the proper medical management of VUR?**
   - **Prophylactic nighttime antibiotics:** The duration of therapy is quite controversial; some authorities recommend treatment until reflux subsides, whereas others stop antibiotics in boys who are free of infection for several years even if the reflux persists.
   - **Surveillance urine cultures** every 2–3 months or more frequently if there are symptoms of a UTI.
   - **Repeat VCUG or RNC** every 2 years to reevaluate VUR. A *renal ultrasound* is done biannually to evaluate renal growth. Imaging studies are continued until the reflux resolves.

159. **When should a patient with VUR be referred to a urologist or nephrologist?**
   - Recurrent UTIs despite adequate antibiotic prophylaxis
   - Noncompliance with medical management
   - Failure of reflux to resolve in a girl by the time of puberty
   - Severity of reflux worsening over time
   - History of a persistent voiding dysfunction

- Progressive renal scarring or deterioration in function of the scarred kidney as documented by renal scan

Garin EH, Orta-Sibu N, Campos A: Primary vesicoureteral reflux in childhood. Adv Pediatr 49:341–357, 2002.

160. **Should asymptomatic siblings of a patient with VUR have urologic imaging done as a screen for reflux?**

The incidence of reflux is thought to be <1% in normal children, but some studies have demonstrated reflux in 33–45% of siblings of patients with reflux. Among identical twins, the rate is 80%. Consequently, many authorities recommend screening siblings who are <7 years old with a radionuclide cystogram. Siblings >7 years old who have a history of previous UTIs should also be screened for reflux. Although the incidence of reflux is higher in siblings, data are still lacking to prove that the screening and treatment of asymptomatic siblings decreases infectious renal scarring.

Hollowell JG, Greenfield SP: Screening siblings for vesicoureteral reflux. J Urol 168:2138–2141, 2002.

ACKNOWLEDGMENT

The editors gratefully acknowledge contributions by Drs. Thomas Kennedy, James Prebis, and Stephen J. Wassner that were retained from the first three editions of *Pediatric Secrets*.

CHAPTER 14

NEUROLOGY

Kent R. Kelley, MD

ANTIEPILEPTIC DRUGS

1. **Should treatment with antiepileptic drugs (AEDs) be started after the first seizure in a child?**

   Children with an isolated, uncomplicated seizure usually do *not* require AED therapy. Epidemiologic studies have shown that nearly 60% of children with an uncomplicated single seizure will not experience a second. "Delaying" treatment until after the second seizure does not adversely affect the long-term chance of epilepsy remission.

   AEDs are not without risks and side effects, both dose-related and idiosyncratic. Other factors, including electroencephalogram (EEG) results, antecedent neurologic history, family history, and imaging (in selective cases) influence the risk of recurrence and should be considered. Risk for recurrent seizures is sharply increased if the seizure was nocturnal, the neurologic status is not normal, there is a positive family history, if no immediate precipitating cause can be identified, and the EEG reveals epileptiform discharges.

   Guerrini R, Arzimanoglou A, Brouwer O: Rationale for treating epilepsy in children. Epileptic Disord 4:S9–S21, 2002.

   Hirtz D, Berg A, Bettis D, et al; Quality Standards Subcommittee of the American Academy of Neurology; Practice Committee of the Child Neurology Society: Practice parameter: Treatment of the child with a first unprovoked seizure: Report of the Quality Standards Subcommittee of the American Academy of Neurology and the Practice Committee of the Child Neurology Society. Neurology 60:166–172, 2003.

   Holmes GL: Overtreatment in children with epilepsy. Epilepsy Res 52:35–42, 2002.

2. **What is the advantage of monotherapy chosen according to the epilepsy syndrome?**
   - Chronic toxicity is directly related to the number of drugs consumed.
   - As compared with monotherapy, intellectual and sensorium impairment is increased for any given AEDs (despite "normal" drug levels).
   - Drug interactions may paradoxically lead to loss of seizure control.
   - It is difficult to identify the cause of an adverse reaction.

   Menkes JH, Sankar R: Paroxysmal disorders. In Menkes JH, Sarnat HB (eds): Child Neurology, 6th ed. Philadelphia, Lippincott Williams & Wilkins, 2000, pp 959–961.

3. **When should blood levels be obtained if seizures are poorly controlled or compliance is questionable?**

   Trough serum drug levels should be obtained to detect subtherapeutic or toxic concentrations. It is most helpful to check the serum level right before the dose, preferably in the morning before any medication is given. An inadequate serum concentration is the most common cause of persistent seizures, but drug toxicity, especially with phenytoin, may also manifest by deteriorating seizure control. There generally will be less variation in blood concentrations with tablets or capsules as compared with liquid preparations; suspensions in particular result in notoriously inconsistent dosages.

   Glauser TA, Pippenger CE: Controversies in blood-level monitoring: Reexamining its role in the treatment of epilepsy. Epilepsia 41:6–15, 2000.

4. **Which AEDs are recommended for primary generalized tonic-clonic seizures in children?**

The "traditional" AEDs (phenobarbital, primidone, phenytoin) are no longer considered the drugs of choice for grand mal seizures for many age groups because of side effects, although **phenobarbital** remains the drug of choice for neonatal seizures. Studies have shown that most of the major anticonvulsants are comparable for reducing or eliminating seizure recurrences.

Class I evidence demonstrates that phenytoin, carbamazepine, phenobarbital, primidone, valproate, topiramate, oxcarbazepine, and lamotrigine are effective for the treatment of primary generalized tonic-clonic seizures. On the basis of efficacy and tolerability, valproate and lamotrigine have emerged as the current drugs of choice for grand mal seizures. In addition, several of the newer AEDs have a broad spectrum of effects and may also be considered.

Faught E: Clinical trials for treatment of primary generalized epilepsies. Epilepsia 44:S44–S50, 2003.

French JA, Kanner AM, Bautista J, et al; Therapeutics and Technology Assessment Subcommittee of the American Academy of Neurology; Quality Standards Subcommittee of the American Academy of Neurology; American Epilepsy Society: Efficacy and tolerability of the new antiepileptic drugs I: Treatment of new onset epilepsy: Report of the Therapeutics and Technology Assessment Subcommittee and Quality Standards Subcommittee of the American Academy of Neurology and the American Epilepsy Society. Neurology 62:1252–1260, 2004.

LaRoche SM, Helmers SL: The new antiepileptic drugs. JAMA 291:605–614, 2004.

5. **What is the drug of choice for absence epilepsy?**

Ethosuximide (Zarontin), **valproate** (divalproex sodium or Depakote), and **lamotrigine** (Lamictal) are all equally effective for eliminating or substantially reducing the number of absence attacks. Ethosuximide is traditionally the drug of choice, for several reasons:

- It works well for many patients. It not only stops the clinical attacks of absence, but it often normalizes the EEG by "erasing" the 3/sec spike-wave discharges.
- It is well tolerated by most patients. Although rare cases of serious bone marrow, liver, or dermatologic disorders have occurred, routine or frequent blood tests are not considered obligatory by most physicians.
- It has a relatively long serum half-life (40 hours). Thus, once- or twice-daily dosing is appropriate and represents a real convenience to the patient.
- It is relatively inexpensive.

Disadvantages are that ethosuximide only protects against absence seizures. Children with coexisting generalized convulsions should be treated with valproate or lamotrigine. Disadvantages of valproate include the risks of idiosyncratic liver toxicity, weight gain, and teratogenicity. Lamotrigine should also be considered, with the relative risk of rash and generally favorable cognitive profile taken into account.

6. **Can AEDs paradoxically cause a worsening of seizures?**

A paradoxic worsening of seizure control by various AEDs has been noted for decades. Mechanisms may include nonspecific effects of drug intoxication. In addition, specific medications may exacerbate specific seizure types. For example, carbamazepine may worsen the absence, myoclonic, and astatic seizures seen in generalized epilepsy syndromes; phenytoin and vigabatrin may also worsen generalized seizures; and gabapentin and lamotrigine may worsen myoclonic seizures.

Perucca E, Gram L, Avanzini G, Dulac O: Antiepileptic drugs as a cause of worsening seizures. Epilepsia 39:5–17, 1998.

7. **What are the typical dose-related side effects of AEDs?**

Dose-related side effects occur somewhat predictably and can be anticipated, particularly as the medication dose is initiated and escalated. Common dose-related side effects include sedation, headache, gastrointestinal irritation, unsteadiness, and dysarthria. Management commonly consists of reducing the dose by 25–50% and waiting approximately 2 weeks for tolerance to develop. In addition, behavioral and cognitive side effects can occur in some patients; these can be more subtle, and controversy exists regarding the relative effects of various AEDs.

Loring DW, Meador KJ: Cognitive side effects of the antiepileptic drugs in children. Neurology 62:872–877, 2004.

8. **What idiosyncratic drug reactions are associated with antiepileptic medications?**

Idiosyncratic reactions occur unpredictably, are potentially fatal, and do not correlate with dose of medication.

- **Carbamazepine:** Leukopenia, aplastic anemia, thrombocytopenia, hepatic dysfunction, rashes
- **Ethosuximide:** Leukopenia, pancytopenia, rashes
- **Phenobarbital:** Rashes, Stevens-Johnson syndrome, hepatic dysfunction
- **Phenytoin:** Hepatic dysfunction, lymphadenopathy, movement disorder, Stevens-Johnson syndrome, fulminant hepatic failure
- **Valproic acid:** Fulminant hepatic failure, hyperammonemia, pancreatitis, thrombocytopenia, rash, stupor

9. **Which children are most susceptible to valproic-acid–induced acute hepatic failure?**

The highest incidences occur in children <2 years old who are receiving polytherapy (1 in 540). In children <2 years old who are receiving valproic acid monotherapy, the rate is reduced to about 1 in 8,000. The complication is unrelated to dosage and typically occurs during the first 3 months of therapy. Up to 40% of individuals who receive valproic acid will have dose-related elevations of liver enzymes, which are transient or resolve with dosage adjustments. However, liver function test monitoring is not helpful for predicting acute hepatic failure. It has been hypothesized that valproic acid may cause carnitine deficiency, hyperammonemia, and hepatotoxicity. Despite a lack of data from clinical trials, some clinicians recommend prophylactic carnitine supplementation.

Bryant AE, Dreifuss FE: Valproic acid hepatic fatalities. Neurology 48:465–469, 1996.

10. **What are the warning signs and symptoms of hypersensitivity syndromes?**

Symptoms often occur early, within the first months of treatment. Families need to be educated about the potential for drug reactions. Concerning symptoms include fever of >40°C, protracted vomiting, lethargy, exfoliation of the skin, mucosal (or palm or sole) lesions, facial edema, swelling of the tongue, confluent erythema, skin pain, palpable purpura, protracted bleeding from minor cuts, lymph-node enlargement, and asthmatic symptoms. Multiple studies have shown that families fail to appreciate evolving symptoms of idiosyncratic reactions and continue to administer the offending agent. Examination may reveal lymphadenopathy, palpable purpura, blisters, and wheezing. Laboratory abnormalities may include eosinophilia, atypical lymphocytosis, and abnormal liver function enzymes. Routine surveillance of blood chemistries and complete blood counts (every 3–6 months) are standard practice, but they are unlikely to identify potentially life-threatening conditions.

Browne TR, Holmes GL: Epilepsy. N Engl J Med 344:1145–1151, 2001.

Stern RS: Improving the outcome of patients with toxic epidermal necrolysis and Stevens-Johnson syndrome. Arch Dermatol 136:410–411, 2000.

11. **What are the suggested dosing guidelines and therapeutic ranges of AEDs?**
See Table 14-1.

TABLE 14-1.	GUIDELINES FOR DOSES OF ESTABLISHED ANTIEPILEPTIC DRUGS IN CHILDREN*		
Drug	Trade name	Standard maintenance dose range (mg/kg/day)	Target plasma drug concentration range (μg/mL)
Carbamazepine	Tegretol/Carbatrol	10–30	4–12
Ethosuximide	Zarontin	15–40	40–120
Gabapentin	Neurontin	30–45	5–15
Lamotrigine (monotherapy)	Lamictal	2–8	2–20
Oxcarbazepine	Trileptal	20–40	5–50
Phenobarbital	Luminal	2–10	10–45
Phenytoin	Dilantin, Fosphenytoin	4–7	10–30
Tiagabine	Gabitril	1–2	5–70
Topiramate	Topamax	5–10	2–25
Valproate	Depakote	30–45	60–120
Zonisamide	Zonegran	4–12	10–40

*Therapeutic ranges are somewhat arbitrary. Levels above "normal" may be maintained to control seizures if side effects do not occur. Conversely, levels in the therapeutic range may have toxic effects. It is important to treat the patient and not the number.

12. **What is Diastat?**
Diazepam rectal gel (Diastat) has been approved for the treatment of status epilepticus and severe recurrent convulsive seizures in children. It is prescribed for home use by parents. Dosages (as they are for most medications in pediatric patients) are based on weight, and the medication is available in various premixed concentrations with syringe applicators.

13. **After what period can AEDs be safely discontinued?**
The withdrawal of antiepileptic drugs should be considered when the child is *free of seizures for 2 years* because well-controlled investigations have shown that the risk of relapse in children whose seizures have been in remission for 2 years is low. Although there is no uniform agreement about factors that are predictive of outcome, the highest remission rate appears to occur in those who are otherwise neurologically normal and in whom the EEG at the time of discontinuation lacks specific epileptiform features and displays a normal background. The prognosis is the worst for children with symptomatic epilepsies, persistently abnormal EEGs, and abnormal neurologic examinations.

Greenwood RS, Tennison MB: When to start and stop anticonvulsant therapy in children. Neurology 56:1073–1077, 1999.
Smith R, Ball R: Discontinuing anticonvulsant medication in children. Arch Dis Child 87:259–260, 2002.

14. **When the decision is made to discontinue AEDs, should the tapering period be long or short?**

In practice, all AEDs should be tapered gradually rather than abruptly discontinued, although there is no actual withdrawal state produced by a "cold turkey" reduction of most AEDs (e.g., phenytoin, carbamazepine, valproate, ethosuximide). By contrast, a withdrawal syndrome of agitation, signs of autonomic overactivity, and seizures follow the sudden elimination of habitually consumed diazepam or short-acting barbiturates (e.g., secobarbital). The long elimination half-life of phenobarbital lessens the risk of withdrawal symptoms after abrupt discontinuation.

In a study of >100 children who had been seizure-free for either 2 or 4 years, the risk of seizure recurrence during tapering and after discontinuation of the AED was no different if the period of taper was 6 weeks or 9 months. Rapid tapering appears to be an acceptable means of discontinuation.

Tennison M, Greenwood R, Lewis D, Thorn M: Discontinuing antiepileptic drugs in children with epilepsy: A comparison of a six-week and a nine-month taper period. N Engl J Med 330:1407–1410, 1994.

CEREBRAL PALSY

15. **How is cerebral palsy (CP) defined?**

CP describes a heterogenous group of static motor and posture disorders of cerebral or cerebellar origin that typically manifest early in life. It is frequently accompanied by epilepsy, sensory impairment, and mental retardation. Note that the definition does not imply etiology; however, known causes include cerebral malformations, infection (both intrauterine and extrauterine), perinatal stroke, multiple pregnancy, hypoxic-ischemic encephalopathy, and trauma. The process is nonprogressive, and the motor function affected reflects the part of the brain that is involved. Although nonprogressive, clinical manifestations often change over time as the expression of the underlying brain is modified by normal brain development and maturation.

16. **What are the Levine (POSTER) criteria for the diagnosis of CP?**

P = Posturing/abnormal movements
O = Oropharyngeal problems (e.g., tongue thrusts, swallowing abnormalities)
S = Strabismus
T = Tone (hyper- or hypotonia)
E = Evolutional maldevelopment (primitive reflexes persist or protective/equilibrium reflexes fail to develop [e.g., lateral prop, parachute reflex])
R = Reflexes (increased deep tendon reflexes/persistent Babinski's reflex)
Abnormalities in four of these six categories strongly point to the diagnosis of CP.

Feldman HM: Developmental-behavioral pediatrics. In Zitelli BJ, Davis HW: Atlas of Pediatric Diagnosis, 4th ed. St. Louis, Mosby, 2002, p 75.

17. **What are the types of CP?**

Clinical classification is determined on the basis of the nature of the movement disorder, muscle tone, and anatomic distribution. A single patient may have more than one type. Spastic CP is the most common, accounting for about two thirds of cases.

1. **Pyramidal (or spastic) CP:** This type is characterized by neurologic signs of upper motor neuron damage with increased "clasp knife" muscle tone, increased deep tendon reflexes, pathologic reflexes, and spastic weakness. Spastic CP is subclassified on the basis of distribution:
   - Hemiparesis: Primarily unilateral involvement, with the arm usually moving more than the leg
   - Quadriparesis: All limbs are involved, with the legs often more involved than the arms

- Diparesis: Legs are much more involved than the arms, which may show no or only minimal impairment
2. **Extrapyramidal (nonspastic or dyskinetic) CP:** This type is characterized by prominent involuntary movements or fluctuating muscle tone, with choreoathetosis as the most common subtype. Distribution is usually symmetric among the four limbs.
3. **Hypotonic CP:** This type manifests as generalized muscle hypotonia that persists with normal or increased deep tendon reflexes. Many patients with this condition develop cerebellar deficits of incoordination and ataxia, and about one third of patients have severe retardation.
4. **Ataxic CP:** Primarily cerebellar signs are seen.
5. **Mixed types**

Murphy N, Such-Neibar T: Cerebral palsy diagnosis and management: the state of the art. Curr Probl Pediatr Adolesc Health Care 33:146–169, 2003.

18. **What proportion of CP is related to birth asphyxia?**
In contrast with popular perception, large clinical epidemiologic and longitudinal studies indicate that perinatal asphyxia is an important—but relatively minor—cause. Estimates range from a low of 3% to a high of 21%. In most cases, the events leading to CP occur in the fetus before the onset of labor or in the newborn after delivery.

Nelson KB: Can we prevent cerebral palsy? N Engl J Med 349:1765–1769, 2003.

19. **How well do Apgar scores correlate with the development of CP?**
In a large study of 49,000 infants, a low Apgar score correlated poorly with the development of CP. Of term infants with scores of 0–3 at 1 or 5 minutes, 95% did not develop CP. Of those with scores of 0–3 at 10 minutes, 84% did not develop CP. If the 10-minute Apgar score improved to 4 or more, the rate for CP was <1%. A low Apgar score (0–3) at 20 minutes, however, had an observed CP rate of nearly 60%. Conversely, nearly 75% of patients with CP had 5-minute Apgar scores of 7–10.

Nelson KB, Ellenberg JH: Apgar scores as predictors of chronic neurologic disability. Pediatrics 68:36–44, 1981.
Papile Lu-Ann: The Apgar score in the 21st century. N Engl J Med 344:519–520, 2001.

20. **Why is CP difficult to diagnose clinically during the first year of life?**
- Hypotonia is more common than hypertonia and spasticity in the first year, which makes the prediction of CP difficult.
- The early abundance of primitive reflexes (with variable persistence) may confuse the clinical picture.
- An infant has a limited variety of volitional movements for evaluation.
- Substantial myelination takes months to evolve and may delay the clinical picture of abnormal tone and increased deep tendon reflexes.
- Most infants who develop CP do not have identifiable risk factors; most cases are not related to labor and delivery events.

Shapiro BK, Capute AJ: Cerebral palsy. In McMillan JA, DeAngelis CD, Feigin RD, Warshaw JB (eds): Oski's Pediatrics, Principles and Practice, 3rd ed. Philadelphia, Lippincott Williams & Wilkins, 1999, pp 1910–1917.

21. **What behavioral symptoms during the first year should arouse suspicion about the possibility of CP?**
- Excessive irritability, constant crying, and sleeping difficulties (Severe colic is noted in up to 30% of babies who are eventually diagnosed with CP.)
- Early feeding difficulties with difficulties in coordinating suck and swallow, frequent spitting up, and poor weight gain

- "Jittery" or "jumpy" behavior, especially at times other than when hungry
- Easily startled behavior
- Stiffness when handled, especially during dressing, diapering, and handwashing
- Paradoxically "precocious" development, such as early rolling (actually a sudden, reflexive roll rather than a volitional one) or the stiff-legged "standing" with support of an infant with spastic diplegia

Bennett FC: Diagnosing cerebral palsy—the earlier the better. Contemp Pediatr 16:65–76, 1999.

22. **What gross motor delays are diagnostically important in the infant with possible CP?**
    - Inability to bring the hands together in midline while in a supine position by the age of 4 months
    - Head lag persisting beyond 6 months
    - No volitional rolling by 6 months
    - Inability to independently sit straight by 8 months
    - No hands-and-knees crawling by 12 months

    Bennett FC: Diagnosing cerebral palsy—the earlier the better. Contemp Pediatr 16:65–76, 1999.

23. **What problems are commonly associated with CP?**
    - **Mental retardation:** Seen in two thirds of total patients; most commonly observed in children with spastic quadriplegia
    - **Learning disabilities**
    - **Ophthalmologic abnormalities:** Strabismus, amblyopia, nystagmus, refractive errors
    - **Hearing deficits**
    - **Communication disorders**
    - **Seizures:** Seen in one third of total patients; most commonly observed in children with spastic hemiplegia
    - **Failure to thrive**
    - **Feeding problems**
    - **Gastroesophageal reflux**
    - **Behavioral and emotional problems:** Especially attention-deficit/hyperactivity disorder and depression)

    Murphy N, Such-Neibar T: Cerebral palsy diagnosis and management: the state of the art. Curr Probl Pediatr Adolesc Health Care 33:146–169, 2003.

KEY POINTS: CEREBRAL PALSY

1. Apgar scores correlate poorly with the ultimate diagnosis of cerebral palsy.

2. During the first year of life, *hypotonia* is more common than *hypertonia* in patients who are ultimately diagnosed with the disease.

3. Keep an eye on the eyes: As many as 75% of children with cerebral palsy have ophthalmologic problems (e.g., strabismus, refractive errors).

4. Spastic hemiplegia is the most common type of cerebral palsy that is associated with seizures.

5. Monitor regularly for hip subluxation, especially in patients with spastic diparesis, because earlier identification assists therapy.

24. **What features in an infant suggest a progressive central nervous system (CNS) disorder rather than CP as the cause of a motor deficit?**
    - **Abnormally increasing head circumference:** Possible hydrocephalus, tumor, or neurodegenerative disorder
    - **Eye anomalies:** Cataracts, retinal pigmentary degeneration, optic atrophy (possible neurodegenerative disease), coloboma, chorioretinal lacuna, optic nerve hypoplasia (possible Aicardi's syndrome or septo-optic dysplasia)
    - **Skin abnormalities:** Vitiligo, café-au-lait spots, nevus flammeus port-wine (possible Sturge-Weber syndrome or neurofibromatosis)
    - **Hepatomegaly and/or splenomegaly** (possible storage disease)
    - **Decreased or absent deep tendon reflexes**
    - **Sensory abnormalities:** Diminished sense of pain, position, vibration, or light touch
    - **Developmental regression or failure to progress:** Rett syndrome or Leigh disease

    Taft LT: Cerebral palsy. Pediatr Rev 16(11):411–418, 1995.

CEREBROSPINAL FLUID

25. **What is normal cerebrospinal fluid (CSF) pressure?**
    CSF pressure as measured during a lumbar puncture varies with age, positional technique, and combativeness of the patient. Normal CSF opening pressure as measured with the patient in the *recumbent lateral* position is up to 50 mm H_2O in neonates, up to 85–110 mm H_2O in young infants, and up to 150 mm H_2O in older children. As measured with the patient in the *flexed lateral* position, CSF pressure is higher, ranging from 100–280 mm H_2O in children. With the patient in the *sitting* position, average pressures are even higher.

    Bonadio WA: The cerebrospinal fluid: Physiologic aspects and alterations associated with bacterial meningitis. Pediatr Infect Dis J 11:423–432, 1992.
    Ellis RW: Lumbar cerebrospinal fluid opening pressure measured in a flexed lateral decubitus position in children. Pediatrics 93:622–623, 1994.

26. **What is the normal CSF volume in an infant, child, and adolescent?**
    Estimates for the volume of the ventricular system are 40–50 mL in a term newborn, 65–100 mL in an older child, and 90–150 mL in a teenager or adult. The choroid plexus actively secretes a distillate of CSF at a rate of 0.3–0.4 mL/min in children and adults, which equals about 20 mL/h or 500 mL/day. This equates to an hourly CSF volume turnover rate of approximately 15%.

27. **What are the common causes of an elevated CSF protein?**
    Elevated CSF protein (>30 mg/dL) is a nonspecific finding that is encountered in various neurologic disorders. Several common etiologies should be considered:
    - **Infection:** Tuberculous meningitis, acute bacterial meningitis (pneumococcal, meningococcal, *Haemophilus influenzae*), syphilitic or viral meningitis, encephalitis
    - **Inflammation:** Guillain-Barré syndrome (GBS), multiple sclerosis, peripheral neuropathy, postinfectious encephalopathy
    - **Tumor** of the cerebral hemispheres or spinal cord
    - **Vascular accidents,** such as cerebral hemorrhage (including subarachnoid hemorrhage, subdural hemorrhage, intracerebral hemorrhages) or stroke as a result of cranial arteritis, diabetes mellitus, or hypertension
    - **Degenerative disorders** involving white-matter disease (e.g., Krabbe's disease)
    - **Metabolic disorders** (e.g., uremia)
    - **Toxins** (e.g., lead)

28. **What CSF findings suggest metabolic disease as a cause of neurologic signs and symptoms?**
    - **Elevated CSF protein concentration** is characteristic of metachromatic leukodystrophy and globoid-cell encephalopathy.
    - **Low CSF glucose concentration** is consistent with hypoglycemia caused by a defect of gluconeogenesis or a defect in the transport of glucose across the blood-brain barrier (GLUT-1 deficiency syndrome).
    - **Low CSF folate concentration** suggests a defect involving folate metabolism.
    - **Presence in the CSF of amino acids, specifically glycine, glutamate, and gamma aminobutyric acid (GABA),** may be diagnostic of nonketotic hyperglycinemia, pyridoxine-dependent epilepsy, or another defect in the GABA shunt.
    - **Lactate** and **pyruvate** values are elevated in CSF disorders of cerebral energy metabolism, including pyruvate dehydrogenase deficiency, pyruvate carboxylase deficiency, numerous disturbances of the respiratory chain, and Menkes' syndrome.
    - **Low CSF lactate** value may be seen in the GLUT-1 deficiency syndrome.
    - **Abnormal CSF biogenic amines** suggest several disorders that are associated with disturbed neurotransmission.

29. **As tests of meningeal irritation, what constitutes a positive Kernig's or Brudzinski's sign?**
    Kernig's sign or the straight-leg-raising sign; it consists of flexing the hip to 90° and attempting to extend the knee. The limitation of knee extension as a result of painful resistance is a positive sign.

    Brudzinski's sign is a positive sign, and it is present if a reflex flexion of the thighs occurs when a patient's neck is passively flexed.

30. **How do the manifestations of increased intracranial pressure differ in an infant as compared with an older child?**
    Infant: Increasing head circumference, delayed closure of the fontanel, suture separation, bulging fontanel, failure to thrive, macrocephaly, setting sun sign, shrill cry
    Older child: Headache (especially in the early morning, awakening the child from sleep, or association with vomiting), nausea, persistent vomiting, personality/mood changes, lethargy, anorexia, fatigue, somnolence, diplopia as a result of sixth-nerve palsy or third-nerve palsy with uncal herniation, papilledema

31. **What comprises Cushing's triad?**
    Cushing's triad consists of the development of slow or irregular respirations, decreased heart rate, and elevated blood pressure (particularly an increased systolic pressure with a widening pulse pressure) resulting from an increase in intracranial pressure (ICP). Cushing's triad may be observed in children with increased ICP or compression of the posterior fossa, which houses the medullary circulatory control center. It is a very late finding of increased ICP.

32. **How is hydrocephalus classified?**
    Communicating hydrocephalus is present if a tracer dye injected into one lateral ventricle appears in the lumbar CSF. This type of hydrocephalus is caused by an inability to normally reabsorb CSF by the arachnoid granulations, which can occur from meningeal scarring as a result of bacterial meningitis or intraventricular hemorrhage.

    Noncommunicating hydrocephalus refers to conditions causing intraventricular obstruction and alteration of the flow of dye into the lumbar CSF. Congenital malformations (especially aqueductal stenosis and Dandy-Walker syndrome with cystic dilatation of the fourth ventricle) and mass lesions (e.g., tumors, arteriovenous malformations) can cause noncommunicating hydrocephalus.

Hydrocephalus ex vacuo describes increases in volume without increased CSF pressure, which is seen in conditions of reduced cerebral tissue (e.g., malformation, atrophy).

33. **What is the normal growth rate of head circumference during the first year of life?**
Head circumference at birth is about 34 cm for the term infant. The head circumference normally grows by 2 cm/month for the first 3 months of life, 1 cm/month for months 4–6, and 0.5 cm/month up to 1 year of life. The measurement of head circumference should be part of the examination of any child and should be plotted at every visit. The head circumference represents brain growth, but it is also influenced by hydrocephalus and subdural or epidural fluid collections.

34. **What are the complications of ventricular shunts?**
Ventricular shunts drain CSF from the ventricles in patients whose normal outflow or absorption has been blocked. The fluid may be drained to a variety of different locations, including the peritoneum, the kidney, or the atrium. Shunts draining CSF have remarkably improved the outcome of children with hydrocephalus, but they are subject to obstruction, infection, or mechanical malfunction. Shunt malfunctions present signs of increased ICP. Children with shunt infections often have a low-grade fever as well as signs of increased ICP. Because it is impossible to know the compliance properties of the ventricular system, children with shunt malfunction or infection are at risk for sudden, catastrophic decompensation. Children suspected of having shunt malfunctions or infection require urgent attention, and they should be closely observed until the shunt has been fully evaluated.

35. **What are the characteristic features of pseudotumor cerebri?**
Pseudotumor cerebri consists of an increased ICP in the absence of a demonstrable mass lesion and with a normal CSF formula. Characteristic features include the following:
- Headache, fatigue, vomiting, anorexia, stiff neck, and diplopia from increased ICP
- Normal neurologic examination except for papilledema or a third- or sixth-nerve palsy
- Normal computed tomography (CT) scan, except sometimes for small ventricles
- Normal CSF profile with the exception of an elevated opening pressure

36. **What causes pseudotumor cerebri?**
Although there are multiple possible causes, >90% of cases are idiopathic. Among the reported causes are the following:
- **Drugs:** Tetracycline, nalidixic acid, nitrofurantoin, corticosteroids, excess vitamin A
- **Endocrine disorders:** Hyperthyroidism, Cushing's syndrome, hypoparathyroidism
- **Thrombosis** of the dural venous sinuses as a result of head trauma, otitis media, mastoiditis, or obstruction of jugular veins in the superior vena cava syndrome

37. **What treatment is recommended for severe cases of pseudotumor cerebri?**
Patients with sustained visual field loss or severe refractory headache are candidates for treatment. Specific treatment depends on the presence of an identifiable precipitant, which should be removed when possible. For example, the cessation of the offending medication (e.g., tetracycline) or weight reduction in obese patients is recommended. Nonspecific treatment includes the administration of acetazolamide, furosemide, or hydrochlorothiazide and, sometimes, corticosteroids. In severe cases, surgical intervention is available via installation of a lumboperitoneal shunt or optic nerve sheath decompression.

38. **Can anything be done to minimize the chance of a post–lumbar-puncture headache?**
- Avoid a head-up posture during the procedure.

- Use the smallest possible needle (22 gauge or smaller), and advance the bevel "up," with the patient in the decubitus position.

There is debate about whether the maintenance of a prone position for several hours after the procedure can prevent the headache.

39. Why may it be dangerous to do a lumbar puncture using a needle with the stylette removed?

The (unproven) theory is that the stylette may prevent nerve roots of the cauda equina from becoming entrapped in the needle and may cause less disruption of the dural sac. Another concern is that, without the stylette, skin cells may enter the core of the needle, where they can be introduced into the subarachnoid space and form an epidermoid tumor.

CLINICAL ISSUES

40. What distinguishes the pediatric neurologic examination?

Observation. The most useful information is often acquired by watching the child move and play. The level of interaction, creativity, and degree of sustained attention can be observed and are all important components of the mental status examination. By observing eye movements, response to sounds, the child's reaction to visual stimuli introduced into the peripheral visual field, and the symmetry of facial movements, most of the cranial nerves can be tested. Persistent asymmetries of spontaneous motor activity (e.g., consistently reaching across midline for an object) are reliable signs of weakness. Inspection of the seated posture and gait of the child provides an assessment of the cerebellum and cerebellar outflow pathways.

41. What are the advantages and disadvantages of CT as compared with MRI for pediatric neurologic evaluations?

CT scan without contrast is the best imaging technique for neurologic emergencies to screen a patient with significant head trauma for skull fractures, signs of herniation, or acute intracranial hemorrhage. It can also be used to screen for acute strokes and subarachnoid hemorrhages. Midline or ventricular shifts caused by masses and cerebral edema or increased ICP can be noted, and it clearly identifies bone. This rapid study allows for routine monitoring and is less expensive than MRI. There is a small but defined risk of radiation from CT scans.

CT scan with contrast uses radiodense contrast material to allow for the better identification of disruptions in the blood-brain barrier or of highly vascular structures, thereby significantly improving the detection of tumors, edema, focal inflammation, hemangiomas, and arteriovenous malformations.

MRI without contrast is the preferred modality for most nonurgent examinations. It defines the structures of the brain more precisely than CT does, especially within the spinal cord, the posterior fossa, and the cisterns. It is more effective for subtle hemorrhages (especially subacute and chronic) and for tumors or masses. Different tissue-specific relaxation constants, called T1 and T2, and proton density allow for the better definition of white and gray matter; it also provides an image in three dimensions. MRI is unreliable for fractures, and the longer testing time may require sedation. Also, monitoring patients is more difficult in closed units. There are no known biologic hazards from MRI, which measures the emission of the radio waves that are released when protons return to a lower-energy state after excitation within characteristic tissue environments. MRI is contraindicated in patients with metallic implants that are ferromagnetic.

MRI with contrast is helpful for defining brain metastases and distinguishing postoperative scarring from other pathology.

Magnetic resonance angiography is a special type of MRI that displays larger arteries and veins without the use of contrast. It is less invasive than traditional arteriograms, and it is useful for defining arterial stenosis and identifying intracranial hemangiomas, arteriovenous malformations, and vascular aneurysms.

Altemeier WA 3rd, Levine C, Rodriguez F: A pediatrician's view. Imaging procedures in pediatric neurological conditions. Pediatr Ann 27:607–609, 1998.

42. **A child presents with progressive left leg weakness and diplopia, especially when looking toward the left. Where is the lesion?**
The above history in combination with an examination showing upper motor neuron nerve dysfunction, long tract signs, brisk reflexes, up-going toe (Babinski's sign), and a contralateral third nerve palsy (down and out) localizes the lesion to **the right pyramidal tract before the decussation** (crossing over) and **involves a lesion of the right third-nerve nucleus.** The progressive course suggests a slow-growing lesion, such as a pontine glioma.

43. **A dilated and unreactive pupil indicates the compression of what structure?**
The third cranial nerve. This may be the result of compression anywhere along the course of the nerve. Uncal herniation is a medial displacement of the uncus of the temporal lobe and may cause this sign.

44. **Pinpoint pupils and respiratory changes indicate the compression of what structure?**
Progressive central herniation of the brain downward through the foramen magnum causes compression of the **pons** and can produce this finding.

45. **How does the presentation of stroke differ between infants and older children?**
Infants usually have a seizure, whereas older children have acute hemiplegia.

Calder K, Kokorowski P, Tran T, Henderson S: Emergency department presentation of stroke. Pediatr Emerg Care 19:320–328, 2003.

46. **What is the differential diagnosis of stroke in children?**
Cerebrovascular disease, or stroke, can be the result of primary vascular disease, bleeding disorder (hemorrhagic stroke), or a variety of secondary problems that lead to thrombotic or embolic occlusions (most commonly of the middle cerebral artery). Diagnostic possibilities include the following:
Cardioembolic: Cyanotic congenital heart disease, atrial myxoma, endocarditis, rheumatic or other valvular heart disease
Hematologic: Hemoglobinopathies (especially sickle cell disease), hypercoagulable states (antithrombin III deficiency, protein C or S deficiency), hyperviscosity (leukemia, hyperproteinemia, thrombocytosis), coagulation disorders (lupus-associated antibodies, hemophilia, thrombocytopenia, factor V abnormalities, hyperhomocystoinomia)
Circulatory: Vasculitis (infectious or inflammatory), occlusive (homocystinuria, arteriosclerosis, fibromuscular dysplasia of the internal carotid artery, posttraumatic carotid scarring), carotid or vertebral artery dissection, moyamoya disease, atrioventricular malformation with steal syndrome, anomalous circulation, posttraumatic air embolism, arterial aneurysm, hemiplegic migraine
Metabolic: Mitochondrial disease

Carlin TM, Chanmugam A: Stroke in children. Emerg Med Clin North Am 20:671–685, 2002.

47. **What is the derivation of "moyamoya" in moyamoya disease?**
Moyamoya, which is Japanese for "puff of smoke," refers to the cerebral angiographic appearance of patients with this primary vascular disease that results in stenosis of the

internal carotid artery. It also occurs in a wide variety of conditions, such as neurofibromatosis type 1, sickle cell disease, Down syndrome, and tuberous sclerosis, in addition to the idiopathic condition that is endemic in Japan. Because it is a chronic condition, fine vascular collaterals can develop, and it is these collaterals that create the "puff of smoke" appearance on angiography.

48. **A child who develops weakness, incontinence, and ataxia 10 days after a bout of influenza likely has what diagnosis?**

    Acute disseminated encephalomyelitis is thought to be a post- or parainfectious process that is targeted against central myelin. Any portion of the white matter may be affected. Multiple lesions with a perivenular lymphocytic and mononuclear cell infiltration and demyelination are seen on pathologic examination. Acute disseminated encephalomyelitis has been associated with mumps, measles, rubella, varicella-zoster, influenza, parainfluenza, mononucleosis, and immunization. An associated transverse myelitis may be acute (developing over hours) or subacute (developing over 1–2 weeks), with both motor and sensory tract involvement. Bladder and bowel dysfunction is often early and severe. CSF examination shows mild increase of pressure and up to 250 cells/mm^3, with a lymphocyte predominance. The MRI shows an increased T2 signal intensity. Prognosis, particularly with the use of intravenous corticosteroids, is good.

49. **In patients with acute injury to the brain, what two types of edema may occur?**

    - **Vasogenic edema** results from increased permeability of the capillary endothelium with resulting exudation. It is more marked in cerebral white matter and occurs as a result of inflammation (meningitis and abscess), focal processes (hemorrhage, infarct, or tumor), vessel pathology, or lead or hypertensive encephalopathy.
    - **Cytotoxic edema** results from the rapid swelling of cells, especially astrocytes, and also from neurons and endothelial cells as a result of dysfunction of the membranes and ionic pumps from energy failure, which may lead to cellular death. Hypoxia caused by cardiac arrest, hypoxic-ischemic encephalopathy (HIE), various toxins, severe infections, status epilepticus, infarct, or increased ICP is also a possible cause.

50. **What are the treatments for increased intracranial pressure?**

    - **Hyperventilation:** The usual goal is to lower the pCO_2 to 25–30 mm. This causes vasoconstriction, which decreases the intracranial vascular volume.
    - **Fluid restriction, osmotic diuretics,** and **hypertonic mannitol solution** all work to shrink brain water content, provided there is an intact blood-brain barrier.
    - **Head elevation** in a midline position to 30° maximizes venous return.
    - **External ventricular drains** are sometimes placed, both to monitor pressure and to allow for a minimal amount of CSF withdrawal.
    - **Normalization of physiologic parameters:** It is important to avoid significant hypotension, hypoxia, hypoglycemia, and hyperthermia.

51. **How is brain death defined?**

    Brain death is defined by an irreversible absence of cortical and midbrain activity. There must be an absence of a reversible etiology (i.e., toxic-metabolic, medication, hypothermia, hypotension, or surgically remediable causes). Spinal cord, peripheral nerve, or reflex muscular activity may persist despite brain death. Decorticate or decerebrate posturing, however, is inconsistent with brain death. The examination must remain unchanged over the time. Other countries have defined brain death as the absence of brain stem function alone, but in the United States, the absence of cortical function also must be demonstrated. The clinical hallmark of brain death is deep, unremitting, unresponsive coma.

Banasiak KJ, Lister G: Brain death in children. Curr Opin Pediatr 15:288–293, 2003.
Wijdicks EFM: The diagnosis of brain death. N Engl JMed 344:1215–1221, 2001.

52. **How is the diagnosis of brain death made?**
Patients with suspected brain death should be observed over 12–24 hours for the following:
- Unresponsive coma and the absence of eye opening, extraocular movements, vocalizations, or other cerebral-generated activity
- The complete absence of brain-stem function, including nonresponsive, midposition, or fully dilated pupils; no spontaneous or reflexive eye movements on oculovestibular testing ("doll's eyes" and calorics); no bulbar muscle function (i.e., corneal, gag, cough, sucking, and rooting reflexes); and no respirations on apnea testing

Supportive testing, if needed, to document brain death can include absent cerebral cortical activity as evidenced by a properly recorded "flat," "isoelectric," or electrocerebral silence (determined by EEG), the absence of blood flow to the hemispheres by cerebral arteriography or radionuclide study, or the presence of ICP that exceeds mean blood pressure for several hours.

Banasiak KJ, Lister G: Brain death in children. Curr Opin Pediatr 15:288–293, 2003.
Wijdicks EFM: The diagnosis of brain death. N Engl JMed 344:1215–1221, 2001.

53. **How do the criteria for the determination of brain death vary by age?**
The Task Force on Brain Death in Children recommends that no determination of brain death be made in neonates <7 days old. In infants who are 7 days to 2 months old, two examinations and EEGs separated by at least 48 hours are recommended. In infants 2 months to 1 year old, two examinations and EEGs separated by at least 24 hours are recommended. A repeat examination and EEG are not required if cerebral blood flow study shows absence of flow. In children >1 year old, if the etiology is irreversible, laboratory testing is not required, and a 12-hour period of observation is recommended. If there is a potentially reversible condition (e.g., HIE), then at least a 24-hour period of observation is recommended.

Report of special task force of the American Academy of Pediatrics Task Force on Brain Death in Children. Guidelines for the determination of brain death in children. Pediatrics 80:298–300, 1987.

54. **Compare the "persistent vegetative state" with the "minimally conscious state."**
- **The persistent vegetative state** is "a form of eyes-open permanent unconsciousness in which the patient has periods of wakefulness and physiological sleep/wake cycles, but at no time is the patient aware of himself or herself or the environment." If this state persists for >3 months in children, the long-term outlook is grim.
- **The minimally conscious state** occurs on emergence from this vegetative state, and a patient must demonstrate a reproducible action in one or more of four types of behavior: (1) simple command following; (2) gestural or verbal "yes/no" responses; (3) intelligible verbalization; or (4) purposeful behaviors.

American Academy of Neurology: Position of the American Academy of Neurology on certain aspects of the care and management of the persistent vegetative state patient. Adopted by the Executive Board, American Academy of Neurology, April 21, 1988, Cincinnati, Ohio. Neurology 39:125–126, 1989.
Giacino JT, Ashwal S, Childs N, et al: The minimally conscious state: Definition and diagnostic criteria. Neurology 58:349–353, 2002.

55. **What is the differential diagnosis of an intracranial bruit?**
An intracranial bruit can be found in normal children. Disorders that may be associated with an intracranial bruit include the following:
- Fever
- Cerebral angioma
- Intracerebral tumors
- Thyrotoxicosis
- Cerebral aneurysm
- Any cause of increased ICP

- Anemia
- Cerebral arteriovenous malformations
- Meningitis
- Cardiac murmurs

Mace JW, Peters ER, Mathies AW, Jr.: Cranial bruits in purulent meningitis in childhood. N Engl J Med 278:1420–1422, 1968.

56. **In a previously normal child who develops acute ataxia, what are the two most common diagnoses?**
    1. **Drug ingestion**, especially antiepileptic drugs, heavy metals, alcohol, and antihistamines
    2. **Acute postinfectious cerebellitis**, most commonly after varicella: This is a diagnosis of exclusion if drug screening, CT or MRI, CSF evaluation, and other tests are negative.

57. **What are the causes of toe walking?**
    - CP (spastic diplegia)
    - Muscular dystrophy
    - Spinal dysraphism
    - Hereditary or acquired polyneuropathies
    - Intraspinal and filum terminale tumor
    - Equinovarus deformity
    - Isolated congenital shortening of the Achilles tendon
    - Variation of normal in early stages of walking
    - Normal development pattern in some toddlers

58. **What is Babinski's response?**
    Stimulation of the lateral aspect of the sole of the foot to the distal metatarsals may elicit a *plantar response* (extension); this indicates a lack of cortical inhibition and aids in the diagnosis of central hypotonia. It is abnormal outside of the neonatal period, when a flexor response develops. The stimulus elicits a numbers of sensory pathways with competing functions (including grip and withdrawal) and is somewhat dependent on the state of the infant and the examiner's technique. Its value as a localizing sign in the neonate is more controversial, but a consistent asymmetry is abnormal.

59. **A 7-year-old child with progressive ataxia, kyphoscoliosis, nystagmus, pes cavus (high arch), and an abnormal electrocardiogram (ECG) likely has what diagnosis?**
    Friedreich's ataxia. This heredodegenerative disease is an autosomal recessive disorder with childhood onset of gait ataxia, absent tendon reflexes, and extensor plantar responses. The spinal cord shows degeneration and sclerosis of the spinocerebellar tracts, the posterior column, and the corticospinal tracts. The condition is rare. The gene for Friedreich's ataxia has been mapped to chromosome 9q13, contains a trinucleotide repeating sequence (GAA), and encodes for a protein called *frataxin*. A deficiency of frataxin leads to the accumulation of iron in the mitochondria and to oxidative stress, which leads to cell death.

Alper G, Narayanan V: Friedreich's ataxia. Pediatr Neurol 28:335–341, 2003.

60. **What clinical features help to distinguish peripheral from central vertigo?**
    Peripheral vertigo implies dysfunction of the labyrinth or vestibular nerve, whereas central vertigo is associated with abnormalities of the brain stem or temporal lobe.
    Peripheral
    - Hearing loss, tinnitus, and otalgia may be associated.
    - Past pointing and falling in the direction of unilateral disease occur.
    - In bilateral disease, ataxia occurs with the eyes closed.
    - Vestibular and positional nystagmus are present.

Central

- Cerebellar and cranial nerve dysfunction are frequently associated.
- No hearing loss is present.
- An alteration of consciousness may be associated.

Fenichel GM: Clinical Pediatric Neurology: A Signs and Symptoms Approach, 4th ed. Philadelphia, W.B. Saunders, 2001, 347–351.

61. **In what settings is hyperacusis noted?**

Hyperacusis, or increased sensitivity to sound, is found in patients with injury to the facial nerve (CN VII), which innervates the stapedius muscle, or in those with injury to the trigeminal nerve (CN V), which innervates the tensor tympani muscle. Exaggerated startle response to sound or vibration occurs in patients with lysosomal storage diseases (e.g., sphingolipidoses such as Tay-Sachs disease, GM_1 gangliosidosis, and Sandhoff's disease), Williams syndrome, hyperkalemia, tetanus, and strychnine poisoning.

62. **What is the most common cause of asymmetric crying facies?**

In this entity, one side of the lower lip depresses during crying (on the normal side), and the other does not. Often misdiagnosed as a facial nerve palsy resulting from forceps delivery, the most common cause is **congenital absence of the depressor anguli oris muscle** of the lower lip. Its occasional association with heart defects warrants ECG and chest x-ray in these patients.

63. **What are the common causes of peripheral seventh-nerve palsy?**

Facial weakness caused by a lesion of the facial nerve (cranial nerve VII) is common. The facial weakness involves both the upper and lower face and affects both emotional and volitional facial movements. Any part of the nerve can be disturbed: the nucleus itself, the axon as it passes through the pons, or the peripheral portion of the nerve. Common etiologies include the following:

- **Trauma**
- **Developmental hypoplasia** or **aplasia,** including the Möbius anomaly
- **Bell's palsy** (usually idiopathic, but may follow nonspecific viral infections)
- **Infections,** including the Ramsay Hunt syndrome (herpes zoster invasion of the geniculate ganglion producing herpetic vesicles behind the ear and painful paralysis of the facial nerve); Lyme disease; local invasion from suppurative mastoiditis or otitis media; mumps, varicella, or enterovirus neuritis; sequelae of bacterial meningitis; and parotid gland infection, inflammation, or tumor
- **GBS** (Guillain-Barré syndrome)
- **Tumor** of the brain stem or cerebellar pontine angle tumors
- **Inflammatory disorders** such as sarcoidosis

64. **During recovery from Bell's palsy, why do the eyes water at mealtime?**

These are *crocodile tears*. The facial nerve supplies autonomic motor function to the lacrimal and salivary glands. Because of aberrant reinnervation during the course of healing from a facial nerve palsy, tasting a meal can trigger tearing rather than salivation. Folklore has it that crocodiles feel compassion for their victims and weep while munching.

65. **When are "doll's eyes" movements considered normal or abnormal?**

The oculovestibular reflex (also called oculocephalic, proprioceptive head-turning reflex, or doll's eyes reflex) is used most commonly as a test of brain-stem function. The patient's eyelids are held open while the head is briskly rotated from side to side. A positive response is contraversive conjugate eye deviation (i.e., as the head rotates to the right, both eyes deviate to the left). Doll's eyes movements are interpreted as follows:

- In healthy awake newborn infants (who cannot inhibit or override the reflex with willful eye movements), the reflex is easy to elicit and is a normal finding. It can be used to test the range of the extraocular movements of infants during the first weeks of life.
- In healthy, awake, mature individuals, normal vision overrides the reflex, which is thus normally absent, and so the eyes follow the head turning.
- In a patient in a coma with preserved brain-stem function, the depressed cortex does not override the reflex, and doll's eyes movements occur in rapid head rotation. Indeed, the purpose of eliciting this reflex in the comatose patient is to demonstrate that the brain stem still functions normally.
- In a patient in a coma with brain-stem damage, the neural circuits that carry out the reflex are impaired, and the reflex is abolished.

66. **How are cold calorics done?**
As a test of brain-stem function in an obtunded or comatose individual, 5 mL of ice cold water is placed in the external ear canal (after ensuring the integrity of the tympanic membrane), with the head elevated at 30°. A normal response occurs with deviation of the eyes to the side in which the water was placed. No response indicates severe dysfunction of the brain stem and the medial longitudinal fasciculus.

67. **What causes pinpoint pupils?**
Pupillary size represents a dynamic balance between the constricting influence of the third nerve (representing the parasympathetic autonomic nervous system) and the dilating influence of the ciliary nerve (which conducts fibers of the sympathetic nervous system). Pinpoint pupils indicate that the constricting influence of the third cranial nerve is not balanced by opposing sympathetic dilation. Etiologies could include the following:
- **Structural lesion in the pons** through which descend the sympathetic pathways
- **Metabolic disorders**
- **Opiates,** such as heroin or morphine
- **Other agents,** including propoxyphene, organophosphates, carbamate insecticides, barbiturates, clonidine, meprobamate, pilocarpine eyedrops, and mushroom or nutmeg poisoning

68. **What is the differential diagnosis of ptosis?**
Ptosis is the downward displacement of the upper eyelid as a result of dysfunction of the muscles that elevate the eyelid. A drooping eyelid may represent *pseudoptosis* caused by swelling of the eyelid as a result of local edema or active blepharospasm. *True ptosis* results from weakness of the eyelid muscles or interruption of its nerve supply. Etiologies include the following:
- **Muscular:** Congenital ptosis, which may occur alone or in the setting of Turner's or Smith-Lemli-Opitz syndrome, myasthenia gravis, botulism, or some muscular dystrophies
- **Neurologic:** Horner syndrome, which results from the interruption of the sympathetic supply to Müller's smooth eyelid muscle, and third-nerve palsy, which innervates the levator palpebral muscle

69. **What does the Marcus Gunn pupil detect?**
An **afferent pupillary defect**. The pupils are normally equal in size (except for patients with physiologic anisocoria) as a result of the consensual light reflex: light entering either eye produces the same-strength "signal" for the constriction of both the stimulated and nonstimulated pupil. Some diseases of the maculae or optic nerves affect one side more than the other. For example, a meningioma may develop on one optic nerve sheath. As a result of unilateral or asymmetric optic nerve dysfunction, a Marcus Gunn pupil may result.

70. **How is the swinging flashlight test done to detect a Marcus Gunn pupil?**
   - The patient is examined in a dim room, and fixation is directed to a distant target. This permits maximal pupillary dilation because of a lack of direct light and accommodation reflexes.
   - Light presented to the "good" eye produces the equal constriction of both pupils. A flashlight is swung briskly over the bridge of the nose to the eye with the "defective" optic nerve. The abnormal pupil remains momentarily constricted from the lingering effects of the consensual light response. However, the impaired eye with its reduced pupillomotor signal soon escapes the consensual reflex and actually dilates, despite being directly stimulated with light. The pupil that paradoxically dilates to direct light stimulation displays the *afferent defect.*

71. **When attending a pediatric conference in London, is it prudent to avoid the meat pies?**
   New-variant Creutzfeldt-Jakob disease and transmissible spongiform encephalopathies (or prion diseases) have achieved some pediatric notoriety, with cases having been described in adolescents. These are a group of clinical syndromes in animals and humans that are characterized by slowly progressive neurodegenerative disease. The increases of bovine spongiform encephalopathy in Great Britain noted during the mid-1980s prompted successful control measures, and the U.S. Centers for Disease Control and Prevention now characterizes the risk of exposure to bovine spongiform encephalopathy in Great Britain as remote.

   Whitely RJ, McDonald N, Ashir DM, American Academy of Pediatrics; Committee on Infectious Disease: Technical report: Transmissible spongiform encephalopathies: A review for pediatricians. Pediatrics 106:1160–1165, 2000.

EPILEPSY

72. **What is epilepsy?**
   Epilepsy describes a syndrome of recurrent, unprovoked seizures. It is derived from the Greek verb *epilepsia* meaning "to seize upon" or "to take hold of." The early Greeks referred to it as the sacred disease, but Hippocrates debunked this notion and argued from clinical evidence that it arose from the brain. Epilepsy is not an entity or even a syndrome but rather a symptom complex arising from disordered brain function that itself may be the result of a variety of pathologic processes.

   Chang BS, Lowenstein DH: Epilepsy. N Engl J Med 349:1257–1266, 2003.

73. **What is the long-term outcome for children with epilepsy?**
   There are many different causes of epilepsy, and, in large part, the outcome relates to the underlying etiology. Children with idiopathic or genetically determined epilepsy have the best prognosis, whereas children with antecedent neurologic abnormalities fare less well. Nearly 75% of children will enter into a sustained remission 3–5 years after the onset of their epilepsy. There is no evidence that antiepileptic medications as they are currently used in clinical practice are neuroprotective or that they alter the long-term outcome of patients. Although there is a favorable prognosis for the remission of seizures, children with epilepsy are at an increased risk for having other long-term challenges, including difficulties achieving social, educational, and vocational goals. Treatment with antiepileptic medications is one important part of the management of the child, but other critical aspects of the physician–patient interaction, including educating, counseling, and advocacy, are equally important.

74. **How often are EEGs abnormal in healthy children?**
   Approximately 10% of "normal" children have mild, nonspecific abnormalities in background activity. About 2–3% of healthy children have unexpected incidental epileptiform (i.e., spikes or sharp wave) patterns. Some may have heritable, familial EEG abnormalities without a clinical

seizure disorder (e.g., centrotemporal spikes seen in benign seizure-susceptibility syndromes such as rolandic epilepsy).

75. **Should an EEG be done on all children who have a first afebrile seizure?**
This is a major controversial issue. Of new-onset seizures in children, about one third do not involve fever. The American Academy of Neurology has recommended that all children with a first seizure without fever undergo an EEG in an effort to better classify the epilepsy syndrome. Others argue that the quantity of expected information from obtaining EEGs for all cases is too low to affect treatment recommendations in most patients. They suggest that a selective approach to EEG use should be pursued, particularly for children with a seizure of focal onset, for children <1 year old, and for any child with unexplained cognitive or motor dysfunction or abnormalities on neurologic examination.

> Gilbert DL, Buncher CR: An EEG should not be routinely obtained after first unprovoked seizure in childhood. Neurology 54:635–641, 2000.
> Hirtz D, Ashwal S, Berg A, et al: Practice parameter: Evaluating a first nonfebrile seizure in children: Report of the Quality Standards Subcommittee of the American Academy of Neurology, the Child Neurology Society, and the American Epilepsy Society. Neurology 55:616–623, 2000.

76. **Which disorders commonly mimic epilepsy?**
Many conditions are characterized by the sudden onset of abnormal consciousness, awareness, reactivity, behavior, posture, tone, sensation, or autonomic function. Syncope, breath-holding spells, migraine, hypoglycemia, narcolepsy, cataplexy, sleep apnea, gastroesophageal reflux, and parasomnias (night terrors, sleep walking, sleep talking, nocturnal enuresis) feature an abrupt or "paroxysmal" alteration of brain function and suggest the possibility of epilepsy. Perhaps one of the most difficult attacks to distinguish is the "nonepileptic" seizure (also called a pseudoepileptic or hysterical seizure).

77. **What are the two key questions for the classification of the epilepsy syndrome?**
   1. **Where does the seizure begin?** If the seizure appears to begin in part of the brain, it is partial or "localization related." Partial seizures (formerly called "focal seizures") are divided into *simple* and *complex* types.
   2. **Is brain development normal?** If the seizure arises from a developmentally normal brain, it is a *primary* or *idiopathic* epilepsy; arising from an abnormal brain makes it a *secondary* or *symptomatic* epilepsy. "Cryptogenic" is the term used to describe seizures in a child who has not had normal neurologic development and in whom the etiology cannot be found.

78. **What are the categories of seizures in children?**
The syndrome classification as codified by the International League Against Epilepsy distinguishes seizure on the basis of type rather than etiology (Table 14-2). Combinations of seizure types may occur in an individual patient.

79. **What are the causes of "symptomatic" seizures?**
Symptomatic seizures are those that are caused by an identifiable injury to the brain, as opposed to idiopathic or cryptogenic epilepsy. The seizures are a sign of underlying disease or pathology that must be managed, if possible, independently of the seizure itself (Table 14-3).

80. **If a previously normal child has an afebrile, generalized tonic-clonic seizure, what should parents be told about the risk of recurrence?**
Studies indicate that the recurrence rate is *between 25% and 50%*. The EEG is an important predictor of recurrence. A subsequent normal EEG reduces the 5-year recurrence risk to 25%. Occurrence of the seizure during sleep increases the risk to 50%. Half of recurrences will occur

during the first 6 months after the first seizure; two thirds will occurs within 1 year, and 90% or more will have occurred within 2 years. The child's age at the time of the first seizure and the duration of the seizure do not affect the recurrence risk.

Shinnar S, Berg AT, Moshe SL, et al: The risk of seizure recurrence after a first unprovoked afebrile seizure in childhood: An extended follow-up. Pediatrics 98:216–225, 1996.

TABLE 14-2. INTERNATIONAL LEAGUE AGAINST EPILEPSY SEIZURE CLASSIFICATION

Partial (focal, local) seizures
Simple partial seizures
With motor signs: Focal motor, Jacksonian, versive, postural, phonatory
With somatosensory or special sensory symptoms (simple hallucinations, e.g., tingling, light flashes, buzzing): somatosensory, visual, auditory, olfactory, gustatory, vertiginous
With autonomic symptoms and signs
With psychic symptoms (disturbances of higher cerebral functions): Dysphasic, dysmnesic, cognitive, affective, illusions, structured hallucinations

Generalized seizures
Absence seizures, with impairment of consciousness, with clonic, atonic, tonic, or autonomic components, or with automatisms occurring alone or in combination
Atypical absences, more pronounced changes of tone than in absence seizures; onset and/or cessation not abrupt
Monoclonic seizures (single or multiple)
Clonic seizures
Tonic seizures
Tonic-clonic seizures
Atonic seizures

Unclassified epileptic seizures
Complex partial seizures (with impairment of consciousness)
Simple partial onset followed by impairment of consciousness
   With no other features
   With simple partial features
   With automatisms
Partial seizures evolving to secondarily generalized tonic-clonic seizures

Adapted from Vedanarayanan VV: Diagnosis of epilepsy in children. Pediatr Ann 28:218–224, 1999.

81. **Should all children with a new-onset afebrile generalized seizure have a CT or MRI evaluation?**
Although most adults with new-onset seizures should have a head imaging study (preferably MRI), the relatively high frequency of idiopathic seizure disorders in children often obviates a

scan in those with generalized seizures, nonfocal EEGs, and normal neurologic examinations. Consider obtaining a cranial imaging study in the following situations:

- Any seizure with focal components (other than mere eye deviation)
- Newborns and young infants with seizures
- Status epilepticus at any age
- Focal slowing or focal paroxysmal activity on EEG

Hirtz D, Berg A, Bettis D, et al; Quality Standards Subcommittee of the American Academy of Neurology; Practice Committee of the Child Neurology Society: Practice parameter: Treatment of the child with a first unprovoked seizure: Report of the Quality Standards Subcommittee of the American Academy of Neurology and the Practice Committee of the Child Neurology Society. Neurology 60:166–175, 2003.

TABLE 14-3. CAUSES OF SYMPTOMATIC SEIZURES

Fever	**Toxins**
Simple febrile seizures	Drugs
Complicated febrile seizures	Drug withdrawal
	Biologic toxins
Trauma	
Impact seizures	**Stroke**
Early posttraumatic seizures	Ischemic stroke
Late posttraumatic seizures	Embolic stroke
	Hemorrhagic stroke
Hypoxia	
Complicated breath-holding spells	**Intracranial hemorrhage**
Hypoxic seizures	Subdural hemorrhage
	Subarachnoid hemorrhage
Metabolic	Intracerebral hemorrhage
Acquired metabolic disorders	Intraventricular hemorrhage
Neurologic effects of systemic disease	
Inborn errors of metabolism	

Adapted from Evans OB: Symptomatic seizures. Pediatr Ann 28:231–237, 1999.

82. **What are the most common inherited seizure or epilepsy syndromes?**
    - Febrile convulsions
    - Rolandic epilepsy, childhood absence epilepsy
    - Juvenile myoclonic epilepsy (of Janz)

83. **What are the clinical features of rolandic epilepsy?**
    Rolandic epilepsy is an idiopathic localization-related epilepsy that represents 10–15% of all childhood seizure disorders.
    - It begins in school-aged children (4–13 years old) who are otherwise healthy and neurologically normal.
    - Seizures are idiopathic or familial (autosomal dominant inheritance with age-dependent penetrance).

- Seizures may be simple or complex and partial or generalized. Classically, there is a history of one-sided facial paresthesias and twitching and drooling that may be followed by hemi-clonic movements or hemitonic posturing. Consciousness is typically preserved. The seizures are primarily nocturnal and may secondarily generalize.
- Often referred to as "benign" because the individual is developmentally normal, seizures are usually rare and nocturnal, and they most often resolve after puberty.

84. **What are the EEG features of rolandic epilepsy?**
Focal spikes and sharp waves localized to the rolandic (central, midtemporal, centrotemporal, or sylvian) regions against a normal background.

85. **What are the types of absence seizures?**
Typical absence
- EEG: 3-Hz spike and wave
- Observations: Abrupt onset and ending (typically 5–10 seconds)
- Subtypes
  1. Simple: Unresponsiveness with no other associated features except minor movements (e.g., lip-smacking or eyelid twitching)
  2. Complex: Unresponsiveness with more prolonged mild atonic, myoclonic, or tonic features or automatisms

Atypical absence (most common in Lennox-Gastaut syndrome)
- EEG: 2-Hz (or slower) spike and wave
- Observations: Gradual onset and ending; frequency is more cyclic; unresponsive with more prolonged and pronounced atonic, tonic, myoclonic, or tonic activity

86. **In a child who is suspected of having absence seizures, how can a seizure be elicited during an examination?**
Hyperventilation for at least 3 minutes is a useful provocative maneuver to precipitate an absence seizure. Young patients may be coaxed into overbreathing by making a game of it. Hold a tissue paper in front of the child's mouth, and then instruct the patient to keep breathing fast enough to keep the tissue aloft.

87. **What percentage of patients with absence seizures also have occasional grand mal seizures?**
About 30–50%.

88. **What is the prognosis for children with absence epilepsy?**
The prognosis for patients with childhood absence epilepsy has been studied prospectively, and nearly 90% of patients who have normal intelligence, normal neurologic examination, normal EEG background activity, no family history of convulsive epilepsy, and no history of tonic-clonic convulsions will become free of seizures. Conversely, the complete absence of favorable factors is associated with a poor prognosis for the cessation of seizures. It may be that absence seizures are expressed on a spectrum from typical childhood absence epilepsy that is genetic in origin to the Lennox-Gastaut syndrome, which is symptomatic of brain injury.

89. **A teenager, like his father, develops brief, bilateral, intermittent jerking of his arms. What seizure disorder is he likely to have?**
Juvenile myoclonic epilepsy, which is also called myoclonic epilepsy of Janz, is a familial form of primary idiopathic generalized epilepsy that typically involves "fast" 3- to 5-Hz spike and wave discharges on EEG ("impulsive petit mal") and autosomal dominant inheritance. The distinctive clinical features of this type of epilepsy include morning myoclonic jerks,

generalized tonic-clonic seizures upon awakening, normal intelligence, a family history of similar seizures, and onset between the ages of 8 and 20 years.

90. What are myoclonic seizures?
These seizures are characterized by rapid, bilateral, symmetric muscle contractions of short duration—"quick jerks." They may be isolated, or they may occur repetitively. Myoclonic seizures may be the sole manifestation of epilepsy, or, more commonly, they may be associated with absence attacks or tonic-clonic attacks.

91. What distinguishes atonic and akinetic seizures?
Atonic seizure involves the sudden and usually complete loss of tone in the limb, neck, and trunk muscles. Muscle control is lost without warning, and the child may be seriously injured. This situation is often aggravated by the occurrence of one or more myoclonic jerks immediately before muscle tone is lost so that the fall is associated with an element of propulsion. Atonic seizures are particularly common in children with static encephalopathies, and they may prove refractory to therapy. In **akinetic seizures**, movement is arrested without a significant loss of muscle tone; this is very rare.

92. What is the classic triad of infantile spasms?
Spasms, **hypsarhythmia**, and **developmental regression**. Infantile spasms are known as West's syndrome, and the condition is named for the physician who first described the condition in his own son in 1841.

93. What characterizes hypsarhythmia?
The term means "mountainous slowing," and it describes the classic interictal EEG of infantile spasms and is characterized by *extremely high-voltage, slow, and disorganized brain waves with multifocal spike activity*. Hypsarhythmia may either precede or follow the onset of infantile spasms. This EEG configuration may appear first or most obviously in non–rapid eye movement sleep and confirms the clinical diagnosis of infantile spasms.

94. How commonly is a cause identified in infantile spasms?
A cause can be identified in *up to 75%* of children with infantile spasms, particularly in those who are symptomatic at the time of the initial seizure. Of identifiable causes, three fourths are prenatal/perinatal, and one fourth are postnatal. All patients with infantile spasms should have detailed neuroimaging and metabolic and genetic studies. Causes, including some possible specific examples, include the following:
- **Prenatal/perinatal:** Neurocutaneous disorders (tuberous sclerosis), brain injury (hypoxic-ischemic encephalopathy), intrauterine infection (cytomegalovirus), brain malformations (lissencephaly, agenesis of the corpus callosum), inborn metabolic errors (nonketotic hyperglycinemia, phenylketonuria, maple syrup urine disease, pyridoxine dependency)
- **Postnatal:** Infectious (herpes encephalitis), hypoxic-ischemic encephalopathy, head trauma

95. What is the prognosis for infants with infantile spasms?
Prognosis in large part depends on the clinical state at the time of the first seizure. In the cryptogenic or idiopathic group (10–15%), development, neurologic examination, and imaging studies are usually normal at the onset. With adrenocorticotropic hormone (ACTH) treatment, 40–65% will have a complete or near-complete recovery. In the symptomatic group (85–90%), neurologic deficits or cranial abnormalities are typically present before the first seizure. In this group, complete or near-complete recovery is achieved by only 5–15%.

Dana Alliance for Brain Initiatives: www.dana.org

96. What is the treatment of choice for infantile spasms?

Currently in the United States, most children with infantile spasms are treated with *ACTH* as the first treatment option; the majority of patients will respond to this medication. *Vigabatrin*, particularly in infants with tuberous sclerosis and those <3 months old, has been found by some studies to be useful. However, Vigabatrin is not approved for use in the United States in part because of its possible side effects of the constriction of peripheral visual fields.

Mackay MT, Weiss SK, Adams-Webber T, et al; American Academy of Neurology; Child Neurology Society: Practice parameter: Medical treatment of infantile spasms. Neurology 62:1668–1681, 2004.

97. What are the side effects that are associated with ACTH?

The potential side effects of ACTH are prodigious. The treatment is associated with approximately 5% mortality in some series as a result of massive *gastric hemorrhage* from ulceration of the mucosa, *sepsis* as a result of immunologic compromise, or *cardiac failure* caused by a dilated cardiomyopathy. Echocardiography can reveal changes in advance of the clinical hypertension and may be a useful screening tool for the latter complication. The routine testing of the stool for occult blood, the regular monitoring of blood pressure, the screening of the urine for glucose, and the institution of a low-salt diet are other appropriate precautions. In addition to these short-term side effects of ACTH, there are other complications that are related to prolonged use, as are seen with other steroid treatments.

98. What is the most likely diagnosis in a child of Ashkenazi descent with stimulus-sensitive seizures, cognitive deterioration, and a cherry red spot?

The classic lysosomal lipid storage disorder presenting symptoms of a progressive encephalopathy during infancy is **Tay-Sachs disease**. The infantile forms of GM_2 gangliosidosis includes Tay-Sachs disease, which is caused by a deficiency of hexosaminidase A, and Sandhoff's disease, which is caused by a deficiency of hexosaminidase A and B. Tay-Sachs is an autosomal recessive disorder that is localized to chromosome 15, with an incidence of 1 in 3,900 in the Ashkenazi Jewish population of Eastern or Central European descent. The enzymatic defect leads to intraneuronal accumulation of GM_2 ganglioside. Normal development is seen until 4–6 months of age, when hypotonia and a loss of motor skills occur, with the subsequent development of spasticity, blindness, and macrocephaly. The classic cherry red spot is present in the ocular fundi of >90% of patients.

99. A patient with seizures, microcephaly, and a low CSF glucose but a normal serum glucose has what likely condition?

The **GLUT-1 deficiency syndrome,** which was previously referred to as the **glu**cose **t**ransporter protein deficiency syndrome, was first described in 1991. The clinical phenotype is variable, but the child usually presents symptoms during the first years of life with seizures and delays of motor and mental development. The head circumference decelerates during the first years of life. The diagnosis should be suspected if CSF reveals low glucose (and lactate) concentrations without evidence of inflammation and blood sugars are normal.

National Institute of Neurological Disorders and Stroke: www.ninds.nih.gov

100. What is the clinical triad of the Lennox-Gastaut syndrome?

Lennox-Gastaut syndrome is characterized by **mental retardation, seizures** of various types, and disorganized **slow spike and wave activity** on an EEG. The seizures usually begin during the first 3 years of life and are characteristically severe and refractory to anticonvulsant drugs. Prognosis is poor, with >80% of children continuing to have seizures into adulthood.

Crumrine PK: Lennox-Gastaut syndrome. J Child Neurol 17:S70–S75, 2002.

101. **How is status epilepticus defined?**
    - More than 30 minutes of continuous seizure activity
    - Recurrent seizures without full recovery of consciousness between seizures

102. **What are the most common precipitants of status epilepticus in children?**
    - Fever/infection (36%)
    - CNS infection (5%)
    - Medication change (20%)
    - Trauma (4%)
    - Unknown (9%)
    - Cerebrovascular (3%)
    - Metabolic (8%)
    - Ethanol/drug-related (2%)
    - Congenital (7%)
    - Tumor (1%)
    - Anoxia (5%)

    Working Group on Status Epilepticus: Treatment of convulsive status epilepticus: Recommendations of the Epilepsy Foundation of America's Working Group on Status Epilepticus. JAMA 270:854–859, 1993.

103. **How should a child who presents with status epilepticus be managed?**
    - **0–5 minutes:** Confirm the diagnosis. Maintain the airway by head positioning or oropharyngeal airway. Administer nasal oxygen. Suction as needed. Obtain and frequently monitor vital signs using pulse oximetry and ECG. Establish an intravenous line. Obtain venous blood for laboratory determinations (e.g., glucose, serum chemistries, hematology studies, toxicology screen, culture, anticonvulsant levels if patient is a known epileptic).
    - **6–9 minutes:** If hypoglycemic (or if a rapid reagent strip for glucose testing is not available), administer 2 mL/kg of $D_{25}W$ or 5 mL/kg of $D_{10}W$. In an infant with no known seizure disorder, give 100 mg of pyridoxine intravenously. Monitor oxygenation by pulse oximetry and vital signs.
    - **10–20 minutes:** Administer lorazepam, 0.1 mg/kg (up to 4 mg) intravenously at 2 mg/min, *or* diazepam, 0.2 mg/kg (up to 10 mg) intravenously at 5 mg/min. Repeat diazepam in 5 minutes if seizure persists. If intravenous access cannot be established, give diazepam, 0.5 mg/kg via the rectum. Intramuscular therapy is not recommended.
    - **21–60 minutes:** If seizures persist, administer fosphenytoin (preferred for children) intravenously at 15–20 mg phenytoin equivalents (PE)/kg loading dose at 150 mg PE/min or 3 mg PE/kg/min. If phenytoin is used, the dose is 15–20 mg/kg at 1 mg/kg/min intravenously while monitoring ECG and blood pressure. The infusion should be slowed if dysrhythmia or QT-interval widening develops.
    - **60 minutes:** If seizures persist for 15 minutes after the use of phenytoin, administer additional doses of fosphenytoin/phenytoin, 5 mg/kg to a maximum of 30 mg/kg total. If seizures persist, give phenobarbital (20 mg/kg) intravenously at 100 mg/min. With the use of phenobarbital after benzodiazepines, the risk of respiratory depression is increased, and the likely need for intubation increases and should be anticipated. If phenobarbital fails to stop the seizure, other measures (e.g., general anesthesia) are usually necessary.

    Hanhan UA, Fiallos MR, Orlowski JP: Status epilepticus. Pediatr Clin North Am 48:683–694, 2001.
    Lowenstein DH, Alldredge BK: Status epilepticus. N Eng J Med 338:979–986, 1998.

104. **What is the most common cause of refractory seizures?**
    An **inadequate serum concentration** of antiepileptic medication is the most common cause of persistent seizures, but other causes should be considered:
    - **Drug toxicity,** especially with phenytoin, may manifest by deteriorating seizure control.

- **Metabolic abnormalities,** particularly in patients with inborn errors of metabolism, may be seen.
- **Medications** may have a paradoxic reaction and exacerbate certain types of seizures, particularly in children with mixed seizure disorders. For example, carbamazepine or phenytoin may control generalized tonic-clonic seizures in patients with juvenile myoclonic epilepsy, but they may aggravate myoclonic and absence seizures.
- **Incorrect identification** of the epilepsy syndrome may be a cause. Partial seizures may masquerade as a generalized form of epilepsy in the very young child (bilateral symmetric tonic posturing may be seen in partial seizures). Conversely, generalized forms of epilepsy may first appear as partial seizures (severe infantile myoclonic epilepsy). Treatment based on an epilepsy syndrome rather than ictal semiology usually improves control in these circumstances.

105. **What is the role of video EEG in the management of intractable epilepsy?**
Epilepsy may be intractable to treatment because of incorrect diagnosis or treatment. Video EEG recordings of a patient's typical spell may clarify diagnosis and help to guide treatment. In a study of the pediatric population, there was an event detection rate of >50%. Of those events, two thirds were epileptic seizures, and one third were nonepileptic phenomena.

Del Giudice E, Crisanti AF, Romano A: Short duration outpatient video electroencephalographic monitoring: The experience of a southern-Italian general pediatric department. Epileptic Disord 4:197–202, 2002.

106. **What is the role of the ketogenic diet for the treatment of seizures?**
The ketogenic diet is effective for the treatment of all seizure types, particularly in children with myoclonic forms of epilepsy. The diet involves supplying the majority of calories through fats with concurrent limitation of carbohydrates and protein. The mechanism of seizure control is unclear, but it is perhaps related to a switch in the cerebral metabolism from the use of glucose to the use of beta-hydroxybutyrate. After 24 hours of fasting, the child is placed on a high-fat diet in which the ratio of fats to carbohydrates and protein combined is 3–4:1. Anticonvulsant drugs may be reduced or eliminated entirely if the diet is effective. The regimen must be followed closely, and parents must understand the demands of close adherence to the diet. A skilled dietitian is instrumental for providing variety and palatability to the diet. It is important to recall that the diet may have adverse effects, including serious, potentially life-threatening complications such as hypoproteinemia, lipemia, and hemolytic anemia.

Nordli D: The ketogenic diet: Uses and abuses. Neurology 58(12 Suppl 7):S21–S24, 2002.
Thiele EA: Assessing the efficacy of antiepileptic treatments: The ketogenic diet. Epilepsia 44 Suppl 7:S26–S29, 2003.

KEY POINTS: EPILEPSY

1. Definition: Repeated, unprovoked seizures

2. Classified as localization-related (focal partial onset) and generalized

3. Most important classification questions:
   - Where does the seizure begin?
   - Is brain development normal?

4. Epilepsy syndromes further subdivided as *idiopathic* (presumed genetic), *symptomatic* (known etiology), and *cryptogenic*

5. Proper classification of epilepsy syndromes guidance of treatment options and prognosis

107. **What is the role of the vagal nerve stimulator in seizure control?**

The vagal nerve stimulator is a surgically implanted device that intermittently stimulates the left vagus nerve; however, why this decreases seizure frequency is not well understood. It is a palliative—not curative—procedure that has been performed in adults and in some children with intractable complex partial seizures or generalized tonic seizures who were thought not to be candidates for definitive surgical cure. The vagal nerve stimulator has been placed in children as young as 2–3 years old, but most of the experience is in older children.

Buchhalter JR, Jarrar RG: Therapeutics in pediatric epilepsy, Part 2: Epilepsy surgery and vagus nerve stimulation. Mayo Clin Proc 78:371–378, 2003.

Wheless JW, Maggio V: Vagus nerve stimulation therapy in patients younger than 18 years. Neurology 59(6 Suppl 4):S21–S25, 2002.

108. **What should a teenager with epilepsy be told about the potential of obtaining a driver's license?**

State requirements vary regarding individuals with epilepsy and the right to drive. The most common requirement is a specified seizure-free period and submission of a physician's evaluation of the patient's ability to drive safely. Many states require the periodic submission of medical reports while the license is active. In addition, many states allow exceptions under which a license may be issued for a shorter seizure-free period (e.g., if a seizure occurred in isolation as a result of medication change or intercurrent illness), or they may issue licenses with restrictions (e.g., daytime driving only). A summary of requirements for each state is available from the Epilepsy Foundation.

Epilepsy Foundation: www.efa.org

109. **When should a child be referred for epilepsy surgery evaluation?**

Although many epilepsy syndromes in childhood have spontaneous remission, 20% of incident epilepsy is intractable, and 5% of patients with intractable epilepsy may benefit from epilepsy surgery. Indications for surgery are intractable disabling seizures and/or deteriorating development. In general, outcome is determined by the completeness of the evaluation and the congruence of the data, the completeness of the resection, and the etiology of the seizures.

Nordli DR, Kelley KR: Selection and evaluation of children for epilepsy surgery. Pediatr Neurosurg 34:1–12, 2001.

FEBRILE SEIZURES

110. **How are febrile seizures defined?**

Febrile seizures are defined as a provoked convulsion caused by a fever that is without evidence of CNS pathology and that occurs in children between the ages of 1 month and 7 years (most commonly between the ages of 6 months and 5 years, with a peak at the end of the second year of life). Children with a history of epilepsy who have an exacerbation of seizures with fever are excluded. Febrile seizures occur in 2–5% of children in this country, and they are more frequent in certain populations. There is often a positive family history of febrile convulsions.

111. **What is the likelihood of recurrence of a febrile seizure?**

The likelihood of recurrence increases with younger age of onset, with a recurrence rate about *1 in 2* if the patient is <1 year old when the initial seizure occurs and *1 in 5* if the patient is >3 years old during the initial seizure. About half of recurrences will occur within 6 months of the first seizure; three fourths will occur within 1 year, and 90% will occur within 2 years. In the younger age group, there is also a 30% chance of multiple recurrences as compared with an 11% risk of multiple recurrences if the first seizure occurred after the age of 1 year. Overall, recurrence rate in the pediatric population is about 30%.

112. **What features make a febrile seizure complex rather than simple?**
    - **Simple febrile seizure:** Relatively brief (<15 minutes long) and occurs as a solitary event (one attack in 24 hours) in the setting of fever not caused by CNS infection
    - **Complex (also called atypical or complicated) febrile seizure:** Focal, extended in duration (>15 minutes long), or occurring more than once in 1 day

113. **Why are complex febrile seizures more worrisome than simple febrile seizures?**
    They suggest a more serious problem. For example, a focal seizure raises concern of a localized or lateralized functional disturbance of the CNS. An unusually long seizure (>15 minutes) also raises the suspicion of primary CNS infectious, structural, or metabolic disease. Repeated seizures within a 24-hour period likewise imply a potentially more serious disorder or impending status epilepticus.

114. **When should a lumbar puncture be performed as part of the evaluation of a young child with a simple febrile seizure?**
    This is often a difficult question when a well-appearing infant or toddler is examined after a febrile seizure, and approaches vary by clinician and textbook. The American Academy of Pediatrics conservatively recommends that, after a seizure with fever in children <12 months old, a lumbar puncture should be *strongly considered* because signs and symptoms associated with meningitis may be minimal or absent in this age group. In children between 12 and 18 months old, a lumbar puncture should be *considered* because signs and symptoms can be subtle. In children >18 months old, when meningeal signs are typically present in meningitis, a lumbar puncture can be *deferred* if such signs are not present. In younger patients who have received prior antibiotic therapy, a lumbar puncture should be *strongly considered,* because treatment can mask the signs and symptoms of meningitis. It should be noted that a seizure as the sole manifestation of bacterial meningitis in febrile children is unusual. In one retrospective study of 503 patients with meningitis, none were noted to have bacterial meningitis manifesting solely as a simple seizure.

    American Academy of Pediatrics: Provisional Committee on Quality Improvement: Practice parameter: The neurodiagnostic evaluation of the child with a first simple febrile seizure. Pediatrics 97:769–775, 1996.
    Green SM, Rothrock SG, Clem KJ, et al: Can seizures be the sole manifestation of meningitis in febrile children? Pediatrics 92:527–534, 1993.

115. **What ancillary testing should be considered in a patient with a complex febrile seizure?**
    Most children with their first atypical febrile seizure should undergo a **CSF examination** to rule out intracranial infection. Children with focal motor seizures or postictal lateralized deficits (motor paresis, unilateral sensory or visual loss, sustained eye deviation, or aphasia) require a **CT scan** to check for a structural abnormality. The immediate performance of an **EEG** offers limited insight into the patient's disease. Prominent generalized postictal slowing is not unexpected. Definite focal slowing suggests a possible structural abnormality. For a simple febrile seizure, an EEG is not indicated because it is not predictive of either the risk of recurrence of febrile seizures or the development of epilepsy.

    American Academy of Pediatrics: Provisional Committee on Quality Improvement: Practice parameter: The neurodiagnostic evaluation of the child with a first simple febrile seizure. Pediatrics 97:769–775, 1996.
    Warden CR, Zibulewsky J, Mace S, et al: Evaluation and management of febrile seizures in the out-of-hospital and emergency department settings. Ann Emerg Med 41:215–222, 2003.

116. **What is the risk of epilepsy after a febrile seizure?**
The risk depends on several variables. In otherwise normal children with a simple febrile seizure, the risk of later epilepsy is about 2%. The risk of epilepsy is higher if any of the following are present:
- There is a close family history of nonfebrile seizures.
- Prior neurologic or developmental abnormalities exist.
- The patient had an atypical or complex febrile seizure, defined as focal seizures, seizures lasting ≥15 minutes, and/or multiple attacks within 24 hours.
One risk factor increases the risk to 3%. If all three risk factors are present, the likelihood of later epilepsy increases to 5–10%.

Waruiru C, Appleton R: Febrile seizures: An update. Arch Dis Child 89:751–756, 2004.

KEY POINTS: FEBRILE SEIZURES

1. Simple: Brief and lasting <15 minutes

2. Complex: Focal, >15 minutes long or recurrence within 1 day

3. Risk of recurrent febrile seizure increases if positive family history or seizure occurs at <1 year of age and/or body temperature of <40°C

4. Risk of developing future nonfebrile seizures is low (only 2% by age 7)

5. Increased risk for developing epilepsy if complex febrile seizure, prior neurologic abnormality, or family history of seizure disorder

117. **What is the long-term outcome for children with febrile seizures?**
In a previously normal child, the risk of death, neurologic damage, or persistent cognitive impairment from a single febrile seizure is near zero. These potential complications are more likely with complex febrile seizures, but the risk is still exceedingly low. Impaired cognition in the latter group is more likely if afebrile seizures subsequently develop. Febrile status epilepticus has a very low mortality with proper treatment in recent years, and the development of mesial temporal sclerosis is less than 1 in 70,000.

Verity CM, Greenwood R, Golding J: Long-term intellectual and behavioral outcomes of children with febrile convulsions. N Engl J Med 338:1723–1728, 1998.

118. **After a febrile seizure, should a child be treated with prophylactic antiepileptics?**
For most children, a simple febrile seizure is an unwanted but transient disruption of their health, and treatment is not necessary. Treatment may be considered in the very young child if febrile seizures recur and in children with preexisting neurologic abnormalities or with complex febrile seizures. Long-term prophylaxis does not improve the prognosis in terms of subsequent epilepsy or motor or cognitive ability.

Baumann RJ, Duffner PK: Treatment of children with simple febrile seizures: The AAP practice parameter. American Academy of Pediatrics. Pediatr Neurol 23:11–17, 2000.
Offringa M, Moyer VA: Evidence based management of seizures associated with fever. BMJ 323:1111–1114, 2001.

119. **Do prolonged febrile seizures result in an increased peripheral white blood cell count?**
A common clinical question in children is whether a leukocytosis, if found, can be explained on the basis of a prolonged seizure as a stress reaction. In a study of 203 children with seizures

and fever, 61% had a normal peripheral white blood cell count. No association was found between blood leukocytosis and febrile seizure duration in children.

van Stuijvenberg M, Moll HA, Steyerberg EW, et al: The duration of febrile seizures and peripheral leukocytosis. J Pediatr 133:557–558, 1998.

HEADACHE

120. **What are the emergency priorities when evaluating a child with a severe headache?**
As with all common presenting symptoms, the main priority is to rule out diagnostic possibilities that may be life-threatening:
- Malignant hypertension
- Increased intracranial pressure (e.g., mass lesion, acute hydrocephalus)
- Intracranial infections (e.g., meningitis, encephalitis)
- Subarachnoid hemorrhage
- Stroke
- Acute angle closure glaucoma (may appear as a headache, but rare in children)

121. **When should neuroimaging be considered in a child with headache?**
- Abnormal neurologic signs
- Headache increasing in frequency and severity
- Headache occurring in early morning or awakening child from sleep
- Headache made worse by straining or by sneezing or coughing (may be a sign of increased ICP)
- Headache associated with severe vomiting without nausea
- Headache worsened or helped significantly by a change in position
- Fall off in linear growth rate
- Recent school failure or significant behavioral changes
- New-onset seizures, especially if seizure has a focal onset (*see* previous discussion)
- Migraine headache and seizure occurring in the same episode, with vascular symptoms preceding the seizure (20–50% risk of tumor or arteriovenous malformation)
- Cluster headaches in any child or teenager

Lewis DW, Ashwal S, Dahl G, et al; Quality Standards Subcommittee of the American Academy of Neurology; Practice Committee of the Child Neurology Society: Practice parameter: Evaluation of children and adolescents with recurrent headaches: Report of the Quality Standards Subcommittee of the American Academy of Neurology and the Practice Committee of the Child Neurology Society. Neurology 59:490–498, 2002.

KEY POINTS: CLASSIC HEADACHE OF INCREASED INTRACRANIAL PRESSURE

1. Awakens patient from sleep at night

2. Pain present upon awakening in the morning

3. Vomiting without associated nausea

4. Made worse by straining, sneezing, or coughing

5. Intensity of pain changes with changes in body position

6. Pain lessens during the day

Halsam RHA: Migraine headaches. In Behrman RE, Kliegman R, Jensen HB (eds): Nelson Textbook of Pediatrics, 16th ed. Philadelphia, W.B. Saunders, 2000, pp 1832–1834.

Schor NF: Brain imaging and prophylactic therapy in children with migraine: Recommendations versus reality. J Pediatr 143:776–779, 2003.

122. **What is the origin of the word *migraine*?**
Ancient Greek physicians recognized a specific type of recurring head pain that was unilateral. The modern word *migraine* is a French modification of the Greek term *hemikrania*.

123. **What are the clinical presentations of migraine headaches in children?**
Migraine is a periodic disorder with symptom-free periods that is characterized by headaches with a throbbing nature, unilateral location, relief after sleep, aura, associated abdominal pain, nausea, or vomiting. Classic migraines are uncommon in younger children, and they may occur with a visual aura, irritability, pallor, nausea, and vomiting that last hours to days. Migraine headaches without an aura are more common in children. The prevalence of migraine in childhood is about 4% and becomes more common in teenage girls and young women. Childhood migraine may appear to be benign paroxysmal vertigo of childhood, ophthalmoplegic migraine, or hemiplegic, confusional, or basilar artery migraines. There may be a history of recurrent vomiting or motion sickness. There is often a family history of migraine, and the genetics may be multifactorial.

Al-Twaijri WA, Shevell MI: Pediatric migraine equivalents: Occurrence and clinical features in practice. Pediater Neurol 26:365–368, 2002.

124. **What are the diagnostic criteria for common migraine?**
Common migraine is also called migraine without aura. Diagnostic criteria from the International Headache Society include the following:
- Five attacks
- Duration of 4–72 hours
- Characteristics (two out of four):
  1. Unilateral
  2. Pulsating
  3. Moderate or severe
  4. Aggravated by physical activity
- Concomitant features (one out of two):
  1. Nausea and/or vomiting
  2. Photophobia/phonophobia

Singer HS: Migraine headaches in children. Pediatr Rev 15:94–101, 1994.

125. **Which physical findings are important during the initial evaluation of possible migraine headache?**
- Height and weight should be normal for age. Pituitary tumor, craniopharyngioma, or partial ornithine transcarbamylase deficiency may all result in growth failure and mimic migraine headache. Head circumference should be normal, thus ruling out hydrocephalus.
- Skin should be checked for abnormalities. Throbbing headaches are common in neurofibromatosis and systemic lupus erythematosus, both of which have easily recognizable skin manifestations.
- Blood pressure should be normal.
- Check for sinus tenderness or pain with head movement (implying cervical spine disease). The patient should be examined for carious teeth, misaligned bite, or disordered chewing and jaw opening (temporomandibular joint dysfunction).
- Auscultation should reveal no cranial bruits (if present, these suggest possible arteriovenous malformation or mass lesion).
- The neurologic examination should be normal.

126. **When do children begin to have migraine headaches?**
About 20% suffer their first headache before the age of 10 years.

127. **Which foods have been associated with the development of migraine headaches?**
Tyramine-rich foods (cheese, red wine), foods with monosodium glutamate (Chinese and Mexican food), nitrate-rich foods (smoked meats, salami), marinated foods, alcoholic beverages, caffeinated beverages, chocolate, citrus fruits, and beans.

128. **What is the most common form of complex migraine in children?**
Complex migraines are those migraine headaches that are accompanied by transient neurologic signs or symptoms. These include hemiplegic migraine, ophthalmoplegic migraine (orbital pain with third nerve palsy), acute confusional state, and the "Alice in Wonderland" syndrome (hallucinations and distortion of object size). The most common form is **basilar artery migraine**, which has a variety of symptoms, including blurred vision, vertigo, ataxia, dysarthria, and loss of consciousness.

129. **What is familial hemiplegic migraine?**
Familial hemiplegic migraine, as its name implies, is an autosomal dominant disorder that is clinically characterized by transient hemiparesis followed by migraine headache. About 20% are affected by permanent cerebellar signs. Mutations in CACNA1A (which encodes a neuronal calcium channel) on chromosome 19 is found in half of affected families.

Ducros A, Denier C, Joutel A, et al: The clinical spectrum of familial hemiplegic migraine associated with mutations in neuronal calcium channel. N Engl J Med 345:17–24, 2001.

130. **What nonpharmacologic therapies are available for the treatment of migraine?**
- Migraine elimination diet
- Normalization of sleep habits
- Discontinuance of possible triggering medications (e.g., analgesic overuse, bronchodilators, oral contraceptives)
- Biofeedback
- Relaxation therapy
- Family counseling (if family stress is a trigger)
- Self-hypnosis

Allen KD: Using biofeedback to make childhood headaches less of a pain. Pediatr Ann 33:241–245, 2004.

131. **What are the best medications to abort a severe migraine attack that has not responded to acetaminophen or nonsteroidal anti-inflammatory drugs?**
Ergotamines, Midrin (isometheptene mucate, dichloralphenazone, acetaminophen), and sumatriptan.

Ueberall MA, Wenzel D: Intranasal sumatriptan for the acute treatment of migraine in children. Neurology 52:1507–1510, 1999.

Winner P, Rothner AD, Saper J, et al: A randomized, double-blind, placebo-controlled study of sumatriptan nasal spray in the treatment of acute migraine in adolescents. Pediatrics 106:989–997, 2000.

132. **Who should be started on prophylactic medication for migraine headaches?**
There are no precise criteria, but generally prophylactic treatment should be considered if any of the following are present:
- Headaches with aura occur frequently
- Headaches with aura are poorly responsive to abortive medication
- School attendance is significantly affected
- Headaches, although infrequent, last for several days

133. **What medications are used in children for the prevention of migraine headaches?**
    - Beta-blockers (especially propranolol)
    - Calcium-channel blockers (especially verapamil)
    - Nonsteroidal anti-inflammatory drugs (especially naproxen)
    - Tricyclic antidepressants (especially amitriptyline)
    - Antiepileptics (especially divalproex sodium)
    - Cyproheptadine

134. **How long are the prophylactic medications continued?**
    The optimal duration of therapy remains unclear, but many authorities suggest a treatment duration of 4–6 months followed by an attempt at weaning. Less than 50% will require the reinitiation of medication.

MOVEMENT DISORDERS

135. **What are the various types of pathologic hyperkinetic movements?**
    - **Tremors:** Rhythmic oscillatory movements, both supination-pronation and flexion-extension, seen in resting state or with activity
    - **Chorea:** Quick dancing movements of proximal and distal muscles with irregular unpredictable random jerks
    - **Athetosis:** Irregular, slow, distal writhing movements
    - **Stereotypy:** Repetitive, purposeless motions (e.g., body rocking, head rolling) that resemble voluntary movements often associated with akathisia (sensory and motor restlessness)
    - **Dystonia:** Slow, twisting, sustained movements; may result in abnormal postures and progress to contractures
    - **Ballismus:** Abrupt, random, violent, flinging movements, often proximal and unilateral
    - **Myoclonus:** Abrupt, brief, jerky contractions of one or more muscles, often stimulus-sensitive
    - **Tics:** Rapid, sudden, repetitive movements or vocalizations

136. **What techniques can be used to elicit abnormal movements (particularly chorea)?**
    Methods of provocative testing include the maintenance of posture in extension against gravity, hyperpronation (or "spooning," especially above the head), tongue protrusion ("trombone tongue"), squeezing the finger of the examiner ("milk-maid's grip"), pouring liquid, and drawing a spiral.

137. **What disorders are commonly associated with the various hyperkinetic movements?**
    - **Tremors, resting:** Primary juvenile Parkinson's disease, secondary Parkinson's disease
    - **Tremors, kinetic:** Essential (familial) tremor, cerebellar disorders, brain-stem tumors, hyperthyroidism, Wilson's disease, electrolyte disturbance (e.g., glucose, calcium, magnesium), heavy-metal intoxication (e.g., lead, mercury), multiple sclerosis
    - **Chorea:** Sydenham's chorea (associated with rheumatic fever), Huntington's disease, hyperthyroidism, infectious mononucleosis, pregnancy, anticonvulsants, neuroleptic drugs, closed head injury, systemic lupus erythematosus, carbon monoxide poisoning, Wilson's disease, hypocalcemia, polycythemia, parainfectious/infectious encephalopathies (e.g., rubeola, syphilis)
    - **Athetosis:** CP, other static encephalopathies, Lesch-Nyhan syndrome, kernicterus

- **Stereotypy:** Autism, Rett syndrome, neuroleptic drugs (i.e., tardive dyskinesia), schizophrenia
- **Dystonia:** Idiopathic primary dystonias (e.g., torsion dystonia), Sandifer's syndrome, spasmus nutans, neuroleptic drugs, static encephalopathy, perinatal asphyxia, familial dystonia (sometimes dopa-responsive)
- **Ballismus:** Encephalitis, closed head injury
- **Myoclonus:** Sleep myoclonus, benign myoclonus of infancy, postanoxic encephalopathy, uremic encephalopathy, hyperthyroidism, urea-cycle defects, side effects of tricyclic therapy, slow virus infections, Wilson's disease, myoclonus-opsoclonus, neuroblastoma, epileptic encephalopathies, mitochondrial disease, prion disease, Tay-Sachs disease, startle disease, sialidosis

138. **What constitutes a tic?**
Tics are brief, sudden, repetitive, stereotyped, involuntary, and purposeless movements or vocalizations. They most commonly involve muscles of the head, neck, and respiratory tract. Their frequency can be increased by anxiety, stress, excitement, and fatigue. They are decreased during sleep and relaxation, during activities involving high concentration, and, at times, through voluntary action. In some cases, premonitory feelings (e.g., irritation, tickle, temperature change) can precipitate the motor or vocal response.

139. **What is the range of clinical tics?**
- **Motor (simple clonic):** Eye blinking, eye jerking, head twitching, shoulder shrugging
- **Motor (simple dystonic):** Bruxism, abdominal tensing, shoulder rotation
- **Motor (complex):** Grunting, barking, sniffing, snorting, throat clearing, spitting
- **Vocal (complex):** Coprolalia (obscene words), echolalia (repeating another's words), palilalia (rapidly repeating one's own words)

140. **What makes a tic tick?**
Transient and chronic tic disorders usually do not have an identifiable cause. However, dyskinesias such as tics can be found in association with a number of other conditions:
- **Chromosomal abnormalities:** Down syndrome, fragile X syndrome
- **Developmental syndromes:** Autism, pervasive developmental disorder, Rett syndrome
- **Drugs:** Anticonvulsants, stimulants (e.g., amphetamines, cocaine, methylphenidate, pemoline)
- **Infections:** Encephalitis, postrubella syndrome

141. **How should simple tics be treated?**
Simple motor tics are common and occur in more than 5–21% of school-aged children. Simple tics generally do not require pharmacologic intervention and can be treated expectantly by developing relaxation techniques, minimizing stresses that exacerbate the problem, avoiding punishment for tics, and decreasing fixation on the problem. Most simple tics self-resolve in 2–12 months.

142. **What comorbidities occur in children with tics?**
The prevalence of tic disorder is higher in younger children and in males and is associated with school dysfunction, obsessive-compulsive disorder, and attention-deficit/hyperactivity disorder. In addition, separation anxiety, overanxious disorder, simple phobia, social phobia, agoraphobia, mania, major depression, and oppositional defiant disorder were found to be significantly more common in children with tics.

Khalifa N, von Knorring AL: Prevalence of tic disorders and Tourette syndrome in a Swedish school population. Dev Med Child Neurol 45:415–419, 2003.
Kurlan R, Como PG, Miller B, et al: The behavioral spectrum of tic disorders: A community-based study. Neurology 59:414–420, 2002.

143. When do tics warrant pharmacologic intervention?

Tics that have a significant disabling impact on a child's educational, social, or psychologic well-being (particularly if they have been present for >1 year) may require intervention. When the complexity of tics increases or the diagnosis of Tourette's syndrome is suspected, pharmacotherapy should also be considered. Most theories point to a hyperdopaminergic state of the basal ganglia as the most likely etiology for unregulated movements. Pharmacologic management includes the administration of dopamine blockers (e.g., fluphenazine, haloperidol) or clonidine (the method and site of action are unclear) or the cessation of any stimulant drugs that can cause dopamine release. Because of the high associated incidence of obsessive-compulsive disorder and attention-deficit/hyperactivity disorder, other medications may be needed, and consultation with a pediatric psychiatrist or neurologist is often warranted.

144. What are the diagnostic criteria for Tourette's syndrome?

In 1885, Gilles de la Tourette described a syndrome of motor tics and vocal tics with behavioral disturbances and a chronic and variable course. *Diagnostic and Statistical Manual of Mental Disorders (DSM IV)* criteria for Tourette's syndrome require the following:

- Multiple motor tics
- One or more vocal tics
- Onset before the age of 21 years
- Waxing and waning course
- Presence of tics for >1 year (usually on a daily basis)
- No identifiable medical etiology

145. What is coprolalia?

Coprolalia is an irresistible urge to utter profanities, occurring as a phonic tic. Only 20–40% of patients with Tourette's syndrome have this phenomenon, and it is not essential for the diagnosis.

KEY POINTS: REQUIREMENTS FOR DIAGNOSIS OF TOURETTE'S SYNDROME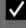

1. Multiple motor tics

2. One or more vocal tics

3. Onset before the age of 21 years

4. Waxing and waning course

5. Presence of tics for >1 year

6. No identifiable medical etiology

146. What behavioral problems are associated with Tourette's syndrome?

- Obsessive-compulsive disorder
- Attention-deficit/hyperactivity disorder
- Severe conduct disorders
- Learning disabilities (particularly math)
- Sleep abnormalities
- Depression, anxiety, and emotional lability

Tourette Syndrome Association: www.tsa-usa.org

147. **Why is the diagnosis of Tourette's syndrome commonly delayed?**
   - Tendency to associate unusual symptoms with attention-getting or psychological problems
   - Incorrect belief that all children with Tourette's syndrome must have severe tics
   - Attribution of vocal tics to upper respiratory infections, allergies, or sinus or bronchial problems
   - Diagnosis of eye blinking or ocular tics as ophthalmologic problems
   - Mistaken belief that coprolalia is an essential diagnostic feature

   Singer HS: Tic disorders. Pediatric Ann 22:22–29, 1993.

148. **What is the cause of tardive dyskinesia?**
   Tardive dyskinesia is a hyperkinetic disorder of abnormal movements, most commonly involving the face (e.g., lip smacking or pursing, chewing, grimacing, tongue protruding). Tardive dyskinesia occurs during treatment with neuroleptics (e.g., chlorpromazine, haloperidol, metoclopramide) or within 6 months of their discontinuance. This disorder is thought to be a result of dopaminergic dysfunction of the basal ganglia because these drugs act as dopamine-receptor blockers.

149. **For a patient taking neuroleptic medication, how long must therapy last before symptoms of tardive dyskinesia can develop?**
   About *3 months* of continuous or intermittent treatment with neuroleptics is needed before the risk of tardive dyskinesia increases.

150. **What is neuroleptic malignant syndrome?**
   Neuroleptic malignant syndrome is a syndrome of movement (rigidity, tremor, chorea, and dystonia), autonomic dysfunction (fever, hypertension, tachycardia, diaphoresis, irregular respiratory pattern, urinary retention), alternation of consciousness, and rhabdomyolysis with an elevation of creatinine kinase. It occurs within weeks of starting neuroleptics, and there is a 20% associated mortality rate in adults.

151. **Which movement disorder in children presents with "dancing eyes and dancing feet"?**
   Opsoclonus-myoclonus (infantile polymyoclonus syndrome or acute myoclonic encephalopathy of infants) is a rare but distinctive movement disorder in children that is seen during the first 1–3 years of life. Opsoclonus is characterized by wild, chaotic, fluttering, irregular, rapid, conjugate bursts of eye movements (saccadomania). Myoclonus is sudden, shock-like muscular twitches of the face, limbs, or trunk. The anatomic site of pathology is the cerebellar outflow tracts. The etiology may be direct viral invasion, postinfectious encephalopathy, or neuroblastoma.

152. **What are the paroxysmal movement disorders?**
   The paroxysmal movement disorders are rare, intermittent, episodic disorders of movement that appear during childhood. They may be sporadic or familial, and the movements include chorea, dystonia, athetosis, and ballismus. Classification schemes are evolving, but they are primarily movement-induced (kinesigenic, exertion-induced), hypnogenic (arising from sleep), and non-kinesigenic. Pathophysiology is unknown, but channelopathies may be involved, and treatment is with AEDS, acetazolamide, and dopamine-modulating therapies.

   Sanger TD: Pediatric movement disorders. Curr Opin Neurol 16:529–535, 2003.

153. **What is alternating hemiplegia?**
   Alternating hemiplegia of childhood is a rare disorder of intermittent, alternating hemiplegia that presents during early childhood and that is characterized by abnormal eye movement and

dystonic episodes followed by hemiplegia. There may be an autonomic prodrome, and recovery takes from hours to days. Children with early onset typically have greater developmental delay and movement disorders.

NEONATAL SEIZURES

154. **How are neonatal seizures classified?**
Although there is no universally accepted standard classification system, one based on clinical criteria is commonly used. It divides neonatal seizures into four types:
1. **Subtle**
2. **Tonic** (partial or generalized)
3. **Clonic** (partial or multifocal)
4. **Myoclonic** (partial, multifocal, or generalized)
   All seizure types are recognized as paroxysmal alterations in behavioral, motor, or autonomic function. Not all clinically observed phenomena, however, are accompanied by associated epileptic surface-EEG activity, and this electroclinical disassociation is increased after AED treatment. Partial clonic, tonic, and myoclonic seizures have been shown to have the most consistent EEG ictal correlate.

155. **What is the most common type of clinical seizure during the neonatal period?**
The so-called *subtle seizure*. Rather than arising as an abrupt dramatic "convulsion" with obvious forceful twitching or posturing of the muscles, the subtle seizure appears as an unnatural, repetitive, stereotyped choreography, featuring oral-buccal-lingual movements, eye blinking, nystagmus, lip smacking, or complex integrated limb movements (swimming, pedaling, or rowing) and other fragments of activity drawn from the limited repertoire of normal infant activity. These neonates frequently have HIE and moderately to markedly abnormal EEGs, and they are at significantly greater risk for mental retardation, CP, and epilepsy.

156. **What are the causes of neonatal seizures?**
   - Hypoxic-ischemic encephalopathy caused by asphyxia
   - Infection
   - Toxins (e.g., inadvertent fetal injection with local anesthetic; cocaine, including withdrawal)
   - Metabolic abnormalities (e.g., hypoglycemia, hypocalcemia, hypomagnesemia, pyridoxine deficiency, inborn errors)
   - CNS malformations
   - Cerebrovascular lesions (e.g., intraventricular, periventricular hemorrhage, subarachnoid hemorrhage, infarction, arterial cerebral occlusion)
   - Benign familial neonatal-infantile seizures (e.g., a sodium channelopathy)

   Zupanc ML: Neonatal seizures. Pediatr Clin North Am 51:961–978, 2004.

157. **In premature and full-term infants, how do the causes of seizures vary with regard to relative frequency and time of onset?**
See Table 14-4.

158. **What is an acceptable work-up in a newborn with seizures?**
The work-up should include a careful prenatal and natal history as well as a complete physical examination. Laboratory studies should include blood for glucose, electrolytes, calcium, phosphorus, and magnesium. A lumbar puncture should be performed to rule out meningitis. Neuroimaging studies (cranial ultrasound, CT scan, or MRI) are mandatory. Additional studies, where warranted, include blood levels for ammonia, lactate, and pyruvate; additional CSF studies (e.g., lactate, pyruvate, glycine, CSF neurotransmitters if metabolic disease is suspected); and urine studies for organic and amino-acid analysis for possible inborn errors of

metabolism. Serial use of EEG polygraphy can document persistent seizures, especially the persistence of electrographic seizures without clinical seizures after initial treatment.

TABLE 14-4. VARIANCE IN RELATIVE FREQUENCY AND TIME OF ONSET OF CAUSES OF SEIZURES

Etiology	Postnatal time of onset		Relative frequency	
	0–3 days	>3 days	Premature	Full-term
Hypoxic-ischemic	+		+++	+++
Intracranial hemorrhage*	+	+	++	+
Hypoglycemia	+		+	+
Hypocalcemia	+	+	+	+
Intracranial infection†	+	+	++	+
Developmental defects	+	+	++	++
Drug withdrawal	+	+	+	+

*Hemorrhages are principally germinal matrix-intraventricular in the premature infant and subarachnoid or subdural in the term infant.
†Early seizures occur usually after intrauterine nonbacterial infections (e.g., toxoplasmosis, cytomegalovirus infection), and later seizures usually occur with herpes simplex encephalitis or bacterial meningitis.
Adapted from Volpe JJ (ed): Neurology of the Newborn, 3rd ed. Philadelphia, W.B. Saunders, 1995, p 184.

159. **In what settings should an inborn error of metabolism be suspected as a cause of neonatal seizures?**
   ■ The onset of seizures is beyond day 1 of life (the exception is pyridoxine deficiency).
   ■ The infant becomes symptomatic after the introduction of enteral or parenteral nutrition.
   ■ The seizures are intractable and do not respond to conventional AEDs.
      Characteristic EEG patterns may be seen in maple syrup urine disease, propionic acidemia, and pyridoxine deficiency.

   Scher MS: Neonatal seizures. In Polin RA, Yoder MC, Burg FD (eds): Workbook in Practical Neonatology, 3rd ed. Philadelphia, W.B. Saunders, 2001, p 359.

160. **How are seizures differentiated from tremors in the neonate?**
      See Table 14-5.

TABLE 14-5. TREMORS VERSUS SEIZURES

Clinical feature	Tremors	Seizures
Abnormality of gaze or eye movement	0	+
Movements are exquisitely stimulus sensitive	+	0
Predominant movement	Tremor	Clonic jerking
Movements cease with passive flexion	+	0
Autonomic changes	0	+

Adapted from Volpe JJ (ed): Neurology of the Newborn, 3rd ed. Philadelphia, W.B. Saunders, 1995, p 182.

161. **What are the treatment options for neonatal seizures?**

Neonatal seizures may be treated with phenobarbital. Studies of the pharmacokinetics of phenobarbital in neonates have indicated that it is most appropriate to load with a full 20 mg/kg rather than smaller fractions. If seizures persist, additional increments of phenobarbital to total loading doses of 40 mg/kg can be given. Continued seizures may be treated with a loading dose of 20 mg/kg of phenytoin (or phenytoin equivalents in the case of fosphenytoin). The usual maintenance dose for phenobarbital is between 3 and 6 mg/kg/day and between 3 and 4 mg/kg/day for phenytoin. Efficacy from either of these two agents is low, with only a third of patients showing an immediate complete response. Even after apparently successful intravenous treatment with phenobarbital and phenytoin with the resolution of clinical seizures, electrographic seizures may continue unabated. The significance of this finding is unclear, and the need to suppress electrographic seizures without clinical accompaniments is controversial.

Levene M: The clinical conundrum of neonatal seizures. Arch Dis Child Fetal Neonatol Ed 86:F75–F77, 2002.

Rennie JM, Boylan GB: Neonatal seizures and their treatment. Curr Opin Neurol 16:177–181, 2003.

162. **What is the treatment for refractory seizures in the neonate?**

Frequent and recurrent seizures are not uncommon in newborns and are especially common in the setting of asphyxia. If seizures are refractory to full dosing of phenobarbital and phenytoin, the addition of drugs in the benzodiazepine family (e.g., diazepam, lorazepam) or of paraldehyde is generally effective. It is important to ensure that no underlying biochemical disturbance is present before the serum levels of anticonvulsants are raised to maximal concentrations. Although pyridoxine-dependent seizures are rare, a trial dose of pyridoxine should be administered intravenously to infants with recurrent seizures of uncertain etiology. If possible, simultaneous EEG recording should be performed to document the cessation of seizure activity and the normalization of the EEG within minutes of pyridoxine treatment. Infants with pyridoxine-dependent epilepsy may have profound autonomic dysfunction (apnea, bradycardia, and hypotension) in response to initial pyridoxine administration and should be monitored carefully.

163. **Of what prognostic value is the interictal EEG in a neonate with seizures?**

This study can have significant prognostic value. Severe interictal EEG abnormalities (e.g., burst-suppression, marked voltage suppression, flat or isoelectric) are highly predictive (90%) of a fatal outcome or severe neurologic sequelae. Conversely, a normal interictal EEG in a term infant with seizures confers a very low (10%) likelihood of significant neurologic impairment. Moderate abnormalities (e.g., voltage asymmetries, immature patterns) have a mixed outcome.

Laroia N, Guillet R, Burchfiel J, McBride MC: EEG background as predictor of electrographic seizures in high risk neonates. Epilepsia 39:545–551, 1998.

164. **After an infant has recovered from a seizure, how long should medication be continued?**

Maintenance therapy typically involves the use of phenobarbital because it is difficult to achieve therapeutic levels of phenytoin with oral administration in infancy, and other medications (e.g., carbamazepine) are less well studied. Although phenobarbital is generally well tolerated, it may have deleterious effects on behavior, attention span, and possibly brain development. It does not prevent the later development of epilepsy. Many authorities recommend discontinuing therapy if the neurologic examination has normalized. In addition, if the neurologic examination is abnormal but an EEG by the age of 3 months reveals no seizure activity, consideration can also be given to stopping phenobarbital.

165. **In patients with neonatal seizures, how does the cause affect the prognosis?**

See Table 14-6.

TABLE 14–6. RELATIONSHIP BETWEEN CAUSE AND PROGNOSIS OF NEONATAL SEIZURE

Etiology	Favorable outcome*	Mixed outcome	Unfavorable outcome*
Toxic-metabolic	Simple late-onset hypocalcemia Hypomagnesemia Hyponatremia Mepivacaine toxicity	Hypoglycemia Early-onset complicated hypocalcemia Pyridoxine dependency	Some aminoacidurias
Asphyxia	—	Mild hypoxic-ischemic encephalopathy	Severe hypoxic-ischemic encephalopathy
Hemorrhage	Uncomplicated subarachnoid hemorrhage	Subdural hematoma Intraventricular hemorrhage (grades I and II)	Intraventricular hemorrhage (grades III and IV)
Infection	—	Aseptic meningoencephalitis; some bacterial meningitides	Herpes simplex encephalitis; some bacterial meningitides
Structural	—	Simple traumatic contusion	Malformations of the central nervous system

*Favorable prognosis implies at least an 85–90% chance of survival and subsequent normal development. Unfavorable prognosis implies a high likelihood (85–90%) of death or serious handicap in survivors.
From Scher MS: Neonatal seizures. In Polin RA, Yoder MC, Burg FD (eds): Workbook in Practical Neonatology, 3rd ed. Philadelphia, W.B. Saunders, 2001, p 366.

NEUROCUTANEOUS SYNDROMES

166. **What are the three most common neurocutaneous syndromes?**
   1. Neurofibromatosis
   2. Tuberous sclerosis complex
   3. Sturge-Weber syndrome

167. **What are the inheritance patterns of the various neurocutaneous syndromes?**

Neurofibromatosis	Autosomal dominant
Tuberous sclerosis complex	Autosomal dominant
von Hippel-Lindau syndrome	Autosomal dominant
Incontinentia pigmenti	X-linked dominant
Sturge-Weber syndrome	Sporadic
Klippel-Trénaunay-Weber syndrome	Sporadic

168. **What is the derivation of the term *phakomatosis*?**
The term *phakomatosis* is derived from the Greek *phakos*, meaning "lentil" or "lens-shaped," and it refers to patchy, circumscribed dermatologic lesions that are the hallmark of this group of disorders. In addition to dermatologic features, these syndromes have hamartomatous involvement of multiple tissues, especially the CNS and the eye. More commonly, the term *neurocutaneous syndrome* is used.

169. **What are the diagnostic criteria for neurofibromatosis-1 (NF1)?**
Two or more of the following:
   - Café-au-lait spots (six or more that are >5 mm in diameter before puberty; six or more that are >15 mm in diameter after puberty)
   - Skinfold freckling (axillary or inguinal region)
   - Neurofibromas (two or more) of any type, or one plexiform neurofibroma
   - Optic glioma
   - Iris hamartomas, also called Lisch nodules (two or more)
   - Characteristic bony lesion (i.e., sphenoid dysplasia, thinning of the cortex of the long bones with or without pseudoarthrosis)
   - First-degree relative(s) with NF1

   Lynch TM, Gutmann DH: Neurofibromatosis type I. Neurol Clin 20:841–865, 2002.

170. **How does NF1 differ from NF2?**
NF1, which is also known as classic von Recklinghausen's disease, is much more common (1 in every 3,000–4,000 births) than NF2 and accounts for up to 90% of cases of neurofibromatosis. NF2 (1 in every 50,000 births) is characterized by bilateral acoustic neuromas, intracranial and intraspinal tumors, and affected first-degree relatives. NF1 has been linked to alterations on chromosome 17, whereas NF2 is linked to alterations on chromosome 22. Dermatologic findings and peripheral neuromas are rare in NF2. Other rarer subtypes of neurofibromatoses (e.g., segmental distribution) have been described.

171. **How common are café-au-lait spots at birth?**
Up to 2% of black infants will have three café-au-lait spots at birth, whereas one café-au-lait spot occurs in only 0.3% of white infants. White infants with multiple café-au-lait spots at birth are more likely than black infants to develop neurofibromatosis. In older children, a single café-au-lait spot that is >5 mm in diameter can be found in 10% of white and 25% of black children.

   Hurwitz S: Neurofibromatosis. In Hurwitz S (ed): Clinical Pediatric Dermatology, 2nd ed. Philadelphia, W.B. Saunders, 1993, pp 624–629.

172. **If a 2-year-old child has seven café-au-lait spots that are >5 mm in diameter, what is the likelihood that neurofibromatosis will develop, and how will it evolve?**
Up to 75% of these children, if followed sequentially, will develop one of the varieties of neurofibromatosis, most commonly type 1. In a study of nearly 1,900 patients, 46% with sporadic NF1 did not meet criteria by the age of 1 year. By the age of 8 years, however, 97% met the criteria, and by the age of 20 years, 100% did. The typical order of appearance of features is café-au-lait spots, axillary freckling, Lisch nodules, and neurofibromas. Yearly evaluation of patients with suspicious findings should include a careful skin examination, ophthalmologic evaluation, and blood pressure measurement.

   DeBella K, Szudek J, Friedman JM: Use of the National Institutes of Health criteria for the diagnosis of neurofibromatosis 1 in children. Pediatrics 105:608–614, 2000.
   Korf BR: Diagnostic outcome in children with multiple café-au-lait spots. Pediatrics 90:924–927, 1992.

173. **What are Lisch nodules?**

Pigmented iris hamartomas (Fig. 14-1). Although these are not usually present at birth in patients with NF1, up to 90% will develop multiple Lisch nodules by the age of 6 years. Hamartomas are focal malformations that are microscopically composed of multiple tissue types, and these can resemble neoplasms. However, unlike neoplasms, they grow at similar rates as normal components and are unlikely to pathologically compress adjacent tissue.

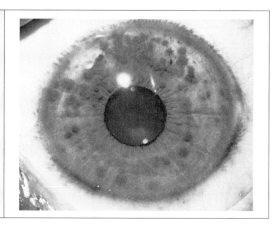

Figure 14-1. Lisch nodules. (From Zitelli BJ, Davis HW: Atlas of Pediatric Physical Diagnosis, 4th ed. St. Louis, Mosby, 2002, p 507.)

174. **How common is a positive family history in cases of NF1?**

Because of the high spontaneous mutation rate for this autosomal dominant disease, only *about 50%* of newly diagnosed cases are associated with a positive family history.

175. **What are the primary diagnostic criteria for tuberous sclerosis complex (TSC)?**

TSC is characterized by hamartomatous growths that occur in multiple tissues. The National Institutes of Health Consensus Conference in 1998 revised the diagnostic criteria for TSC on the basis of major or minor features. Definite TSC consisted of two major features *or* one major and two minor features; probable and possible TSC had fewer features. No single finding was considered pathognomonic for TSC. Two gene site abnormalities, *TSC1* (chromosome 9) and *TSC2* (chromosome 16), have been identified. Genetic testing is now available.

Major features	Minor features
Facial angiofibromas	Dental enamel pits
Nontraumatic ungual or periungual fibroma	Bone cysts
Hypomelanotic macules (more than 3)	Hamartomatous rectal polyps
Shagreen patch	Gingival fibromas
Multiple retinal nodular hamartomas	Cerebral white matter migration tracts
Cortical tuber	
Subependymal nodule or giant cell astrocytoma	
Cardiac rhabdomyoma, single or multiple	

Hyman MH, Whittemore VH: National Institutes of Health Consensus Conference: Tuberous sclerosis complex. Arch Neurol 57:662–665, 2000.

176. **What is the classic triad of TSC?**

1. Seizures
2. Mental retardation
3. Facial angiofibroma (adenoma sebaceum)

However, less than a third of patients will develop these classic features.

177. **What is the most common presenting symptom of TSC?**
Seizures. About 85% of patients have seizures, and infantile spasms are the most common. Tonic and atonic seizures are also seen. Complex partial seizures are frequently seen in conjunction with other seizure types. Mental retardation is especially common with the onset of seizures before the age of 2 years. Autism and other behavioral disturbances are also frequently seen in children with TSC.

178. **What are skin findings in patients with tuberous sclerosis?**
See Table 14-7.

TABLE 14-7. SKIN FINDINGS IN TUBEROUS SCLEROSIS		
Age at onset	**Skin findings**	**Incidence**
Birth or later	Hypopigmented macules	80%
2–5 years	Angiofibromas	70%
2–5 years	Shagreen patches	35%
Puberty	Periungual and gingival fibromas	20–50%
Birth or later	Café-au-lait spots	25%

179. **Why is the term *adenoma sebaceum* a misnomer when used to describe patients with tuberous sclerosis?**
On biopsy, these papules are actually *angiofibromas*. They have no connection to sebaceous units or adenomas. This rash occurs in about 75% of patients with tuberous sclerosis, usually developing on the nose and central face between the ages of 5 and 13 years. It is red, papular, and monomorphous, and it is often mistaken for acne (Fig. 14-2). The diagnosis of tuberous sclerosis should be entertained in children who develop a rash that is suggestive of acne well before puberty.

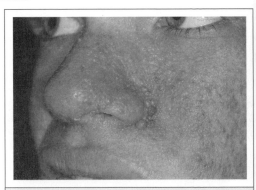

Figure 14-2. Adenoma sebaceum in patient with tuberous sclerosis. (From Sahn EE: Dermatology Pearls. Philadelphia, Hanley and Belfus, 1999, p 86.)

180. **What is the "tuber" of tuberous sclerosis?**
These 1- to 2-cm lesions consist of small stellate neurons and astroglial elements that are thought to be primitive cell lines resulting from abnormal differentiation. They may be located in various cortical regions. They are firm to the touch, like a small potato or tuber.

181. **What is the tissue type of a shagreen patch?**
A shagreen patch is an area of cutaneous thickening with a pebbled surface that, on biopsy, is a **connective tissue nevus.** The term *shagreen* derives from a type of leather that is embossed by knobs during the course of processing.

182. **Which types of facial port-wine stains are most strongly associated with ophthalmic or CNS complications?**

Port-wine stains can occur as isolated cutaneous birthmarks or, particularly in the areas underlying the birthmark, in association with structural abnormalities in the following areas: (1) the choroidal vessels of the eye, thereby leading to glaucoma; (2) the leptomeningeal vessels of the brain, thus leading to seizures (Sturge-Weber syndrome); and (3) hemangiomas in the spinal cord (Cobb syndrome). Glaucoma or seizures are most often associated with port-wine stains in children demonstrating the following:

- Involvement of the eyelids
- Bilateral distribution of the birthmark
- Unilateral involvement of all three branches (V_1, V_2, V_3) of the trigeminal nerve
  Ophthalmologic assessment and radiologic studies (CT or MRI) are indicated for children exhibiting these findings.

  Tallman B, Tan OT, Morelli JG, et al: Location of port-wine stains and the likelihood of ophthalmic and/or central nervous system complications. Pediatrics 87:323–327, 1991.

  Thomas-Sohl KA, Vaslow DF, Maria BL: Sturge-Weber syndrome: a review. Pediatr Neurol 30:303–310, 2004.

183. **What is unique to the genetics of epidermal nevus syndrome?**

The *complete absence of vertical transmission* and the *exclusively partial character* of the epidermal nevus syndrome support the hypothesis that the syndrome is caused by an autosomal dominant lethal mutation with expression from a partial somatic mutation. It involves the eye, the bone, and the brain. The central nervous system abnormalities consist of hemimegencephaly, mental retardation, seizures, and stroke caused by cerebrovascular dysplasia. Dermatologic findings include verrucous, hyperkeratotic papules in a linear array (often widespread), hemangiomas, café-au-lait spots, and areas of hypopigmentation.

184. **What are the three stages of incontinentia pigmenti?**

Incontinentia pigmenti is an X-linked dominant disorder that is associated with seizures and mental retardation. The condition is presumed to be lethal to boys in utero because nearly 100% of cases are female.

Stage 1—Vesicular stage: Lines of blisters are present on the trunk and extremities of the newborn that disappear in weeks or months. They may resemble herpetic vesicles. Microscopic examination of the vesicular fluid demonstrates eosinophils.

Stage 2—Verrucous stage: Lesions develop in the patient around age 3–7 months of age that are brown and hyperkeratotic, resembling warts; these disappear over 1–2 years.

Stage 3—Pigmented stage: Whorled, swirling (marble-cake–like), macular, hyperpigmented lines develop. These may fade over time, leaving only remnant hypopigmentation in late adolescence or adulthood (which is sometimes considered a fourth stage).

NEUROMUSCULAR DISORDERS

185. **How can the anatomic site responsible for muscle weakness be determined clinically?**

See Table 14-8.

186. **What are the causes of acute generalized weakness?**

- **Infectious/postinfectious conditions:** Acute infectious myositis, GBS, enteroviral infection
- **Metabolic disorders:** Acute intermittent porphyria, hereditary tyrosinemia

TABLE 14-8. CLINICAL DETERMINATION OF ANATOMIC SITE RESPONSIBLE FOR MUSCLE WEAKNESS

	Upper motor neuron	Anterior horn cell	Neuromuscular junction	Peripheral nerve	Muscle
Tone	Increased (may be decreased acutely)	Decreased	Normal, variable	Decreased	Decreased
Distribution	Pattern (e.g., hemiparesis, paraparesis) Distal > proximal	Variable, asymmetric	Fluctuating, cranial nerve involvement	Nerve distribution	Proximal > distal
Reflexes	Increased (may be decreased early)	Decreased to absent	Normal (unless severely involved)	Decreased to absent	Decreased
Babinski	Extensor	Flexor	Flexor	Flexor	Flexor
Other	Cognitive dysfunction, atrophy only very late	Fasciculations, atrophy, no sensory involvement	Fluctuating course	Sensory nerve involvement, atrophy, rare fasciculations	No sensory deficits; may te tenderness and signs of inflammation

Adapted from Packer RJ, Berman PH: Neurologic emergencies. In Fleisher GR, Ludwig S (eds): Textbook of Pediatric Emergency Medicine, 3rd ed. Baltimore, Williams & Wilkins, 1993, p 584.

- **Neuromuscular blockade:** Botulism, tick paralysis
- **Periodic paralysis:** Familial (hyperkalemic, hypokalemic, normokalemic)

  Fenichel GM: Clinical Pediatric Neurology: Signs and Symptoms Approach, 4th ed. Philadelphia, W.B. Saunders, 2001, pp 192–197.

187. **If a child presents with weakness, what aspects of the history and physical examination suggest a myopathic process?**

History

- Gradual rather than sudden onset
- Proximal weakness (e.g., climbing stairs, running) rather than distal weakness (more characteristic of neuropathy) predominates
- Absence of sensory abnormalities, such as "pins-and-needles" sensations
- No bowel and bladder abnormalities

Physical examination

- Proximal weakness is greater than distal weakness (except in myotonic dystrophy)
- Positive Gower sign (patient arises from a sitting position by pushing the trunk erect by bracing the arms against anterior thigh as a result of weakness of the pelvic girdle and the lower extremities)
- Neck flexion weaker than neck extension
- During the early stages, reflexes normal or only slightly decreased
- Normal sensory examination
- Muscle wasting but no fasciculations
- Muscle hypertrophy seen in some dystrophies

  Weiner HL, Urion DK, Levitt LP: Pediatric Neurology for the House Officer. Baltimore, William & Wilkins, 1988, pp 136–138.

188. **How does electromyography help to differentiate between myopathic and neurogenic disorders?**

Electromyography measures the electrical activity of resting and voluntary muscle activity. Normally, the action potentials are of standardized duration and amplitude, with two to four distinguishable phases. In **myopathic** conditions, the durations and amplitudes are shorter than expected; in **neuropathies**, they are longer. In both conditions, extra phases (i.e., polyphasic units) are usually noted.

189. **How is pseudoparalysis distinguished from true neuromuscular disease?**

Pseudoparalysis (hysterical paralysis) or weakness may be seen in conversion reactions (i.e., emotional conflicts presenting as symptoms). In conversion reactions, sensation, deep tendon reflexes, and Babinski's response are normal; movement may also be noted during sleep. *Hoover's sign* is also helpful in cases of unilateral paralysis. With the patient lying supine on the table, the examiner places a hand under the heel of the unaffected limb and asks the patient to raise the plegic limb. In pseudoparalysis, no pressure is felt under the heel on the unaffected side.

190. **Why is it important to localize the cause of hypotonia?**

Localization of the level of the lesion is critical for determining the nature of the pathologic process. In the absence of an acute encephalopathy, the differential diagnosis of hypotonia is best approached by asking the question, "Does the patient have normal strength despite the hypotonia, or is the patient weak and hypotonic?" The combination of weakness and hypotonia usually points to an abnormality of the anterior horn cell or the peripheral neuromuscular apparatus, whereas hypotonia with normal strength is more characteristic of brain or spinal cord disturbances.

KEY POINTS: HYPOTONIA

1. Localization of lesion is critical for determining pathologic process.

2. Most important question: Is strength normal or abnormal?

3. Hypotonia *with weakness:* Think abnormality in anterior horn cell or peripheral neuromuscular apparatus.

4. Hypotonia *without weakness:* Think brain or spinal-cord disturbance.

191. How can you detect myotonia clinically?
Myotonia is a painless tonic spasm of muscle that follows voluntary contraction, involuntary failure of relaxation, or delayed muscle relaxation after a contraction. It can be elicited by grip (e.g., handshake), forced eyelid closure (or delayed eye opening in crying infants), lid lag after upward gaze, or percussion over various sites (e.g., thenar eminence, tongue).

192. How do the presentations of the two forms of myotonic dystrophy differ?
The presentation of **congenital** myotonic dystrophy is during the immediate newborn period. Symptoms include hypotonia, facial diplegia with "tenting" of the upper lip, and, frequently, severe respiratory distress as a result of intercostal and diaphragmatic weakness, especially in the right hemidiaphragm. Feeding problems as a result of poor suck and gastrointestinal dysmotility are also present. The **juvenile** presentation of this condition is during the first decade of life. This form is characterized by progressive weakness and atrophy of the facial and sternocleidomastoid muscles and shoulder girdle, impaired hearing and speech, and excessive daytime sleepiness. Clinical myotonia is more likely, and there may be mental retardation.

193. In a newborn with weakness and hypotonia, what obstetric and delivery features suggest a diagnosis of congenital myotonic dystrophy?
A history of spontaneous abortions, polyhydramnios, decreased fetal movements, delays in second-stage labor, retained placenta, and postpartum hemorrhage all raise the concern for congenital myotonic dystrophy. Because the mother is nearly always affected in congenital myotonic dystrophy (although previously diagnosed in only half the cases), a careful clinical and electromyographic evaluation of the mother is essential.

194. Why is myotonic dystrophy an example of the phenomenon of "anticipation"?
Genetic studies have shown that the defect in myotonic dystrophy is an expansion of a trinucleotide (CTG) in a gene on the long arm of chromosome 19 that codes for a protein kinase. The gene product was named myotonin-protein kinase, and it is thought to be involved in sodium- and chloride-channel function. In successive generations, this repeating sequence has a tendency to increase, sometimes into the thousands (normal is <40 CTG repeats), and the extent of repetition correlates with the severity of the disease. Thus, each succeeding generation is likely to get more-extensive manifestations and earlier presentations of the disease (i.e., the phenomenon of *anticipation*).

195. How does the pathophysiology of infant botulism differ from that of food-borne and wound botulism?
- **Infant botulism** results from the ingestion of *Clostridium botulinum* spores that germinate, multiply, and produce toxin in the infant's intestine. The source of the spores is often

unknown, but it has been linked to honey in some cases, and spores have been found in corn syrups. Therefore, these foods are not advised for infants <1 year old.

- **Food-borne botulism** involves cases in which preformed toxin is already present in the food. Improper canning and anaerobic storage permits spore germination, growth, and toxin formation, which result in symptoms if the toxin is not destroyed by proper heating.
- **Wound botulism** occurs if spores enter a deep wound and germinate.

196. **What is the earliest indication for intubation in an infant with botulism?**
Intubation is indicated if there is *a loss of protective airway reflexes*. This occurs before respiratory compromise or failure, because diaphragmatic function is not impaired until 90–95% of the synaptic receptors are occupied. An infant with hypercarbia or hypoxia is at very high risk for imminent respiratory failure.

   Schreiner MS, Field E, Ruddy R: Infant botulism: A review of 12 years' experience at the Children's Hospital of Philadelphia. Pediatrics 87:159–165, 1991.

197. **In an infant with severe weakness and suspected botulism, why is the use of aminoglycosides relatively contraindicated?**
The botulism toxin acts by irreversibly blocking acetylcholine release from the presynaptic nerve terminals. Aminoglycosides, tetracyclines, clindamycin, and trimethoprim also interfere with acetylcholine release; therefore they have the potential to act synergistically with the botulinum toxin to worsen or prolong neuromuscular paralysis.

198. **What are the two most common symptoms in children with juvenile myasthenia gravis?**
Ptosis and **diplopia.** Myasthenia gravis is characterized by a highly variable clinical course of fluctuating weakness (characteristically with increasing contractions) that initially involves muscles that are innervated by the cranial nerves. It is caused by a defect in neuromuscular transmission that is caused by an autoimmune antibody-mediated attack on the acetylcholine receptors.

199. **What are the risks to a neonate who is born to a mother with myasthenia gravis?**
Passively acquired neonatal myasthenia develops in about 10% of infants born to myasthenic mothers because of the transplacental transfer of antibody directed against acetylcholine receptors (AChR) in striated muscle. Signs and symptoms of weakness typically arise within the first hours or days of life. Pathologic muscle fatigability commonly causes feeding difficulty, generalized weakness, hypotonia, and respiratory depression. Ptosis and impaired eye movements occur in only 15% of cases. The weakness virtually always resolves as the body burden of anti-AChR immunoglobulins diminishes. Symptoms typically persist for about 2 weeks but may require several months to disappear completely. General supportive treatment is usually adequate, but oral or intramuscular neostigmine may help to diminish symptoms.

200. **How does the pathophysiology of juvenile versus congenital myasthenia gravis differ?**
Juvenile (and adult) myasthenia gravis is caused by *circulating antibodies* to the AChR of the postsynaptic neuromuscular junction. Occurrence is rare before the age of 2 years. **Congenital myasthenia gravis** is a *nonimmunologic process.* It is caused by morphologic or physiologic features affecting the pre- and postsynaptic junctions, including defects in ACh synthesis, endplate acetylcholinesterase deficiency, and endplate AChR deficiency. *Neonatal myasthenia gravis* refers to the transient weakness that occurs in infants of mothers with myasthenia gravis.

201. **How is the edrophonium (Tensilon) test done?**
Edrophonium is a rapid-acting anticholinesterase drug of short duration that improves symptoms of myasthenia gravis by inhibiting the breakdown of ACh and increasing its concentration in the neuromuscular junction. A test dose of 0.015 mg/kg is given intravenously; if it is tolerated, the full dose of 0.15 mg/kg (up to 10 mg) is given. If measurable improvement in ocular muscle or extremity strength occurs, myasthenia gravis is likely. Because edrophonium may precipitate a cholinergic crisis (e.g., bradycardia, hypotension, vomiting, bronchospasm), atropine and resuscitation equipment should be available.

202. **Does a negative antibody test exclude the diagnosis of juvenile myasthenia gravis?**
No. Up to 90% of children with juvenile myasthenia have measurable anti-AChR antibodies, but, in the other 10%, continued clinical suspicion is necessary because their symptoms are usually milder (e.g., ocular muscle weakness, minimal generalized weakness). In these children, other tests (e.g., edrophonium, electrophysiologic studies, single-fiber electromyography) may be needed to make the diagnosis.

203. **What are the four characteristic features of damage to the anterior horn cells?**
Weakness, fasciculations, atrophy, and hyporeflexia.

204. **What processes can damage the anterior horn cells?**
   - **Degenerative** (spinal muscular atrophy): Werdnig-Hoffman, Kugelberg-Welander
   - **Metabolic:** Tay-Sachs disease (hexosaminidase deficiency), Pompe's disease, Batten disease (ceroid-lipofuscinosis), hyperglycinemia, neonatal adrenoleukodystrophy
   - **Infectious:** Poliovirus, coxsackievirus, echoviruses

205. **How are the inherited progressive spinal muscular atrophies distinguished?**
See Table 14-9.

206. **What are muscular dystrophies?**
A muscular dystrophy is an inheritable myopathy that affects limbs or facial muscles and that is progressive, with pathologic evidence of degeneration or regeneration without any abnormal storage material.

207. **What is the clinical importance of dystrophin?**
Dystrophin is a muscle protein that is presumed to be involved in anchoring the contractile apparatus of striated and cardiac muscle to the cell membrane. As a result of a gene mutation, this protein is completely missing in patients with Duchenne's muscular dystrophy. On the other hand, muscle tissue from patients with Becker's muscular dystrophy contains reduced amounts of dystrophin or, occasionally, a protein of abnormal size.

208. **How are Duchenne's and Becker's muscular dystrophies distinguished?**
See Table 14-10.

209. **Is corticosteroid therapy effective for the treatment of Duchenne's muscular dystrophy?**
Several studies have documented an improvement in strength with an optimal dose of prednisone of 0.75 mg/kg/day. The strengthening effect lasts for up to 3 years while the steroid is continued. Appropriate timing and duration of treatment have not been established, and side effects (weight gain and increased susceptibility to infection) may outweigh the benefits in many cases.

TABLE 14-9. PROGRESSIVE SPINAL MUSCULAR ATROPHIES

Disorder	Inheritance	Age of onset	Clinical features
Acute infantile SMA (Werdnig-Hoffmann disease, SMA type 1)	Autosomal recessive	In utero to 6 months	Frog-leg posture; areflexia; tongue atrophy and fasciculations progressive swallowing and respiratory problems; survival <4 years
Intermediate SMA (chronic Werdnig-Hoffmann disease, SMA type 2)	Autosomal recessive; rarely autosomal dominant	3 months to 15 years	Proximal weakness; most sit unsupported; decreased or absent reflexes; high incidence of scoliosis, contractures; survival may be up to 30 years
Kugelberg-Welander disease (SMA type 3)	Autosomal recessive; rarely autosomal dominant	5–15 years	May be part of the spectrum of SMA 2; hip girdle weakness; calf hypertrophy; decreased or absent reflexes; may be ambulatory until fourth decade

SMA = spinal muscular atrophy.
Adapted from Parke JT: Disorders of the anterior horn cell. In McMillan JA, DeAngelis CD, Feigin RD, Warshaw JB (eds): Oski's Pediatrics. Principles and Practice, 3rd ed. Philadelphia, J.B. Lippincott, 1999, p 1959.

210. **What is the most likely diagnosis in a child with progressive walking difficulties evolving over several days?**
GBS is an acute demyelinating neuropathy that is characterized by ascending, acute, progressive peripheral and cranial nerve dysfunction and paresthesias. In younger children (<6 years), it may be heralded by pain. It is frequently preceded by a viral respiratory or gastrointestinal illness, immunizations, or surgery. The disease is characterized by the presence of multifocal areas of the inflammatory demyelination of nerve roots and peripheral nerves. As a result of the loss of the healthy myelin covering, the conduction of nerve impulses (action potentials) may be blocked or dispersed. The resulting clinical effects are predominantly motor (i.e., the evolution of flaccid, areflexic paralysis). There is a variable degree of motor weakness. Some individuals have mild brief weakness, whereas fulminant paralysis occurs in others. Autonomic signs (e.g., tachycardia, hypertension) and sensory symptoms (e.g., painful dysesthesias) are not uncommon, but they are overshadowed by the motor signs. More than half of these patients develop facial involvement, and mechanical ventilation may be required. The *Miller Fisher variant* is characterized by gait ataxia, areflexia, and ophthalmoparesis.

Newswanger DL, Warren CR: Guillain-Barré syndrome. Am Fam Physician 69:2405–2410, 2004.

211. **What CSF findings are characteristic of GBS?**
The classic CSF finding is the **albuminocytologic dissociation.** Most common infections or inflammatory processes generate an elevation of white blood cell count *and* protein. The CSF

profile in GBS includes a normal cell count with elevated protein, usually in the range of 50–100 mg/dL; however, at the onset of disease, the CSF protein concentration may be normal.

TABLE 14-10.	DUCHENNE'S VERSUS BECKER'S MUSCULAR DYSTROPHY		
	Genetics	**Diagnosis**	**Manifestations**
Duchenne's	1 in 3,500 male births X-linked Several different deletions/point mutations in dystrophin gene result in a completely nonfunctional protein New mutations occur Carrier females may have mild weakness or cardiomyopathy	Whole blood DNA may reveal a deletion in ~65%; otherwise, EMG and muscle biopsy studies are definitive	Clinically evident at 3–5 years of age Regular, stereotyped course of progressive proximal weakness Calf hypertrophy Loss of ambulation by 9–12 years Worsening scoliosis and contractures Eventual dilated cardiomyopathy and/or respiratory failure Life expectancy of 16–19 years
Becker's	1 in 20,000 male births X-linked Various mutations in dystrophin gene result in reduced amount of or partially functional protein	More benign clinical course Reduced dystrophin levels in muscle cells (by immunostaining) or abnormal dystrophin	Clinically evident during early second decade Milder, slower course as compared with Duchenne's Calf pseudohypertrophy Pes cavus Cardiac and CNS involvement unusual Ambulatory until 18 years or beyond Life expectancy twice as long as compared with Duchenne's

Adapted from Tsao VY, Mendell JR: The childhood muscular dystrophies: Making order out of chaos. Semin Neurol 19:9–23, 1999.

212. **Outline the management of acute GBS.**

Early clinical monitoring is focused on the development of bulbar or respiratory insufficiency. Bulbar weakness manifests as unilateral or bilateral facial weakness, diplopia, hoarseness, drooling, depressed gag reflex, or dysphagia. Frank respiratory insufficiency may be preceded by air hunger, dyspnea, or a soft muffled voice (hypophonia). The autonomic nervous system is occasionally involved, and this is signified by the presence of labile blood pressure and body temperature. The management of GBS includes the following:

- Observation in an intensive care unit is critical, with frequent monitoring of vital signs.
- The early institution of plasmapheresis or intravenous immunoglobulin shortens the clinical course and lessens long-term morbidity; the value of corticosteroid therapy is controversial.
- If bulbar signs are present, the patient should receive nothing orally and the mouth is suctioned frequently. Hydration is maintained intravenously, and nutritional support is provided by nasogastric feedings.
- The vital capacity (VC) is measured frequently. In children, the normal VC may be calculated as VC = 200 mL × age in years. If the VC falls below 25% of normal, endotracheal intubation is performed. Careful pulmonary toilet is conducted to minimize atelectasis, aspiration, and pneumonia.
- Meticulous nursing care includes careful patient positioning to prevent pressure sores, compression of peripheral nerves, and venous thrombosis.
- Physical therapy is conducted to prevent the development of contractures by passive range-of-movement exercises and splinting to maintain physiologic hand and limb postures until muscle strength returns.

213. **What is the prognosis for children with GBS?**
Children seem to recover more quickly and more fully than adults. Fewer than 10% have significant residual deficits. In rare cases, the neuropathy may recur as a chronic inflammatory demyelinating polyneuropathy.

214. **How do syndromes of ascending paralysis compare in the clinical presentation?**
See Table 14-11.

215. **How does multiple sclerosis appear during childhood?**
Multiple sclerosis is extremely rare in childhood (0.2–2.0% of all cases). Studies of affected children demonstrate a variable predominance of boys during early childhood and females during adolescence. Ataxia, muscle weakness, and transient visual or sensory symptoms are relatively common presentations. CSF examination may demonstrate mild (<25 cells/mm^3) mononuclear pleocytosis with an increasing probability of oligoclonal bands with each recurrence. MRI is the single most useful diagnostic test: the presence of multiple, periventricular white matter plaques (bright areas on T2 images) confirms the diagnosis.

Sluder JA, Newhouse P, Fain D: Pediatric and adolescent multiple sclerosis. Adolesc Med 13:461–485, 2002.

SPINAL CORD DISORDERS

216. **Which spinal segments do each of the common reflexes test?**
See Table 14-12.

217. **How common are asymptomatic spinal anomalies in normal children?**
Up to 5% of children have spina bifida occulta, an incomplete fusion of the posterior vertebral arches, which is usually noted as an incidental radiographic finding. The defect most commonly involves the lower lumbar lamina of L5 and S1.

218. **When should an occult spinal dysraphism be suspected?**
Occult spinal dysraphism (or malformation) should be suspected in children who have the following dorsal midline features:

TABLE 14-11. FEATURES OF FOUR SIMILAR SYNDROMES OF ASCENDING PARALYSIS

Feature	Tick paralysis	Guillain-Barré syndrome	Spinal cord lesion	Poliomyelitis
Ataxia	Present	Absent	Absent	Absent
Rate of progression	Hours to days	Days to weeks	Gradual or abrupt	Days to weeks
Muscle-stretch reflexes	Absent	Absent	Variable	Absent
Babinski's sign	Absent	Absent	Present	Absent
Sensory loss	None	Mild	Present	None
Meningeal signs	Absent	Rare	Absent	Present
Fever	Absent	Rare	Absent	Present
Cerebrospinal fluid				
Protein level	Normal	High	Normal or high	High
White cell count (per mm^3)	<10	<10	Variable	>10
Time to recovery	<24 hours after tick removal	Weeks to months	Variable, depending on cause	Months to years or no recovery (permanent paresis)

Adapted from Felz MW, Smith CD, Swift TR: A six-year-old girl with tick paralysis. N Engl J Med 342:90–94, 2000.

- An abnormal collection of hair
- Cutaneous abnormalities (e.g., hemangioma, pigmented nevi)
- Cutaneous dimples or tracts or abnormal gluteal folds
- Subcutaneous mass (lipoma, fluid, or bone) on the lower back

In 80–90% of cases, there is an associated vertebral abnormality. Almost all of the signs and symptoms of spinal cord malformation involve the lower extremities, the bowel and bladder, and the spine. In older individuals, sexual function may be affected. The diagnosis should also be suspected in patients with symptoms of progressive lower extremity weakness or sensory loss, atrophy, gait abnormalities, foot deformities, pressure sores, incontinence and urinary tract infections, and scoliosis.

219. **What is the recurrence rate of open neural-tube defects?**
Open neural-tube defects (myelomeningocele or spina bifida and anencephaly) are usually have multifactorial causes, but, in some cases, they may be the result of Mendelian recessive inheritance. The general recurrence rate is 2.5% for mothers of affected children, sisters of the mother of an affected child, and female children born to individuals with spina bifida. Daily folic acid intake of 400 μg reduces the risk of spina bifida by as much as 70%. Serum and amniotic alpha-fetoprotein can detect open neural-tube defects, and ultrasound is also a useful tool.

TABLE 14-12. SPINAL SEGMENTS AND COMMON REFLEXES

Deep tendon reflex	Superficial reflex	Peripheral nerve	Segmental organization
	Pupillary	Optic/oculomotor	CNII–III
Jaw jerk		Trigeminal	CNV
	Corneal	Trigeminal/facial	CNV–VII
	Gag	Glossopharyngeal/vagal	CNIX–X
Biceps		Musculocutaneous	C5–C6
Brachioradialis		Radial	C5–C6
Triceps		Radial	C6–C8
Finger flexion		Median/ulnar	C7–T1
Abdominal reflex		Thoracic	T8–12
	Umbilical	Thoracic	T8–12
	Cremasteric	Genitofemoral	L1–L2
Adductor		Femoral/obturator	L2–L4
Quadriceps		Femoral	L2–L4
	Plantar reflex	Sciatic	S1–S2
	Anal wink	Pudendal	S3–S5

220. **What differentiates the various Chiari's malformations?**

Chiari's malformations are characterized by cerebellar elongation and protrusion of the foramen magnum into the cervical spinal cord. Anatomic anomalies of the hindbrain and skeletal structure result in different positioning of the various structures relative to the upper cervical canal and foramen magnum with different clinical features.

Type I is clinically the least severe and is generally asymptomatic during childhood. The presentation of a Chiari I malformation may be insidious, and it is associated with mental retardation. Epilepsy is found in a small minority of these patients. There may be paroxysmal vertigo, drop attacks, vague dizziness, and headache, which may be increased by the Valsalva maneuver. Occipital headache precipitated by exertion may progress to torticollis, downgaze nystagmus, periodic nystagmus, and oscillopsia. MRI findings in patients with Chiari I malformations include malformations of the base of the skull and of the upper cervical spine, including hydromyelia, syringomyelia, and syrinx.

Type II is the most common of those diagnosed during childhood. Medulla and cerebellum, together with part or the entire fourth ventricle, are displaced into the spinal canal. A variety of cerebellar, brain stem, and cortical defects can occur. This type is strongly associated with noncommunicating hydrocephalus and lumbosacral myelomeningocele.

Type III comprises any of the features of types I and II, but the entire cerebellum is herniated throughout the foramen magnum, with a cervical spina bifida cystica. Hydrocephalus is a common feature.

Type IV is cerebellar hypoplasia without a connection with the other malformations (this designation was made by Chiari).

Menkes JH, Sarnat HB: Malformations of the central nervous system. In Menkes JH, Sarnat HB (eds): Child Neurology, 6th ed. Philadelphia, Lippincott Williams & Wilkins, 2000, pp 324–326.

KEY POINTS: EARLY CLUES TO SPINAL-CORD COMPRESSION

1. Scoliosis producing sustained poor posture

2. Back or abdominal pain beginning abruptly during sleep

3. Increased sensitivity of spinal column to local pressure or percussion

4. Bowel or bladder dysfunction

5. Diminished sensation in the anogenital region and lower limbs

221. **What is the full anatomic expression of myelomeningocele?**
Children with myelomeningocele have a complex, multifaceted, congenital disorder of structure that represents a dysraphic state (i.e., a defective closure of the embryonic neural groove). In its full expression, it is typified anatomically by the following:
- The presence of unfused or excessively separated vertebral arches of the bony spine (spina bifida)
- Cystic dilation of the meninges that surround the spinal cord (meningocele)
- Cystic dilation of the spinal cord itself (myelocele)
- Hydrocephalus and the spectrum of congenital cerebral abnormalities

222. **If the diagnosis of myelomeningocele is made prenatally, should delivery be done by cesarean section?**
This remains controversial. A 1991 study of infants delivered by cesarean section before the onset of labor had significantly less paralysis at the age of 2 years than did infants with comparable lesions who were delivered vaginally after a period of labor. On the basis of this study, many centers adopted a policy of elective cesarean section for uncomplicated fetal myelomeningocele. Others have criticized this study and continued vaginal deliveries without detecting any differences in short-term and long-term outcomes of these infants.

    Lewis D, Tolosa JE, Kaufmann M, et al: Elective cesarean delivery and long-term motor function or ambulation status in infants with meningomyelocele. Obstet Gynecol 103:469–473, 2004.
    Luthy DA, Wardinsky T, Shurtleff DB, et al: Cesarean section before the onset of labor and subsequent motor function in infants with meningocele diagnosed antenatally. N Engl J Med 324:662–666, 1991.
    Merrill DC, Goodwin P, Burson JM, et al: The optimal route of delivery for fetal meningomyelocele. Am J Obstet Gynecol 179:235–240, 1998.

223. **What is the likelihood that a patient with myelomeningocele will have hydrocephalus?**
Hydrocephalus is seen in 95% of children with thoracic or high lumbar myelomeningocele. The incidence decreases progressively with more caudal spinal defects to a minimum of 60% if the myelomeningocele is located in the sacrum.

224. **What is the usual cause of stridor in a child with myelomeningocele?**
The stridor is usually caused by **dysfunction of the vagus nerve**, which innervates the muscles of the vocal cords. In their resting position, the edges of the cords meet in the midline; during speech, they move apart. Hence, in bilateral vagal nerve palsies, the free edges of the vocal cords are closely opposed and obstruct air flow, thereby resulting in stridor. In symptomatic patients, the motor nucleus of the vagus nerve may be congenitally hypoplastic or aplastic. More commonly, the vagal dysfunction is believed to arise from a mechanical traction injury

caused by hydrocephalus, which produces progressive herniation and inferior displacement of the abnormal hindbrain. Shunting the hydrocephalus may alleviate the traction and improve the stridor. Sometimes the later recurrence of stridor indicates the reaccumulation of hydrocephalus as a result of ventriculoperitoneal shunt failure.

225. **What are the principal options for managing urinary incontinence in patients with myelomeningocele?**
About 80% of patients have a neurogenic bladder, which most commonly manifests as a small, poorly compliant bladder and an open and fixed sphincter. Options include the following:
- Clean intermittent catheterization, which results in more complete emptying than simple Credé's maneuvers
- Artificial urinary sphincter to increase outlet resistance
- Surgical urinary diversion (e.g., suprapubic vesicostomy), which is uncommonly used
- Augmentation cystoplasty to increase bladder capacity in combination with the use of oxybutynin (a smooth-muscle antispasmodic)

   Blum RW, Pfaffinger K: Myelodysplasia in childhood and adolescence. Pediatr Rev 15:480–488, 1994.

226. **How frequently is myelomeningocele associated with mental retardation?**
Only *15–20%* of patients have associated mental retardation. Hydrocephalus per se does not cause the mental retardation that is associated with this syndrome. (Recall that children with appropriately treated congenital hydrocephalus caused by simple aqueductal stenosis usually have normal psychomotor development.) Only severe hydrocephalus with a very thick cortical mantle predicts lower intelligence. Mental retardation is usually attributed to acquired secondary CNS infection or subtle microscopic anomalies of neuronal migration and differentiation, which may coexist with the macroscopically visible malformation of the hindbrain.

227. **In an infant born with myelomeningocele, how does the initial evaluation predict long-term ambulation potential?**
The level of motor function—and not the level of the defect—is most predictive of ambulation.
- **Thoracic:** No hip flexion is noted. Almost no younger children will ambulate, and only about a third of adolescents will ambulate with the aid of extensive braces and crutches.
- **High lumbar (L1, L2):** The patient is able to flex the hips, but there is no knee extension. About a third of children and adolescents will ambulate, but only with extensive assistive devices.
- **Mid lumbar (L3):** The patient is able to flex the hips and extend the knee. The percentage of those able to ambulate is midway between those with high and low lumbar lesions.
- **Low lumbar (L4, L5):** The patient is able to flex the knee and dorsiflex the ankle. Nearly half of younger children and nearly all adolescents will ambulate, with varying degrees of braces or crutches.
- **Sacral (S1–S4):** The patient is able to plantar flex the ankles and move the toes. Nearly all children and adolescents will ambulate, with minimal or no assistive devices.

ACKNOWLEDGMENT

The editors and the author gratefully acknowledge contributions by Drs. Douglas R. Nordli, Jr., Peter Bingham, and Robert R. Clancy that were retained from the first three editions of *Pediatric Secrets*.

CHAPTER 15

ONCOLOGY

Richard Aplenc, MD, MCSE, Jeffrey Skolnik, MD, and Peter C. Adamson, MD

CHEMOTHERAPY/RADIATION THERAPY

1. **What was the first cytotoxic chemotherapeutic agent used for the treatment of children with leukemia?**
   In 1948, Sidney Farber reported success using aminopterin (4-aminopteroyl-glutamic acid) in 16 children with acute leukemia. Aminopterin was a precursor to the antifolate drug methotrexate, which is commonly used today.

   Farber S, Diamond LK, Mercer RD, et al. Temporary remissions in acute leukemia in children produced by folic acid antagonist, 4-amino-pteroylglutamic acid (aminopterin). N Engl J Med 238:787–793, 1948.

2. **Name the common cytotoxic chemotherapeutic drug classes.**
   Chemotherapeutic drugs are usually classified by their primary site and mechanism of action or source. The most common are the **alkylators**, **antimetabolites**, **antitumor antibiotics**, and **plant toxins**.

3. **Where are the sites of action of various anticancer drugs?**
   See Table 15-1.

TABLE 15-1.	**MECHANISM OF ACTION OF CHEMOTHERAPEUTIC DRUGS COMMONLY USED IN PEDIATRIC PATIENTS**	
Drug class	**Examples**	**Mechanism of action**
Alkylating agents		Cross-link DNA, thereby preventing replication of DNA and transcription of RNA
	Mechlorethamine, cyclophosphamide, ifosfamide, melphalan, nitrogen mustard	DNA cross-linking via classic covalent bond of alkyl group to DNA template
	Carmustine, lomustine (nitrosoureas)	DNA cross-linking and inhibition of DNA repair
	Cisplatin, carboplatin	DNA cross-linking by platination
	Busulfan, thiotepa, dacarbazine, procarbazine	DNA cross-linking
Antimetabolites		Structural analogs of key molecules involved in DNA/RNA synthesis

Drug class	Examples	Mechanism of action
TABLE 15-1.	MECHANISM OF ACTION OF CHEMOTHERAPEUTIC DRUGS COMMONLY USED IN PEDIATRIC PATIENTS	

Drug class	Examples	Mechanism of action
	Methotrexate	Structural analog of folic acid; inhibits dihydrofolate reductase, depleting tetrahydrofolate and precursors for the synthesis of purines and thymidine
	6-Mercaptopurine, 6-thioguanine	Purine analogs that compete with endogenous purine bases
	Cytarabine	Pyrimidine analog (deoxycytosine); incorporates into DNA and inhibits DNA polymerase, leading to chain termination
Antitumor antibiotics		Naturally occurring products with various mechanisms
	Doxorubicin, daunomycin, idarubicin (anthracyclines)	DNA intercalation and inhibition of topoisomerases, altering the three-dimensional shape of DNA/RNA during replication and transcription, leading to double- and single-stranded breaks; free-radical formation; interaction with cell membranes
	Dactinomycin	DNA intercalation and inhibition of topoisomerase II
	Bleomycin	Induction of DNA strand breaks by free radicals
Plant alkaloids		Derived from plant extracts
	Vincristine, vinblastine (vinca alkaloids)	Inhibitors of mitosis; bind to tubulin, interfering with microtubule assembly and formation of the mitotic spindle
	Etoposide (epipodophyllotoxin)	Topoisomerase II inhibitor
Miscellaneous	Prednisone, dexamethasone (corticosteroids)	Lympholysis, probably via binding of steroid receptor complex; also used as anti-inflammatory, immuno-suppressant, and antiemetic
	L-Asparaginase	Enzyme that depletes asparaginase in cells

From Weiner MA, Cairo MS: Pediatic Hematology/Oncology Secrets. Philadelphia, Hanley & Belfus, 2002, p 95.

4. **Which chemotherapeutic agents are cell cycle-dependent? In which phase are they most active?**
See Fig. 15-1.

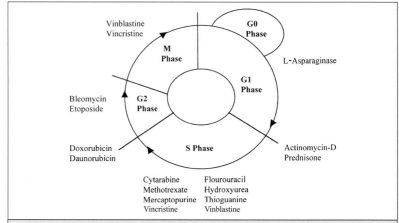

Figure 15-1. Phases in which cell-cycle-dependent chemotherapy agents are most active. G0 = resting phase (nonproliferation), G1 = gap1 (pre-DNA synthesis with diploid RNA and protein synthesis), S = DNA synthesis, G2 = gap2 (post-DNA synthesis), M = mitosis. (From Weiner MA, Cairo MS: Pediatric Hematology/Oncology Secrets. Philadelphia, Hanley & Belfus, 2000, p 96).

5. **What is the difference between adjuvant and neoadjuvant chemotherapy?**
Adjuvant chemotherapy is administered *after* the primary treatment of a tumor (surgical resection or radiation therapy), when there is no remaining gross tumor that can be assessed for response to the chemotherapy.
   Neoadjuvant chemotherapy is administered *before* the delivery of definitive local treatment and then continues afterwards in the adjuvant setting. For children with solid tumors, several cycles of neoadjuvant chemotherapy are often administered to improve the chances of achieving complete surgical resection and improved local control of a primary tumor.
   www.cancereducation.com
   www.oncolink.upenn.edu

6. **Why are most chemotherapeutic drug dosages based on body surface area (BSA)?**
In theory, BSA correlates better than body weight with cardiac output and hence hepatic and renal perfusion. Because most drug clearance occurs via hepatic and renal mechanisms, anti-cancer drugs that have a very narrow therapeutic index are usually dosed in a manner that is normalized to BSA. The exception is made for infants, who have a very high BSA-to-body-weight ratio; infants receive chemotherapy based on body weight. BSA can be estimated using height and weight. One estimate can be obtained with the following formula:

$$\text{BSA (m}^2) = \sqrt{[(\text{Weight} \times \text{Height})/3{,}600]}$$

7. **What is a cycle of chemotherapy?**
A cycle of chemotherapy starts with a period of drug administration (usually 1–5 days) that is followed by a 2–3-week interval of recovery. Most cycles last 3–4 weeks.

8. **What is the difference between pharmacokinetics and pharmacodynamics?**
   Pharmacokinetics refers to the effect of the body on the drug. It is the study of how drugs are absorbed, distributed, metabolized, and eliminated from the body. Common parameters include elimination half-life, peak concentration, clearance, and area under the concentration-time curve.

   Pharmacodynamics refers to the effect of the drug on the body. A pharmacodynamic effect can be a toxicity measurement (decrease in blood counts) or an anticancer measurement (decrease in the size of a tumor) after chemotherapy.

9. **What are the phases of a clinical trial?**
   - **Phase I:** *The dose determination phase.* This phase is designed primarily to recommend a dose for further testing in children, usually the maximum tolerated dose. Pharmacokinetic studies are performed during phase I trials to help learn whether children handle a drug differently than adults. Phase 1 trials typically enroll 18–30 children.
   - **Phase II:** *The efficacy phase.* Usually a group of children with the same diagnosis are studied, and the percentage of patients in whom the drug causes a tumor to decrease in size is determined. Phase II trials enroll from 30–150 children, depending on how many different tumor types are being studied.
   - **Phase III:** *The comparative phase.* This phase studies whether a new drug (or a new combination of drugs) that was found to be efficacious in a phase 2 trial can improve therapy relative to the best current therapy. Phase III trials are randomized and can enroll hundreds to thousands of children.

   Shah S, Weitman S, Langevin AM, et al: Phase I therapy trials in children with cancer. J Pediatr Hematol Oncol 20:431–438, 1998.

10. **What is the major dose-limiting toxicity for the alkylating agents?**
    Myelosuppression. Alkylating agents are chemically reactive compounds that covalently add an alkyl group; this is most important with regard to macromolecules involved in DNA synthesis, damaging templates, and inhibiting synthesis. Agents include the nitrogen mustards, oxazaphosphorines (including cyclophosphamide and ifosfamide), busulfan, and cisplatin.

11. **What are the common side effects of methotrexate?**
    Myelosuppression and **mucositis.** In high doses, the drug can be nephrotoxic and cause dermatitis, hepatitis, and mucositis. Most importantly, toxicity is primarily a function of duration of exposure. Because methotrexate can collect within fluid compartments (e.g., pleural or peritoneal effusions), it should be avoided in patients with significant third-space fluid collections.

12. **From what drug does leucovorin provide rescue?**
    Methotrexate. Leucovorin is a reduced form of folic acid, which is a treatment for the toxicity of methotrexate. Methotrexate inhibits the enzyme dihydrofolate reductase, which depletes cells of a major pathway that synthesizes reduced folates.

13. **If one had to choose a single laboratory test before administering high-dose methotrexate, which one should it be?**
    Determination of serum creatinine is essential before administering high-dose methotrexate. The kidneys eliminate >90% of methotrexate. In the presence of abnormal renal function, high-dose methotrexate carries a high risk of severe or fatal toxicity.

14. **Which class of drugs can be a cause of long-term cardiotoxicity?**
    Anthracyclines. Doxorubicin (Adriamycin) and daunorubicin (daunomycin) are antitumor antibiotics called anthracyclines. Cumulative doses of anthracyclines increase the risk of late cardiotoxicity; to avoid this effect, the total lifetime dose should usually not exceed 450 mg/m^2.

15. **Which anticancer drugs are vesicants?**
A *vesicant* is an agent that produces a vesicle; in oncology, it is a chemotherapeutic drug that can cause a severe burn if the drug infiltrates around the intravenous catheter. The **anthracyclines** (doxorubicin, daunorubicin), **dactinomycin**, and the **vinca alkaloids** (vincristine, vinblastine) are all vesicants. These drugs must be administered either through a central venous catheter or through a newly placed, free-flowing intravenous catheter that does not cross over a joint space.

16. **Which chemotherapeutic agent used in the treatment of Hodgkin's disease causes pulmonary toxicity?**
Bleomycin, a mixture of low molecular weight peptides isolated form the fungus *Streptomyces verticillus*, is part of the ABVD (Adriamycin, bleomycin, vinblastine, dacarbazine) regimen that is used for the treatment of Hodgkin's disease. Subacute or chronic pneumonitis progressing to interstitial fibrosis is its primary toxicity. Exposure to high concentrations of oxygen (e.g., in the operating room) can exacerbate bleomycin's pulmonary toxicity and must be avoided in any patient who has received the drug.

17. **Which antileukemic drugs can produce hyperglycemia as a side effect?**
Corticosteroids and **asparaginase** can both result in hyperglycemia. If hyperglycemia develops during induction chemotherapy, these drugs are not stopped. Instead, doses of insulin can be administered.

18. **What are the most effective antiemetics for the prevention and treatment of chemotherapy-induced vomiting?**
The serotonin-receptor antagonists **ondansetron** and **granisetron** are the most effective agents for chemotherapy-associated emesis. They work less well for delayed emesis, for which combinations of antihistamines and phenothiazines may be used. Dexamethasone is a useful adjunct when administering highly emetogenic chemotherapy.

> Dupuis LL, Nathan PC: Options for the prevention and management of acute chemotherapy-induced nausea and vomiting in children. Pediatr Drugs 5:597–613, 2003.

19. **What drug, made famous in Frank Capra's 1944 film about two sweet old ladies, is making a dramatic comeback in the treatment of one form of leukemia?**
The remedy used by the ladies in *Arsenic and Old Lace* is making an encore performance. In the early 1990s, investigators in China reported that arsenic, an ancient remedy, was found to be highly effective in the treatment of patients with acute promyelocytic leukemia. Arsenic appears to trigger an apoptotic response in promyeloblasts, but its precise mechanism of action is still under investigation.

20. **Who develops the "somnolence syndrome"?**
Transient symptoms attributed to *temporary demyelination* have been observed 6–8 weeks following completion of central nervous system (CNS) radiation, most commonly for CNS prophylaxis for acute lymphoblastic leukemia (ALL). Children who develop the "somnolence syndrome" have lethargy, headache, and anorexia that last for about 2 weeks. Computed tomography and cerebrospinal fluid studies show no consistent abnormality, but an electroencephalogram will often reveal a slow-wave activity consistent with diffuse cerebral disturbance. The use of steroids during irradiation appears to minimize the occurrence of the syndrome.

21. **A patient has received 40 Gray (Gy) of radiation. What does Gray mean?**
Gray is the basic unit of measurement used to quantify the energy of the amount of radiation received, and it is a measure of joules per kilogram of body weight. The gray is named in honor of L. H. Gray, an English radiation scientist, and 100 centigray (cGy) equals 1 Gy. Historically, cGy were referred to as *rads*.

22. **What is radiation recall?**
Radiation recall is a delayed effect that results from the interaction of certain chemotherapeutic agents (doxorubicin, daunorubicin, or actinomycin-D) with radiation. After radiation therapy, an erythematous rash in the previous radiation field develops. The rash is geographic, usually precisely following the outline of the radiation field. Many of these occur months after the radiation treatment.

23. **What is a "fraction" of radiation?**
Radiation therapy is coordinated so that a patient receives a maximally tolerated total amount of Gy. However, exposure to large amounts of radiation in one instance does not necessarily result in optimal cellular destruction, and it may have significant side effects. As a result, radiation is "fractionated" into smaller doses. Patients may receive up to dozens of individual fractions to achieve total radiation doses. For solid tumors, radiation is delivered over 2–6 weeks.

24. **Why are patients transfused frequently when undergoing radiation therapy?**
Ideally, patients undergoing radiation therapy should have a minimum hemoglobin concentration of 10 gm/dL to allow for tissue oxidization and electron transformation.

25. **What are the long-term sequelae of chemotherapy and irradiation?**
A variety of problems can ensue, depending on the age of the patient and the types of treatment. Four areas of prime concern include *cognitive deficits* (particularly in children <5 years old), *cardiac disease* (especially with the intensive use of anthracyclines), *endocrinopathies* (especially hypopituitarism, thyroid abnormalities, and gonadal end-organ failure), and *second malignancies*.

    Friedman DL, Meadows AT: Late effects of childhood cancer therapy. Pediatr Clin North Am 49:1083–1106, 2002.
    Oberfield SE, Sklar CA: Endocrine sequelae in survivors of childhood cancer. Adolesc Med 13:161–169, 2002.

CLINICAL ISSUES

26. **A patient has a central venous catheter and develops a fever. What should be done?**
The risk of bacteremia is increased in patients with central venous catheters. As such, any patient with an indwelling central venous catheter and a fever (usually 38.5°C or above) should have a blood culture obtained from each lumen of the catheter and intravenous antibiotics administered until evidence of a negative blood culture is provided.

27. **A patient is neutropenic and has a fever. What should be done?**
Because neutropenic patients are at risk of invasive bacterial infections, patients who are neutropenic (absolute neutrophil count <500/mm^3 or <1,000/mm^3 and falling) and without localizing features on examination should have blood cultures obtained and should receive broad-spectrum antibiotics. Antibiotic coverage should include both gram-negative and gram-positive organisms, including antibiotics that are active against *Pseudomonas aeruginosa*. Broad-spectrum antibiotics are continued until neutrophil counts show definitive signs of recovery.

28. **A patient remains febrile and neutropenic despite appropriate antibacterial antibiotics for several days. Is there cause for concern?**
Patients who are persistently neutropenic are at increased risk of invasive *fungal* infections. Neutropenic individuals who remain febrile despite appropriate antibiotics or who become febrile while receiving more than 5–7 days of broad-spectrum antibacterials are suspected to

have developed invasive fungal infection. They should be empirically treated with an antifungal agent.

29. **When should you consider removing a central venous catheter?**
Catheters colonized with fungi will not be cleared with antifungal therapy; these catheters must be removed. In addition, catheters colonized with bacteria that fail to clear despite proper antimicrobial treatment must be removed as well. Finally, catheters are occasionally removed in acute situations if patients are experiencing cardiovascular decompensation in the face of overwhelming sepsis and bacteremia (e.g., patients with a suspected central line infection).

30. **How should a patient who has oral candidiasis/esophageal candidiasis be treated?**
Candida species of yeast are a common cause of oral or esophageal infections in immunocompromised hosts. Topical antifungals (e.g., nystatin) may be tried in cases of simple oral candidiasis, and these can be added to regimens to treat esophageal candidiasis. However, systemic therapy is usually indicated in cases of esophageal candidiasis. Fluconazole is the first-line agent that can be used against candidal mucosal infections.

31. **After receiving broad-spectrum antibiotic therapy for 4 days for fever and neutropenia, a patient develops a new fever that is associated with abdominal cramps and bloody diarrhea. What is the most likely diagnosis?**
The patient most likely has *Clostridium difficile colitis* brought on by treatment with broad-spectrum antibiotics. The diagnosis should be confirmed by detection of the *C difficile* toxins in the stool, and either metronidazole or oral vancomycin should be initiated promptly.

32. **Why do patients on chemotherapy receive trimethoprim-sulfamethoxazole?**
Trimethoprim-sulfamethoxazole is used to prevent *Pneumocystis carinii* pneumonia. Prophylaxis can be obtained with 2–3 days of consecutive-day dosing per week.

33. **What paraneoplastic syndromes can occur in childhood?**
Paraneoplastic signs or symptoms are those that are unrelated to a malignancy but that can herald cancer. They occur more commonly in adults than children. However, unexplained high calcium, watery diarrhea, polymyositis, dermatomyositis, unexplained high hemoglobins, hypertension, precocious puberty, and opsoclonus/myoclonus can be associated with childhood malignancies.

de Graaf JH, Tamminga RY, Kamps WA: Paraneoplastic manifestations in children. Eur J Pediatr 153:784–791, 1994.

34. **What is the triad of tumor lysis syndrome?**
Hyperuricemia, hyperkalemia, and **hyperphosphatemia**. These metabolic complications occur as a result of the rapid lysis of a large tumor burden, especially in Burkitt's lymphoma and T-cell leukemia/lymphoma. Secondary renal failure and symptomatic hypocalcemia can also occur.

35. **What factors can contribute to renal failure in tumor lysis syndrome?**
- **Uric acid nephropathy:** The degradation of nucleic acids leads to increases in serum uric acid, which is soluble at physiologic pH but can precipitate in the acid milieu of the collecting tubules.
- **Calcium-phosphate crystallization:** Lymphoblasts (which contain four times the phosphate of lymphocytes) release phosphate, and, if the calcium-phosphate product exceeds 60, crystals can form in the renal microvasculature.

- **Tumor burden:** The tumor itself may contribute to preexisting renal problems by parenchymal involvement, obstructive uropathy, and venous stasis.

36. **Which patients are at highest risk for tumor lysis syndrome?**
The patients at highest risk are those with the most rapidly dividing tumors. The highest risk is with **Burkitt's lymphoma/leukemia,** followed by T-lineage acute lymphoblastic leukemia and T-cell lymphoblastic lymphoma.

37. **Why is bicarbonate used in the initial management of tumor lysis syndrome?**
The mainstay of tumor lysis therapy is aggressive hydration with alkalinization (with diuresis when necessary). Uric acid is relatively insoluble in the acidic pH of the urine, but this solubility increases with increased urine pH. Bicarbonate increases the pH and solubility of uric acid. After the uric acid normalizes and allopurinol is being administered, alkalinization is stopped.

38. **What do you do for a chemotherapy patient whose sister develops chickenpox?**
Immunocompromised patients are at high risk for disseminated varicella infections. Exposed seronegative patients (or patients with low-titer antivaricella antibody) should receive varicella zoster immune globulin within 96 hours of the exposure. Patients who develop an active varicella infection should be treated with intravenous acyclovir. All exposed patients, even if they receive varicella zoster immune globulin, should be isolated from other immunocompromised patients for 28 days after exposure.

39. **A child undergoing induction chemotherapy for leukemia develops right lower quadrant pain and tenderness. What diagnosis should be considered?**
Typhlitis. Although patients with cancer or those receiving chemotherapy may develop appendicitis, typhlitis is a severe necrotizing infection of the ileocolonic junction that occurs in neutropenic patients.

40. **What is the differential diagnosis of a lack of response to platelet transfusion?**
Patients who fail to respond to platelet transfusions may have developed an *alloantibody*, most often an HLA antibody, to donor platelets. This antibody binds to and causes the removal of the platelet from the circulation. Patients with veno-occlusive disease of the liver after receiving certain chemotherapeutic agents or after undergoing a bone marrow transplant may also be refractory to platelet transfusions.

41. **What is the difference between a Broviac and a Port-A-Cath?**
Children who require repeated blood draws or intravenous medications often have a semipermanent central venous catheter placed.
- A **Broviac catheter** is tunneled through the subcutaneous tissues of the chest and emerges as a thin plastic tube, usually at the level of the second or third rib.
- A **Port-A-Cath** contains a subcutaneous reservoir and is implanted under the skin of the chest. It is not visible, but it must be accessed by inserting a small needle through the skin and into the reservoir.

42. **What is the differential diagnosis of an anterior mediastinal mass?**
The five "Ts" can be used to remember the differential diagnosis of an anterior mediastinal mass: **t**eratoma (germ-cell tumor), **t**hymoma, **t**hyroid tumor, **T**-cell leukemia, and **t**errible lymphoma.

43. **What is superior mediastinal syndrome? How is it managed?**
Superior mediastinal syndrome results from the presence of an anterior mediastinal mass that compresses the trachea and the superior vena cava. Patients have a cough and dyspnea,

particularly when supine, and they have swelling of the head and upper extremities as a result of venous compression. Patients with a large mediastinal mass must not be anesthetized because of the risk of complete airway obstruction and vascular collapse. The optimal management of a mediastinal mass is prompt diagnosis and the initiation of appropriate treatment. Irradiation of the mass may provide emergent relief while the diagnosis is being made.

44. **Which tumors most commonly cause superior vena cava syndrome?**
In childhood, the most common primary cause is **non-Hodgkin's lymphoma**. Less-frequent causes are Hodgkin's disease, neuroblastoma, and sarcomas. Nonmalignant infectious causes are unusual but can include histoplasmosis or tuberculosis. The most frequent cause in children, however, is **iatrogenic**, resulting from vascular thrombosis after surgeries for congenital heart disease, shunting procedures for hydrocephalus, or central catheterization for venous access.

45. **Why is a generous mediastinal shadow on x-ray much more worrisome in a teenager as compared with an infant?**
Among infants, the incidence of Hodgkin's disease is extremely low. The thymus normally has a distinctive shape with flaring at the base and indentations from the ribcage ("sail sign"), which can usually be delineated on plain film. In teenagers, thymic enlargement has a higher likelihood of malignancy, particularly Hodgkin's disease, which is usually accompanied by lymphadenopathy in other areas of the mediastinum, particularly the paratracheal, tracheobronchial, and hilar regions.

46. **Which neoplasms are associated with hemihypertrophy?**
Wilms' tumor, hepatoblastoma, and **adrenal cortical carcinoma** are associated with hemihypertrophy either as part of Beckwith-Wiedemann syndrome or in isolation. Between 1% and 3% of Wilms' tumor patients have hemihypertrophy.

47. **Which cancers are often associated with splenomegaly?**
Acute leukemia, chronic myeloid leukemia, chronic myelomonocytic leukemia, Hodgkin's disease, and non-Hodgkin's lymphoma. Solid tumors rarely metastasize to the spleen to the point of causing splenomegaly.

48. **What are the predictors of malignancy in the pediatric patient with peripheral lymphadenopathy?**
A common clinical problem is determining which patients with enlarged lymph nodes require biopsy for diagnosis. In a study of 60 patients, risk of malignancy increased with increasing size (>1 cm), increasing number of adenopathy sites, and increasing ages (≥8 years old). Supraclavicular location, abnormal chest x-ray, and fixed nodes were also significantly predictive of malignancy.

Nield LS, Kamat D: Lymphadenopathy in children: When and how to evaluate. Clin Pediatr 43:25–33, 2004.

Soldes OS, Younger JG, Hirschl RB: Predictors of malignancy in childhood peripheral lymphadenopathy. J Pediatr Surg 34:1447–1452, 1999.

49. **When are transfusions necessary?**
Although there are no absolute criteria, in most centers, packed red blood cells are given when a patient has a hemoglobin level of <8.0 gm/dL. Platelets are empirically administered for a platelet count of <10,000–20,000/mm^3 in an otherwise well patient; a higher threshold may be used if there is active bleeding, disseminated intravascular coagulation (DIC), or a planned procedure. Granulocyte transfusions may be effective in neutropenic patients with a refractory infection caused by a gram-negative organism. Transfusions with plasma may be used for the treatment of coagulopathies.

50. **Why are blood products irradiated and leukocyte-depleted?**
Irradiation of blood products prevents transfusion-associated graft-versus-host disease (GVHD), which occurs when small numbers of T cells in the blood product are transferred into an immunocompromised patient. **Leukocyte-depletion** removes other white blood cells that would increase the risk of febrile transfusion reactions, alloimmunization, and the transmission of cytomegalovirus.

51. **What are the most common symptoms experienced by oncology patients who are receiving only palliative care at the end of life?**
Fatigue, pain, and dyspnea. Parents report that these symptoms are managed effectively in less than one third of children. As compared with adults, twice as many children die in hospitals during the final stages of disease, and half of them are on a ventilator. Insufficient attention to palliative care is a large problem.

Berde CB, Sethna NE: Analgesics for the treatment of pain in children. N Engl J Med 347:1094–1103, 2002.

Himelstein BP, Hilden JM, Boldt AM, et al: Pediatric palliative care. N Engl J Med 350:1752–1762, 2004.

Wolfe J, Grier HE, Klar N, et al: Symptoms and suffering at the end of life in children with cancer. N Engl J Med 342:326–333, 2000.

EPIDEMIOLOGY

52. **What are the frequencies of relative incidence of the childhood cancers in the United States?**

Leukemias	27%	Soft-tissue tumors	6%
CNS tumors	21%	Bone tumors	5%
Lymphomas	11%	Retinoblastoma	3%
Neuroblastoma	7%	Other tumors	14%
Wilms' tumor	6%		

Gurney JG, Severson RK, Davis S, et al: Incidence of cancer in children in the United States. Sex-, race-, and 1-year age-specific rates by histologic type. Cancer 75:2186–2195, 1995.

53. **How do the types of malignancies compare between infants and adolescents?**
See Figs. 15-2 and 15-3.

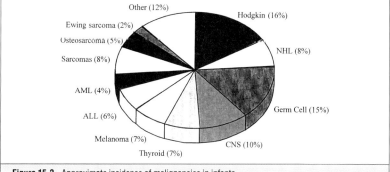

Figure 15-2. Approximate incidence of malignancies in infants.

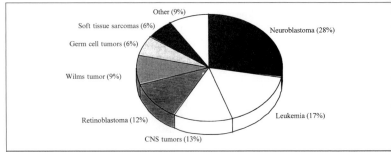

Figure 15-3. Approximate incidence of malignancies in adolescents.

54. **Is cancer the most common cause of death in children <15 years old?**
Cancer ranks a distant second, accounting for 10% of deaths in children <15 year old.
Accidents account for nearly 45% of deaths among this age group; congenital anomalies rank
third, with 8%, and homicide ranks fourth, with 5%.

55. **What is the most common neoplasm of childhood?**
ALL. Approximately 4 in 100,000 children <15 years old develop this neoplasm annually
(i.e., about 2,000 cases per year in the United States).

> Pui A-H: Acute lymphoblastic leukemia. N Engl J Med 350:1535–1548, 2004.

56. **What are the relative risks for children to develop leukemia?**
See Table 15-2.

TABLE 15-2. RELATIVE RISK FOR CHILDREN TO DEVELOP LEUKEMIA	
Population at risk	**Estimated risk**
U.S. white children	1 in 2,800
Siblings of a child with leukemia	1 in 700
Identical twin of a child with leukemia	1 in 5
Children with:	
Down syndrome	1 in 75
Fanconi syndrome	1 in 12
Bloom syndrome	1 in 8
Ataxia-telangiectasia	1 in 8
Exposures:	
Atom bomb within 100 m	1 in 60
Ionizing radiation	?
Benzene	1 in 960
Alkylating agents	1 in 2,000?

Data from Mahoney DH, Jr.: Neoplastic diseases. In McMillan JA, DeAngelis CD, Felgin RD, Warshaw JB
(eds): Oski's Pediatrics, Principles and Practice, 3rd ed. Philadelphia, J.B. Lippincott, 1999, p 1494.

57. **What are the risks of the Li-Fraumeni syndrome?**

Li-Fraumeni syndrome is an autosomal dominant condition caused by heritable mutations in the *p53* tumor-suppressor gene. The *p53* gene is located on chromosome 17 and plays a central role in controlling progression through the cell cycle. Patients with a heritable mutation in one *p53* allele are at high risk of malignancy if they develop a spontaneous mutation in the second allele. Patients with Li-Fraumeni syndrome are predisposed to many cancers, including rhabdomyosarcoma, brain tumors, acute leukemia, adrenocortical cell carcinoma, and premenopausal breast cancer. Members of such families have an estimated *50% probability of developing an invasive cancer* by the age of 30.

Padakasama S, Tomlinson GE: Genetic predisposition and screening in pediatric cancer. Pediatr Clin North Am 49:1393–1415, 2002.

58. **Which cancers have a significant racial predilection?**

Wilms' tumor has a higher incidence among black female infants. **Ewing's tumor** is about 30 times more common in whites than in blacks. **Hodgkin's disease** is rare in those of East Asian descent.

59. **What cancers are most commonly associated with a second neoplasm?**

See Table 15-3.

TABLE 15-3. CANCERS MOST COMMONLY ASSOCIATED WITH A SECOND NEOPLASM	
Primary tumors	**Secondary tumors**
Retinoblastoma	Osteosarcoma
	Pinealoblastoma
Hodgkin's disease	Acute nonlymphoblastic leukemia
	Non-Hodgkin's lymphoma
	Sarcoma (in radiation field)
	Thyroid carcinoma
	Breast carcinoma (in radiation field)
Acute lymphoblastic leukemia	Brain tumors
	Non-Hodgkin's lymphoma
Sarcomas	Sarcomas

60. **Are any childhood cancers associated with an increased alpha-fetoprotein?**

Increased alpha-fetoprotein is associated with germ-cell tumors, including endodermal sinus tumors of the ovary, testicular yolk-sac carcinoma, hepatocellular tumors, and retinoblastoma. Normally, alpha-fetoprotein is synthesized in the liver, yolk sac, and gastrointestinal tract of the fetus. Synthesis usually stops at birth; it disappears with a half-life of 3.5 days. Elevated serum levels are most commonly seen with nonmalignant liver disease. Levels remain elevated for 5–7 weeks after resection of the tumor, but persistence beyond that time is suggestive of residual disease.

61. **Are there any known transplacental carcinogens?**

Diethylstilbestrol, which was used to prevent spontaneous abortion, has been associated with an increased risk of vaginal cancer in the female offspring. It has also been reported that there is a 10-fold increased risk of monoblastic leukemia in the infants of mothers who smoke marijuana. It has been suggested that sedatives and a number of nonhormonal drugs are transplacental carcinogens, but this is not proven. It also has not been proved that cigarette smoke and the use of oral contraceptives are transplacental carcinogens.

62. **Is prenatal ultrasound associated with a risk of leukemia later in childhood?**
No. In vitro, ultrasound has been shown to cause cell membrane changes and thus concern has been expressed regarding potential effects on embryogenesis and pre- and postnatal development. However, in a study of all deaths from leukemia in Swedish children over a 16-year period, no association with prenatal ultrasound was found. Of note, the only known association of prenatal ultrasound with alterations in development has been a preference for left-handedness.

> Kieler H, Ahlsten G, Haglund B, et al: Routine ultrasound screening in pregnancy and aspects of the children's subsequent neurological development. Obstet Gynecol 91:750–756, 1998.
> Naumburg E, Bellocco R, Cnattingius S, et al: Prenatal ultrasound examinations and risk of childhood leukaemia: Case-control study. BMJ 320:282–283, 2000.

63. **Do children living near electrical power lines have an increased risk of developing cancer?**
Although a few small studies have suggested an association between power lines and an increased risk of ALL, the largest and best designed study as reported by Linet did *not* find evidence to support this hypothesis. Since that time, additional overseas studies have not demonstrated a significant risk.

> Draper G, Vincent T, Kroll ME, Swanson J: Childhood cancer in relation to distance from high-voltage power line in England and Wales: A case-control study. BMJ 330:1290–1293, 2005.
> UK Childhood Study Investigators: Exposure to power-frequency magnetic fields and the risk of childhood cancer. Lancet 354:1925–1931, 1999.

LEUKEMIA

64. **What are the most common clinical findings in the initial presentation of ALL?**
- **Hepatosplenomegaly:** 70% (10–15% of children have marked enlargement of the liver or spleen to a level below the umbilicus)
- **Fever:** 40–60%
- **Lymphadenopathy:** 25–50% with moderate or marked enlargement
- **Bleeding:** 25–50% with petechiae or purpura
- **Bone/joint pain:** 25–40%
- **Fatigue:** 30%
- **Anorexia:** 20–35%

65. **What are the typical hematologic findings noted during the presentation of ALL?**
Leukocyte count (mm^3)
- <10,000   45–55%
- 10,000–50,000   30–35%
- >50,000   20%

Hemoglobin (gm/dL)
- <7.5   45%
- 7.5–10.0   30%
- >10   25%

Platelet count (mm^3)
- <20,000   25%
- 20,000–99,000   50%
- >100,000   25%

KEY POINTS: ACUTE LYMPHOBLASTIC LEUKEMIA

1. Most common childhood malignancy

2. Increased risk: Patients with Down Syndrome, congenital immunodeficiency syndrome, exposure to ionizing radiation; sibling of patient with acute lymphoblastic leukemia

3. Chemotherapy phases: Induction (to achieve remission), delayed intensification, maintenance

4. Survival (if in standard risk group) >80% at 5 years after completion of therapy

5. Most common sites of relapse: Bone marrow, central nervous system, testis

66. **What studies of tumor cells are useful for determining a patient's prognosis?**
The **cytogenetics/DNA index** is a determination of the number and structure of the chromosomes/chromosomal material in tumor cells and comparing this with normal rates. More than 50 chromosomes or a DNA index of >1.16 is favorable. Certain chromosomal translocations are unfavorable. **Immunophenotyping** is also useful and involves the determination of B- or T-cell lineage, with maturity or immaturity of cells.

Pui C-H, Relling MV, Downing JR: Acute lymphoblastic leukemia. N Engl J Med 350:1535–1548, 2004.

67. **Why do children with ALL who are <1 year old have poorer prognoses?**
The great majority of infants with ALL in this age group often have a full complement of unfavorable features: high white blood cell count, CNS leukemia, bulky extramedullary disease, and t(4;11) (a translocation associated with poor response to therapy). By contrast, the prognosis for infants with acute myelogenous leukemia (AML) is not necessarily less favorable than that of older children.

68. **Why do boys with ALL fare more poorly than girls?**
In boys, after a full course of chemotherapy with remission, testicular involvement is a common site of relapse, occurring in up to 10% of cases. In older boys and teenage males, there is a higher incidence of T-cell disease than in girls. T-cell disease is associated with adverse prognostic factors (high white blood cell count, hepatosplenomegaly, and mediastinal masses) and alone carries a poorer prognosis. In girls, ovarian relapse is very rare, although it is difficult to diagnose after bone marrow relapse.

69. **Is ethnicity related to treatment outcome in patients with acute leukemia?**
Ethnicity appears to be related to outcome in both ALL and AML in children. In both leukemias, African-American ethnicity is associated with a poorer outcome. Although the reasons are not known, these differences may be the result of either host or leukemia characteristics.

70. **What are the known risk factors for the development of childhood ALL?**
   ▪ Down syndrome
   ▪ Ataxia telangiectasia
   ▪ High-dose radiation

71. **In addition to leukemia, what other diagnoses should be considered when evaluating a child who shows symptoms of pancytopenia?**
   ▪ Aplastic anemia
   ▪ Viral-induced suppression
   ▪ Drug-induced suppression
   ▪ Metastatic disease to the bone marrow

- Hemophagocytic syndromes
- Disseminated histoplasmosis
- Transfusion-associated GVHD

72. **Although many prognostic factors have come and gone for childhood ALL, which two have remained significant for the past 40 years?**
The two most consistent prognostic factors are *age* and *elevation of presenting white blood cell count*. Children <1 year old or >10 years old have a worse prognosis, as do those with a presenting white blood cell count of ≥50,000/mm³. Prognostic factors are important because, although 95% of ALL patients achieve remission (less than 5% lymphoblasts in bone marrow), 25% relapse. Identifying patients at higher risk is important so that more aggressive or novel therapy can be considered.

73. **Other than age at diagnosis and white blood count, what other factor has the greatest prognostic impact on long-term survival?**
A better prognosis is seen in patients who have a brisk initial response to therapy. This has been defined differently in separate studies. The Children's Cancer Group found an improved prognosis in patients with <5% blasts in the bone marrow after 7 days of chemotherapy. The Berlin-Frankfurt-Münster group found a similar prognosis in patients who had <1,000 blasts/mm³ in the peripheral blood after 7 days of prednisone.

KEY POINTS: HIGHER-RISK GROUPS WITH POORER PROGNOSIS OF PATIENTS WITH ALL

1. Age: <1 year and >10 years
2. White blood cell count: >50,000/mm³
3. Chromosomal translocation abnormalities, specifically t(8;14), t(9;22), and t(4;11)
4. Hypoploidy (<45 chromosomes)
5. Malignant cells, with mature B-cell or T-cell immunophenotyping
6. Central nervous system involvement
7. African-American and Hispanic patients
8. Males

74. **What is the prognostic value of minimal residual disease?**
Polymerase chain reaction technology can identify children with minimal residual disease after the completion of induction therapy by identifying residual leukemic cells (i.e., those beyond the detection capabilities of conventional microscopic evaluation) in patients in remission. Leukemia-associated immunophenotyping is another technique that can detect their presence. The presence of minimal residual disease was associated with much higher and faster rates of relapse.

75. **What is the acute risk of a very elevated blast count noted at the time of the initial diagnosis of leukemia?**
An elevated blast count at diagnosis may cause *CNS leukostasis* and *stroke*. The risk is higher in patients with AML, because myeloblasts are larger in size and may have procoagulant activity that increases the risk of stroke or hemorrhage. Leukocytapheresis is sometimes used to reduce the blast count before initiating therapy, but its impact on improving outcome remains unproven.

76. **What are the most common sites of extramedullary relapse of ALL?**
The most common is the *CNS*, and this is followed by *testicular* relapse. Testicular disease is accompanied by painless testicular swelling (usually unilateral). The diagnosis must be confirmed by biopsy. Patients with testicular disease require irradiation in addition to intensive retreatment with chemotherapy.

77. **What are the long-term side effects of cranial radiation administered for the prevention of CNS leukemia?**
A number of endocrinologic complications can occur, including growth hormone deficiency, hypothyroidism, hypogonadism, impaired fertility, and premature ovarian failure. Children are also at risk for deficits in attention, memory, and intelligence quotient. Less commonly, leukoencephalopathy may occur. Finally, children receiving cranial radiation are at risk of developing a second malignant neoplasm.

78. **What distinguishes leukemia from lymphoma?**
The distinction is often difficult, because ALL can resemble non-Hodgkin's lymphoma. Cytomorphologically, there is little difference between T-cell lymphoblastic lymphoma and ALL or between the B cells of Burkitt's lymphoma and mature B-cell ALL. As an arbitrary rule, the presence of ≥25% blast cells in the bone marrow defines leukemia.

79. **What is a chloroma?**
A chloroma is a tumor that is formed by a coalescence of AML blasts. It may appear in bones, skin, soft tissue, or other sites. Its name is derived from its green appearance on its cut surface.

Downing JR, Burnett A: Acute myeloid leukemia. N Engl J Med 341:1051–1062, 1999.

80. **What is the significance of the Philadelphia chromosome?**
The Philadelphia chromosome, discovered in Philadelphia in 1960 by Nowell and Hungerford, was the first clonal cytogenetic abnormality (a balanced translocation between chromosomes 9 and 22) described in leukemia. The result is a new fusion gene that codes for a tyrosine kinase with increased enzymatic activity. The Philadelphia chromosome is seen in >90% of patients with chronic myelogenous leukemia (CML) but also in ≤5% of children with ALL (20% of adult ALL) and in ≤2% of children with AML. Different isoforms of the fusion gene may be present in ALL. Ph+ ALL has a much poorer prognosis.

Arico M, Valsecchi MG, Camitta B, et al: Outcome of treatment in children with Philadelphia chromosome-positive acute lymphoblastic leukemia. N Engl J Med 342:998–1006, 2000.

81. **What is the appropriate treatment for CML?**
The *definitive* treatment for CML is **allogeneic stem-cell transplantation**. However, for patients who do not have an appropriate stem-cell donor, treatment with interferon-alpha may reduce the white blood cell count, and it may occasionally result in a cytogenetic remission. Hydroxyurea may also be employed to reduce the peripheral white blood cell count, but it is not curative. Gleevec, a tyrosine kinase inhibitor, is highly effective for inducing remission. However, resistance to Gleevec may develop, and thus, in children, stem-cell transplantation currently remains the definitive therapy for CML.

Goldman JM, Melo JV: Chronic myeloid leukemia—Advances in biology and new approaches to treatment. N Engl J Med 349:1451–1464, 2003.

82. **In children who have very elevated white blood cell counts, why are CNS hemorrhagic complications more likely in patients with AML than in those with ALL?**
As compared with lymphocytes, leukocytes (especially promyelocytes and monoblasts) contain compounds with *procoagulant* activity that are released as the cells lyse, and this may lead to microthrombi formation, disseminated intravascular coagulation, and hemorrhage.

LYMPHOMA

83. **What is the malignant cell of Hodgkin's disease?**
    The Reed-Sternberg cell. Its normal cell of origin remains unclear, with the predominance of evidence indicating a B or T lymphocyte. However, the cells alone are not pathognomonic of Hodgkin's disease and may be seen in infectious mononucleosis, non-Hodgkin's lymphoma, carcinomas, and sarcomas.

84. **How is Hodgkin's disease staged?**
    Hodgkin's lymphoma, like non-Hodgkin's lymphoma, is classified according to the stage of disease and histology, as in the Ann Arbor System. It is also staged according to whether there are symptoms. Patients with no symptoms are referred to as having *A* disease. Patients with documented fever, involuntary weight loss of >10%, or night sweats are considered to have *B* disease. Intractable pruritus may also be a symptom, but it is not among the B symptoms used for staging.

    Stage is determined both clinically and pathologically. Location of lymph node regions is the critical factor: I (single region), II (regions on the same side of the diaphragm), III (regions on both sides of the diaphragm), or IV (diffuse disease). **Clinical staging** refers to staging that is done without histologic proof. **Pathologic staging** refers to biopsy-proven disease in a given region and usually involves a staging laparotomy and splenectomy to determine the extent of disease.

85. **What are B symptoms?**
    Fever, *night sweats*, and *weight loss*. Their presence carries a poorer prognosis for patients with Hodgkin's disease.

86. **What is the histologic classification of Hodgkin's disease?**
    See Table 15-4.

TABLE 15-4. THE RYE, NEW YORK, HISTOLOGIC CLASSIFICATION*

	Lymphocytes	Reed-Sternberg cells	Other	Incidence
Lymphocyte predominant	Many	Few	Histiocytes	10–15%
Nodular sclerosing	Many	Few or many	Bands of refractile fibrosis	40–70%
Mixed cellularity	Many	Few or many	Eosinophils, histiocytes	20–30%
Lymphocyte depletion	Few	Many	No refractile fibrosis	<5%

*Based on the relative number of lymphocytes and Reed-Sternberg cells.

87. **What is the prognosis for the various stages of Hodgkin's disease?**
    The prognosis for children with Hodgkin's disease is excellent in that most are cured. For stages I and IIA, the 5-year relapse-free survival is >80% for patients treated with radiation only, and it may be >90% for patients treated with radiation and chemotherapy. For stage IIB,

prognosis is not as good, especially if there is a massive mediastinal tumor, but 5-year survival is still >80%. The same survival figures pertain to stage IIIA disease, but treatment generally is more extensive than that for a limited stage II disease. For stage IV disease, 5-year relapse-free survival is 70–90%.

88. How are non-Hodgkin's lymphomas classified?

Non-Hodgkin's lymphomas include a heterogeneous group of malignant solid tumors that are of lymphoid origin. Their classification is still disputed. In general, these lymphomas are divided according to the **extent of spread** in the body and histology. The disease is either local-ized or disseminated. Localized tumors are limited to either a node or an area (e.g., the appen-dix, a tonsil) and may include some regional surrounding nodes. Disease can also originate in bone. The tumor cells may spread to the bone marrow or spinal fluid (much like leukemia), or they may disseminate throughout the abdomen and pleural space.

Histology is divided into *lymphoblastic* and *nonlymphoblastic* types. The most common type of lymphoblastic lymphoma occurs in the mediastinum and probably originates in the thymus. Disease is virtually always disseminated at diagnosis. Nonlymphoblastic lymphomas include Burkitt's lymphoma and peripheral T-cell lymphomas. Burkitt's lymphoma often occurs in the retroperitoneum and is usually disseminated. The classification of the Non-Hodgkin's lymphomas of childhood is very different from that of adults.

Sandlund JT, Downing JR, Crist WM: Non-Hodgkin's lymphoma in childhood. N Engl J Med 334:1238–1248, 1996.

89. What second malignancies are common among patients treated for Hodgkin's disease?

The type of second malignancy depends in part on the treatment used for the primary tumor. Depending on the field included in primary treatment, *radiation* increases the risk of skin, bone, and breast cancer. Chemotherapy with alkylating agents increases the risk of AML.

Hudson MM, Donaldson SS: Hodgkin's disease. Pediatr Clin North Am 44:891–906, 1997.

90. What are the common types of lymphoma in children?

As compared with adults, aggressive, high-grade lymphomas occur more frequently in children. The three most common types are *Burkitt's lymphoma, lymphoblastic lymphoma,* and *large-cell lymphoma.*

91. What is the common cytogenetic abnormality in Burkitt's lymphoma?

t(8;14) fuses the c-myc oncogene to the immunoglobulin heavy chain gene. This *translocation* is found in both endemic and sporadic forms, although the breakpoints differ.

92. What is an eosinophilic granuloma?

Eosinophilic granuloma is a lytic tumor of bone that is accompanied by pain and sometimes swelling. Its histology is identical to that of Langerhans cell histiocytosis, with which it is now classified. Biopsy of an isolated eosinophilic granuloma is often curative, although lesions may also regress spontaneously.

93. What are the features of Langerhans cell histiocytosis (LCH)?

LCH is a multifaceted disorder and replaces the diseases grouped under the term "histiocytosis X." The presenting symptoms of LCH may be isolated bone lesions (eosinophilic granuloma), bone lesions together with exophthalmos and diabetes insipidus (Hand-Schüller-Christian disease), or with disseminated disease (Letterer-Siwe disease). Other features include skin rashes that resemble seborrheic dermatitis, chronic otitis externa, lymphadenopathy, hepatosplenomegaly, pancytopenia, neurologic deficits, and pulmonary disease. Mild forms of the disease tend to wax and wane even without treatment, whereas disseminated disease is often resistant to therapy.

NERVOUS SYSTEM TUMORS

94. **How are CNS tumors classified?**
Most are typically classified on the basis of histology:
- **Glioma:** Arises from supportive tissue (astrocytes)
- **Ependymoma:** Arises from the ependymal cells that line the ventricles
- **Germ cell tumor:** Arises from totipotent germ cells
- **Rhabdoid:** Arises from an unknown cell type
- **Craniopharyngioma**

95. **Where is the most common area for each tumor to occur?**
- **Glioma:** Cerebellum and optic pathway (more commonly benign and low grade); cerebrum or brainstem (more commonly malignant and higher grade)
- **Ependymoma:** Fourth ventricle; less commonly the spinal cord
- **Germ cell tumor:** Pineal or supracellar region
- **Primitive neuroectodermal tumor (PNET) medulloblastoma:** Midline of the cerebellum
- **Rhabdoid:** Posterior fossa
- **Craniopharyngioma:** Choroid plexus

96. **What are the most common supratentorial brain tumors? What are their symptoms?**
Supratentorial tumors include tumors of the cerebrum, basal ganglia, thalamus, and hypothalamus. They can be gliomas, ependymomas, PNETs, germ-cell tumors, choroid-plexus tumors, or craniopharyngiomas. These tumors can show signs of increased intracranial pressure, such as headache and vomiting. In addition, these tumors may be accompanied by focal deficits, such as memory loss, weakness, and visual changes.

97. **What are the most common infratentorial tumors? What are their symptoms?**
Infratentorial tumors include tumors of the cerebellum and brainstem. They can be astrocytomas, medulloblastomas, ependymomas, or gliomas. If infratentorial tumors block cerebrospinal fluid outflow, headache and vomiting may be the presenting sign; they can also become apparent with localizing signs such as cranial nerve palsies or ataxia.

98. **With regard to the primary site of origin, how do childhood brain tumors contrast with those of adults?**
Approximately 50% of brain tumors in children are *infratentorial*, with three fourths of these located in the cerebellum or fourth ventricle. By contrast, the majority of brain tumors in adult patients are *supratentorial* in location.

99. **Which cranial nerve abnormality is most common in children showing signs of increased intracranial pressure as the result of a posterior fossa tumor?**
Inability to abduct one or both eyes (**cranial nerve VI palsy**) may result from an elevation in intracranial pressure and can be a false localizing sign for the primary brain tumor.

100. **What are the three Es of the diencephalic syndrome?**
Diencephalic syndrome is the constellation of symptoms that result from the presence of a hypothalamic tumor: **e**uphoria, **e**maciation, and **e**mesis.

101. **What is Parinaud's syndrome?**
Parinaud's syndrome is the result of increased intracranial pressure at the dorsal midbrain, causing downgaze, papillary dilation, and nystagmus.

102. **What is Cushing's triad?**

Cushing's triad represents the body's attempt to compensate for increased intracranial pressure and consists of **bradycardia**, **hypertension**, and **abnormal respiratory pattern**.

103. **What are the key evaluations for a child with a newly diagnosed medulloblastoma?**

Medulloblastomas may spread contiguously to the cerebellar peduncle, to the floor of the fourth ventricle, into the cervical spine, or above the tentorium. In addition, medulloblastomas may disseminate via the cerebrospinal fluid. Every patient should thus be evaluated with diagnostic imaging (magnetic resonance imaging) of the spinal cord and of the whole brain. Examination of cerebrospinal fluid should be performed after resection of the primary tumor.

104. **What is a "dropped met"?**

Most brain tumors do not metastasize; they are fatal because of local invasion. A *dropped metastasis* occurs when a primary brain tumor spreads via cerebrospinal fluid pathways, thereby resulting in meningeal deposits along the spinal cord. These metastases have "dropped" from their original site down to the spinal cord or cauda equina.

105. **What is the difference between a glioma, an astrocytoma, and glioblastoma multiforme?**

- A **glioma** (from the Greek word *glia* for glue and the suffix -*oma* for tumor) is a neoplasm that is derived from one of the various types of cells that form the interstitial tissue of the central nervous system, such as astrocytes, oligodendria, and ependymal cells. Of the gliomas, astrocytomas of variable malignancy are the most prevalent.
- **Astrocytomas** are subdivided into categories (grades) on the basis of the degree of tumor anaplasia and the presence or absence of necrosis. The juvenile pilocytic and subependymal astrocytoma are low-grade gliomas. Anaplastic astrocytomas (grade 3) grow more rapidly than the more differentiated astrocytomas.
- **Glioblastoma multiforme** is the highest-grade astrocytoma (grade 4).

  Ullrich NJ, Pomeroy SL: Pediatric brain tumors. Neurol Clinics 21:897–913, 2003.

106. **What is a PNET?**

A **primitive neuroectodermal tumor**. The term refers to tumors that are composed primarily of undifferentiated neuroepithelial cells, and it has come to describe supratentorial tumors of neuroectodermal origin (sPNET) and cerebellar neuroectodermal tumors (medulloblastoma).

107. **Why is the prognosis for children with brainstem gliomas so poor?**

A basic tenet of CNS tumors is that a gross total resection is necessary to achieve the greatest chance of long-term cure. Brainstem tumors most commonly are fully intrinsic to the pons and unresectable. Although radiation can improve symptoms, there currently is no known curative therapy for the very large majority of children with brainstem gliomas.

108. **What are neuroblastomas?**

Tumors of the postganglionic central nervous system. They are the most common malignant tumor among infants.

09. **Why can neuroblastoma arise in a spectrum of locations in children?**

Neuroblastomas are tumors of the neural crest tissue. Abnormal migration of neural crest cells, which are destined for the adrenal medulla or the para-aortic sympathetic ganglia, form pockets of immature neuroma. Thus tumors arise anywhere along the neuroaxis and in the adrenal glands.

110. **What are the most common presentations of neuroblastoma?**
Children with **disseminated** neuroblastoma are irritable and ill, and they often have exquisite bone pain, proptosis, and periorbital ecchymoses. Seventy percent of neuroblastomas arise in the abdomen; half of these arise in the adrenal gland, and the other half arise in the parasympathetic ganglia and are distributed throughout the retroperitoneum and the paravertebral area in the chest and neck. The tumor produces and excretes catecholamines, which can on occasion cause systemic symptoms such as sweating, hypertension, diarrhea, and irritability. Children with **localized** neuroblastoma may have symptoms referable to a mass.

111. **What is Horner syndrome?**
Ptosis, miosis (with unequal pupils), and anhidrosis. The syndrome can occur from congenital brachial plexus injury, but acquired Horner syndrome requires evaluation for cervical, intrathoracic, or intracranial pathology, particularly neuroblastoma.

KEY POINTS: CENTRAL NERVOUS SYSTEM TUMORS

1. Second most common neoplasm of childhood, after leukemia

2. Older children (>1 year): Most tumors are infratentorial (cerebellar or brainstem)

3. Younger children (<1 year): Most tumors are supratentorial

4. Gold standard for diagnosis: Magnetic resonance imaging with and without gadolinium enhancement

5. Back pain, extremity weakness, and/or bowel/bladder dysfunction suggestive of spinal cord lesions/metastases

112. **Where does neuroblastoma tend to metastasize?**
Neuroblastoma spreads to the liver, the bone, the bone marrow, and, less commonly, to the skin.

113. **What is meant by "dancing eyes-dancing feet?"**
"Dancing eyes-dancing feet" is a descriptive term for **opsoclonus-myoclonus**, a condition in which children with neuroblastoma develop horizontal nystagmus and involuntary lower extremity muscle spasm. These symptoms are thought to arise from a nonspecific antibody reaction to neuroblastoma that cross-reacts with the motor end plate. These symptoms do not always improve, despite appropriate neuroblastoma therapy.

114. **What urinary test aids in the diagnosis of neuroblastoma?**
Urinary concentrations of catecholamines and metabolites, including dopamine, homovanillic acid, and vanillylmandelic acid, are often increased (>3 standard deviations above the mean per milligram creatinine for age) in children with neuroblastoma.

115. **Why would a toddler with neuroblastoma be treated with Accutane?**
Retinoic acid (isotretinoin, also called Accutane) has been shown in vitro to promote neuroblast differentiation and maturation. Clinical studies have found that children with advanced-stage neuroblastoma who receive Accutane at the completion of their cancer therapy have a somewhat improved likelihood of cure.

16. What does the S stand for in stage IVS neuroblastoma?
Stage IVS is a "**s**pecial" type of neuroblastoma that is found only in children <1 year old. Along with a primary tumor, these infants may have bone marrow, liver, and skin disease as well. Even without therapy, these cancers spontaneously regress and disappear over time. Treatment is only indicated if the patient is symptomatic from the underlying disease (e.g., large abdominal mass, liver disease).

17. How does the prognosis for patients with neuroblastoma vary by stage?
- **Stage I or II:** 90% chance of cure with surgery alone. Children whose disease is not controlled with surgery frequently have unfavorable biologic features, such as unfavorable histology (i.e., many mitotic figures and/or karyorrhexis) and elevated serum ferritin, amplified N-*myc* cellular oncogene, or both.
- **Stage III:** 50% chance of cure with surgery, radiation, and chemotherapy. Biologic features at diagnosis also determine the prognosis of these patients.
- **Stage IV:** 20% chance of long-term survival. Age is an especially important prognostic variable in that those <1 year old have a considerably better outlook.
- **Stage IV-S:** >80% chance of long-term survival with supportive care alone. Infants <6 weeks old may die of liver failure or mechanical problems related to a big liver. Few patients with stage IVS disease actually progress to typical stage IV disease with bone and extensive marrow involvement.

KEY POINTS: NEUROBLASTOMA

1. Most common pediatric extracranial solid tumor

2. Most common malignant tumor among infants

3. Majority of children <4 years old

4. Poorer prognosis: >1 year old, metastatic disease, *MYCN* amplification

5. Most metastatic at diagnosis

6. Paraneoplastic syndromes: VIP syndrome (diarrhea as a result of increased **v**asoactive **i**ntestinal **p**eptide), opsoclonus-myoclonus ("dancing eyes, dancing feet"), and catecholamine excess (with flushing, sweating, headache, hypertension)

18. How can the site of spinal cord compression be clinically localized?
Spinal tenderness on percussion correlates with localization in up to 80% of patients. In addition, neurologic evaluation of strength, sensory level changes, reflexes, and anal tone can help to pinpoint the location in the spinal cord, the conus medullaris (the terminal neural portion of the spinal cord), or the cauda equina. Progression is rapid with spinal cord compression but may be rapid or variable with compression of the conus medullaris or the cauda equina. The levels of the spine most frequently affected are summarized in Table 15-5.

19. What is leukokoria?
Leukokoria, or white pupil, can be obvious, or it can be a subtle asymmetry on pupillary red reflex evaluation. Although other diagnoses can accompany leukokoria, the one that is most feared is retinoblastoma.

TABLE 15-5.	FREQUENCY OF INVOLVEMENT OF CERVICAL, THORACIC, AND LUMBOSACRAL SPINE
Spinal level	**Involvement**
Cervical	10%
Thoracic	70%
Lumbar	20%

From Gates RA, Fink RM: Oncology Nursing Secrets, 2nd ed. Philadelphia, Hanley & Belfus, 2001, p 470.

120. **What is the heredity of retinoblastoma?**
Although the majority of cases are sporadic, retinoblastoma can be inherited as an autosomal dominant trait with nearly complete penetrance. Of all cases, 60% are nonhereditary and unilateral, 15% are hereditary and unilateral, and 25% are hereditary and bilateral. Families of patients with retinoblastoma should have genetic counseling.

121. **What is the "two-hit" hypothesis of cancer, particularly retinoblastoma?**
Alfred Knudson's "two-hit" hypothesis is a basic tenet of malignant transformation. In 1971, Knudson calculated the genetic probabilities of developing retinoblastoma and hypothesized that patients with bilateral disease first inherited a *germline mutation* and then underwent a second *somatic mutation* to develop the disease. Patients with unilateral or sporadic disease developed two somatic mutations during early childhood. The identification of the genes associated with the first of the "two hits" correctly predicted the presence of tumor suppressor genes.

 Knudson A: Two genetic hits (more or less) to cancer. Nat Rev Cancer 1:157–162, 2001.

122. **In what age group does retinoblastoma usually occur?**
Retinoblastoma most often occurs in younger children, with 80% of cases diagnosed before the age of 5 years. Retinoblastoma is usually confined to the eye, with >80% of children being cured with current therapy.

 Shields CL, Shields JA: Recent developments in the management of retinoblastoma. J Pediatr Ophthalmol Strabismus 36:8–18, 1999.

123. **For what other tumors are retinoblastoma patients at increased risk?**
Patients with the hereditary type of retinoblastoma have a markedly increased frequency of second malignant neoplasms. The cumulative incidence is about 26 ±1 0% in nonirradiated patients and 58 ± 10% in irradiated patients by 50 years after diagnosis of retinoblastoma. Most of the second malignant neoplasms are **osteosarcomas**, **soft-tissue sarcomas**, and **melanomas.**

OTHER SOLID NON-CNS TUMORS

124. **What are the peak ages of incidence of the most common solid tumors of childhood?**
Neuroblastoma and **Wilms' tumor** are tumors of early childhood. **Ewing's sarcoma** and **osteosarcoma** are more prevalent during adolescence. **Rhabdomyosarcoma** occurs throughout childhood and the teenage years.

125. **What factors contribute to the relapse of solid tumors?**

Even in the best centers with treatment delivered in an optimal manner for curable tumors, relapses occur for reasons that remain unexplained and that are probably intrinsic to the biology of the tumor. However, the following variables may contribute to treatment failure:

- Suboptimal treatment that is not given according to a recognized protocol or that is administered by an inexperienced physician
- Failure to control the primary tumor with surgery and irradiation
- Metastatic spread of tumor at presentation
- Tumor that is resistant to chemotherapy

126. **What is a Wilms' tumor?**

A primary malignant renal tumor of large histologic diversity. The age at which a child is most commonly diagnosed with Wilms' tumor is summarized in Figure 15-4.

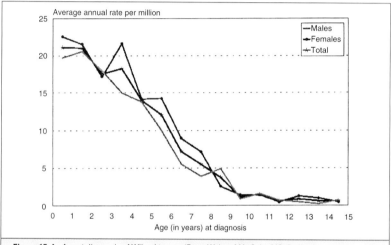

Figure 15-4. Age at diagnosis of Wilms' tumor. (From Weiner MA, Cairo MS: Pediatric Hematology/Oncology Secrets. Philadelphia, Hanley & Belfus, 2000, p 157.)

127. **What are the three histologic components of a Wilms' tumor?**

Wilms' tumors are considered triphasic, consisting of a *blastemal* (immature) component, an *epithelial* (tubular) component, and a *stromal* (muscular) component.

128. **How is Wilms' tumor distinguished radiographically from neuroblastoma?**

- **Wilms' tumor:** Computed tomography images will show *intrinsic* distortion of the kidney parenchyma and the collecting system. Only 10% of children with Wilms' tumor have calcifications.
- **Neuroblastoma:** This is almost always is *extrarenal* and causes displacement—not distortion—of the renal parenchyma and collecting system. Calcifications are seen in >50% of children with abdominal neuroblastoma.

129. **Where does Wilms' tumor metastasize?**

Locally, Wilms' tumor can grow through the renal capsule, invade the renal veins, extend into the vena cava, and even progress into the chambers of the heart. The lungs are a common site of metastasis. Spread also occurs into the regional lymph nodes.

130. **What is a stage V Wilms' tumor?**

 Bilateral Wilms' tumor is known as a stage V tumor. Each tumor is staged independently; prognosis with bilateral disease is not necessarily poor.

131. **What is WAGR syndrome?**

 The constellation of **W**ilms tumor, **a**niridia, **g**enitourinary abnormalities, and mental **r**etardation.

132. **"Small, round, blue-cell tumor" is often used in the description of which childhood tumors?**

 Neuroblastoma, rhabdomyosarcoma, Ewing's sarcoma, lymphoblastic leukemia, and lymphoma. All appear as small, round, blue cells on low-power microscopic examination. High-power microscopic examination, usually in combination with a panel of immunohistochemical stains and molecular diagnostics, is required for definitive diagnosis.

133. **Which solid tumors metastasize to the bone marrow?**

 Neuroblastoma, lymphoma, alveolar rhabdomyosarcoma, Ewing's sarcoma/PNET, and retinoblastoma.

134. **What is Ewing's sarcoma?**

 A family of poorly differentiated primary tumors of nonosseous cell origin that includes Ewing's sarcoma of bone, extraosseous Ewing's sarcoma, and PNET of bone or soft tissue.

135. **Where are the most common locations of Ewing's sarcoma?**

 The pelvis, leg, upper arm, and rib. These tumors arise in extraskeletal (soft-tissue) locations and can locally invade the bone.

136. **What are the two most common sites of metastases for patients with Ewing's sarcoma?**

 Ewing's sarcoma often metastasizes to the **lungs** and somewhat less frequently to other **bones**. In general, lymph nodes are not involved, which suggests that dissemination of this tumor is primarily hematogenous.

137. **What is osteosarcoma?**

 A malignant spindle cell tumor in which the cells produce neoplastic osteoid. It is the most common primary malignancy of bone in children.

138. **Osteosarcoma generally arises in which part of the bone?**

 The *metaphyses* of long bones of the extremities. Between 60% and 80% of tumors are located in the metaphyses of the knee (i.e., the proximal tibia or the distal femur).

139. **Do all patients with osteosarcoma require surgical resection of the primary tumor?**

 Surgical resection of the primary tumor is a requirement for curative treatment of osteosarcoma. By contrast with Ewing's sarcoma, osteosarcoma is a relatively radiation-resistant tumor, and thus surgical resection after neoadjuvant chemotherapy is a mainstay of treatment.

140. **For patients with localized osteosarcoma, what factor is most predictive of a favorable outcome?**

 Patients with >95% necrosis of the primary tumor (as determined by pathologic examination) after neoadjuvant chemotherapy have a better prognosis than those with lesser amounts of necrosis.

41. What do Ewing's sarcoma and osteosarcoma have in common?
Both are treated with neoadjuvant chemotherapy, which is an initial 2–3 month period of chemotherapy, followed by local control with surgery. For select cases of Ewing's sarcoma, radiation therapy is also used. Both tumors can develop distant metastases in the lungs and in other bones, and both tumors are cancers of adolescence. Although both Ewing's sarcoma and osteosarcoma appear to be soft-tissue tumors arising in bone, only osteosarcoma is truly a tumor of bone, whereas Ewing's sarcoma is a primitive neuroectodermal tumor.

42. In what solid tumor has the surgical resection of pulmonary metastases been shown to result in long-term cure?
Although many pediatric sarcomas metastasize to the lungs, only surgical resection of pulmonary metastases from osteosarcoma has been definitively shown to contribute to cure, and only, in general, when the metastases are few in number. The role of the surgical resection of pulmonary metastases arising from other sarcomas (e.g., rhabdomyosarcoma, Ewing sarcoma) is less clear and is only undertaken in select circumstances.

43. What is a limb-salvage procedure?
In an attempt to save as much natural tissue as possible, patients with soft-tissue sarcomas often undergo a "limb-salvage" surgery, in which cancerous tumor is removed from the bone without amputation. Because of the proximity of osteosarcomas to the knee joint, this often results in the removal of the joint itself as well. Patients who undergo a limb-salvage procedure will require a prosthesis or crutches to ambulate.

44. What is a rhabdomyosarcoma?
A soft-tissue tumor that arises from cells that give rise to striated skeletal muscle. It is the most common soft-tissue tumor of childhood.

45. Where do rhabdomyosarcomas usually arise?
The four most common areas are as follows: (1) the head and neck; (2) the genitourinary region; (3) the extremities; and (4) the orbit. The survival rate for those with tumors in other areas is dependent on the amount, if any, of tumor left after resection and the presence or absence of metastatic disease.

46. What sites of disease are associated with the best outcomes for children with rhabdomyosarcoma?
Favorable locations include the orbit, the head and neck (except for parameningeal tumors), the vagina, and the biliary tract. Unfavorable locations include the bladder, the prostate, and the parameninges.

> Crist WM, Anderson JR, Meza JL, et al: Intergroup rhabdomyosarcoma study-IV: Results for patients with nonmetastatic disease. J Clin Oncol 15:3091–3102, 2001.

47. What are the two major histologic subtypes of rhabdomyosarcoma?
Alveolar rhabdomyosarcoma, a name derived from its superficial appearance histologically to lung tissue, tends to occur in older children and adolescents. The majority of these tumors carry the t(2;13) translocation, and they carry a higher risk of recurrence. **Embryonal rhabdomyosarcomas** tend to occur in younger children, and they are the predominant histology associated with favorable site tumors.

48. Which germ-cell tumor is usually seen in young children?
The majority of germ-cell tumors that appear in young children are **benign teratomas** occurring in the sacrococcygeal region. In general, patients with mature teratomas are managed by surgical resection, with care taken for sacrococcygeal tumors to be sure that the entire coccyx is removed.

149. **Virilization may be associated with which childhood cancer?**
Tumors that cause virilism are most commonly those that produce large quantities of dehydroepiandrosterone, a 17-ketosteroid. Tumors that produce testosterone may also cause virilization. Most commonly these are benign tumors of the adrenal gland; rarely are they malignant. However, the distinction between carcinoma and benign adenoma is frequently difficult. Occasionally males with primary hepatic neoplasms may become virilized because of the production of androgens by the tumor.

150. **How great is the risk of malignant transformation in undescended testes?**
The risk of malignancy may be *5–10 times higher* in the undescended testis than in a normal testis. The risk in the contralateral testis may also be increased. Orchidopexy decreases, but does not eliminate, the risk of subsequent malignant transformation.

151. **What are the most common primary liver tumors of childhood?**
Hepatoblastoma and **hepatocellular carcinoma.** Hepatoblastomas usually develop in infants and young children, whereas hepatocellular carcinomas develop throughout childhood. Infection with hepatitis B and C virus are the greatest risk factors for the occurrence of hepatocellular carcinoma.

152. **Which tumor marker is most likely to be elevated in children with hepatic tumors?**
The majority of patients with either hepatoblastoma or hepatocellular carcinoma have an elevated concentration of alpha-fetoprotein that parallels disease activity. Lack of a significant decrease of alpha-fetoprotein with treatment may signify a poor response to therapy. Occasionally hepatoblastomas produce beta-human chorionic gonadotropin and can result in isosexual precocity.

153. **What factors predispose children to the development of hepatocellular carcinoma?**
Hepatitis B and C infection, especially in children with perinatally acquired virus. By contrast with adults, the incubation period from hepatitis virus infection to the development of hepatocellular carcinoma may be extremely short in children.

STEM-CELL TRANSPLANTATION

154. **Identify the three types of stem-cell transplantation.**
   - **Allogenic:** The transfer of bone marrow, peripheral blood stem cells, or umbilical cord blood from a donor to another individual
   - **Autologous:** The use of a person's own bone marrow or peripheral blood stem cells
   - **Syngeneic:** The transfer of bone marrow, peripheral blood stem cells, or umbilical cord blood from a genetically identical donor (i.e., identical twins)

155. **What is conditioning?**
Conditioning is the preparative process, performed by either chemotherapy or chemoradiotherapy, that is designed to destroy residual malignant cells, to provide immunosuppression to minimize the chance of rejection, and to create space in the marrow itself for the transplantation (bone-marrow ablation).

156. **What are the major side effects from total body irradiation used in conditioning?**
In the **short term,** total body irradiation may cause interstitial pneumonitis and nephritis. Over the **long term,** total body irradiation may lead to cataracts, growth retardation, hypothyroidism, other endocrine dysfunction, infertility, and secondary malignancies. The long-term

effects of total body irradiation on pulmonary, cardiac, and neuropsychiatric function continue to be studied.

157. **Do all transplant patients require complete ablation of their recipient bone marrow?**

No. Stem-cell transplants that do not ablate the recipient bone marrow are called nonmyeloablative transplants. Such transplants require vigorous immune suppression to maintain the donor graft as well as a disease that does not require intensive chemotherapy or full donor engraftment for success. Thus, patients with leukemias that respond well to a graft-versus-leukemia effect may benefit from the decreased morbidity and mortality of a reduced-intensity preparative regimen.

158. **What is the chance of siblings having the same human leukocyte antigen (HLA) type?**

The HLAs, which are located on chromosome 6, approximate simple Mendelian inheritance, with two siblings having a 1 in 4 chance of having the same typing. A 1% crossover of material may also occur during meiosis. The larger the family, the more likely a match becomes, as shown by the formula $[1 - (0.75)^n]$, with n being the number of siblings. Thus, a child with five brothers and sisters has a 76% chance of having a sibling with an HLA match.

159. **What is the chance of finding an HLA-matched unrelated donor?**

Although in theory the number of possibilities would equal or even exceed the world's population, thereby making a match astonishingly unlikely, HLA types cluster in individuals of similar genetic and racial backgrounds. In one estimate of persons of European ancestry, approximately 200,000 individuals would need to be screened to reach a 50% chance of finding a match.

Gahrton G: Bone marrow transplantation with unrelated volunteer donors. Eur J Cancer 27:1537–1539, 1991.

160. **How are tumor cells purged from a marrow or peripheral blood stem-cell specimen?**

- Immunologic methods using monoclonal antibodies
- Ex vivo use of chemotherapy
- Selective binding of tumor cells to lectins
- Treatment of marrow with antisense cDNA
- Selective culture of normal cells
- Selection of normal hematopoietic progenitor cells (e.g., CD34+ cells)

161. **What are the different sources of stem cells for transplantation?**

Stem cells may be obtained either from the peripheral blood, the bone marrow itself, or from the umbilical cord blood of a newborn. Peripheral blood stem cells are collected by leukocytapheresis, whereas bone marrow stem cells are collected by multiple bone marrow aspirates. Cord blood is harvested from the placenta at the time of delivery. Stored placental/cord blood is a useful source for patients without a related histocompatible donor because of less GVHD.

Rubenstein P, Corrier C, Scaradvou A, et al: Outcome among 562 recipients of placental-blood transplants from unrelated donors. N Engl J Med 1565–1577, 1998.

162. **What are the advantages and disadvantages of umbilical cord blood as the source for a stem-cell transplantation?**

Advantages

- No risk to mother or infant
- Available on demand after cryopreservation
- Can target minority families
- Donors not lost as a result of age, illness, or relocation

Disadvantages

- Limited number of stem cells in collection
- Possible lack of availability of additional donor cells if graft failure or relapse occurs
- Undiagnosed medical condition may be present in newborn

KEY POINTS: GRAFT-VERSUS-HOST DISEASE

1. Multiorgan inflammatory process caused by donor T lymphocytes

2. Primarily affects the skin, intestine, and liver

3. May cause functional asplenia

4. Mortality usually related to infection

5. Chronic patients at higher risk for bacterial sepsis (particularly pneumococcal), Pneumocystis, and fungal infections

163. **What is the most common worldwide reason for stem-cell transplantation?**
Beta-thalassemia.

164. **Which prophylactic measures should be taken after stem-cell transplantation?**
Patients may receive antibiotics for gut decontamination. An oral antifungal agent such as fluconazole is also frequently administered. Patients should receive *Pneumocystis carinii* prophylaxis and the replacement of immunoglobulins with IVIG. Acyclovir may also be administered.

165. **What are the major features of acute GVHD?**
Acute GVHD typically begins with a fever that is followed by a salmon-colored rash on the palms of the hands and the soles of the feet. The rash may be pruritic and may desquamate. Hepatitis (with jaundice and transaminase elevation) and gastroenteritis (with diarrhea, weight loss, and abdominal pain) may also occur.

166. **How is GVHD managed?**
Doses of methotrexate, cyclosporine, or tacrolimus during the immediate posttransplant period may be given in an attempt to prevent the development of acute GVHD. T-cell depletion of the bone-marrow graft also decreases the incidence of GVHD. For the treatment of acute GVHD, steroids, cyclosporine, or tacrolimus may be used alone or in combination, depending on the extent of donor-recipient mismatch and the severity of GVHD.

167. **After stem-cell infusion, what is the expected time course of engraftment and return of normal hematopoiesis?**
Patients generally recover leukocytes first; this is followed by red cells and then platelets. Evidence of white-cell engraftment generally occurs 8–14 days after the infusion of donor cells. Red-cell transfusion independence typically occurs during the first 6 weeks after the transplant. Complete recovery may take up to 6 months, although chronic GVHD may significantly impair recovery.

168. **How are acute GVHDs of the skin, gut, and liver graded?**
See Table 15-6.

TABLE 15-6. GRADING OF ACUTE GRAFT-VERSUS-HOST DISEASE OF SKIN, GUT, AND LIVER

	Grade I	Grade II	Grade III	Grade IV
Skin (area involved)	<25%	25–50%	>50%	Desquamation or blood loss
Gut (diarrhea L/d)	<0.5	0.5–1.0	1.0–1.5	Ileus, bloody diarrhea
Liver (bilirubin mg/dL)	<3	3–6	6–15	>15 or ↑ALT or AST

169. **What is the clinical grading of chronic GVHD?**
    - **Limited chronic GVHD** involves localized skin involvement (loss of elasticity, pigmentation changes, loss of sweat gland or hair follicles) or hepatic dysfunction; it is usually controlled with immunosuppressive agents.
    - **Extensive chronic GVHD** has either generalized skin involvement or local skin involvement with other organ system damage, including hepatic dysfunction, eye involvement (keratoconjunctivitis), mucosal involvement (sicca syndrome), or the involvement of any other organ. It is more difficult to control than limited chronic GVHD. Patients with extensive chronic GVHD are at high risk for infectious complications, which are the leading cause of morbidity and mortality among these patients.

170. **A 3-year-old patient who was given cyclophosphamide before receiving a bone-marrow transplant 7 days ago and who now receives cyclosporine for GVHD prophylaxis develops a seizure. What is the likely cause?**
    Although high-dose cyclophosphamide may cause fluid retention that can result in hyponatremia and seizures, this more commonly occurs during or immediately after cyclophosphamide administration. Seven days after transplant, cyclosporine is the more likely etiology of the seizures. Appropriate laboratory studies include a cyclosporine level as well as serum sodium, calcium, magnesium, and glucose levels. Toxic levels of cyclosporine would require decreases in the cyclosporine dose.

ACKNOWLEDGMENT

The editors gratefully acknowledge contributions by Dr. Peter Langmuir that were retained from the first three editions of *Pediatric Secrets*.

CHAPTER 16

ORTHOPEDICS

Joshua E. Hyman, MD

CLINICAL ISSUES

1. **What causes Sprengel's deformity?**
   Sprengel's deformity (congenital elevation of the scapula) results from the failure of normal scapular descent during fetal life, thereby resulting in an elevated, hypoplastic scapula. The affected side of the neck appears shorter and broader and may give the appearance of torticollis. A fibrocartilaginous band or omovertebral bone may bridge the space between the medial upper scapula and the spinous process of a cervical vertebra. Abduction of the ipsilateral arm is usually limited, but this limitation may not be clinically significant. Sprengel's deformity may be associated with congenital scoliosis and renal anomalies.

2. **What is torticollis?**
   Combined head tilt and rotatory deformity.

3. **What is the differential diagnosis for torticollis?**
   - **Osseous:** Atlanto-occipital anomalies, unilateral absence of C1, Klippel-Feil syndrome (fusion of cervical vertebrae), atlantoaxial rotatory displacement, basilar impression
   - **Nonosseous:** Congenital muscular torticollis, Sandifer's syndrome (severe gastroesophageal reflux), central nervous system tumors, syringomyelia, Arnold-Chiari malformation, ocular dysfunction (strabismus, oculogyric crisis), infections (cervical adenitis, retropharyngeal abscess), abnormal skin webs (pterygium colli)

4. **When does the mass of congenital muscular torticollis disappear?**
   In the presence of congenital muscular torticollis, a soft nontender mass may appear in the sternocleidomastoid muscle on the affected side. The mass reaches its maximal size at 1 month of age and usually disappears by 4–6 months. Histologically, it consists of dense fibrous tissue and may represent prenatal venous obstruction and muscle damage to the sternocleidomastoid muscle. Congenital muscular torticollis may be associated with developmental dysplasia of the hips.

5. **Are stretching exercises helpful for congenital muscular torticollis?**
   Studies have shown that conservative management with stretching—particularly when initiated at an early age—is very advantageous and lessens the potential need for surgical correction.

   Cheng JC, Wong MW, Tang SP, et al: Clinical determinants of the outcome of manual stretching in the treatment of congenital muscular torticollis in infants. A prospective study of eight hundred and twenty-one cases. J Bone Joint Surg 83-A:679–687, 2001.

6. **What is infantile cortical hyperostosis?**
   Caffey's disease (or syndrome), which usually occurs before 6 months of age, is a condition of unknown etiology that consists of tender, nonsuppurative, cortical swellings of the shafts of bone, most commonly the mandible and clavicle. It remits spontaneously, but exacerbations may persist for several years. In severe cases, corticosteroids may be helpful. Infantile cortical

hyperostosis is a rare condition. The presence of periosteal reaction, especially if asymmetric, should raise the suspicion of battered child syndrome.

7. **What is rickets?**
Rickets is the failure of osteoid to calcify in a growing child, and this is most commonly caused by a lack of vitamin D. The adult equivalent is osteomalacia.

8. **Why is rickets reappearing?**
   - There has been an increase in exclusive breast feeding for prolonged periods without vitamin D supplementation. Human milk is low in vitamin D, and the American Academy of Pediatrics recommends vitamin supplementation for breast-fed infants.
   - Reduced maternal sunlight exposure for cultural, societal, or personal reasons has become more common.
   - Immigrant groups who have increasingly migrated to more temperate regions have more children with this condition; reasons remain unclear for the increased incidence among these groups.

   Gordon CM, Bachrach LK, Carpenter TO, et al: Bone health in children and adolescents: A symposium at the annual meeting of the Pediatric Academic Societies/Lawson Wilkins Pediatric Endocrine Society, May 2003. Curr Probl Pediatr Adolesc Health Care 34:226–242, 2004.
   Wharton B, Bishop N: Rickets. Lancet 362:1389–1400, 2003.

9. **What is the best x-ray view to obtain for evaluating possible rickets?**
Anterior view of the knee, incorporating femoral and tibial metaphyses and epiphyses. Bone growth is most rapid in this area, and rachitic changes are seen earliest at this location.

10. **What x-ray changes are noted in patients with rickets?**
    - Cupping, fraying, and irregularity of the metaphyses
    - Widening of the physis as a result of increased osteoid
    - Loss or increased separation of the zone of provisional calcification
    - Periosteal reaction (appears to separate from diaphysis as a result of increased osteoid)
    - Coarsening of trabeculae
    - Loss of bone density
    - Bowing of long bones

11. **What are the physical signs that are suggestive of rickets?**
The anatomic abnormalities of rickets result primarily from the inability to normally mineralize osteoid; the bones become weak and subsequently distorted. Signs of rickets include the following:
    - Craniotabes
    - Femoral and tibial bowing
    - Delayed suture and fontanel closure
    - "Pigeon breast" (sternal protrusion as a result of use of accessory muscles)
    - Frontal thickening and bossing
    - Defective tooth enamel
    - Harrison's groove (a rim of rib indentation at the insertion of the diaphragm)
    - Palpably widened physes at wrists and ankles
    - "Rachitic rosary" (enlarged costochondral junctions)

12. **Which growth sites are known to develop aseptic necrosis?**
The **osteochondroses** are a group of disorders in which aseptic necrosis of growth centers (epiphyses and apophyses) occurs, with subsequent fragmentation and repair (Table 16-1). The exact cause is unknown. The patient usually has pain at the affected site.

TABLE 16-1. TYPICAL AGE OF ONSET OF OSTEOCHONDROSES		
Location	**Eponym**	**Typical Age of Onset (years)**
Tarsal navicular bone	Köhler's disease	6
Capitellum of distal humerus	Panner's disease	9–11
Carpal lunate	Kienböck's disease	16–20
Distal lunar epiphysis	Burns' disease	13–20
Head of femur	Legg-Calvé-Perthes disease	3–5
Second metatarsal head	Freiberg's disease	12–14
Calcaneal Achilles tendon insertion	Sever's disease	8–9

13. **What are the skeletal dysplasias?**

The skeletal dysplasias are a group of disorders that are characterized by an intrinsic abnormality in the growth and remodeling of cartilage and bone. These generalized disturbances in the development of the skeleton affect the skull, spine, and extremities to varying degrees. Children with this condition frequently have disproportionate short stature and dysmorphic facial features.

14. **Discuss the inheritance pattern and clinical features of osteogenesis imperfecta.**

Of the several types of osteogenesis imperfecta, the most common is type IV, which occurs in 1 in 30,000 live births. The clinical features vary and depend on the severity of the condition (Table 16-2).

TABLE 16-2. TYPES OF OSTEOGENESIS IMPERFECTA		
Type	**Inheritance**	**Clinical Features**
I	Autosomal dominant	Bone fragility, blue sclerae, onset of fractures after birth (most at preschool age)
Type A		Without dentinogenesis imperfecta
Type B		With dentinogenesis imperfecta
II	Autosomal recessive	Lethal in perinatal period, dark blue sclerae, concertina femurs, beaded ribs
III	Autosomal recessive	Fractures at birth, progressive deformity, normal sclerae and hearing
IV	Autosomal dominant	Bone fragility, normal sclerae, normal hearing
Type A		Without dentinogenesis imperfecta
Type B		With dentinogenesis imperfecta

15. **McCune-Albright syndrome is associated with what skeletal abnormalities?**

Polyostotic fibrous dysplasia (i.e., fibrous tissue replacing bones). The fibrous dysplasia occurs most commonly in the long bones and the pelvis and may result in deformity and/or increased thickness of bone. There is associated precocious puberty and café-au-lait spots.

16. **What are the causes of in-toeing gait (pigeon toeing)?**
The condition may be due to problems anywhere in the lower extremity.

Foot:	Metatarsus adductus
	Metatarsus varus
	Talipes equinovarus (clubfoot)
	Pes planus (flat feet)
Leg:	Tibial torsion (internal)
	Genu valgum (knock knees)
	Tibia vara (Blount disease)
	Bow legs
Hip:	Femoral anteversion (medial femoral torsion)
	Paralysis (polio, myelomeningocele)
	Spasticity (cerebral palsy)
	Maldirected acetabulum

Tunnessen WW, Jr.: Signs and Symptoms in Pediatrics, 3rd ed. Philadelphia, Lippincott Williams & Wilkins, 1999, pp 693–695.

17. **A 15-year-old with tibial pain (which is worse at night and relieved by aspirin) has a small hypodense area surrounded by reactive bone formation on x-ray. What is the likely diagnosis?**
Osteoid osteoma, which is a benign bone-forming tumor. It is typically seen in older children and adolescents and exhibits a male predominance (male-to-female ratio, 2:1). Most children complain of localized pain, usually in the femur and tibia; however, arms and vertebrae may also be involved. Radiographs and computed tomography scans demonstrate an osteolytic area surrounded by densely sclerotic reactive bone, and bone scans reveal "hot spots." The site is usually <1 cm in diameter and arises at the junction of old and new cortex. Pathologically, the lesion is highly vascularized fibrous tissue with an osteoid matrix and poorly calcified bone spicules surrounded by a dense zone of sclerotic bone. Treatment is surgical excision.

18. **What is the clinical significance of limb-length discrepancy?**
A significant portion of the population has mild limb-length discrepancy. Limb-length discrepancies of <2 cm in a skeletally mature individual usually require no treatment. In addition to quantitating leg discrepancy in a skeletally immature child, it is important to estimate what the limb-length discrepancy will be at skeletal maturity. This can be done by periodically measuring leg-length discrepancy radiographically and using charts, such as the Green and Anderson "growth-remaining graph" or the Moseley "straight-line graph," to calculate anticipated leg-length discrepancy at skeletal maturity. Assessment of skeletal age is based on the bone age from an anteroposterior hand and wrist radiograph.

19. **What are the possible causes of a limb-length discrepancy?**
   - **Congenital anomalies:** Congenital short femur, proximal femoral focal deficiency, congenital absence of fibula, posteromedial bowing of tibia, tibial hypoplasia, congenital hemihypertrophy
   - **Tumors:** Neurofibromatosis, fibrous dysplasia, enchondromatosis, hereditary multiple exostosis, Klippel-Trénaunay-Weber syndrome
   - **Trauma:** Physeal injuries, fracture
   - **Infection:** Septic arthritis, osteomyelitis
   - **Inflammation:** Juvenile rheumatoid arthritis

20. **What are the long-term effects of uncorrected limb-length discrepancy?**
Equinus contracture of the ankle, scoliosis, low-back problems, and late degenerative arthritis of the hip.

21. **What are the general management principles for a limb-length discrepancy?**
    - **0–2 cm:** No treatment
    - **2–6 cm:** Shoe lift, epiphysiodesis
    - **6–20 cm:** Limb lengthening
    - **>20 cm:** Prosthetic fitting

    There is flexibility in these guidelines to account for factors such as environment, motivation, intelligence, compliance, emotional stability, patient and parent wishes, and associated pathology in the limbs.

    Guidera KJ, Helal AA, Zuern KA: Management of pediatric limb length inequality. Adv Pediatr 42:501–543, 1995.

22. **What is a nursemaid's elbow?**
    Also known as a "pulled elbow," a nursemaid's elbow is a subluxation of the radial head resulting from axial traction applied to the extended arm of a young child. The child is typically unwilling to move the affected limb, and there is tenderness directly over their radial head. Radiographs are normal in this condition. The diagnosis is made by history and physical examination. Discomfort is relieved by reducing the subluxation; this is accomplished by the forceful supination of the extended forearm followed by flexion of the forearm. An audible and palpable click is occasionally present. After successful reduction, the child begins to use the arm spontaneously. If symptoms persist, the child should be reassessed for a possible fracture.

23. **Why have many Little Leagues banned the throwing of a curve ball?**
    To minimize the cases of Little League elbow, which is a medial epicondylitis that results from overuse and flexor-pronator strain. The throwing of a curve ball puts extra stress on the ulnar collateral ligament of the medial aspect of the elbow. Severe strain can result in partial separation of the apophysis, and, occasionally, bony avulsions can occur.

24. **What signs and symptoms suggest a serious cause of back pain in a child that warrants further evaluation?**
    - **Symptoms:** Pain in children <4 years old; interference with daily activities in school, play, or athletics; pain persistence of >4 weeks; night pain (associated with tumor); radiation down the leg (suggests herniated disc or apophysis)
    - **Signs:** Concurrent fever; postural changes; neurologic abnormalities; reproducible point tenderness; limitation of motion on forward bending

    Thompson GH: Back pain in children. J Bone Joint Surg Am 75:928–937, 1993.

25. **What is the differential diagnosis of back pain in children?**
    - **Infectious:** Discitis, vertebral osteomyelitis, vertebral tuberculosis
    - **Developmental:** Scheuermann's kyphosis, scoliosis, spondylolysis, spondylolisthesis
    - **Traumatic:** Herniated disc, muscle strain, fractures, slipped vertebral apophysis
    - **Inflammatory:** Juvenile rheumatoid arthritis, ankylosing spondylitis
    - **Neoplastic:** Eosinophilic granuloma, osteoid osteoma, aneurysmal bone cyst, leukemia, lymphoma, Ewing's sarcoma, osteosarcoma
    - **Visceral:** Urinary tract infection, hydronephrosis, ovarian cysts, inflammatory bowel disease

26. **Do school backpacks contribute to back pain?**
    This is controversial, but some experts suggest that the limits of maximum loads lifted by children should be 10–15% of body weight. In some studies, more than a third of students carried more than 30% of their body weight at least once during the school week. With an apparent increasing incidence of back pain in children and adolescents (particularly those with open epiphyses), the bulging backpack may be one contributing cause.

    Sheir-Neiss GI, Kruse RW, Rahman T, et al: The association of backpack use and back pain in adolescents. Spine 28:922–930, 2003.

    Siambanes D, Martinez JW, Butler EW, Haider T: Influence of school backpacks on adolescent back pain. J Pediatr Ortho 24:211–217, 2004.

27. **Which sports injuries are the most common in school-aged children and adolescents?**

Some 75% of injuries in school-aged children involve the lower extremities, and a majority of injuries to the knee and ankle are reinjuries as a result of incomplete healing from a previous problem. Contusions and sprains are the most common types of injury, with fractures and dislocations accounting for an additional 10–20%. Cranial injuries are the most common cause of sports fatality.

Adolescent boys who participate in contact team sports, particularly football and wrestling, are at the highest risk for injuries. Among girls, softball and gymnastics have the highest injury rate.

Only 10% of sports injuries are caused by an opponent; most injuries are caused by stumbling, falling, or misstepping. The latter finding suggests that improving intrinsic factors (e.g., raising the level of physical fitness, avoiding overuse, and strengthening joint stability) may be more important for the prevention of injuries than external factors (e.g., the choice of equipment).

28. **What entities most commonly constitute orthopedic emergencies?**

Open fracture, impending compartment syndrome, dislocation of major joints (i.e., knee, hip, spine), septic arthritis, and major arterial injury.

KEY POINTS: PEDIATRIC ORTHOPEDIC EMERGENCIES— NO DELAY!

1. Open fracture

2. Impending compartment syndrome

3. Dislocation of major joints

4. Septic arthritis

5. Arterial injury

FOOT DISORDERS

29. **Do infants and children need shoes?**

Barefoot is the natural state of the foot. Individuals who spend most of their lives unshod have stronger feet and fewer foot deformities than those who wear shoes. Before they begin walking, infants do not need foot coverings other than to keep their feet warm. Once the child begins to walk, shoes will offer protection from the cold and from sharp objects.

30. **What advice should be given to a parent about buying shoes for a toddler?**

The best shoe is one that simulates the barefoot:
- The shoe should easily flex.
- The bottom of the shoe should be flat. Heels should be avoided because they tend to force the foot forward and cramp the toes.
- The shoe should be foot-shaped and generously fitted. The toe box should be wide and high to properly accommodate the toddler's pudgy feet.
- The sole should have the same friction as the skin on the bottom of the child's foot.

31. **What is the most common congenital foot abnormality?**
    Metatarsus adductus. In patients with this condition, the front part of the foot (the forefoot) is turned inward as a result of adduction of the metatarsi at the tarsometatarsal joints associated with normal alignment of the hindfoot and midfoot (Fig. 16-1). Most cases are mild and flexible, with the foot easily dorsiflexed and the lateral aspect easily straightened by passive stretching. A simple test to determine if the kidney-shaped curvature is within normal limits is to draw a line that bisects the heel. When extended, this line normally falls between the second and third toe space. If it falls more laterally, metatarsus adductus is present. In utero positioning is the suspected cause of the condition. It is seen more frequently in first-born children, presumably because primigravida mothers have stronger muscle tone in the uterine and abdominal walls.

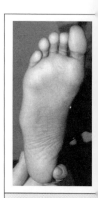

Figure 16-1. Metatarsus adductus. (From Jay RM: Foot and Ankle Pearls. Philadelphia, Hanley & Belfus, 2002, p 52.)

32. **How is metatarsus adductus treated?**
    If the foot can be passively abducted beyond neutral, the prognosis is excellent for a spontaneous correction without any therapeutic intervention. In those feet that are stiffer, a program of passive stretching is in order. The parents are taught to hold the heel in a neutral position and manually abduct the forefoot using their thumb placed over the cuboid as a fulcrum. This exaggerated position should be held for a few seconds and the stretching repeated 10 times each session. These sessions should occur with bathing and diaper changing.

33. **How do congenital metatarsus adductus and congenital metatarsus varus differ?**
    Both deformities are types of kidney-shaped feet in which the forefoot becomes adducted as a result of varying degrees of intrauterine compression. In **metatarsus adductus**, there is no bone abnormality, and the curvature can be readily corrected by passive stretch. In **metatarsus varus**, there is subluxation of the tarsometatarsal joints when the foot is dorsiflexed. Physical examination usually reveals a deep medial cleft, prominence of the base of the fifth metatarsal, and an inability to correct the forefoot passively to align with the heel. Making the distinction is important, because metatarsus adductus usually resolves spontaneously, whereas metatarsus varus gradually worsens without treatment.

    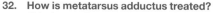
    Craig CL, Goldberg MJ: Foot and leg problems. Pediatr Rev 14:395–400, 1993.

34. **How is clubfoot distinguished from severe metatarsus varus?**
    Clubfoot, or talipes equinovarus congenita, is distinguished pathologically by a combination of forefoot and hindfoot abnormalities (e.g., malrotation of the talus under the calcaneus and plantar flexion or equinus of the ankle). As a rule, clubfoot is a rigid deformity, whereas metatarsus is more flexible. If the ankle can be dorsiflexed to neutral or beyond, metatarsus is a much more likely diagnosis.

35. **How are clubfeet treated?**
    Many clubfeet respond well to serial casting. The casts should be applied as soon after birth as possible, and they are changed weekly. Over the course of 2–3 months, significant improvement in the shape of the foot can be seen. About 80% of the feet that are corrected with casting will require an Achilles tenotomy to correct the equinus deformity. Those feet that are not adequately corrected with casting will require surgical release.

36. **What is a calcaneovalgus foot?**
    This common deformity is the result of an in utero "packaging defect" and is considered a normal variant. The foot lies in an acutely dorsiflexed position, with the top of the foot in contact

with the anterolateral surface of the leg. The heel is in severe valgus, and the forefoot is markedly abducted. Overall the foot is flexible, and both the heel and the forefoot can be corrected into varus. Spontaneous correction is the norm. However, having parents passively stretch the foot is often beneficial.

37. **What foot abnormality results in the appearance of a "Persian slipper" foot?**
Also called "rocker bottom foot," this abnormality is due to **congenital vertical talus**. Lateral radiographs reveal a vertically oriented talus with dislocation of the talonavicular joint. On examination, the forefoot is markedly dorsiflexed, and the heel is rigid and points downward, giving the sole the characteristic convex or boat-shaped appearance. Serial casting and subsequent surgical reversion are the usual treatments. The syndrome most commonly associated with this deformity is trisomy 18.

38. **What should be suspected when pes cavus is noted on examination?**
Pes cavus, or high-arched feet (often associated with claw toes), can result from contractures or disturbed muscle balance (Fig. 16-2). A neurologic cause should be suspected. The differential diagnosis includes normal familial variant, Charcot-Marie-Tooth disease, spina bifida, cauda equina lesion, peroneal muscle atrophy, Friedreich's ataxia, Hurler's syndrome, and polio.

39. **Should children with flexible flat feet be given corrective shoes?**
Flexible flat feet (**pes planovalgus**) is a common finding in infants and children and ≤15% of adults. During weight-bearing activity, the medial longitudinal arch is depressed toward the ground formation, and the heel is in valgus (outward) position. There are no radiographic parameters that define a flat foot; it is felt to be a normal variant that results from ligamentous laxity. Children do not complain of pain, and an arch can be created easily by having the child stand on his/her toes or by dorsiflexing the great toe. This condition is distinguished from pathologic flat feet in which lack of weight bearing

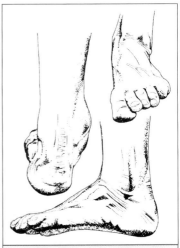

Figure 16-2. Pes cavus. (From Mellion MB, Walsh WM, Shelton GL: The Team Physician's Handbook, 2nd ed. Philadelphia, Hanley & Belfus, 1997, p 603.)

does not lessen the flatness and rigidity is present on physical examination. Prospective studies have shown that corrective shoes or plastic insets (orthotics) are not necessary in children with flexible flat feet because the arch spontaneously develops during the first 8 years of life.

Wenger DR, Mauldin D, Speck G, et al: Corrective shoes and inserts as treatment for flexible flat feet in infants and children. J Bone Joint Surg 71:800–810, 1989.

40. **How does the cause of foot pain vary by age?**
- **0–6 years:** Ill-fitting shoes, foreign body, occult fracture, osteomyelitis, juvenile rheumatoid arthritis (if other joints are involved), rheumatic fever (hypermobile flat foot)
- **6–12 years:** Ill-fitting shoes, foreign body, accessory navicular bone, occult fracture, tarsal coalition (peroneal spastic flat foot), ingrown toenail, Ewing's sarcoma (hypermobile flat foot)
- **12–19 years:** Ill-fitting shoes, foreign body, ingrown toenail, pes cavus, hypermobile flat foot with tight Achilles tendon, ankle sprains, stress fracture, Ewing's sarcoma, synovial sarcoma

Gross RH: Foot pain in children. Pediatr Clin North Am 33:1395–1409, 1986.

41. **A 10-year-old boy with recurrent ankle sprains and painful flat feet should be evaluated for what possible diagnosis?**

Tarsal coalition. Fusion of various tarsal bones via fibrous or bony bridges can result in a stiff foot that inverts with difficulty. When inversion of the foot is done during an examination, tenderness occurs on the lateral aspect of the foot, and peroneal tendons become very prominent. Thus, the condition is also referred to as "peroneal spastic flat foot." Unless the condition is very severe and warrants surgery, corrective shoes are usually adequate treatment. Other possible causes of a rigid flat foot include rheumatoid arthritis, septic arthritis, posttraumatic arthritis, neuromuscular conditions, and congenital vertical talus.

FRACTURES

42. **What are the most common types of fractures in children?**

Physeal and **metaphyseal** fractures are the most common in children, and they are unique to pediatrics. These are sites where children's bones are weakest and ossification is not yet complete. Buckle (compression) and greenstick (incomplete) fractures are also common.

43. **Where are the most frequent sites of fractures among children?**
- Clavicle
- Distal radius
- Distal ulna

44. **What is an open fracture?**

The fracture site is communicated with the external environment. Open fractures have higher incidence of developing infection and a higher degree of soft-tissue damage as compared with closed fractures.

45. **What is a toddler fracture?**

A toddler fracture is a fracture of the tibia in a child 9 months to 3 years old as a result of low-energy forces. Typically, these fractures have a spiral appearance and are not displaced. The fibula is rarely fractured. The child will have a limp or an inability to bear weight. Immobilization in a splint or cast for 3 weeks is the usual treatment.

46. **How are growth-plate fractures classified?**

The **Salter-Harris classification** of growth-plate (physis) injuries (Fig. 16-3) was devised in 1963:
- **Type I:** Epiphysis and metaphysis separate; usually no displacement occurs as a result of the strong periosteum; radiograph may be normal; tenderness over the physis may be the only sign; normal growth after 2–3 week cast immobilization
- **Type II:** Fragment of metaphysis splits with epiphysis; usually closed reduction; casting is for 3–6 weeks (longer for lower extremity than upper extremity); growth usually not affected, except distal femur and tibia

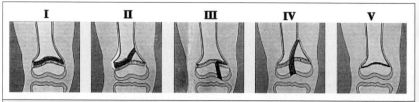

Figure 16-3. Salter-Harris classification. (From Katz DS, Math KR, Groskin SA (eds): Radiology Secrets. Philadelphia, Hanley & Belfus, 1998, p 403.)

- **Type III:** Partial plate fracture involving a physeal and epiphyseal fracture to the joint surface; occurs when growth plate is partially fused; closed reduction more difficult to achieve
- **Type IV:** Extensive fracture involving epiphysis, physis, metaphysis, and joint surface; high risk for growth disruption unless proper reduction (usually done operatively) is obtained
- **Type V:** Crush injury to the physis; high risk for growth disruption

47. What are the sequelae of growth-plate fractures?

Most growth-plate fractures heal without incidence. If there is an injury to the growth plate, a growth disturbance may occur; these are caused by the formation of a bony bridge or bar at the site of physeal damage. If there is damage to the entire physis, premature physeal closure occurs, with resulting longitudinal growth arrest. Asymmetric closure leads to angular deformity of the limb.

48. What is the most common cause of a pathologic fracture?

Also called **secondary fractures**, these are fractures through a bone that is weakened by a pathologic process. The most common such fracture is through unicameral bone cysts (simple bone cysts). These cysts usually occur in the metaphysis of a long bone, most frequently the humerus. They occur predominantly in males, are usually asymptomatic (until a fracture occurs), are centrally located in the bone, and are often quite large.

49. In a patient with suspected fracture, what are the key points on physical examination?

Assess "the five Ps" in the affected extremity:

- **P**ain and point tenderness
- **P**ulse (distal to the fracture)
- **P**allor
- **P**aresthesia (distal to the fracture)
- **P**aralysis (distal to the fracture)

Examine for pain above and below the suspected injury site; multiple fractures are known to occur. The involved extremity should also be carefully examined for deformity, swelling, crepitus, discoloration, and open wounds. A primary concern in any evaluation is a distal neurovascular compromise, which may require immediate surgical intervention.

50. What are the signs of compartment syndrome?

The five Ps noted in the preceding question are seen in impending or established compartment syndrome in which swelling is causing distal ischemia. Among these signs, significant pain with passive stretching of the digits (either flexion or extension) raises suspicion. After the nerve is severely damaged, the patient does not complain of pain. Compartment syndrome is often unrecognized in unconscious patients. A high index of suspicion must be maintained in patients with severe injuries and an altered mental status. In addition, a frightened young child or infant may be very difficult to examine. If there is any concern about compartment syndrome, the compartment pressures must be measured.

51. What is the treatment of compartment syndrome?

Compartment syndrome is an emergency. Compartment pressures can be lowered by incision of the skin and fascia of the involved compartments (e.g., anterior, lateral, deep posterior, superficial posterior in the leg). The wound is left open and covered with sterile dressing until swelling decreases. Dressing changes and partial wound closure are usually done in the operating room. Skin grafts may be necessary.

52. How do you treat a simple clavicular fracture?

These fractures are best managed with a sling and activity restriction. Union occurs in 2–4 weeks, but the sling may be removed once the child is comfortable. The residual bump (fracture callus) may take up to 2 years to smooth out (remodel). Surgery is only necessary if the fracture is open, if there is a neurovascular injury, or if the vascularity of the skin is compromised from significant displacement.

53. **A teenager who punches a wall in anger typically incurs what fracture?**
Boxer fracture. This is a fracture of the distal fifth metacarpal, usually with apical dorsal angulation (Fig. 16-4). Up to 35% of dorsal angulation can be accepted without compromise of function. Reduction often requires pin fixation.

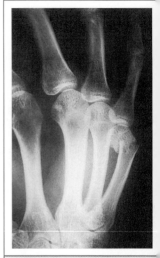

54. **Children who fall on outstretched arms often suffer what type of fractures?**
Colles' fractures. This is a group of complete fractures of the distal radius with varying displacement of the distal fragment. The fall, with the hand outstretched, wrist dorsiflexed, and forearm pronated, often results in a classic "dinner-fork" deformity of the wrist on examination.

55. **What does the presence of the posterior fat pad on an elbow x-ray suggest?**
Of the two fat pads that overlie the elbow joint, only the anterior one is visible on a lateral x-ray. If fluid accumulates in the joint space, as it does in cases involving bleeding, inflammation, or fracture, the fat pads are displaced upward and outward. The position of the anterior pad changes, and the posterior pad becomes visible. If acute trauma has occurred, a fracture should be suspected, and immobilization should be continued, with follow-up studies as needed.

Figure 16-4. Boxer fracture with fracture of fifth (and fourth) metacarpal with volar displacement of the distal fragments after a punching injury. (From Katz DS, Math KR, Groskin SA (eds): Radiology Secrets. Philadelphia, Hanley & Belfus, 1998, p 440.)

56. **In a teenager with wrist trauma, why is palpation of the anatomic "snuff box" a critical part of the physical sign?**
The anatomic snuff box (the inpouching formed by the tendons of the abductor pollicis longus and extensor pollicis longus when the thumb is abducted [in hitchhiker fashion]) sits just above the scaphoid (carpal navicular) bone. The scaphoid is the carpal bone that is most commonly fractured, and these fractures are at higher risk for nonunion or avascular necrosis. Snuff box tenderness, pain on supination with resistance, and pain on longitudinal compression of the thumb should increase suspicion for fracture of the scaphoid bone. Even when an x-ray is negative, if there is significant snuff box tenderness, a fracture should be suspected and the wrist and thumb immobilized. A repeat x-ray in 2–3 weeks may better reveal a fracture. If very high clinical suspicion exists, magnetic resonance imaging can identify a fracture when the plain film is negative.

57. **Name the eight carpal bones of the wrist.**
Disdaining some of the classic (mostly obscene) mnemonics, remember what will happen if a wrist fracture is missed:
Sinister **L**awyers **T**ake **P**hysicians **T**o **T**he **C**ourt **H**ouse
In order of proximal to distal, lateral to medial: **S**caphoid, **l**unate, **t**riquetrum, **p**isiform, **t**rapezium, **t**rapezoid, **c**apitate, and **h**amate.

58. **In pediatric fractures, what amount of angulation is acceptable before reduction is recommended?**
Acceptable angulation or displacement varies with a child's age. Younger children have remarkable healing potential to remodel with minimal to no residual deformity or limitation of rotation. As a rule, in children up to 8 years old, as much as 30° of angulation will heal satisfactorily without reduction. In older children, percentages are lower. In general, fractures that are in the metaphysis or growth plate remodel more completely than midshaft fractures. Rotational malalignment will not remodel.

59. **In which fractures will remodeling of bone *not* occur?**
Bony deformities in children (angulation, displacement, and shortening) can remodel as bone is removed from the tension side and placed on the compression side of the deformity by the redirection of physeal growth. Factors that favor remodeling include young age, proximity of the fracture to the physis, and angulation in the plane of motion of the adjacent joint. The following fractures have a low chance of remodeling and may require closed or open reduction: intra-articular fractures; fractures with excessive shortening, angulation, or rotation; displaced epiphyseal plate fractures; and midshaft or diaphyseal fractures.

60. **How long should fractures be immobilized?**
Children's fractures generally heal more quickly than their counterparts in adults. The length of immobilization, however, depends on several variables, including the child's age, the location of the fracture, and the type of treatment. As a rule of thumb, physeal, epiphyseal, and metaphyseal fractures heal more rapidly than diaphyseal fractures. On average, epiphyseal, physeal, and metaphyseal fractures heal in children within 3–5 weeks, whereas diaphyseal fractures may heal within 4–6 weeks.

www.castroom.com

61. **How long do fractured clavicles and femurs take to heal?**
- **Newborn:** Clavicle, 10–14 days; femur, 3 weeks
- **16-year-old child:** Clavicle, 6 weeks; femur, 6–10 weeks

62. **When is open reduction of a fracture indicated?**
An open reduction is an operative reduction of a fracture. Open reduction may be combined with internal fixation with pins, plates, or screws. Indications include the following:
- Failed closed reduction (often in older children with displaced fractures)
- Displaced intra-articular fractures
- Displaced Salter-Harris III and IV fractures (to prevent premature growth plate closure)
- Unstable fractures in patients with head trauma
- Open fractures (for irrigation and débridement)

HIP DISORDERS

63. **Why has DDH replaced CHD?**
The term *developmental dysplasia of the hip* (DDH) has replaced *congenital hip dislocation* (CHD) to reflect the evolutionary nature of hip problems in infants during the first months of life. About 2.5–6.5 infants per 1,000 live births develop problems, and a significant percentage of these are not present on neonatal screening examinations. Clearly, the overt pathologic process may not be present at birth, and periodic examination of the infant's hip is recommended at each routine well-baby examination until the age of 1 year.
   DDH also refers to the entire spectrum of abnormalities involving the growing hip, ranging from dysplasia to subluxation to dislocation of the hip joint. Unlike CHD, DDH refers to alter-

ations in the hip growth and stability in utero, during the newborn period, and during the infant period. DDH also refers to hip disorders associated with neurologic disorders (e.g., myelomeningocele), connective tissue disorders (e.g., Ehlers-Danlos syndrome), myopathic disorders (e.g., arthrogryposis multiplex congenital), and syndromic conditions (e.g., Larsen's syndrome).

Bauchner H: Developmental dysplasia of the hip (DDH): an evolving science. Arch Dis Child 83:202, 2000.

64. **What are the Ortolani and Barlow maneuvers?**
The most reliable clinical methods of detection remain the Ortolani reduction and the Barlow provocative maneuvers. The infant should be lying quietly supine. Both examinations begin with the hips flexed to 90°. To perform the **Ortolani maneuver**, the hip is abducted, and the trochanter is gently elevated. This allows a dislocated femoral head to glide back into the acetabulum (Fig. 16-5, *A*). The **Barlow maneuver** is performed by adducting the flexed hip and gently pushing the thigh posteriorly in an effort to dislocate the femoral head (Fig. 16-5, *B*).

KEY POINTS: THE FOUR FS OF INCREASED RISK FOR DEVELOPMENTAL DISLOCATION OF THE HIP

1. First born

2. Female

3. Funny presentation (breech)

4. Family history (positive for developmental dysplasia of the hip)

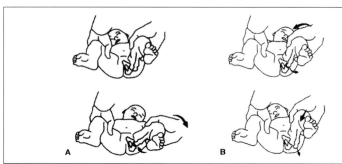

Figure 16-5. *A*, Ortolani maneuver. *B*, Barlow maneuver. (From Staheli LT (ed): Pediatric Orthopedic Secrets. Philadelphia, Hanley & Belfus, 1998, p 166.)

65. **What is the significance of a "hip click" in a newborn?**
A hip click is the high-pitched sensation felt at the very end of abduction when testing for development dysplasia of the hip with the Barlow and Ortolani maneuvers; it occurs in ≤10% of newborns. Classically, it is differentiated from a hip "clunk," which is heard and felt as the hip goes in and out of joint. Although a debatable point, the hip click is felt to be benign. Its cause is unclear and may be the result of movement of the ligamentum teres between the femoral head and the acetabulum or the hip adductors as they slide over the cartilaginous greater trochanter. Worrisome features that might warrant evaluation (e.g., hip ultrasound, hip x-ray) include late

onset of the click, associated orthopedic abnormalities, and other clinical features suggestive of developmental dysplasia (e.g., asymmetric skin folds/creases, unequal leg length).

Witt C: Detecting developmental dysplasia of the hip. Adv Neonatal Care 3:65–75, 2003.

66. **What is the most reliable physical finding for DDH in the older child?**
Limited hip abduction. This is the result of shortening of the adductor muscles.

67. **What other diagnostic signs are suggestive of DDH?**
- **Asymmetry of the thigh and gluteal folds:** However, these may be present in ≤10% of normal infants.
- **Galeazzi test:** With the hips flexed at 90°, the knees may be at different levels as a result of apparent femoral shortening on one side in asymmetric dislocation.
- **Allis test:** With the hips flexed and the heels on the table, uneven knee level suggests hip dislocation.
- **Waddling gait, hyperlordosis of lumbar spine:** This is seen in older patients with bilateral dislocations.

68. **What radiographic studies are most valuable for diagnosing DDH during the newborn period?**
In infants <6 months old, the acetabulum and the proximal femur are predominantly cartilaginous and thus not visible on plain x-ray. In this age group, these structures are best visualized with **ultrasound**. In addition to morphologic information, ultrasound provides dynamic information about the stability of the hip joint.

Weintroub S, Grill F: Ultrasonography in developmental dysplasia of the hip. J Bone Joint Surg 82-A:1004–1018, 2000.

69. **Should all infants be routinely screened by ultrasound for DDH?**
Because physical examination is not completely reliable and the incidence of late-diagnosed DDH has not declined, some investigators have recommended routine ultrasonographic screening. However, others argue that ultrasonography can lead to overdiagnosis and treatment. At present, the issue remains controversial. Universal screening is more commonly done in Europe, whereas in the United States selective screening on the basis of risk factors and physical examination findings is more the norm.

American Academy of Pediatrics: Clinical practice guideline: Early detection of developmental dysplasia of the hip. Pediatrics 105:896–905, 2000.

70. **Who is at a higher risk for DDH?**
Dislocated, dislocatable, and subluxable hip problems occur in about 1–5% of infants. However, 70% of dislocated hips occur in girls, and 20% occur in infants born in breech position. Other risk associations include the following:
- Congenital torticollis
- Skull or facial abnormalities
- First pregnancy
- Positive family history of dislocation
- Metatarsus adductus
- Calcaneovalgus foot deformities in infants <2500 gm
- Amniotic fluid abnormalities (especially oligohydramnios)
- Prolonged rupture of membranes
- Large birthweight

MacEwen GD: Congenital dislocation of the hip. Pediatr Rev 11:249–252, 1990.

71. **How is DDH treated?**
The first goal is to obtain a reduction and maintain that reduction to provide an optimal environment for femoral head and acetabular development. This is accomplished by keeping the

legs abducted and the hips and knees flexed. The most commonly used devices are the Pavlik harness, the Frejka pillow, and the van Rosen splint. Triple diapers have no role in the treatment of DDH; they provide the parents with a false sense of security and do not provide reliable stabilization or positioning.

Wenger DR, Bomar JD: Human hip dysplasia: Evolution of current treatment concepts. J Ortho Sci 8:264–271, 2003.

72. **What is the natural history of untreated DDH?**

A child with *unilateral* DDH may have a leg-length discrepancy and painless (Trendelenburg) limp throughout childhood and young adulthood. Osteoarthritis of the hip joint may develop during the fifth decade of life. Hip fusion and total hip arthroplasty are surgical treatment options for the symptomatic hip in young adults. Children with *bilateral* DDH often have no leg-length inequality and no appreciable limp. They tend to walk with hyperextension of the lumbar spine (hyperlordosis) and have a waddling gait. As with patients with unilateral DDH, these patients tend to develop early osteoarthritis. Total hip arthroplasty is the treatment of choice for adults with symptomatic bilateral DDH.

Some recent studies suggest that a high percentage of newborns with DDH may spontaneously improve without treatment.

Bialik V, Bialik GM, Blazer S, et al: Developmental dysplasia of the hip: A new approach to incidence. Pediatrics 103:93–99, 1999.

73. **What is the significance of a positive Trendelenburg test?**

If a normal individual stands on one leg, ipsilateral hip abductors (primarily the gluteus medius) prevent the pelvis from tilting, and balance is maintained (Fig. 16-6). Children >4 years old can usually stand this way for at least 30 seconds. If the opposite side of the pelvis does tilt or the trunk lurches to maintain balance, this is a positive Trendelenburg sign. It may be an indicator of muscle weakness (as a result of muscular or neurologic pathology) or of hip instability (e.g., acetabular dysplasia).

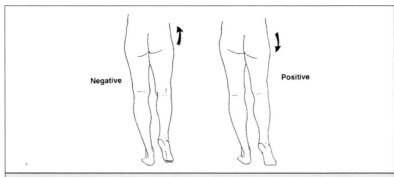

Figure 16-6. Trendelenburg sign. The pelvis tilts toward the normal hip when weight is borne on the affected side. (From Goldstein B, Chavez F: Applied anatomy of the lower extremities. Phys Med Rehabil State Art Rev 10:601–603, 1996.)

74. **What is a Trendelenburg gait?**

A Trendelenburg gait results from functionally weakened hip abductor muscles. It is commonly seen in children with a dislocated hip. With a dislocated hip, the abductor muscles are at a mechanical disadvantage and are effectively weakened, which makes it difficult for them to support the child's body weight. As a result, the pelvis tilts away from the affected hip. In an effort to minimize this imbalance during the stance phase of gait, children lean over the affected hip.

75. **What is the most common cause of a painful hip in a child <10 years old?**
Acute transient synovitis; this condition has also been called toxic synovitis, irritable hip, and coxitis fugax. This is a self-limited inflammatory condition that occurs before adolescence, has no known cause, and generally has a benign clinical outcome. However, it can cause considerable anxiety among physicians and family members during its clinical course, because it can mimic other, more sinister, conditions such septic arthritis, soft-tissue injury, osteomyelitis, Legg-Calvé-Perthes (LCP) disorder, juvenile rheumatoid arthritis, slipped capital femoral epiphysis, and tumor. It may occur anytime from the toddler age group to the late juvenile years, but the peak age of onset is between 3 and 6 years, and it is more common among boys. Acute transient synovitis remains a diagnosis of exclusion. Treatment consists of rest and reduction of the synovitis with anti-inflammatory agents. Most patients experience complete resolution of their symptoms within 2 weeks of onset; the remainder may have symptoms of lesser severity for several weeks.

   Do TT: Transient synovitis as a cause of painful limps in children. Curr Opin Pediatr 12:48–51, 2000.

76. **How can transient synovitis be differentiated from septic arthritis?**
See Table 16-3.

TABLE 16–3.	TRANSIENT SYNOVITIS VERSUS SEPTIC ARTHRITIS	
	Transient Synovitis	**Septic Arthritis**
History	Preceding upper respiratory infection ± low-grade fever	Fever
		Usually large joint involvement (hip,
	Hip or referred knee pain	ankle, knee, shoulder, elbow)
	Limp	
Physical	Refusal to bear weight	Exquisite pain, swelling, warmth
	Can delicately elicit range of motion in affected hip joint	Marked resistance to mobility
Laboratory	ESR normal or mildly elevated	ESR markedly elevated
	Mild peripheral leukocytosis	Leukocytosis with left shift
	Negative blood culture	Often positive blood culture
	Joint fluid cloudy	Joint fluid purulent
	Negative Gram stain	Often positive Gram stain
Radiographs	Occasionally shows fluid in joint space	Possible associated bony findings (early osteomyelitis)

ESR = Erythrocyte sedimentation rate.

77. **What is LCP disease?**
LCP disease is a disorder of the femoral head of unknown etiology that is characterized by ischemic necrosis, collapse, and subsequent repair (Fig. 16-7). Children typically present with pain and/or a limp. The pain may be localized to the groin or may be referred to the thigh or knee.

78. **What are the pathologic stages of LCP disease?**
LCP is a condition of aseptic necrosis of the femoral head involving children primarily between the ages of 4 and 10 years.

- **Incipient or synovitis stage:** Lasting 1–3 weeks, this first stage is characterized by an increase in hip-joint fluid and a swollen synovium associated with reduced movement.
- **Avascular necrosis:** Lasting 6 months–1 year, the blood supply stops to part (or all) of the head of the femur. That portion of the bone essentially dies, but the contour of the femoral head remains unchanged.
- **Fragmentation or regeneration and revascularization:** In the last and longest pathologic stage of LCP, which lasts 1–3 years, the blood supply returns and causes both the resorption of necrotic bone and the laying down of new immature bone. Permanent hip deformity can occur during this last stage.

It is important to note that plain radiographs may lag behind the progression of the disorder by as much as 3–6 months. Radionuclide bone scans are much better, because early ischemia and avascular necrosis are depicted as decreased localizations of isotope.

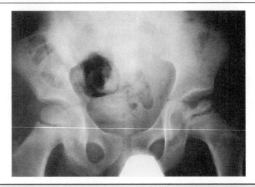

Figure 16-7. Anteroposterior view of the pelvis demonstrates fragmentation and irregularity of the left femoral head in a patient with Legg-Calvé-Perthes disease. The right hip is normal. (From Katz DS, Math KR, Groskin SA (eds): Radiology Secrets. Philadelphia, Hanley & Belfus, 1998, p 405.)

79. **What is the prognosis for children with LCP disease?**
    The two main prognostic factors for LCP disease include the age of the child and the amount of epiphyseal involvement. Children <6 years old tend to have a more favorable prognosis, and those with less epiphyseal involvement also tend to have a better prognosis. Epiphyseal involvement has been classified by Salter into type A (those with <50% epiphyseal involvement) and type B (those with >50% head involvement).

80. **Which conditions are associated with coxa vara?**
    Coxa vara is a condition of a decreased femur shaft-neck angle. The three most common associations are developmental coxa vara, avascular necrosis of the femoral head, and cleidocranial dysostosis.

81. **What condition does the child in Fig. 16-8 have?**
    This is **femoral anteversion** (or medial femoral torsion), which is a common cause of in-toeing in

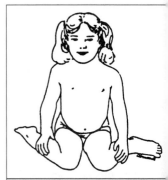

Figure 16-8. Reverse tailor position.

younger children. The child is demonstrating the reverse tailor position, which is a sign of the internally rotated hip.

Staheli LT: Torsional deformity. Pediatr Clin North Am 33:1382, 1986.

82. **How is the extent of femoral anteversion measured?**
With the child lying prone and knees flexed at 90°, the hip normally cannot be rotated internally (i.e., feet pushed outward) more than 60° (angle A in Fig. 16-9, *A*). In addition, external rotation (angle B in Fig. 16-9, *B*) should exceed 20°. A normal child averages approximately 35°. Abnormal results indicate that the cause of in-toeing is likely the result of physiologic femoral anteversion (or, less commonly, hip capsular contractions as are seen in patients with cerebral palsy).

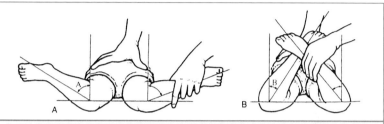

Figure 16-9. Measurement of femoral anteversion. (From Dormans JP: Orthopedic management of children with cerebral palsy. Pediatr Clin North Am 40:650, 1993.)

83. **What symptoms do children with slipped capital femoral epiphysis (SCFE) have?**
SCFE involves progressive displacement with external rotation of the femur on the epiphyseal growth plate. The patient has intermittent or constant hip, thigh, or knee pain that has often lasted weeks to months. In 25%, the pain is bilateral. A limp, a lack of internal rotation, and a hip flexion contracture may be noted. If the patient's hip is flexed, the thigh tends to fall into external rotation. It is important to realize that any patient with knee pain may have underlying hip pathology.

84. **What systemic conditions are associated with SCFE?**
Children with SCFE tend to have delayed skeletal maturation and obesity and usually present between the ages of 8–14 years. This suggests that hormonal factors may lessen the bone's ability to resist shearing forces, thereby resulting in a pathologic fracture through the proximal femoral physis. Systemic factors associated with SCFE include hypothyroidism, panhypopituitarism, hypogonadism, rickets, and irradiation.

INFECTIOUS DISEASES

85. **What percentage of septic arthritis is "culture negative"?**
Several studies have established that 30–60% of patients with clinically apparent septic arthritis have negative cultures of joint fluid. Reasons (both postulated and confirmed) for this observation include the fastidious nature of some less common etiologies of infectious arthritis (e.g., *Kingella kingae*), the loss of viability of some organisms on transport to the laboratory (e.g., *Neisseria* species), and perhaps a substance or cell population in the aspirate fluid that is bacteriostatic during in vitro culture conditions. Prompt processing of specimens and the use of several culture techniques (e.g., solid media plus liquid-culture systems such as those used for blood cultures) can increase the yield of joint fluid cultures.

86. **Which patients with septic arthritis warrant open drainage?**

There is debate regarding the relative merits of open surgical drainage versus repeated needle aspiration. Three settings warrant consideration for surgical intervention:

1. Septic arthritis of the hip (and possibly of the shoulder)
2. Large amounts of fibrin, debris, or loculation within the involved joint space
3. Lack of improvement in 3 days by medical treatment alone

> Dagan R: Management of acute hematogenous osteomyelitis and septic arthritis in the pediatric patient. Pediatr Infect Dis J 12:88–93, 1993.

87. **Where does acute hematogenous osteomyelitis most commonly localize in children?**

Lower extremity (femur, tibia, fibula)	70%
Upper extremity (humerus, radius, ulna)	15%
Foot	4%
Pelvis	4%
Vertebrae, skull, ribs, sternum, scapulae	2%

> Gold R: Diagnosis of osteomyelitis. Pediatr Rev 12:292–297, 1991.

88. **What are the most common bacterial agents found in patients with osteomyelitis?**

Neonates	**Children**
Staphylococcus aureus	*Staphylococcus aureus*
Group B streptococci	Group A streptococci
Enterobacteriaceae (*Salmonella, Escherichia coli,*	*Haemophilus influenzae*
Pseudomonas, Klebsiella)	

The incidence of *H. influenzae* osteomyelitis has significantly declined as a result of immunization.

89. **How helpful is a screening white blood count (WBC) for the diagnosis of osteomyelitis?**

Not very. In two thirds of patients, the total WBC is normal (although in half of these, the differential is shifted to the left). In the other one third, the WBC is elevated, usually with a left shift. The erythrocyte sedimentation rate (ESR) is more sensitive, with 95% of cases having an ESR >15 mm/h with an average rate of 70 mm/h.

90. **How often are blood cultures positive in patients with osteomyelitis?**

Only 50% of the time or less. Because this rate is relatively low, direct bone aspiration should be strongly considered. Aspiration raises the yield to 70–80% and greatly facilitates antibiotic therapy.

91. **As osteomyelitis progresses, how soon do x-ray changes occur?**

- **3–4 days:** Deep-muscle plane shifted away from periosteal surface
- **4–10 days:** Blurring of deep-tissue muscle planes
- **10–15 days:** Changes in bone occur (e.g., osseous lucencies, punched-out lytic lesions, periosteal elevation)

92. **What is the best way to confirm the diagnosis of osteomyelitis?**

Bone infections in children are typically accompanied by fever, local pain, and decreased use of the affected body part (e.g., limp or failure to bear weight). Although point tenderness is often elicited, plain radiographs may appear normal during the first 7–10 days of infection, until a sufficient portion of cortex is damaged. Early during the course of infection, other imaging studies (bone scintigraphy or magnetic resonance imaging) or direct aspiration with Gram stain and culture can be of use for confirming the diagnosis.

93. When treating osteomyelitis, which serum bactericidal level is a better indicator of successful outcome: peak or trough?

Both may be important. Peak titers (i.e., those found at approximately 20–30 minutes after infusion) are associated with successful treatment in acute osteomyelitis if they are ≥1:8 and in chronic osteomyelitis if they are ≥1:16. Trough titers are predictive of a good outcome if they are ≥1:2 in acute osteomyelitis and if they are ≥1:4 in chronic osteomyelitis.

94. When is treatment of osteomyelitis with oral antibiotic agents appropriate?

- An identified organism
- Available oral antibiotic against the organism
- Adequate surgical débridement
- Improving clinical course when receiving intravenous antibiotics
- Patient without vomiting or diarrhea
- Adequate serum levels can be obtained with oral therapy
- Reliable parents and/or patient

Nelson J: Skeletal infections in children. Adv Pediatr Infect Dis 6:59–78, 1991.

95. How long should antibiotics be continued in patients with osteomyelitis and septic arthritis?

The precise answer is unclear, but infections caused by *Staphylococcus aureus* or enteric gram-negative bacteria must be treated for longer periods than those caused by *Haemophilus influenzae, Neisseria meningitidis,* or *Streptococcus pneumoniae*. A minimum of 4–6 weeks is likely necessary for the former group, and 2–3 weeks are needed for the latter. If diagnosis has been delayed, if initial clinical response is poor, or if the ESR remains elevated, longer durations may be needed.

96. When is open surgical drainage indicated in cases of osteomyelitis?

- Abscess formation in the bone, subperiosteum, or adjacent soft tissue
- Bacteremia persisting >49–72 hours after the initiation of antibiotic treatment
- Continued clinical symptoms (e.g., fever, pain, swelling) after 72 hours of therapy
- Development of a sinus tract
- Presence of a sequestrum (i.e., detached piece of necrotic bone)

Darville T, Jacobs RF: Management of acute hematogenous osteomyelitis in children. Ped Infect Dis J 23:255–257, 2004.

97. Why are treatment failures more common in osteomyelitis than in septic arthritis?

- Antibiotic concentrations are much greater in joint fluid than in inflamed bone. Concentrations in joint fluid may actually exceed peak serum concentrations, whereas those in bone may be significantly less than serum concentrations.
- Devitalized bone may serve as an ongoing nidus for infection.
- Diagnosis of osteomyelitis is more likely to be delayed than that of septic arthritis.

98. How do the features of osteomyelitis in the neonate differ from those seen in the older child and adult?

- Neonatal osteomyelitis almost invariably follows hematogenous dissemination.
- Multiple foci of infection are frequently seen.
- Septic arthritis is a frequent association, probably reflecting the spread of infection via blood vessels penetrating the epiphyseal plates.
- The pathogens causing neonatal osteomyelitis are the same as those responsible for sepsis neonatorum.

99. Why are young children more susceptible to infectious discitis than adolescents or adults?

Increased susceptibility in younger children is to the result of differing anatomy of the spine. In children <12 years old, blood vessels extend from the vertebral body through hyaline cartilage to supply nutrition directly to the intervertebral disc and nucleus pulposus. These vessels slowly regress until the adult picture is reached (age 12), at which time nutrition to the nucleus pulposu is supplied primarily by diffusion. The extra blood vessels during early life may facilitate the hematogenous spread of infection or the direct extension of early vertebral osteomyelitis.

KEY POINTS: OSTEOMYELITIS

1. The most common causative organisms in healthy children are *Staphylococcus aureus* and beta-hemolytic streptococci.

2. In children (unlike adults), spread of bacteria to bone is hematogenous rather than by local trauma.

3. In children with a puncture wound and osteomyelitis, think *Pseudomonas aeruginosa*.

4. Because of intravascular sludging and infarction, patients with sickle cell disease are at increased risk, especially for *Salmonella* infections.

5. Bone changes on x-ray may not occur for 10–15 days.

6. Up to 50% of patients with osteomyelitis may have a normal total white blood cell count.

100. How is the diagnosis of discitis established?

Discitis, which is the infection and/or inflammation of the intervertebral disc, most commonly occurs in children between the ages of 4 and 10 years. The etiology is often unclear, but a bacterial cause (particularly *Staphylococcus aureus*) is identified by blood cultures in about 50% of cases. The diagnosis can be difficult because of varied accompanying symptoms, including generalized back pain with or without localized tenderness, refusal to stand or walk, back stiffness with loss of lumbar lordosis, abdominal pain, and unexplained low-grade fever.

As with osteomyelitis, a most helpful laboratory test is an elevated ESR. WBCs may often b normal, and early x-rays (<2–4 weeks of symptoms) may not show changes. Technetium-99 bone scans will demonstrate abnormalities early during the course of illness. Magnetic resonance imaging studies can help distinguish between discitis and vertebral osteomyelitis.

Treatment consists of 3–6 weeks of antistaphylococcal antibiotics, with variable amounts o immobilization and bracing, depending on severity of symptoms. Persistent or atypical cases may require biopsy to identify the etiology.

Early SD, Kay RM, Tolo VT: Childhood diskitis. J Am Acad Orthop Surg 11:413–420, 2003.

101. When is bone scintigraphy used for the evaluation of children with obscure skeletal pain?

When correlated with clinical findings, the results of bone scintigraphy can help localize an abnormality in the bones, joints, or soft tissues. Additional unrelated asymptomatic lesions may also be identified. The bone scan is very sensitive but not very specific. Often, other diagnostic tests are needed to establish the exact etiology of the pain. A bone scan should only be considered after a careful history and physical examination have been performed and plain x-rays of the abnormal area are obtained. The scan is most useful for establishing or ruling ou occult infection or bone tumor.

Kothari NA, Pelchovitz DJ, Meyer JS: Imaging of musculoskeletal infections. Radiol Clin North Am 39:653–671, 2001.

02. What are the phases of a bone scan?
The phases are generally demarcated by the time elapsed since injection of the radionuclide dye.

- **Phase I—Angiographic phase:** During the first few seconds, the dye passes through the large blood vessels and provides early assessment of regional vascularity and perfusion.
- **Phase II—Blood pool phase:** Usually obtained during the first minutes after an injection, this phase highlights the movement of the dye into the extracellular spaces of soft tissue and bone.
- **Phase III—Delayed phase:** By 1.5–3 hours after injection, the dye localizes in the bone with minimal soft-tissue imaging.
- The three-phase process is used to differentiate soft tissue from bony abnormalities. At times a **Phase IV** study may be done by rescanning for the same dye at 24 hours, which further minimizes soft-tissue background activity.

KNEE, TIBIA, AND ANKLE DISORDERS

03. What is the difference between valgus and varus deformities?
Some things seem to be destined to be learned, forgotten, and relearned many times as a rite of passage: the Krebs cycle is one; this is another. The terms refer to angular deformities of the musculoskeletal system. If the distal part of the deformity points toward the midline, the term is *varus*. If the distal part points away from the midline, it is *valgus*. For example, in patients with knock knees, the lower portion of the deformity points away, so the term is *genu valgum*.

Another method is to consider the body in the supine (anatomic) position. Draw a circle around the body. All angles conforming to the curve of the circle are varus; all angles going against the circle are valgus. Bowleggedness conforms to the circle around the body and is, therefore, *genu varum*.

04. Are children normally knock-kneed or bowlegged?
It varies by age. If you use the tibiofemoral angle (the angle formed by the tibia and the femur) as a guide, most children at birth are bowlegged (genu varum) up to 20°, but this tendency progressively diminishes until about 24 months, when the trend toward knock knees (genu valgum) begins. Knock knees continue to the age of 3 years (up to 15°) and then begin to diminish. At about the age of 8 years, most children are—and will remain—knock-kneed at about 7° (Fig. 16-10).

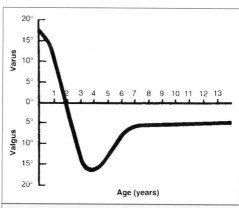

Figure 16-10. Development of the tibiofemoral angle during growth. (From Bruce RW, Jr: Torsional and angular deformities. Pediatr Clin North Am 43:875, 1996.)

05. Which bowlegged infants or toddlers require evaluation?
Radiographs should be considered if bowleggedness demonstrates any of the following features:

- Present after 24 months (the time of normal progression to physiologic genu valgum)
- Worse after age 1 as the infant begins to bear weight and walk

- Unilateral
- Visually >20° (tibiofemoral angle)

106. **What are the causes of pathologic genu varum (bowleggedness) or genu valgus (knock knees)?**

Genu varum	Genu valgum
Physiologic bow legs	Hypophosphatemic rickets
Infantile tibia vara	Previous metaphyseal fracture of the proximal tibia
Hypophosphatemic rickets	Multiple epiphyseal dysplasia
Metaphyseal chondrodysplasia	Pseudoachondroplasia
Focal fibrocartilaginous dysplasia	

Sass P, Hassan G: Lower extremity abnormalities in children. Am Fam Physician 68:461–468, 2003.

107. **Which children are more likely to develop Blount disease?**
Tibia vara, or Blount disease, is a medial angulation of the tibia in the proximal metaphyseal region as a result of a growth disturbance in the medial aspect of the proximal tibial epiphysis. In the infantile type, the child is usually obese and an early walker, and he or she develops pronounced bowlegs during the first year of life. Black females are particularly at risk for severe deformity. In the adolescent variety, the onset occurs during late childhood or early adolescence, and the deformity is usually unilateral and mild. Correction of severe deformity often requires surgical intervention.

108. **How does tibial torsion change with age?**
Tibial torsion, which is the most common cause of in-toeing in children between the ages of 1 and 3 years, gradually rotates externally with age. For excessive internal rotation, bracing was used extensively in the past, but its efficacy is questionable because the natural history of the condition is self-resolution. Measurement is done by noting the thigh–foot angle with the knee flexed to 90°.

109. **How effective is the Denis Browne splint for the treatment of tibial torsion?**
The splint consists of a metal bar connected to shoes or strings about the feet; the bar provides varying degrees of external rotation. The splint has been used in children with tibial torsion in whom spontaneous correction is not occurring. However, there is no scientific evidence that this device alters the natural history of tibial torsion.

110. **What is the most likely diagnosis if a 15-year-old basketball player has painful swelling below both knees?**
Osgood-Schlatter disease. A traction apophysitis, the condition results from repetitive microtrauma to the immature tibial tubercle, which is the site of the insertion of the knee extensor mechanism on the proximal tibia. It is related to the adolescent growth spurt and the level of physical activity. Physical examination reveals tenderness to palpation and swelling over the tibial tubercle. The pain is exacerbated with resisted knee extension.

Appropriate clinical management includes the judicious use of anti-inflammatory medications, restricted activities, quadriceps stretching and strengthening, and cross training. The condition is usually self-limited and resolves with skeletal maturity. Immobilization, which may lead to disuse atrophy, is rarely necessary.

111. **What painful condition is snowshoeing likely to produce?**
Shin splints. This term describes the pain and cramping felt in the compartments of the lower leg after strenuous exercise. It is rare in children but may be seen in teenagers who exercise (especially running on hard surfaces) after extended periods of inactivity. The pain results from muscle strain and inflammation of the musculotendinous units. Swelling and cramping occur,

particularly in the flexor digitorum longus muscle, which flexes the lateral four toes and plantar-flexes the foot at the ankle joint. The muscle swelling may contribute to ischemia. Snowshoeing may be the ultimate test of the anterior tibial muscles.

12. **Which long bone is most frequently absent congenitally?**
The **fibula**. Absence of the fibula may be partial or complete and is usually unilateral. The involved leg is shortened and commonly demonstrates bowing of the tibia and slight shortening of the femur. The foot usually shows a severe deformity with equinus and valgus deformities with absence or abnormal development of the lateral toes.

13. **Why are ligamentous injuries unusual in children?**
In children, ligaments are stronger than growth plates and thus the growth plate will fail (i.e., fracture) before the ligament tears.

14. **How are ankle sprains graded?**
Between 80% and 90% of ankle sprains are the result of excessive inversion and/or plantar-flexion resulting in injury to the lateral ligaments (anterior talofibular and calcaneofibular). The anterior ankle drawer sign is a test of ankle stability (particularly the anterior talofibular ligament). It is accomplished by immobilizing the lower tibia with one hand and, with the ankle at 90°, moving the heel and foot forward with the other hand. If there is marked laxity with a poor endpoint, a complete tear or *third-degree sprain* is likely. Moderately increased laxity as compared with the other ankle indicates a partial tear or *second-degree sprain*. No laxity indicates a *first-degree sprain*.

15. **Which ankle sprains should be evaluated with an x-ray?**
More than 5,000,000 radiographs are estimated to be taken annually in children and adults for ankle injuries, yet there are no widely accepted guidelines. One set of guidelines (the Ottawa Ankle Rules) suggests obtaining an x-ray if there is malleolar pain and one or both of the following conditions is present: (1) the inability to bear weight for four steps immediately after the injury and during office or emergency room evaluation; and/or (2) bone tenderness at the posterior edge or tip of either malleolus. When these simple criteria were used in studies involving children and adults, no fractures were missed, and unnecessary x-rays were reduced by 25%.

Clark KD, Tanner S: Evaluation of the Ottawa Ankle Rules in children. Pediatr Emerg Care 19:73–78, 2003.

16. **Should ankle sprains be casted?**
If inversion ankle sprains are not complicated by a fracture or peroneal tendon dislocation, casting is not warranted. It has no benefit over early immobilization with a wrap, such as commercially available air stirrups. Additionally, complete immobilization may delay rehabilitation.

17. **How should knee pain be evaluated?**
Evaluation by history and physical examination should focus not only on the offending knee but also the hip and the contralateral knee. The history should seek information regarding the mechanism of injury, the onset and duration of pain, the change in pain with activities and rest, and the presence of night pain. The precise location of the pain is crucial to making the correct diagnosis. The effects of previous treatments, presence of swelling, locking, or giving way are also pertinent points. For the examination, the patient should be in shorts or a gown. Always examine both knees; the uninjured knee will serve as a normal control. Begin with an evaluation of gait, lower-extremity weight-bearing alignment, muscle definition, leg lengths, swelling, and ligaments. Next, test for range of motion (active/passive), effusion, tenderness

(joint line, physis, patella, tibial tubercle, collateral ligaments), strength, patella tracking, and stability.

118. **What is the most significant mistake made during the evaluation of knee pain?**
Failure to evaluate the hip as a source of the pain. Hip pathology frequently masquerades as knee pain (e.g., Perthes' disease, slipped capital femoral epiphysis).

119. **If a ninth-grade soccer player with knee swelling "felt a pop" while scoring a goal, what are three possible diagnoses?**
A pop or snap sensation in the setting of acute knee injury is usually associated with the following:
1. Anterior cruciate ligament injury
2. Meniscal injury
3. Patellar subluxation

120. **In acute injury, what are the main causes of blood in the knee joint?**
Acute hemarthrosis is most commonly the result of the following:
- Rupture of the anterior or posterior cruciate ligaments
- Peripheral meniscal tears
- Intratrabecular fracture
- Major disruption or tear in the joint capsule

121. **How common are meniscal tears in younger children?**
Meniscal tears rarely occur before the age of 12 years. A discoid meniscus is a congenitally abnormal meniscus and can appear at almost any age. Meniscal tears in youths are typically associated with significant injuries that arise from a memorable event. They produce pain, swelling, and limping. There is often an associated injury to the anterior cruciate ligament.

122. **A 5-year-old boy with a painless swelling in the back of his knee has what likely condition?**
Popliteal cyst. Also called Baker cysts, these are occur more frequently in boys, are usually found on the medial side of the popliteal fossa, and are painless. In children, the cysts are rarely associated with intra-articular pathology. The natural history is for the cyst to disappear spontaneously after 6–24 months. A prolonged period of observation is recommended before considering surgical excision. Atypical findings (e.g., tenderness, firmness, history of rapid enlargement, pain) are justification for further diagnostic evaluation.

> Seil R, Rupp S, Jochum P, et al: Prevalence of popliteal cysts in children. A sonographic study and review of the literature. Arch Orthop Trauma Surg 119:73–75, 1999.

123. **A teenager has chronic knee pain, swelling, and occasional "locking" of the knee joint, and his x-ray reveals increased density and fragmentation at the medial femoral condyle. What condition does he likely have?**
Osteochondritis dissecans. In this avascular necrosis syndrome, focal necrosis of articular cartilage and underlying bone occurs. The cause is unknown, but antecedent trauma is common. The section of bone may detach and lodge in the contiguous joint. Males are more commonly affected, and pain occurs, especially with strenuous activity. Associated findings may include stiffness, swelling, clicking, and occasional locking. A plain radiograph can reveal the diagnosis, but magnetic resonance imaging is more sensitive when findings are equivocal. Extended immobilization is the primary treatment. Continued pain or locking of the joint warrants the consideration of arthroscopy to search for intra-articular fragments. Long-term complications can include degenerative arthritis.

124. **What predisposes a child or teenager to recurrent dislocation of the patella?**
- **Orthopedic conditions:** Genu valgum, patella alta, hypoplasia of the lateral femoral condyle, laterally located tibial tubercle, vastus medialis insufficiency, abnormal attachment of the iliotibial tract
- **Syndromes of generalized ligamentous laxity:** Down syndrome, Ehlers-Danlos syndrome, Marfan's syndrome, Turner's syndrome

Mizuta H, Kubota K, Shiraishi M, et al: Recurrent dislocation of the patella in Turner syndrome. J Pediatr Orthop 14:74–77, 1994.

125. **Who manifests the apprehension sign?**
Individuals with acute or subacute *subluxation* or *dislocation of the patella.* With the patient's knee supported at 30°, the examiner applies pressure to the medial border of the patella. If the patient displays impending distress or apprehension, the test is positive. No discomfort makes patellar pathology less likely. The apprehension sign is also seen in individuals with *shoulder instability* (especially glenohumeral problems) who fear dislocation when certain maneuvers are performed. For anterior instability, the arm is placed in maximal external rotation and abduction (similar to an overhand throw position). For posterior instability, the shoulder is placed at 90° of forward flexion and internal rotation.

126. **How does patellofemoral stress syndrome occur?**
This major cause of chronic knee pain in teenagers results from malalignment of the extensor mechanism of the knee as a result of a variety of causes. It is most commonly seen as an "overuse" entity in sports that involve running and full-knee flexion (e.g., track, soccer). It has been inappropriately called *chondromalacia patella,* which is a specific pathologic diagnosis of an abnormal articular surface that occurs in a minority of these patients. The patella serves as the fulcrum on which the various muscles of the quadriceps extend the knee. Forces may act asymmetrically, thereby causing greater stress on the lateral aspect of the patella, especially in individuals with anteversion of the femur, external torsion of the patella, high (alta) patella, abnormally developed quadriceps, excessive flattening of the femoral groove, or a wide Q angle. Treatment consists of ice, rest, nonsteroidal anti-inflammatory drugs, quadriceps strengthening, hamstring stretching, and possibly patellar-stabilizing braces.

127. **What is the Q angle?**
Draw a line from the anterior-superior iliac spine through the center of the patella, and then draw a line from the center of the patella to the tibial tubercle. The resultant angle is the Q angle, also called the quadriceps angle. For teenage males, the average Q angle is 14°, and, for females, it is 17°. Angles of >20° predispose individuals (particularly runners) to chronic knee pain because of patellar strain.

SPINAL DISORDERS

128. **What is the differential diagnosis for scoliosis?**
Scoliosis is a lateral curvature of the spine (i.e., coronal plane deformity). *Kyphosis* and *lordosis* are posterior and anterior curvatures, respectively (i.e., sagittal plane deformity). About 1–2% of the pediatric population have a spinal deformity, but very few are severe enough to require treatment: 85% of cases are idiopathic; 5% are congenital (including hemivertebrae and vertebral fusions); 5% are neuromuscular (cerebral palsy, polio, spinal muscular atrophy, muscular dystrophy); and 5% are miscellaneous (e.g., Marfan's syndrome, Ehlers-Danlos syndrome, tumors).

Ahn UM, Ahn NU, Nallamshetty L, et al: The etiology of adolescent idiopathic scoliosis. Am J Ortho 31:387–395, 2002.

129. **How is screening for spinal deformity performed?**
The child should be undressed or dressed only in underwear or a gown (open from the back). From the back and side, the child is examined standing, flexed forward at the hips, and sitting (to eliminate leg-length inequality). The head and arms hang down unsupported. The contour of the back is observed from the side, the rear, and the front for the following signs that can suggest scoliosis:
- Shoulder or scapular asymmetry
- Visible deformity of spinous processes
- Asymmetry of paraspinal muscles or rib cage in the thoracic spine while bending (>0.5 cm in lumbar region and >1.0 cm in thoracic region; a scoliometer may be used for this determination)
- Sagittal plane deformity when viewed from the side
- Waist-crease asymmetry that does not disappear when sitting (most waist-crease asymmetries are the result of minor leg-length discrepancies)
- Excessive thoracic kyphosis during forward-bending when viewed from the side

130. **What constitutes an abnormal scoliometric measurement?**
The scoliometer (also called an inclinometer) is a type of protractor used to measure the vertebral rotation and rib humping that is seen in scoliosis with the forward-bending test. An angle of ≤5° is usually insignificant; an angle of ≥7° warrants consideration of standing posteroanterior and lateral radiographs for more precise assessment of curvature.

131. **Are males or females more likely to have scoliosis?**
Females are five times more likely than males to have scoliosis.

132. **How valuable are school-based screening programs for scoliosis?**
This is controversial. About 26 states in the United States mandate school scoliosis screening. Experts in favor of these programs contend that reliable screening procedures exist and that early identification will lead to earlier nonoperative care and the prevention of progression and of the need for surgical intervention. Opponents argue that the low incidence of children requiring treatment, the low positive-predictive value of screening programs, and high numbers of children unnecessarily referred do not justify the programs. The U.S. Preventive Services Task Force now recommends against the routine screening of asymptomatic adolescents for idiopathic scoliosis.

U.S. Preventive Services Task Force: Screening for idiopathic scoliosis in adolescents: Recommendation statement. Am Fam Physician 71:1975–1976, 2005.

133. **How is scoliosis measured by the Cobb method?**
This is the standard technique used to quantify scoliosis in posteroanterior or lateral radiographs. One line is drawn along the vertebra tilted the most at the top of the curve, and another is drawn at the bottom of the curve. The curvature is represented by angle "a," which can be measured in two ways, as illustrated in Fig. 16-11.

134. **Why is Risser staging important when evaluating patients with scoliosis?**
Risser staging is a method of estimating bone growth potential on the basis of the appearance of the iliac crest on radiographs that are taken for scoliosis. Scoliosis progresses most during the rapid growth phase of adolescence. The **iliac apophysis** is the secondary ossification center that develops laterally to the iliac crest and that can be used to quantify the remaining growth potential. Stage I begins shortly after puberty, and stage IV indicates that spinal growth is nearly complete. Stage V, which is seen in adults, indicates complete fusion. If a patient has entered stage IV or V, progression of scoliosis is unlikely. Earlier stages indicate that careful follow-up examinations must be done because of increased risk of progression.

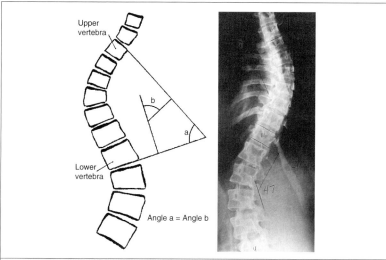

Figure 16-11. Measurement of the Cobb angle. (From Kaz DS, Math KR, Groskin SA (eds): Radiology Secrets. Philadelphia, Hanley & Belfus, 1998, p 321.)

35. **What is the recommended treatment of scoliosis?**
    - Observation with serial examinations every 4–6 months if the patient is mature and the curvature is <25°
    - Bracing if the curvature is 25–40° with >2 years of growth remaining
    - Surgery if the curvature is >40°

KEY POINTS: SCOLIOSIS

1. Scoliosis of >10° is relatively common (1–2%), but progression to ≥25° and required treatment is rare.

2. Bracing will not eliminate curvature, but it may prevent progression.

3. Establishing the maturity level of bone is important because the risk of progression is increased with immaturity.

4. Progressive curves are seven times more likely to appear in girls than in boys.

5. All scoliosis is not idiopathic: assess for limb-length discrepancy, neurocutaneous signs, and neurologic abnormalities, especially reflexes.

36. **What is the differential diagnosis of disc-space narrowing seen on a radiograph?**
    Disc-space infection, posttraumatic changes, congenital abnormalities, and tumor. If the patient has disc-space narrowing and a history of pain, the diagnosis of acute disc-space infection is likely. Asymptomatic patients with isolated findings of disc-space infection may have congenital abnormalities (e.g., congenital kyphosis, failure of segmentation).

137. **What diagnosis should you consider in a teenage male with very poor posture that is not self-correctable?**

     Scheuermann's kyphosis. This is a wedge-shaped deformity of the vertebral bodies of unclear etiology that causes juvenile kyphosis (abnormally large dorsal thoracic or lumber curves). Common in teenagers (up to 5–8%), it is distinguished from simple bad posture ("postural round-back deformity") by its sharp angulation and lack of correction by active or passive maneuvers. X-ray studies reveal anterior vertebral body wedging and irregular erosions of the vertebral endplate. Treatment consists of exercise, bracing, and, rarely, surgical correction (for severe deformities).

138. **How does spondylolysis differ from spondylolisthesis?**

     Spondylolysis is a condition in which there is a defect in the pars interarticularis (vertebral arch) of a vertebra that is most common at L5 in children and adolescents. **Spondylolisthesis** is a condition (usually resulting from spondylolysis) that is characterized by forward slippage of one vertebra on the lower vertebrae. Pain is the most common presenting symptom for both conditions. The etiology is unclear, but various theories relate it to hereditary factors, congenital predisposition, trauma, posture, growth, and biomechanical factors. Treatment includes watchful waiting, limitation of activity, exercise therapy, bracing, casting, and surgery, depending on the patient's age, the magnitude of the slippage, the extent of pain, and the predicted likelihood of progression of the deformity.

     Kraft DE: Low back pain in the adolescent athlete. Pediatr Clin North Am 49:643–654, 2002.

ACKNOWLEDGMENT

The editors gratefully acknowledge contributions by Drs. Francis Y. Lee, John P. Dormans, Richard S. Davidson, Mark Magnusson, and David P. Royce that were retained from the first three editions of *Pediatric Secrets*.

CHAPTER 17

PULMONOLOGY

Robert Wilmott, MD

ALLERGIC RHINITIS

1. **How common is allergic rhinitis?**
   Very common. Between 10% and 40% of children experience rhinitis as the most common manifestation of allergic disease.

2. **In addition to chronic congestion, what features on physical examination suggest chronic allergic rhinitis?**
   - "Allergic facies": Open mouth, midface hypoplasia
   - "Allergic salute": Nasal crease on bridge of nose as a result of chronic upward rubbing with the palm of the hand
   - Diminished sense of taste and smell
   - Dental malocclusion
   - Allergic "shiners" (dark circles under the eyes)
   - Increased infraorbital folds
   - Cobblestoning of conjunctiva/posterior oropharynx

3. **What are the major risk factors for allergic rhinitis?**
   - Positive family history
   - Heavy maternal cigarette smoking during the first year of life
   - Early introduction of solid foods
   - Individuals born during pollen season
   - Higher serum immunoglobulin E (IgE) levels (>100 IU/mL before 6 years of age)
   - Atopic dermatitis

   Gentile DA, Shapiro GG, Skono DP: Allergic rhinitis. In Leung DYM, Sampson HA, Geha RS, Szefler SJ: Pediatric Allergy: Principles and Practice. St. Louis, Mosby, 2003, p 288.

4. **How does the time of year help identify the potential cause of allergic rhinitis?**
   Tree pollen is usually associated with the onset of the growing season. After local tree pollination, *grass pollens* appear; this may occur earlier in locales where there are short winters. *Weed pollen* is associated with the late-summer pollen peak, and ragweed is the primary weed pollen in eastern and central North America. *Fungal* aeroallergens span the growing season. Relative concentrations of household *animal allergens, dust mites*, and *indoor fungi* generally increase when doors and windows are closed. However, dust mites proliferate in areas of high humidity and may cause perennial symptoms.

   Naclerio R, Solomon W: Rhinitis and inhalant allergens. JAMA 278:1842–1848, 1997.

5. **Which variables affect allergy skin testing in children?**
   - **Test site:** The forearm is less reactive than the back. The lower back is less reactive than the mid and upper back.
   - **Patient age:** Wheals on skin testing increase in size from infancy on and then often decline after 50 years of age. Infants react primarily with a small wheal and a large erythematous flare.

- **Seasonality:** Allergen skin test sensitivity is increased after the pollen season and then declines until the next season.
- **Medications:** These can inhibit allergen skin test response for various lengths of time: cetirizine (3–10 days), loratadine (3–10 days), diphenhydramine (1–3 days), chlorpheniramine (1–3 days), and hydroxyzine (1–10 days).
- **Test technique:** Prick skin tests are more specific than intradermal skin tests.

   Demoly P, Michel FB, Bousquet J: In vivo methods for study of allergy skin tests, techniques, and interpretation. In Middleton E, Reed CE, Ellis EF, et al: Allergy: Principles and Practice. St. Louis, Mosby, 1998, pp 430–439.

6. **What is RAST?**
   The radioallergosorbent test (RAST) is an in vitro laboratory method used to quantify the amount of allergen-specific IgE. The test allergen is bound to solid-phase particles with which the patient's serum is then incubated. If the patient's serum contains the antigen-specific IgE, then the patient's IgE will bind to the RAST antigen. Nonspecific IgE is removed by washing. Radiolabeled anti-IgE is then added and binds to the IgE-antigen complex. Quantification of radioactivity (which correlates with the quantity of antigen-specific IgE) is determined using a gamma counter.

7. **Summarize the pros and cons of skin testing versus in vitro testing (e.g., RAST) for allergies.**
   In vitro tests
   - No risk of anaphylaxis
   - Results not influenced by medications, dermatographism, or extensive dermatologic disease
   - More costly

   Skin testing
   - Less costly
   - More sensitive than in vitro tests
   - Results immediately available

8. **What are the recommended treatments for children with chronic allergic rhinitis?**
   - Environmental control measures for allergen avoidance
   - Pharmacotherapy (including antihistamines, leukotriene receptor antagonists, intranasal steroids, and topical cromolyn)
   - Immunotherapy for individuals suboptimally controlled by above measures or those with severe symptoms

   American Academy of Allergy, Asthma and Immunology: www.aaaai.org

9. **What are the major indoor allergens?**
   Dust mite, animal dander, cockroach, and mold.

10. **How can you rid the home of cat allergen?**
    - Remove upholstered furniture, carpet, and other sources harboring the allergen.
    - Obtain new bedding or impermeable bedding covers.
    - The cat's roaming areas should be limited, particularly the bedroom. The bedroom is the most important room to maintain as free of cat allergen as possible. Keeping the cat outside is an option for some.
    - Use high-efficiency particulate air filters or electrostatic air cleaners.
    - Consider a felinectomy.

KEY POINTS: ALLERGIC RHINITIS

1. History (family, environmental, associated symptoms) is key to diagnosis.

2. With two atopic parents, the risk to the child is 50–70%.

3. Radioallergosorbent testing is indicated in patients with severe skin disorders or a risk of severe reaction to skin testing.

4. Sensitivity of testing: Intradermal > skin prick > radioallergosorbent.

5. Allergic features: Shiners (dark circles under eyes), increased infraorbital folds, transverse nasal bridge crease, cobblestoning of conjunctiva/posterior oropharynx.

6. Immunotherapy: Consider this when allergen avoidance and pharmacotherapy have produced suboptimal results.

11. **How can house dust mite (HDM) concentrations be minimized?**

Allergens from HDM are extremely important triggers of allergic rhinitis and asthma. They are airborne during and immediately after disturbance. Individuals often sleep or sit on surfaces containing high concentrations of HDM, such as the bed, pillow, or sofa. The following methods may help control HMD allergen:

- Replace mattress and pillow encasements.
- Wash bedding every 1–2 weeks, preferably in hot water (>130°F).
- Eliminate stuffed animals, books, and other sources that harbor HDM from the bedroom.
- Regularly dust hard surfaces and vacuum carpeted surfaces.
- Reduce indoor relative humidity (<45%).

Wood RA: Environmental control. In Leung DYM, Sampson HA, Geha RS, Szefler SJ: Pediatric Allergy: Principles and Practice. St. Louis, Mosby, 2003, p 270.

12. **Which children should be considered for immunotherapy?**

Immunotherapy is the treatment of choice for hymenoptera venom sensitivity—in carefully selected patients—to prevent life-threatening allergic reactions. Immunotherapy should be considered as treatment for IgE-mediated diseases (e.g., allergic rhinitis, allergic asthma) when allergen avoidance and adjunctive pharmacotherapy have produced suboptimal results. Although allergen immunotherapy may be helpful in patients whose asthma is difficult to control, allergen immunotherapy is contraindicated in patients with unstable asthma in those individuals whose FFV_1 levels are <70% of the predicted value.

Golden DBK: Insect allergy. In Adkinson NF, Yunginger JW, Basse WW, et al: Middleton's Allergy: Principles and Practice, 6th ed. St. Louis, Mosby, 2003, pp 1475–1486.

Matsui EC, Eggleston PA: Immunotherapy for allergic disease. In Leung DYM, Sampson HA, Geha RS, Szefler SJ: Pediatric Allergy: Principles and Practice. St. Louis, Mosby, 2003, pp 277–285.

13. **How common is exercise-induced bronchospasm in children with allergic rhinitis?**

Up to 40% of patients with allergic rhinitis but no history of asthma have abnormal pulmonary function tests in response to exercise.

Bierman EW: Incidence of exercise-induced asthma in children. Pediatrics 56:847–850, 1975.

ASTHMA

14. **When does asthma usually have its onset of symptoms?**

    Approximately 50% of childhood asthma develops before the age of 3 years, and nearly all has developed by the age of 7 years. The signs and symptoms of asthma, including chronic cough, may be evident much earlier than the actual diagnosis but may be erroneously attributed to recurrent pneumonia or "wheezy bronchitis."

    American Lung Association: www.lungusa.org

15. **Is asthma more common in males or females?**

    Asthma is two to three times more common in boys than girls until the onset of puberty, and it then equalizes during adolescence. When onset is in adulthood, it is more common among females.

16. **Which children with wheezing at an early age are likely to develop chronic asthma?**

    Although about one third of children will have an episode of wheezing before they are 3 years old, most (60%) do not develop persistent wheezing. Risks factors for persistence include the following:
    - Positive family history of asthma (especially maternal)
    - Increased IgE levels
    - Atopic dermatitis
    - Rhinitis not associated with colds
    - Secondhand smoke exposure

    Martinez FD, Wright AL, Taussig LM, et al; for The Group Medical Associates: Asthma and wheezing in the first six years of life. N Engl J Med 332:133–138, 1995.

17. **What historical points are suggestive of an allergic basis for asthma?**
    - Seasonal nature with concurrent rhinitis (suggesting *pollen*)
    - Symptoms worsen when visiting a family with pets (suggesting *animal dander*)
    - Wheezing occurs when carpets are vacuumed or bed is made (suggesting *mites*)
    - Symptoms develop in damp basements or barns (suggesting *molds*)

18. **How common is exercise-induced bronchospasm (EIB) in children?**

    Very common, and it is often overlooked. Significant symptoms (e.g., cough, chest tightness, wheezing, dyspnea) are noted after exercise in approximately 80% of asthmatic children, although abnormal pulmonary function tests can be found in nearly 100% of these patients. Among atopic children, the incidence of EIB has been estimated to be as high as 40%.

19. **How is EIB diagnosed?**

    EIB is likely if the peak flow rate or FEV_1 drops by 15% after 6 minutes of vigorous exercise. This exercise can include jogging on a motor-driven treadmill (15% grade at 3–4 mph), riding a stationary bicycle, or running up and down a hallway. Peak flow can then be measured with simple peak flow meters or a spirometer every 2–3 minutes, although peak flows are not as reliable as spirometry. The greatest reduction in EIB is usually seen 5–10 minutes after exercise. As further verification of the diagnosis, if the patient has developed a decreased peak flow (and possibly wheezing), two puffs of a $beta_2$-agonist should be administered to reverse the bronchospasm.

    Sheth KK: Activity-induced asthma. Pediatr Clin North Am 50:697–716, 2003.

20. **What mechanisms lead to airway obstruction during an acute asthma attack?**

    The main causes of airflow obstruction in acute asthma are *airway inflammation*, including edema, *bronchospasm*, and increased *mucus* production. Chronic inflammation eventually results in airway remodeling, which may not be clinically apparent.

    Bousquet J, Jeffery PK, Busse WW, et al: Asthma. From airway bronchoconstriction to airways inflammation and remodeling. Am J Respir Crit Care Med 161:1720–1745, 2000.

21. **All that wheezes is not asthma. What are the other noninfectious causes?**
    - **Aspiration pneumonitis:** Especially in a neurologically impaired infant or an infant with gastroesophageal reflux, and especially if there is coughing, choking, or gagging with feedings. If there is a clear association with feedings, consider the possibility of tracheoesophageal fistula.
    - **Bronchiolitis obliterans:** Chronic wheezing often after adenoviral infection.
    - **Bronchopulmonary dysplasia:** Especially if there has been prolonged oxygen therapy/ventilatory requirement during the neonatal period.
    - **Ciliary dyskinesia:** Especially if recurrent otitis media, sinusitis, or situs inversus is present.
    - **Congenital malformations:** Including tracheobronchial anomalies, tracheomalacia, lung cysts, and mediastinal lesions.
    - **Cystic fibrosis:** If wheezing is recurrent, failure to thrive, chronic diarrhea, or recurrent respiratory infections.
    - **Congenital cardiac anomalies:** Especially lesions with large left-to-right shunts.
    - **Foreign-body aspiration:** If associated with an acute choking episode in an infant >6 months old.
    - **Vascular rings, slings, or compression.**

22. **How is the severity of an acute asthma attack estimated?**
    See Table 17-1.

TABLE 17-1. SEVERITY OF AN ASTHMA ATTACK

Sign or Symptom	Mild	Moderate	Severe
PEFR*	70–90% predicted of personal best	50–70% predicted of personal best	<50% predicted of personal best
Respiratory rate, resting or sleeping	Normal to 30% increase above the mean	30–50% increase above the mean	Increase over 50% above the mean
Alertness	Normal	Normal	May be decreased
Dyspnea[†]	Absent or mild; speaks in complete sentences	Moderate; speaks in phrases or partial sentences; infant's cry softer and shorter, infant has difficulty suckling and feeding	Severe; speaks only in single words or short phrases; infant's cry softer and shorter, infant stops suckling and feeding
Pulsus paradoxus[†]	<10 mm Hg	10–20 mm Hg	20–40 mm Hg
Accessory muscle use	No intercostal retraction to mild retractions	Moderate intercostal retraction with tracheosternal retractions; use of sternocleidomastoid muscles; chest hyperinflation	Severe intercostal retractions, tracheosternal retractions with nasal flaring during inspiration; chest hyperinflation

Continued

TABLE 17-1.	SEVERITY OF AN ASTHMA ATTACK—CONT'D		
Sign or Symptom	**Mild**	**Moderate**	**Severe**
Color	Good	Pale	Possibly cyanotic
Auscultation	End expiratory wheeze only	Wheeze during entire expiration and inspiration	Breath sounds becoming inaudible
Oxygen saturation	>95%	90–95%	<90%
P_{CO_2}	<35	<40	>40

*Peak expiratory flow rate (PEFR) assessed for children 5 years of age or older.
†Parents' or physician's impression of degree of child's breathlessness.
‡Pulsus paradoxus does not correlate with phase of respiration in small children.
Within each category, the presence of several parameters, but not necessarily all, indicates the general classification of the exacerbation.
Gentile DA, Michaels MG, Skones DP: Allergy and Immunology. In Zitelli BJ, Davis HW (eds): Atlas of Pediatric Physical Diagnosis, 4th ed. St. Louis, Mosby, 2002, p 98.

23. **Is a chest x-ray necessary for all children who wheeze for the first time?**
    A chest x-ray should be considered for a first-time wheezing patient in the following situations:
    - Findings on physical examination that suggest other diagnoses
    - Marked asymmetry of breath sounds
    - Suspected pneumonia
    - Suspected foreign-body aspiration
    - Hypoxemia or marked respiratory distress
    - Older child with no family history of asthma or atopy
    - Suspected congestive heart failure
    - History of trauma (e.g., burns, scalds, blunt or penetrating injury)

24. **What are the usual findings on arterial blood gas sampling during acute asthma attacks?**
    The most common finding is **hypocapnia** (i.e., low CO_2) because of hyperventilation. Hypoxemia may also be present unless the child is being treated with oxygen. Therefore, hypercapnia is a serious sign that suggests that the child is tiring or becoming severely obstructed. This finding should prompt reevaluation and consideration of admission to a high-acuity unit.

25. **What are indications for hospital admission in patients with asthma?**
    After therapy in the emergency department, admission is advisable if a child has any of the following:
    - Depressed level of consciousness
    - Incomplete response with moderate retractions, wheezing, peak flow <60% predicted, pulsus paradoxus >15 mmHg, SaO_2 ≤90%, pCO_2 ≥42 mmHg
    - Breath sounds significantly diminished
    - Evidence of dehydration
    - Pneumothorax
    - Residual symptoms and history of severe attacks involving prolonged hospitalization (especially if intubation was required)
    - Parental unreliability

An equally difficult (and very unpredictable) challenge relates to predicting which patients will relapse after responding to therapy and subsequently require hospitalization. This is a major problem because rates of relapse can approach 20–30%.

26. **Is a nebulizer more effective than a metered-dose inhaler (MDI) with a spacer for the treatment of asthma?**

    For the treatment of exacerbations of asthma, nebulizers are primarily used in children <2 years old because of the ease of administration. Although an MDI with a spacer is used more commonly among older children, several studies indicate that they are equally or more effective than nebulizers among young children, even those with moderate or severe acute asthma. Furthermore, the MDI with a spacer requires less treatment time and has fewer side effects, and it is often preferred by patients and parents.

    Castro-Rodriguez JA, Rodrigo GJ: Beta-agonists through metered-dose inhaler with valved holding chamber versus nebulizer for acute exacerbation of wheezing or asthma in children under 5 years of age: A systematic review with meta-analysis. J Pediatr 145:776–779, 2004.

    Hsu JT, Parker S: Are inhalers with spacers better than nebulizers for children with asthma? J Fam Pract 53:55–57, 2004.

    Rubin BK, Fink JB: The delivery of inhaled medication to the young child. Pediatr Clin North Am 50:717–732, 2003.

27. **List the possible acute side effects of albuterol and other beta-agonists.**

    - **General:** Hypoxemia, tachyphylaxis
    - **Renal:** Hypokalemia
    - **Cardiovascular:** Tachycardia, palpitations, premature ventricular contractions, atrial fibrillation
    - **Neurologic:** Headache, irritability, insomnia, tremor, weakness
    - **Gastrointestinal:** Nausea, heartburn, vomiting

28. **Are anticholinergics useful for the treatment of pediatric asthma?**

    The precise role of anticholinergics (including ipratropium bromide and atropine sulfate) in pediatrics remains ill-defined as a result of potential side effects and the paucity of studies of their efficacy for both acute and chronic asthma management. However, some evidence suggests that multiple doses of anticholinergics may be of value during the initial management of pediatric patients with severe exacerbations of asthma ($\leq$55% of predicted FEV_1). For mild to moderate disease, evidence does not suggest a benefit.

    Plotnick LH, Ducharme FM: Should inhaled anticholinergics be added to b_2 agonists for treating acute childhood and adolescent asthma? A systematic review. BMJ 317:971–977, 1998.

    Qureshi F, Pestian J, Davis P, Zaritsky A: Effect of nebulized ipratropium on the hospitalization rates of children with asthma. N Engl J Med 339:1013–1020, 1998.

29. **Why has theophylline fallen from grace as a treatment for asthma?**

    As a result of concerns about its potential toxicity (e.g., vomiting, tachycardia, seizures), side effects (e.g., behavioral changes, impaired school performance), and questionable efficacy, theophylline is no longer considered part of routine therapy. Its use may be considered in an acute setting if a patient is becoming fatigued and developing respiratory failure. Some practitioners still use it in chronic settings, particularly for nocturnal asthma.

    Fotinos C, Dodson S: Is there a role for theophylline in treating patients with asthma? J Fam Pract 51:744, 2002.

30. **How is chronic asthma severity classified among teenagers and children >5 years old?**

    The National Asthma Education and Prevention Program categorizes asthma on the basis of daytime and nighttime symptoms and frequency of exacerbations. Extent of short-acting beta-agonist use can also be considered.

Intermittent

Symptoms ≤2 times per week

Asymptomatic between exacerbations
Exacerbations brief (a few hours to a few days)

Nocturnal symptoms: ≤2 times per month
beta-agonist use: ≤2 times/week

Mild persistent

Symptoms >2 times per week but <1 time per day
Exacerbations may affect activity
Nocturnal symptoms: 3–4 times per month
beta-agonist use: >2 times per week, but <1 time per day

Moderate Persistent

Daily symptoms
Exacerbations affect activity
Exacerbations >2 times per week; may last days
Nocturnal symptoms 5–9 times per month

beta-agonist use: daily

Severe persistent

Continual symptoms
Limited physical activity
Frequent exacerbations
Nocturnal symptoms: ≥10 times per month
beta-agonist use: 4 times per day; does not completely relieve symptoms

Bacharier LB, Strunk RC: Asthma in older children. In Leung DYM, Sampson HA, Geha RS, Szefler SJ (eds): Pediatric Allergy: Principles and Practice. St. Louis, Mosby, 2003, pp 414–415.

31. **What is the treatment of choice for patients with *persistent* asthma?**
Inhaled corticosteroids. Daily administration significantly improves symptoms, reduces exacerbations, and allows healing of the chronic inflammatory changes that have taken place in the airways over time. Dosing and the use of adjunctive medications (e.g., long-acting inhaled beta$_2$-agonists) depend on the severity of the persistence.

32. **What is the role of other daily medications for the treatment of chronic asthma in children?**
Leukotriene-receptor antagonists, such as montelukast (Singulair) and zafirlukast (Accolate), are nonsteroidal anti-inflammatory agents. Their precise role (i.e., primary therapy versus "sparing" drugs for steroid use) remains under evaluation, particularly in such areas as EIB. The role of nedocromil, a nonsteroidal anti-inflammatory medication with mechanisms of action similar to those of cromolyn, remains to be elucidated in children.

Childhood Asthma Research and Education Network: www.asthma-carenet.org.

33. **Do inhaled steroids affect growth in children?**
Results are conflicting but tend to indicate that mild growth suppression occurs among children receiving moderate to high doses, particularly in more severe asthmatics and primarily during the first year of therapy. However, asthma per se can also inhibit growth, and inhaled steroid therapy does not appear to affect eventual adult height. It is important that children who require the extended use of inhaled steroids are monitored for height and height velocity and cataracts.

Berger WE, Shapiro GG: The use of inhaled corticosteroids for persistent asthma in infants and young children. Ann Allergy Asthma Immunol 92:387–402, 2004.
De Benedictis FM, Selvaggio D: Use of inhaler devices in pediatric asthma. Pediatr Drugs 5:629–638, 2003.

34. **What is anti-IgE treatment for asthma?**
Omalizumab (Xolair) is a recombinant monoclonal antibody that was originally developed by immunizing mice with human IgE. This antibody forms a complex with unbound IgE, interferes with its binding with cell receptors, and thus prevents the subsequent release of inflammatory and chemical mediators, including histamine. It has shown great promise for the treatment of moderate to severe asthma in pediatric patients, and it has an excellent safety profile.

Lanier BQ: Newer aspects in the treatment of pediatric and adult asthma: Monoclonal anti-IgE. Ann Allergy Asthma Immunol 90:13–15, 2003.

35. **Is there a role for complementary and alternative medicines in the treatment of asthma?**
    There is no clear direction or guidelines for the use of complementary and alternative medicines for children with asthma, although these therapies are often independently used by families. Hypnosis, yoga, relaxation techniques, and massage have shown benefit in some studies, but a recent review of studies involving mind-body techniques, relaxation, manual therapies, and diet has found a tendency to little or no significant difference between placebo and sham therapy.

    Markham AW, Wilkinson JM: Complementary and alternative medicines (CAM) in the management of asthma: an examination of the evidence. J Asthma 41:131–139, 2004.

36. **How useful are pulmonary function tests when evaluating and following children with asthma?**
    Pulmonary function tests are very useful for the longitudinal evaluation of outpatients with asthma, for demonstrating a satisfactory response to therapy, and for identifying the severely obstructed, hyperinflated asymptomatic patient who has a poor prognosis if unrecognized. Home peak flow meters to measure the peak expiratory flow rate on a daily or as-needed basis can also be helpful. A baseline predicted or personal-best value can be obtained and home therapy initiated when the peak expiratory flow rate falls.

KEY POINTS: ASTHMA

1. This is the most common chronic disease of childhood.

2. Typical abnormalities on spirometry include the following: decreased FEV_1 and FEV_1/FVC ratio; *increase* in FEV_1 (>15%) with bronchodilator or *decrease* in FEV_1 (>15%) with methacholine or histamine.

3. Classification is based on frequency of symptoms, nighttime symptoms, and lung function—mild intermittent, mild persistent, moderate persistent, and severe persistent.

4. $PaCO_2$ measurements that are normal (40 mmHg) or rising in an asthmatic with tachypnea or significant respiratory distress are worrisome for evolving respiratory failure.

5. Signs of impending respiratory failure include severe retractions, accessory muscle use (especially sternocleidomastoids), decreased muscle tone, and altered mental status.

37. **What proportion of childhood asthmatics "outgrow" their symptoms?**
    Popular pediatric teaching has been that most children with asthma outgrow their symptoms. However, studies suggest that this is erroneous and that only 30–50% become free of symptoms, primarily those with milder disease. Many children who "outgrow" symptoms have recurrences during adulthood. Studies also indicate that many infants who wheeze with viral infections and are asymptomatic between illnesses tend to "outgrow" their asthma. Children whose initial wheezing occurs later in life, with allergen sensitization as a major factor, tend to have more persistence of recurrent bronchospasm. Although the overall trend is for asthma to become milder, a large percentage of adults have persistent obstructive disease, both recognized and unrecognized.

    Sears MR, Greene JM, Willan AR, et al: A longitudinal, population-based, cohort study of childhood asthma followed to adulthood. N Engl J Med 349:1414–1422, 2003.

BRONCHIOLITIS

38. What is the most important cause of lower respiratory tract disease among infants and young children?

Respiratory syncytial virus (RSV). Up to 100,000 children are hospitalized annually in the United States as a result of this pneumovirus, which is different from—but closely related to—the paramyxoviruses. Disease most commonly occurs during outbreaks in winter or spring in the United States and during the winter months of July and August in the Southern Hemisphere.

39. What other agents cause bronchiolitis?

Although RSV is estimated to cause 50–90% of cases, other agents responsible for bronchiolitis include metapneumovirus (second most-common cause), parainfluenza virus, influenza virus types A and B, and adenovirus. Human metapneumovirus was recently recognized as a significant cause of acute bronchiolitis.

McIntosh K, McAdam AJ: Human metapneumovirus—an important new respiratory virus. N Engl J Med 350:431–433, 2004.

Williams JV, Harris PA, Tollefson SJ, et al: Human metapneumovirus and lower respiratory tract disease in otherwise healthy infants and children. N Engl J Med 350:443–450, 2004.

40. What are the best predictors of the severity of bronchiolitis?

The single best predictor at an initial assessment appears to be **oxygen saturation**, which can be determined by pulse oximetry. SaO_2 <95% correlates with more severe disease; low SaO_2 is often not clinically apparent, and objective measurements are necessary. An arterial blood gas with PaO_2 of ≤65 or $PaCO_2$ >40 mmHg is particularly worrisome. Other predictors of increased severity include the following:

- An ill or "toxic" appearance
- History of prematurity (gestational age, <34 weeks)
- Atelectasis on chest x-ray
- Respiratory rate of >70 breaths per minute
- Infant <3 months old

41. What are the typical findings on chest x-ray in a child with bronchiolitis?

The picture is varied. Most commonly, there is hyperinflation of the lungs. Bilateral interstitial abnormalities with peribronchial thickening are common. Up to 20% of children may have lobar, segmental, or subsegmental consolidation that can mimic bacterial pneumonia. With the possible exception of atelectasis, the chest x-ray findings do not correlate well with the severity of the disease.

42. How common is apnea in patients with RSV bronchiolitis?

About 20% of hospitalized infants develop apnea. Infants at highest risk include former premature infants (particularly those who are <44 weeks postconception), the very young (1–4 months), and those with chronic lung disease. A large number of infants with RSV infection who require assisted ventilation do so because of severe recurrent apnea rather than respiratory failure. The mechanisms leading to apnea are unclear, but it tends to resolve within a few days. Hospitalized high-risk infants should be monitored. Of note is that sudden infant death syndrome (SIDS) has not been clearly associated with RSV infection.

43. Is the use of steroids justified for bronchiolitis?

Although corticosteroids have been used by clinicians for many years for the treatment of bronchiolitis, the preponderance of multiple controlled studies has shown no immediate or long-term advantage with their use, either by the systemic or inhaled route. However, their value or lack thereof continues to be debated, and papers continue to be published with conflicting findings.

Csonka P, Kaila M, Laippala P, et al: Oral prednisolone in the acute management of children age 6 to 35 months with viral respiratory infection-induced lower airway disease: A randomized, placebo-controlled trial. J Pediatr, 143:725–730, 2003.

Schuh S, Coates AL, Binnie R, et al: Efficacy of oral dexamethasone in outpatients with acute bronchiolitis. J Pediatr 140:27–32, 2002.

Garrison MM, Christakis DA, Harvey E, et al: Systemic corticosteroids in infant bronchiolitis: A meta-analysis. Pediatrics 105:E44, 2000.

44. **Are bronchodilators such as albuterol effective as a therapy for bronchiolitis?**
The use of bronchodilator therapy for bronchiolitis is controversial. Between 30% and 50% of infants with RSV bronchiolitis will have a positive response to inhalation therapy, and infants with a strong family history of asthma are most likely to respond. In infants with significant wheezing, a trial of albuterol may be indicated.

King VJ, Viswanathan M, Bordley WC, et al: Pharmacologic treatment of bronchiolitis in infants and children: A systematic review. Arch Pediatr Adolesc Med 158:1217–1237, 2004.

Steiner RWP: Treating acute bronchiolitis associated with RSV. Am Fam Physician 69:325–330, 2004.

45. **Is there a vaccine to prevent RSV infection?**
No, there is not yet a safe and effective vaccine against RSV. However, palivizumab (Synagis), a monoclonal antibody directed against RSV, is effective for prophylaxis of RSV infection in premature infants. It is given intramuscularly and must be given once per month during the RSV season. This drug is not indicated for the treatment of RSV infection. However, vaccines for RSV are in development.

KEY POINTS: BRONCHIOLITIS

- The most common causes are respiratory syncytial virus and metapneumoviruses.

- The illness severity is greatest between 2 and 6 months of age.

- Atelectatic changes on chest x-ray are common.

- In most cases, supportive care is all that is needed.

- In more severe cases, the value of bronchodilators and corticosteroids is debated.

46. **Does infection with RSV confer lifelong protection?**
No. In fact, reinfection is very common. In day-care centers, ≤75% of infants who acquire RSV infections during the first year of life are reinfected during the subsequent 2 years. Primary infections tend to be the most severe episodes, with subsequent illnesses being more muted. In older children and adults, RSV infections present the same symptoms as "colds," and reinfection is also common.

47. **If a 5-month-old child is hospitalized as a result of RSV bronchiolitis, what should the parents be told about the likelihood of future episodes of wheezing?**
In follow-up studies, 40–50% of these infants have subsequent recurrent episodes of wheezing, usually during the first year after illness. Subclinical pulmonary abnormalities may also persist. The question of whether the pulmonary sequelae are the result of the bronchiolitis or of a genetic predisposition to asthma remains unclear. Factors such as pulmonary abnormalities before the illness, passive cigarette-smoke exposure, atopic diathesis, and immunologic responses of virus-specific IgE determine the risk of recurrence.

48. **How is bronchiolitis distinguished from asthma in a wheezing infant?**
Asthma is a clinical diagnosis in all age groups that is characterized by reversible airway obstruction with hyperresponsiveness to various stimuli, including viral infections. However, the viral infections themselves—rather than underlying bronchial pathology—can be responsible for the wheezing in an infant with acute symptoms. Differentiating between the two diseases at the time of presentation can be virtually impossible. The infant wheezing from bronchiolitis generally has other symptoms (e.g., fever, rhinorrhea), and RSV antigen testing may be positive. If repeated episodes of reversible wheezing occur, especially if they are not during the RSV season, asthma is likely. Other diagnoses (e.g., cystic fibrosis, gastroesophageal reflux) must also be considered.

CLINICAL ISSUES

49. **How is hemoptysis differentiated from hematemesis?**

	Hemoptysis	Hematemesis
Color	Bright red and frothy	Dark red or brown
pH	Alkaline	Acid
Consistency	May be mixed with sputum	May contain food particles
Symptoms	Preceded by gurgling	Preceded by nausea
	Accompanied by coughing	Accompanied by retching

Rosenstein BJ: Hemoptysis. In Hilman BC (ed): Pediatric Respiratory Disease. Philadelphia, W.B. Saunders, 1993, p 533.

50. **What are the indications for surgical repair of pectus excavatum?**
This is still an area of considerable controversy. Children with pectus excavatum (Fig. 17-1) tend to have reduced total lung capacity, reduced vital capacity, increased residual volume, and reduced stroke volume during maximum exercise. However, most patients are still in the normal range for these values. The most common complaints relate to poor self-image and decreased exercise tolerance. Counseling is often sufficient for the cosmetic aspects, but many older patients report an improvement in exercise tolerance following repair, despite what seem to be minor changes in cardiac function. Whether the reason is cosmetic or to improve maximum exercise, operative repair should be delayed until the child is >6 years old to decrease the risk of recurrence during the pubertal growth spurt.

Malek MH, Fonkalsrud EW, Cooper CB: Ventilatory and cardiovascular responses to exercise in patients with pectus excavatum. Chest 124:870–882, 2003.

Haller JA, Loughlin GM: Cardiorespiratory function is significantly improved following corrective surgery for severe pectus excavatum. J Cardiovasc Surg 41:125–130, 2000.

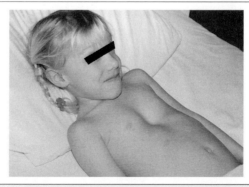

Figure 17-1. Pectus excavatum. (From James EC, Corry RJ, Perrry JF: Principles of Basic Surgical Practice. Philadelphia, Hanley & Belfus, 1987, p173.)

51. **What is the most common cause of chronic cough?**
Postnasal drip, acting alone or with other conditions. The differential diagnosis of chronic cough is very long and includes congenital anomalies, infectious or postinfectious cough, asthma-related cough, gastroesophageal reflux, aspiration, physical and chemical irritation, and psychogenic cough.

52. **When should the diagnosis of psychogenic cough be considered?**
A psychogenic cough should be considered in those children with a persistent dry, barklike, explosive daytime cough that disappears with sleep or pleasant activity. It often starts after an upper respiratory infection. The patient complains of a tickle or something in the throat. Physical examination and laboratory work are normal, and conventional therapies are ineffective. Behavior management is the preferred treatment, although, in some cases, psychological intervention is required.

53. **What medications are most effective for cold symptoms in children?**
Multiple studies have failed to show benefit over placebo of any particular medication, including dextromethorphan, diphenhydramine, codeine, and echinacea. Supportive care with patience and self-resolution of symptoms remain the mainstay of treatment.

Committee on Drugs: Use of codeine- and dextromethorphan-containing cough remedies in children. Pediatrics 99:918–919, 1997.
Paul IM, Yoder KE, Crowell KR, et al: Effect of dextromethorphan, diphenhydramine, and placebo on nocturnal cough and sleep quality for coughing children and their parents. Pediatrics 114:e85–e90, 2004.
Taylor JA, Weber W, Standish L, et al: Efficacy and safety of echinacea in treating upper respiratory tract infections in children. JAMA 290:2824–2830, 2003.

54. **What constitutes passive cigarette smoke?**
Passive cigarette smoke consists of both the smoker's exhalation (mainstream smoke, about 15% of total) and the more noxious sidestream (the unfiltered burning end of the cigarette, about 85% of total). This has been the subject of much study.

55. **What are the possible risks of passive cigarette smoke exposure?**
- Decreased fetal growth
- Increased incidence of sudden infant death syndrome
- Increased incidence of middle ear effusions
- Increased frequency of upper and lower respiratory tract infections
- Appearance of asthma at an earlier age with more frequent exacerbations
- Impaired lung function

Longer-term issues of increased cancer rates and cardiovascular disease remain under study. In addition, if a parent smokes, a child is twice as likely to become a smoker.

DiFranza JR, Lew RA: Morbidity and mortality in children associated with the use of tobacco products by other people. Pediatrics 97:560–568, 1996.

56. **How is clubbing diagnosed?**
Digital clubbing is the presence of increased amounts of connective tissue under the base of the fingernail. This may be determined by the following:
- **Rock the nail** on its bed between the examiner's finger and thumb. In patients with clubbing, the nail seems to be floating.
- **Visual inspection** reveals that the distal phalangeal depth (DPD), which is the distance from the top of the base of the nail to the finger pad, exceeds the interphalangeal depth (IPD), which is the distance from the top of the distal phalangeal joint to the underside of the joint. Normally, the DPD/IPD ratio is <1, but in patients with clubbing it is >1.
- The **diamond (or Schamroth's) sign:** Normally, if the nails of both index fingers or any other two identical fingers are opposed, there is a diamond-shaped window present between the nail bases (Fig. 17-2); this window disappears in patients with clubbing.

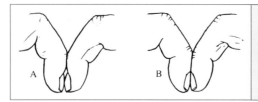

Figure 17-2. *A,* Normal child with a diamond-shaped window between the nail bases when the fingers are opposed. *B,* In digital clubbing, the diamond-shaped window is obliterated by the increased amount of soft tissue under the base of the nail.

57. **What are the causes of digital clubbing?**
- **Pulmonary:** Bronchiectasis (as in cystic fibrosis, bronchiolitis obliterans, ciliary dyskinesia), pulmonary abscess, empyema, interstitial fibrosis, malignancy, pulmonary atrioventricular fistula
- **Cardiac:** Cyanotic congenital heart disease, chronic congestive heart failure, subacute bacterial endocarditis
- **Hepatic:** Biliary cirrhosis, biliary atresia, alpha$_1$-antitrypsin deficiency
- **Gastrointestinal:** Crohn's disease, ulcerative colitis, chronic amebic and bacillary diarrhea, polyposis coli, small bowel lymphoma
- **Endocrine:** Thyrotoxicosis, thyroid deficiency
- **Hematologic:** Thalassemia, congenital methemoglobinemia (rare)
- **Idiopathic:** May be a variation of normal and not indicative of underlying disease
- **Hereditary:** May be a variation of normal and not indicative of underlying disease

   Modified from Hilman BC: Clinical assessment of pulmonary disease in infants and children. In Hilman BC (ed): Pediatric Respiratory Disease. Philadelphia, W.B. Saunders, 1993, p 61.

58. **What is the pathophysiology of clubbing?**
The answer is unclear. The increased connective tissue under the nail beds that causes digital clubbing may be caused by the presence of vasoactive substances that are increased because of hypoxia; increased production in chronic inflammatory disease; or by decreased lung clearance. Another theory proposes that digital clubbing is caused by the local release of platelet-derived growth factor.

59. **Nasal polyps are associated with which conditions?**
- **Children:** Nasal polyps are very rare in children except as a manifestation of cystic fibrosis (Fig. 17-3). Approximately 3% of children with cystic fibrosis have nasal polyps, which are often a recurrent problem. A sweat test is essential in these patients.
- **Adolescents:** There is a wider range of possible diagnoses, including cystic fibrosis, allergic rhinitis, chronic sinusitis, malignancy, "triad asthma" (asthma, nasal polyps, aspirin sensitivity), and ciliary dyskinesia syndrome (e.g., Kartagener's syndrome).

60. **A patient with chronic sinusitis and recurrent pulmonary infections has a chest x-ray that demonstrates a right-sided cardiac silhouette. What diagnostic test should be considered next?**
Bronchial or nasal turbinate mucosal biopsy for electron microscopic evaluation of cilia.
Kartagener's syndrome is one of the ciliary dyskinesia (or immotile cilia) syndromes. The presenting symptoms are a constellation of recurrent pulmonary infections, chronic sinusitis, recurrent otitis media, situs inversus, and infertility (in males). Structural ciliary abnormalities (most common are absent dynein arms) result in abnormal ciliary beat and decreased clearance of respiratory secretions, thereby predisposing the patient to infection. In addition, because spermatozoa have tails with the same ultrastructural abnormalities as respiratory cilia, they move less well. The cause of the situs inversus (Fig. 17-4) is not fully understood, but it occurs in approximately 50% of individuals with primary ciliary dyskinesia. It has been sug-

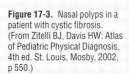
Figure 17-3. Nasal polyps in a patient with cystic fibrosis. (From Zitelli BJ, Davis HW: Atlas of Pediatric Physical Diagnosis, 4th ed. St. Louis, Mosby, 2002, p 550.)

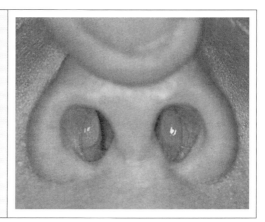

gested that cilia are important for proper organ orientation during embryonic development and that dysfunctional cilia make organ orientation a random event, leading to situs inversus 50% of the time.

61. **What percentage of children snore?**
Between 5% to 10% of preadolescent children are reported by their parents to snore at night.

> www.Kids-ENT.com

62. **In which children who snore should obstructive sleep apnea (OSA) be suspected?**
At night, the child with OSA may have persistent snoring interrupted by periods of silence during which respiratory efforts are made, but there is no air movement. Increased work of breathing, with retractions; prominent mouth breathing; unusual sleep postures; frequent nighttime awakenings; enuresis; and night sweats are symptoms of OSA. During the day, there may be excessive daytime sleepiness, learning problems, morning headaches, or personality changes.

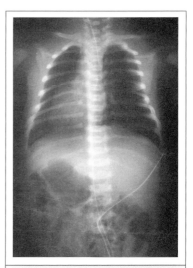
Figure 17-4. Dextrocardia with situs inversus. (From Clark DA: Atlas of Neonatology. Philadelphia, W.B. Saunders, 2000, p 115.)

63. **What evaluations should be performed on a child with suspected OSA?**
- **Physical examination:** Mouth breathing while awake, dysphagia, midface or mandibular hypoplasia, tonsillar hypertrophy, cleft palate, palatal deformity caused by adenoidal hypertrophy, failure to thrive (FTT), or obesity
- **Lateral airway radiograph:** One of the easiest and most direct means of assessing upper airway caliber
- **Nasal endoscopy:** Useful for dynamic assessment of the upper airway and larynx
- **Detailed nocturnal polysomnography** (overnight sleep study or polysomnogram [PSG]): Until consistent clinical correlates can be found, the gold standard for the definitive diagnosis of OSA

- **Cardiologic assessment** (chest x-ray, electrocardiogram, and echocardiography): Used for children with documented OSA and severe or sustained oxygen desaturation

Erler T, Paditz E: Obstructive sleep apnea in children: a state-of-the-art review. Treat Resp Med 3:107–122, 2004.

64. What are the potential long-term consequences of OSA?

The most severe complications of OSA in children are right ventricular hypertrophy, hypertension, polycythemia, compensatory metabolic alkalosis, life-threatening cor pulmonale, and respiratory failure. Later in life, OSA is associated with an increased risk of cardiovascular morbidity and mortality. It is strongly implicated in the development of hypertension, ischemic heart disease, arrhythmias, and sudden death (in individuals with coexisting ischemic heart disease); it also contributes to the risk for stroke.

Chan J, Edman JC, Koltai PJ: Obstructive sleep apnea in children. Am Fam Physician 69:1147–1154, 2004.

65. What is the most common cause of infantile stridor?

Congenital laryngomalacia occurs as a result of prolapse of the poorly supported supraglottic structures: the arytenoids, the aryepiglottic folds, and the epiglottis. Stridor is loudest after crying or exertion, but it typically does not interfere with feeding, sleep, or growth. Symptoms usually resolve at the latest by the time the infant is 18 months old.

66. How can you clinically distinguish bilateral from unilateral vocal cord paralysis in an infant?

Normally, the vocal cords are tonically abducted, with voluntary adduction resulting in speech. With unilateral paralysis, one cord is ineffective for speech, and hoarseness results. The infant's cry may be weak or absent. Stridor is usually minimal but may be positional (e.g., sleeping on the side with the paralyzed cord up may allow it to fall to midline and produce obstructive sounds). With bilateral paralysis, hoarseness is less apparent and the cry remains weak, but stridor (both inspiratory and expiratory) is usually quite prominent; in addition, the infant is more likely to have symptoms of frank pulmonary aspiration.

67. What is the most common cause of chronic hoarseness in children?

Screamer nodes. These are vocal cord nodules caused by vocal abuse, such as repetitive screaming, throat clearing, and coughing. They are the cause of a hoarse voice in >50% of children when hoarseness persists for >2 weeks.

68. Which clinical features are suggestive of foreign-body aspiration?

Symptoms and history	Signs
Child <4 years old	Fixed, localized wheeze
Boys twice as common as girls	Wheezing in a child who has no history of asthma
Coughing	Reduced breath sounds over one lung, one lobe, or
Hemoptysis	one segment
Respiratory infection not resolving	Mediastinal shift
with treatment	One nipple higher than other as a result
History of choking	of unilateral hyperinflation
Difficulty breathing	Stridor

69. Are chest x-rays useful for evaluating a foreign-body aspiration?

Unfortunately, only about 10–15% of aspirated foreign bodies are radiopaque. Thus, inspiratory films are often normal. Features suggesting a foreign-body aspiration are as follows:

- Expiratory chest x-ray showing asymmetry in lung aeration as a result of obstructive emphysema (the foreign body often acts as a ball-valve mechanism, allowing air in but not out)
- Decubitus films that show the same asymmetry (these views are often used in uncooperative children who cannot or will not exhale on command)
- Obstructive atelectasis

70. **What are the possible mechanisms for the development of lung abscesses in children?**
   - **After pneumonia:** Particularly *Staphylococcus aureus, Haemophilus influenzae, Streptococcus pneumoniae,* and *Klebsiella pneumoniae*
   - **Hematogenous spread:** Especially if an indwelling central catheter or right-sided endocarditis is present
   - **Penetrating trauma**
   - **Aspiration:** Especially in neurologically compromised patients
   - **Secondary to infection of an underlying pulmonary anomaly:** Such as a bronchogenic cyst

   Campbell PW: Lung abscess. In Hilman BC (ed): Pediatric Respiratory Disease. Philadelphia, W.B. Saunders, 1993, pp 257–262.

71. **What are the typical clinical findings in patients with bronchiectasis?**
   Bronchiectasis is the progressive dilation and possible eventual destruction of bronchi, most likely from acute and/or recurrent obstruction and infection. It may result from a variety of infections (e.g., adenoviral, rubeola, pertussis, tuberculosis), and it is often associated with underlying pulmonary susceptibility (e.g., cystic fibrosis, ciliary dyskinesia syndromes, immunodeficiencies). Clinical findings can be variable but usually include persistent cough, production of purulent sputum, recurrent fevers, and digital clubbing. Inspiratory crackles are often heard over the affected area. Hemoptysis and wheezing can occur but are uncommon.

72. **A novice teenage mountain-climber develops headache, marked cough, and orthopnea at the end of a rapid, 2-day climb. What is the likely diagnosis?**
   Acute mountain sickness with high-altitude pulmonary edema. This condition results from insufficient time to adapt to altitude changes above 2,500–3,000 meters, with resultant alveolar and tissue hypoxia as a result of pulmonary hypertension and pulmonary edema. In severe cases, cerebral edema can result. Treatment consists of returning the patient to a lower altitude and administering oxygen. If decent and supplemental oxygen are not available, portable hyperbaric chambers and nifedipine should be used until descent is possible.

   Bartsch P, Mairbaurl H, Swenson ER, Maggiorini M: High altitude pulmonary edema. Swiss Med Wkly 133:377–384, 2003.
   Gallagher SA, Hackett PH: High-altitude illness. Emerg Med Clin North Am 22:329–355, 2004.

73. **What is the likely diagnosis of a child with diffuse lung disease, microcytic anemia, and sputum that contains hemosiderin-laden macrophages?**
   Pulmonary hemosiderosis. This condition, the presenting symptoms of which can include chronic respiratory problems or acute hemoptysis, is characterized by alveolar hemorrhage and microcytic hypochromic anemia with a low serum iron level. Hemosiderin ingested by alveolar macrophages can often be detected in sputum or gastric aspirates after staining with Prussian blue. Most commonly, the condition is idiopathic and isolated, but it can be associated with cow's milk hypersensitivity (Heiner's syndrome), glomerulonephritis with basement membrane antibodies (Goodpasture's syndrome), and collagen vascular disease.

74. **How should a child with a spontaneous pneumothorax be managed?**
   If the pneumothorax is small and the child is asymptomatic, observation alone is appropriate. Administration of 100% oxygen may speed resorption of the free air, but this technique is less effective in children in older age groups. If the pneumothorax is >20% (as measured by the [diameter of pneumothorax]^3/[diameter of hemithorax]^3) and/or the patient has evolving respiratory symptoms, insertion of a thoracostomy tube and application of negative pressure should be considered. Signs of tension pneumothorax (e.g., marked dyspnea, tachypnea and tachycardia, unilateral thoracic hyperresonance with reduced breath sounds, tracheal shift) necessitate emergent aspiration and tube placement. Children and adolescents with spontaneous pneumothoraces have a high recurrence rate because of the

common association with subpleural blebs. As a follow-up measure, many authorities recommend chest computed tomography scanning with contrast because significant blebs can be treated by surgical pleurodesis.

75. **Describe the clinical and radiographic features of a tension pneumothorax.**
    - **Clinical:** Increasing respiratory distress, hypoxemia, hypercarbia, hypotension
    - **Radiographic:** Shifting of the mediastinum, flattening of the diaphragm, widening of the intercostal spaces (Fig. 17-5)

76. **In children with pleural effusions, how are exudates distinguished from transudates?**
    Exudative pleural effusions meet a least one of the following criteria:
    - Pleural fluid protein/serum protein ratio >0.5
    - Pleural fluid lactate dehydrogenase (LDH)/serum LDH >0.6
    - Pleural fluid LDH >⅔ of the serum value
    If none of these criteria are met, then the patient has a transudative pleural effusion.

77. **What pediatric diseases are associated with exudative and transudative pleural effusions?**

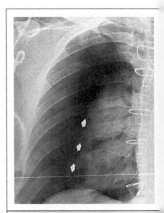

Figure 17-5. Tension pneumothorax. (From Katz DS, Math KR, Groskin SA (eds): Radiology Secrets. Philadelphia, Hanley & Belfus, 1998, p 61.)

Exudative	Transudative
Pneumonia	Congestive heart failure
Tuberculosis	Cirrhosis
Malignancy	Nephrotic syndrome
Chylothorax	Upper airway obstruction

In children, the most common cause for a pleural effusion is pneumonia ("parapneumonic"), whereas, in adults, the most common etiology is congestive heart failure.

78. **What is the value of chest physiotherapy in patients with pediatric pulmonary disease?**
    The main function of chest physiotherapy is to assist with the removal of tracheobronchial secretions to lessen obstruction, reduce airway resistance, enhance gas exchange, and reduce the work of breathing. Its use has been advocated in patients with chronic sputum production (e.g., cystic fibrosis), primary pneumonia, bronchiolitis, asthma, and atelectasis; for intubated neonates; and for postextubation and postoperative patients. Clinical benefits in each category—with the exception of diseases of chronic sputum production—remain highly anecdotal and understudied. Limited evidence does not support a role in bronchiolitis and asthma.

    American Association for Respiratory Care: www.aarc.org.
    Lannefors L, Button BM, McIlwaine M: Physiotherapy in infants and young children with cystic fibrosis: Current practice and future developments. J R Soc Med 97 Suppl 44:S8–S25, 2004.

79. **Who was Ondine, and what was her curse?**
    Ondine was a legendary water nymph who fell in love with Hans, a mortal. She put a curse on him with the stipulation that, should he ever betray her, he would suffocate by not breathing when he fell asleep. Unfortunately, Hans fell for the greater charms of Bertha, and he eventually succumbed to the curse while dozing. The term *Ondine curse* has been used to describe the syndrome of sleep apnea as a result of reduced respiratory drive, although the term *central*

hypoventilation syndrome (CHS) is used more correctly. This rare condition is often associated with other abnormalities of brain-stem function. CHS can be idiopathic, or it can be a complication of an earlier insult to the developing brain. In some families, it is genetic. Children with CHS are initially treated by tracheostomy and mechanical ventilation during sleep. Results with phrenic nerve pacing have been good in older infants and children.

CYSTIC FIBROSIS

80. **What is the basic defect in patients with cystic fibrosis (CF)?**
A defect in the CF transmembrane conductance regulator *(CFTR)* protein. This is a key ion channel that regulates chloride and sodium transfer across the apical membrane of epithelial cells. In patients with CF, chloride is poorly secreted into the airway lumen, and there is increased absorption of sodium from the luminal surface of the airway or duct, thereby resulting in respiratory and pancreatic secretions that are relatively dehydrated and viscid. These hyperviscous secretions obstruct pancreatic ducts, resulting in steatorrhea from exocrine pancreatic insufficiency, and they interfere with pulmonary mucociliary clearance, thereby causing chronic respiratory disease. In the sweat gland, CFTR is involved in the reabsorption of chloride, and abnormal CFTR function in patients with CF leads to the production of sweat with increased sodium and chloride concentrations. Hundreds of mutations of the gene that codes for this protein have been identified.

Rowe SM, Miller S, Sorscher EJ: Cystic fibrosis. N Engl J Med 352:1992-2001, 2005.

81. **What is the incidence of CF in various ethnic groups?**
- **Whites:** 1 in 3,300 live births
- **Hispanics:** 1 in 9,500 live births
- **Native Americans (in the United States):** 1 in 11,200 live births
- **Blacks (in the United States):** 1 in 15,300 live births
- **Asians:** 1 in 32,100 live births

Cystic Fibrosis Foundation: North American CF Registry. Bethesda, Maryland, 1996.
Cystic Fibrosis Foundation: www.cff.org.

82. **What are the presenting signs and symptoms of CF?**
These can be remembered with the acronym **CF PANCREAS:**
- **C** = **C**hronic cough and wheezing
- **F** = **F**ailure to thrive
- **P** = **P**ancreatic insufficiency (signs of malabsorption, including bulky, foul stools)
- **A** = **A**lkalosis and hypotonic dehydration
- **N** = **N**eonatal intestinal obstruction (meconium ileus) and **n**asal polyps
- **C** = **C**lubbing of the fingers and **c**hest radiographs with changes
- **R** = **R**ectal prolapse
- **E** = **E**lectrolyte elevation in sweat (salty skin)
- **A** = **A**bsence or congenital atresia of the vas deferens
- **S** = **S**putum with *Staphylococcus* or *Pseudomonas* (mucoid)

Schidlow DV: Cystic fibrosis. In Schidlow DV, Smith DS (eds): A Practical Guide to Pediatric Respiratory Diseases. Philadelphia, Hanley & Belfus, 1994, p 76.

83. **How is the diagnosis of CF made?**
It is made on the basis of the following:
- Result of a sweat test
- Mutational analysis in the presence of clinical characteristics of CF (this is performed if the sweat test is equivocal)

84. **What constitutes an abnormal sweat test?**
    Sweat gland secretions should be obtained by pilocarpine iontophoresis. A level of sweat chloride >60 mEq/L is abnormal; 40–60 mEq/L is borderline; and <40 mEq/L is normal.

85. **How are newborns screened for CF?**
    Newborns with CF have elevated levels of immunoreactive cationic trypsinogen, which is a precursor of trypsin. If the initial screen for this compound is elevated, mutational analysis of DNA and sweat testing follow in an attempt to confirm the diagnosis.

86. **What are the mainstays of pulmonary therapy for children with CF?**
    - Airway clearance techniques (e.g., chest physiotherapy, mechanical vests, flutter valve)
    - Mucolytic agents (e.g., recombinant human DNAse, acetylcysteine)
    - Anti-inflammatory agents (e.g., ibuprofen, inhaled corticosteroids)
    - Bronchodilators (e.g., beta$_2$-agonists)
    - Antibiotics (oral, inhaled, and intravenous)

    Ratjen F, Doring G: Cystic fibrosis. Lancet 362:681–689, 2003.

KEY POINTS: CYSTIC FIBROSIS

1. This is the most common lethal inherited disease in whites.

2. Cystic fibrosis gene: There are hundreds of known mutations; ΔF508 is the most common in North America (75%).

3. Key to diagnosis: Sweat test (sweat chloride >60 meq/L is abnormal).

4. Chronic obstructive pulmonary disease.

5. Gastrointestinal manifestations can include pancreatic insufficiency, bowel obstruction, rectal prolapse, intussusception, gastroesophageal reflux, and cholelithiasis.

6. Pulmonary colonization with *Pseudomonas* or *Burkholderia* is a poor prognostic sign.

87. **What are the two most common causes of abdominal pain in school-aged children with CF?**
    - **Inadequate intake of pancreatic enzyme supplements:** A dietary and stool pattern history will often reveal changes that are suggestive of poorly controlled fat malabsorption. The adjustment of enzyme therapy can correct the problem.
    - **Constipation** (meconium ileus equivalent): A fecal mass may be noted on examination, and abdominal x-ray can confirm the findings.
      Treatment involves adjusting enzyme therapy and the use of stool softeners and cathartics.

88. **Which features of CF have prognostic significance?**
    - **Gender:** Males have better survival rates than females, although the gap is narrowing.
    - **Colonization with virulent bacteria:** *Pseudomonas aeruginosa* and *Burkholderia* (formerly *Pseudomonas*) *cepacia* are more serious pathogens, which are often resistant to multiple drugs and difficult to clear after the patient becomes persistently infected. *Stenotrophomona maltophilia* is an emerging problem; patients who are chronically colonized with these organisms have significantly poorer survival rates than other patients with CF.
    - **Diabetes mellitus** is a negative prognostic factor that is associated with increased rates of decline in pulmonary function.
    - **Malnutrition** is also associated with increased rates of decline in pulmonary function.

- **Cor pulmonale** is one of the late complications of CF, because progressive obstructive airway disease leads to the development of pulmonary hypertension and respiratory failure. The patient's prognosis is poor after the development of cor pulmonale.
- **Pneumothorax** is associated with moderate to advanced lung disease in patients with CF. Therefore, air leak has traditionally been regarded as a poor prognostic sign. The prognosis has been improving now that pneumothoraces are being managed aggressively.
- **Worsening pulmonary function tests:** Patients with an FEV_1 level of <30% of predicted have an increased 2-year mortality rate.

Goss CH, Rubenfeld GD, Otto K, Aitken ML: The effect of pregnancy on survival in women with cystic fibrosis. Chest 124:1460–1468, 2003.

Kulich M, Rosenfeld M, Goss CH, Wilmott R: Improved survival among young patients with cystic fibrosis. J Pediatr 142:631–636, 2003.

PNEUMONIA

89. **What agents cause pneumonia in children?**
The etiology of community-acquired pneumonia in pediatrics is highly dependent on the age of the child. Most studies cannot determine an etiology in about 50% of patients. Determining an infectious organism can be very difficult, especially in younger children. From the newborn period to 3 months of age, group B streptococcus, gram-negative bacilli, *Chlamydia trachomatis,* and *Ureaplasma urealyticum* are common, and so are RSV and other viruses.

	3 months–5 years	5–10 years	10–15 years
Bacterial	33%	30%	30%
Viral	33%	15%	3%
Mycoplasma pneumoniae	5%	20%	40%
Chlamydia pneumoniae	2%	8%	25%

Lichenstein R, Suggs AH, Campbell J: Pediatric pneumonia. Pediatr Clin North Am 21:437–451, 2003.

Michelow IC, Olsen K, Lozano J, et al: Epidemiology and clinical characteristics of community-acquired pneumonia in children. Pediatrics 113:701–707, 2004.

90. **What are the important trends in the etiology of pneumonia?**
- A **bacterial etiology** is common in all three age groups studied and does not change from infancy to adolescence. The most common bacterial etiology after 3 months of age is *Streptococcus pneumoniae.*
- A **viral etiology** is more common in younger age groups, and it is most frequently RSV. Viruses can be associated with pneumonia in school-aged children, but these become less common with age. Human metapneumovirus is a newly described common pathogen. In older children, influenza is one of the more common etiologies, especially during epidemics.
- **Atypical pneumonia** caused by *Mycoplasma pneumoniae* and *Chlamydia pneumoniae* is uncommon in preschool-aged children. Both *Mycoplasma* and *Chlamydia* become more prevalent in school-aged children and are the most common etiology for pneumonia in the older child.

Williams JV, Harris PA, Tollefson SJ, et al: Human metapneumovirus and lower respiratory tract disease in otherwise healthy infants and children. N Engl J Med 350:443–450, 2004.

91. **Are throat or nasopharyngeal cultures helpful for the diagnosis of pneumonia?**
As a rule, the correlation between throat and nasopharyngeal bacterial cultures and lower respiratory tract pathogens is poor and of limited value. Healthy children may be colonized with a wide variety of potentially pathologic bacteria (e.g., *Staphylococcus aureus, Haemophilus influenzae*), which can be considered part of the normal flora; *Bordetella pertussis* is an exception. Cultures or antigen detection systems to identify respiratory viruses or chlamydia, however, are highly informative because these organisms are rarely carried asymptomatically.

92. **How often are blood cultures positive in children with suspected bacterial pneumonia?**
    10% of the time or less. This number is an estimate, because the true denominator in the equation (the number of true bacterial pneumonias) is difficult to ascertain as a result of the difficulty with making a definitive diagnosis. The low rate of positive blood cultures does suggest that most bacterial pneumonias are not acquired by hematogenous spread.

93. **How often are pleural fluid cultures positive in children with suspected bacterial pneumonia?**
    Between 60% and 85% are positive if antibiotics have not already been initiated. This high yield emphasizes the importance of recognizing a pleural effusion in patients with pneumonia and the value of early thoracentesis before starting antibiotic therapy.

94. **How common is an occult pneumonia in a febrile child with leukocytosis?**
    In a search for a focus of infection, the chest is always a suspect. In a study of children <5 years old without clinical evidence of pneumonia but a temperature of ≥39°C and a total white blood cell count of ≥20,000, the chest x-ray was positive in 19% of cases.

    Bachur R, Perry H, Harper MB: Occult pneumonias: Empiric chest radiographs in febrile children with leukocytosis. Ann Emerg Med 33:166–173, 1999.

95. **Can a chest x-ray reliably distinguish between viral and bacterial pneumonia?**
    No. Viral infections more commonly have perihilar, peribronchial, or interstitial infiltrates; hyperinflation; segmental atelectasis; and hilar adenopathy; however, there can be considerable overlap with bacterial (and chlamydial and mycoplasmal) pneumonia. Bacterial pneumonia more commonly results in an alveolar infiltrate, but the sensitivity and specificity of this finding are not very high.

    Donnelly LF: Maximizing the usefulness of imaging in children with community-acquired pneumonia. Am J Roentgenol 172:505–512, 1999.
    Swingler GH: Radiologic differentiation between bacterial and viral lower respiratory infection in children: A systematic literature review. Clin Pediatr 39:627–633, 2000.

96. **What are indications for hospital admission in children with pneumonia?**
    - All who appear toxic, dyspneic, or hypoxic
    - Suspected staphylococcal pneumonia (e.g., pneumatocele on chest x-ray)
    - Significant pleural effusion
    - Suspected aspiration pneumonia (because of the higher likelihood of progression)
    - Children who cannot tolerate oral medications or who are at significant risk for dehydration
    - Suspected bacterial pneumonia in very young infants, especially with multilobar involvement
    - Poor response to outpatient therapy after 48 hours
    - Those whose family situation and chances for reliable follow-up are suboptimal

97. **What clinical clues suggest atypical pneumonia?**
    These infections tend to start gradually, have minimal or a nonproductive cough, and have frequent constitutional signs (e.g., headache, rash, pharyngitis). Chest radiographs tend to show patchy, peribronchial infiltrates with only occasional lobar consolidation.

98. **What are the causes of "afebrile infant pneumonia" syndrome?**
    The syndrome is usually the result of *Chlamydia trachomatis*, cytomegalovirus, *Ureaplasma urealyticum*, or *Mycoplasma hominis*. Affected infants develop progressive respiratory distress over several days to a few weeks, along with failure to thrive. A maternal history of a sexually transmitted disease is common. Chest x-rays reveal bilateral diffuse infiltrates with hyperinfla-

tion. There may be eosinophilia and elevated quantitative immunoglobulins (IgG, IgA, IgM). The causes overlap clinically, although a history of conjunctivitis suggests chlamydia.

99. How likely is an infant to develop infection if he or she is born to a mother with positive cervical cultures for *Chlamydia trachomatis*?

Up to 50% of infants demonstrate an inclusion conjunctivitis, and 5-20% develop pneumonia. Prevalence of the organism in pregnant women varies from 6–12%, but it can be as low as 2% or as high as 37% in adolescents. Up to 30,000 infants develop chlamydial pneumonia annually, making it the most common cause of pneumonia in children <6 months old.

00. What are the clinical characteristics of chlamydial pneumonia in infants?

- Illness occurs between 2 and 19 weeks after birth. Most infants show symptoms by 8 weeks of age.
- Onset is gradual, with upper respiratory prodromal symptoms lasting >1 week.
- Nearly 100% of patients are afebrile.
- Less than half have inclusion conjunctivitis.
- Respiratory signs and symptoms include the following: staccato cough, tachypnea, diffuse crackles, and occasional wheezing.
- Chest x-ray reveals bilateral hyperexpansion and symmetric interstitial infiltrates.
- Seventy percent have an elevated absolute eosinophil count (>400/mm^3).
- More than 90% have increased quantitative immunoglobulins (IgG, IgM).

01. How helpful are cold agglutinins in the diagnosis of *Mycoplasma pneumoniae* infections?

Cold agglutinins are IgM autoantibodies that are directed against the I antigen of erythrocytes, which agglutinate red cells at 4°C. Up to 75% of patients with mycoplasmal infections will develop them, usually toward the end of the first week of illness, with a peak at 4 weeks. A titer of 1:64 supports the diagnosis. Other infectious agents, including adenovirus, cytomegalovirus, Epstein-Barr virus, influenza, rubella, *Chlamydia*, and *Listeria* can also give a positive result. A single cold agglutinin titer of 1:64 is therefore suggestive but not conclusive evidence of infection with *M pneumoniae*. Because culture and serologic studies are time consuming, rapid diagnosis will await the availability of a sensitive and specific polymerase chain reaction test for *M pneumoniae*.

Waites KB: New concepts of *Mycoplasma pneumoniae* infections in children Pediatr Pulmonol 36:267–278, 2003.

02. When do the radiologic findings of pneumonia resolve?

Although there is a wide range, as a rule, most infiltrates that result from *Streptococcus pneumoniae* resolve in 6–8 weeks, and those that are caused by RSV resolve in 2–3 weeks. However, with some viral infections (e.g., adenovirus), it may take up to 1 year for x-rays to normalize. If significant radiologic abnormalities persist for >6 weeks, there should be a high index of suspicion for a possible underlying problem (e.g., unusual infection, anatomic abnormality, immunologic deficiency).

Regelmann WE: Diagnosing the cause of recurrent and persistent pneumonia in children. Pediatr Ann 22:561–568, 1993.

03. Do children with pneumonia need follow-up x-rays to verify resolution?

Generally, no. Exceptions would include children with pleural effusions, those with persistent or recurrent signs and symptoms, and those with significant comorbid conditions (e.g., immunodeficiency).

Wacogne I, Negrine RJ: Are follow-up chest x-ray examinations helpful in the management of children recovering from pneumonia? Arch Dis Child 88:457–458, 2003.

104. What are the causes of recurrent pneumonia?

- **Aspiration susceptibility:** Oropharyngeal incoordination, vocal cord paralysis, gastroesophageal reflux
- **Immunodeficiency:** Congenital, acquired
- **Congenital cardiac defects:** Atrial septal defect, ventricular septal defect, patent ductus arteriosus
- **Abnormal secretions** or **reduced clearance of secretions:** Asthma, cystic fibrosis, ciliary dyskinesia
- **Pulmonary anomalies:** Sequestration, cystic adenomatoid malformation, tracheoesophageal fistula
- **Airway compression** or **obstruction:** Foreign body, vascular ring, enlarged lymph node, malignancy
- **Miscellaneous:** For example, sickle cell disease, sarcoidosis

Owayed AF, Campbell DM, Wang EE: Underlying causes of recurrent pneumonia in children. Arch Pediatr Adolesc Med 154:190–194, 2000.

KEY POINTS: PNEUMONIA

1. Treatment is most commonly outpatient, but follow-up is key.

2. Effusion or pneumatocele suggest a bacterial cause.

3. Radiographic findings in patients with mycoplasmal infections are highly variable.

4. In half of patients with chlamydial pneumonia, conjunctivitis precedes pneumonia.

5. Hilar adenopathy suggests tuberculosis.

105. How does the pH of a substance affect the severity of disease in aspiration pneumonia?

A low pH is more harmful than a slightly alkaline or neutral pH, and it is more likely to be associated with bronchospasm and pneumonia. The most severe form of pneumonia is seen when gastric contents are aspirated; symptoms may develop in a matter of seconds. If the volume of aspirate is sufficiently large and the pH is <2.5, the mortality may exceed 70%. The radiographic picture may be that of an infiltrate or pulmonary edema. Unilateral pulmonary edema may occur if the child is lying on one side.

106. How should children with aspiration pneumonia be managed?

Acute aspiration can often be treated supportively without antibiotics, because the initial process is a chemical pneumonitis. If secondary signs of infection occur, then antibiotics should be started after appropriate cultures; either penicillin or clindamycin is a reasonable choice to cover the oropharyngeal anaerobes that predominate. If the aspiration is nosocomial then antibiotic coverage should be extended to include Gram-negative organisms as well.

PULMONARY PRINCIPLES

107. In addition to underlying immunologic immaturity, why are infants more susceptible to an increased severity of respiratory disease?

- Very compliant chest wall (allows passage through birth canal, but limits inspiratory effort as it distorts with increased respiratory loading)

- Respiratory muscles more easily fatigued as a result of decreased muscle mass and fewer type I muscles fibers (slow twitch, high oxidative fibers)
- Chest wall elastic recoil is low in infancy (airway closure occurs at a higher relative lung volume)
- High airway compliance facilitates airway collapse and air trapping
- Collateral ventilation poorly developed, thus increasing likelihood of atelectasis during illness
- Higher airway mucous gland concentration in infants than in adults

08. At what age do alveoli stop increasing in number?

Although extra-acinar airway development is complete by 16 weeks of gestation, alveolar multiplication continues after birth. Early studies suggested that postnatal alveolar multiplication ends at 8 years of age. However, more recent studies have shown that it is terminated by 2 years of age and possibly between 1 and 2 years of age. After the end of alveolar multiplication, the alveoli continue to increase in size until thoracic growth is completed.

09. What is the normal respiratory rate of a child?

Rates in a child who is awake can be widely variable, depending on the psychological state and activity. Rates while sleeping are much more reliable and are a good indicator of pulmonary health. As a general rule, the sleeping rate in *infants* is usually <35 breaths per minute; in *toddlers,* it is <30 breaths per minute; in *older children,* it is <25 breaths per minute; and in *adolescents,* it is <20 breaths per minute. However, fever and metabolic acidosis can lead to an increased respiratory rate in the absence of pulmonary disease.

10. What is normal oxygen saturation in healthy infants who are <6 months old?

In a longitudinal study using pulse oximetry, baseline saturation was >95% (normal was 98%, with lower 10th percentile at 95%). However, acute desaturations are common; almost all are associated with brief episodes of apnea while sleeping.

Hunt CE, Corwin MJ, Lister G, et al: Longitudinal assessment of hemoglobin saturation in healthy infants during the first six months of life. J Pediatr 134:580–586, 1999.

11. What is the difference between Kussmaul, Cheyne-Stokes, and Biot types of breathing patterns?

- **Kussmaul:** Deep, slow, regular respirations with prolonged exhalation; seen in diabetic ketoacidosis and salicylate ingestion
- **Cheyne-Stokes:** Crescendo-decrescendo respirations alternating with periods of apnea (no breathing); causes include heart failure, uremia, central nervous system trauma, increased intracranial pressure, and coma
- **Biot** (also known as ataxic breathing): Characterized by unpredictable irregularity; breaths may be shallow or deep and stop for short periods; causes include respiratory depression, meningitis, encephalitis, and other central nervous system lesions involving the respiratory centers

12. Why a sigh?

A sigh is just a sigh in Casablanca, but it is also a very effective anti-atelectatic maneuver. By definition, it is a breath that is more than three times the normal tidal volume.

13. Is there a respiratory basis for yawning?

Although a respiratory function for yawning is frequently suggested, scientific support for this belief is minimal. Increasing the concentration of CO_2 in inspired air increases the respiratory rate but does not change the rate of yawning. Relief of hypoxia and opening areas of microatelectasis are other theories that are not supported by scientific studies. Some studies hypothesize that yawning may be an arousal reflex.

114. **What are "coarse" breath sounds?**

In a patient with coarse breath sounds, the loudness of expiration equals the loudness of inspiration on auscultation. In large airways, expiratory breath sounds are louder than inspiratory breath sounds as a result of turbulence. Coarse breath sounds can be physiologic (as when listening just below the center of the clavicle to primarily bronchial sounds) or pathologic (if interposed fluid allows for the transmission of large airway sounds or if airways are widened [e.g., bronchiectasis]).

115. **At what concentration is inspired oxygen toxic?**

In addition to atelectasis, high oxygen concentration can cause alveolar injury with edema, inflammation, fibrin deposition, and hyalinization. The precise level of hyperoxia that results in injury is unclear and varies by age and underlying lung pathology, but a reasonable rule is to assume that a concentration of >80% for >36 hours is likely to result in significant ongoing damage; 60–80% is likely to be associated with more slowly progressive injury. An inspired oxygen concentration of 50%, even when administered for extended periods of time, is unlikely to cause pulmonary toxicity.

Jenkinson SG: Oxygen toxicity. J Intensive Care Med 3:137–152, 1988.

116. **Why is a child who is receiving 100% oxygen more likely to develop atelectasis than one who is breathing room air?**

Nitrogen is more slowly absorbed than oxygen by alveoli. In room air (with its 78% nitrogen), alveolar collapse is minimized by the continued presence and pressure of nitrogen gas (the "nitrogen stint"). In 100% oxygen, however, the more rapid absorption of oxygen can lead to absorption atelectasis with intrapulmonary shunting.

117. **At what PaO_2 does cyanosis develop?**

Cyanosis develops when the concentration of desaturated (i.e., reduced) hemoglobin is at least 3 gm/dL centrally or 4–6 gm/dl peripherally. However, multiple factors affect the likelihood that a given PaO_2 will result in clinically apparent cyanosis: anemia (less likely), polycythemia (more likely), reduced systemic perfusion or cardiac output (more likely), and hypothermia (more likely). Cyanosis is generally a sign of significant hypoxia. In a patient with adequate perfusion and a normal hemoglobin, central cyanosis is commonly noted when the PaO_2 is approximately 50 mmHg.

118. **What are the causes of a reduced PaO_2 associated with an increased $A\text{-}aDO_2$?**

- **Right-to-left shunting:** Intracardiac, abnormal arteriovenous connections; intrapulmonary shunts that result from perfusion of airless alveoli (e.g., pneumonia, atelectasis), often referred to as ventilation-perfusion mismatching
- **Maldistribution of ventilation:** Asthma, bronchiolitis, atelectasis, etc.
- **Impaired diffusion:** An uncommon mechanism, because many of the conditions previously thought to have a "diffusion block" (e.g., respiratory distress syndrome) also have a major component of shunting; may be seen when interstitial edema affects the septal walls (e.g., in early pulmonary edema and interstitial pneumonia)
- **Decreased central venous oxygen content:** As a result of a sluggish circulation (e.g., shock) or increased tissue oxygen demands (e.g., sepsis)

119. **How does the pulse oximeter work?**

The key principle behind pulse oximetry is that oxygenated hemoglobin allows for more transmission of red light than does reduced hemoglobin. By contrast, transmission of infrared light is unaffected by the amount of oxyhemoglobin present. A light source of red and infrared wavelengths is applied to an area of the body thin enough that the light can traverse a pulsating capillary bed and be detected by a light detector on the other side. Each pulsation increases the distance the light has to travel, which increases the amount of light absorption.

A microprocessor derives the arterial oxygen saturation by comparing absorbencies at baseline and during the peak of a transmitted pulse.

20. What are the disadvantages or limitations of pulse oximetry?
- Patient movement disturbs measurements.
- Poor perfusion states affect accuracy.
- Fluorescent or high-intensity light can interfere with results.
- It is unreliable if abnormal hemoglobin is present (e.g., methemoglobin).
- It is unable to detect hypoxia until the PaO_2 decreases below 80 mmHg.
- Accuracy diminishes with arterial saturations below 70–80%.

21. In infants with unilateral lung disease, should the good lung be up or down?
The good lung should be up. This is another example of why children are not simply small adults. It is well established that adults with unilateral lung disease treated in a decubitus position will have an increase in oxygen saturation when the good lung is placed down; this occurs because of an increase in ventilation to the dependent lung. Studies have shown that the opposite occurs in infants and children, because ventilation is preferentially distributed toward the uppermost lung. This positional redistribution of ventilation seems to change to an adult pattern during the late teenage years.

Davies H, Helms P, Gordon I: Effect of posture on regional ventilation in children. Pediatr Pulmonol 12:227–232, 1992.

ACKNOWLEDGMENT

The editors gratefully acknowledge contributions by Drs. Ellen R. Kaplan, Carlos R. Perez, William D. Hardie, Barbara A. Chini, and Cori L. Daines that were retained from the first three editions of *Pediatric Secrets*.

CHAPTER 18

RHEUMATOLOGY

Carlos D. Rosé, MD, Balu H. Athreya, MD, Elizabeth Candell Chalom, MD, and Andrew H. Eichenfield, MD

CLINICAL ISSUES

1. **What is an ANA profile?**
   Antinuclear antibody (ANA) is made up of circulating gammaglobulins directed against several known and unknown nuclear proteins. At last count, ANA is directed against at least 33 different proteins. Because it is measured by an immunofluorescent technique, it is also called *FANA*. It is now possible to identify several of the specific antigens against which this antibody is directed by using enzyme-linked immunosorbent assay (ELISA), immunodiffusion, and immunoelec-trophoresis; this is the *ANA profile*.

   American College of Rheumatology: www.rheumatology.org

2. **What is the significance of the various antibodies included in the ANA profile?**

Antibody	Associated illness
Anti-double-stranded DNA	Systemic lupus erythematosus (SLE)
Antihistone	Drug-induced lupus
Anti-Ro (also called anti-SS A)	Sjögren's syndrome and neonatal lupus
Anti-La (also called anti-SS B)	Sjögren's syndrome and neonatal lupus

3. **What is the significance of a positive ANA test?**
   ANA is a *sensitive* but *nonspecific* test for the recognition of autoimmune diseases in general and for SLE in particular (sensitivity ~96%); it is used as a first-step diagnostic test when SLE is suspected. In the case of SLE, this has to be followed by a specific test—anti-double-stranded DNA antibody and ANA profile—to confirm the diagnosis.

4. **A 6-year-old girl with a 2-month history of joint pain (onset after a viral illness) has a normal physical examination, complete blood cell count, and erythrocyte sedimentation rate (ESR) but a positive ANA titer of 1:160. What are some of the possible explanations for this positive ANA?**
   - Laboratory variation
   - Nonspecific response to viral illness
   - Preclinical state of SLE (least likely)
   - Normal population frequency (~8% at that titer)
   - Other autoimmune/paraneoplastic conditions

   Tan EM, Feltkamp TE, Smolen JS, et al: Range of antinuclear antibodies in "healthy" individuals. Arthritis Rheum 40:1601–1611, 1997.

5. **Is Raynaud's phenomenon a disease?**
   In 1874, Maurice Raynaud, while still a medical student, described a triad of episodic pallor, cyanosis, and erythema after exposure to cold stress; the term *Raynaud's phenomenon* describes this clinical triad. When this phenomenon is associated with a disease such as scleroderma or lupus, it is called *Raynaud's syndrome;* when the phenomenon is seen as an isolated condition without any other rheumatic disorder, it is called *Raynaud's disease,* although some patients on

long-term follow-up may develop an associated disease (e.g., CREST syndrome [a limited form of systemic sclerosis]). Rheumatologists are commonly consulted for adolescents with blue dusky hands and feet. If there is no pallor, it is probably benign acrocyanosis (Crocq's disease), a benign variant of no clinical relevance. It may occur in association with weight loss in athletes or children treated with amphetamine derivatives for attention-deficit hyperactivity disorder.

Nigrovic PA, Fuhlbrigge RC, Sundel RP: Raynaud's phenomenon in children: A retrospective review of 123 patients. Pediatrics 111:715–721, 2003.

6. **When is a child considered to have hypermobile joints?**
The presence of three of the following features suggests true hypermobility:
- Apposition of the thumb to the flexor aspect of the forearm (Fig. 18-1)
- Hyperextension of the fingers so that they lie parallel to the dorsum of the forearm
- Hyperextension at the elbow of greater than 10°
- Knee hyperextension of greater then 10°
- Ability to touch the floor with the heel and also with the palms of the hands from a standing position without flexing the knee

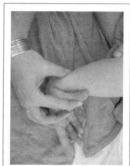

7. **Which children can demonstrate Gorlin's sign?**
Gorlin's sign is the ability to touch the tip of the nose with the tongue. It is seen in conditions associated with hypermobility syndromes, such as Ehlers-Danlos syndrome.

8. **In what settings can reactive arthritis occur?**
Reactive arthritis in its broadest sense refers to a pattern of arthritis associated with a nonarticular (remote) infection. By definition, it is an inflammatory arthritis, but a live organism cannot be isolated by culture of synovial fluid or synovial biopsy. A restricted definition of the syndrome includes arthritis after enteric (e.g., *Salmonella, Shigella, Yersinia, Campylobacter, Giardia*) or genitourinary infections (e.g., chlamydia).

Figure 18-1. Abnormal contact between the thumb and forearm in a young girl with benign hypermobility joint syndrome.

Flores D, Marquez J, Garza M, Espinoza LR: Reactive arthritis: Newer developments. Rheum Dis Clin North Am 29:37–59, 2003.

9. **What conditions are associated with gastroenteritis and arthritis?**
Noninfectious
- Ulcerative colitis
- Crohn's disease
- Behçet's disease
- Henoch-Schönlein purpura
- Celiac disease

Infectious
- *Salmonella*
- *Shigella*
- *Yersinia*
- *Campylobacter*
- Tuberculosis
- Whipple's disease
- Giardiasis

10. **How do synovial fluid characteristics help to determine the diagnosis of arthritis?**
See Table 18-1.

TABLE 18-1. SYNOVIAL FLUID CHARACTERISTICS IN VARIOUS ARTHRITIDES

Group/ Condition	Synovial comple- ment	Color/ clarity	Visco- sity	Mucin clot	White blood cell count (μL)	Polymorphonuclear neutro- phil count (%)	Miscella- neous findings
Noninflam- **matory**							
Normal	N	Yellow, clear	↑↑	G	<200	<25	
Traumatic arthritis	N	Yellow, turbid	↑	F–G	<2,000	<25	Debris
Inflam- **matory**							
Rheumatic fever	N–↑	Yellow, cloudy	↓	F	5,000	10–50	
JRA	N–↓	Yellow, cloudy	↓	Poor	15,000– 30,000	75	
Pyogenic							
Tuberculous arthritis	N–↑	Yellow- white, cloudy	↓	Poor	25,000	50–60	Acid-fast bacteria
Septic arthritis	↑	Serosan- guineous, turbid	↓	Poor	30,000– 50,000	>75	Low glucose, bacteria

11. **One week after mild trauma an 8-year-old girl has pain and tenderness in the right foot and leg, both of which are cold, exquisite, and tender to the touch, with mottled discoloration. What is the likely diagnosis?**

Complex regional pain syndrome, type 1. More commonly called *reflex sympathetic dystrophy,* this poorly understood entity is often confused with arthritis because of localized severe pain in one of the extremities. However, there are several features that separate it from arthritis. The pain is not confined to a single joint; it is regional in nature, involving portions of an extremity, and it often follows minor trauma. The pain is very severe, and even light touch causes pain (i.e., hyperesthesia). Several dysautonomic changes (e.g., mottling, color changes, sweating) may occur. Laboratory findings are normal. Autonomic dysfunction can be confirmed by thermography or by technetium scan, which demonstrates reduced blood flow. Regional osteopenia as a result of disuse may develop.

Because the role of the sympathetic nervous system is unclear and dystrophy may not occur in all cases, the terminology change has been advised by the International Association for the Study of Pain. In type 1, all of the features of the complex are present without definable nerve injury. In type 2, a definable nerve injury is present.

Sherry DD, Malleson PN: The idiopathic musculoskeletal pain syndromes in childhood. Rheum Dis Clin North Am 28:669–685, 2002.

12. **How is complex regional pain syndrome managed?**

Although many children are casted because of suspected hairline fractures, immobilization is contraindicated. Treatment is aimed at providing pain relief using analgesics and other nonmedical modalities. A good explanation of the mechanism of pain and assurance that this condition is controllable are essential when managing these children and their families. A physical therapy program should be started immediately, with emphasis on passive and active range of motion exercises and the maintenance of function. Aquatherapy is particularly useful in these children to initiate therapy. Desensitization of the painful area using one of several modalities (e.g., biofeedback, transcutaneous electrical nerve stimulation, visualization, acupuncture) should be part of the program. A positive attitude on the part of physicians and therapists is essential. In extreme situations, sympathetic blockade may be needed. Newer therapies also include electrical stimulation of the spinal cord and the use of intrathecal baclofen (a gamma-aminobutyric acid-receptor agonist that inhibits sensory input to the neurons of the spinal cord).

van Hilten BJ, van de Beek WJ, Hoff JI, et al: Intrathecal baclofen for the treatment of dystonia in patients with reflex sympathetic dystrophy. N Engl J Med 343:625–630, 2000.

13. **Do children develop fibromyalgia?**

Children as young as 9 years old have been described as having this syndrome. Fibromyalgia is a condition that is characterized by musculoskeletal aches and pains, fatigue, disturbed sleep patterns, and tenderness over various parts of the body. These tender points are specific for the diagnosis (Fig. 18-2). There should be tenderness over at least four of these 11 points for proper classification of individuals. In addition, there should be no tenderness over nonspecific sites such as the forehead or the pretibial region.

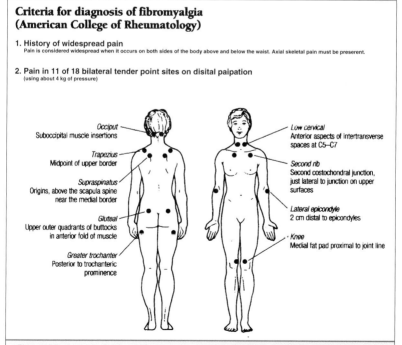

Criteria for diagnosis of fibromyalgia (American College of Rheumatology)

1. **History of widespread pain**
   Pain is considered widespread when it occurs on both sides of the body above and below the waist. Axial skeletal pain must be preserent.

2. **Pain in 11 of 18 bilateral tender point sites on disital paipation**
   (using about 4 kg of pressure)

Occiput
Suboccipital muscle insertions

Trapezius
Midpoint of upper border

Supraspinatus
Origins, above the scapula spine near the medial border

Gluteal
Upper outer quadrants of buttocks in anterior fold of muscle

Greater trochanter
Posterior to trochanteric prominence

Low cervical
Anterior aspects of intertransverse spaces at C5–C7

Second rib
Second costochondral junction, just lateral to junction on upper surfaces

Lateral epicondyle
2 cm distal to epicondyles

Knee
Medial fat pad proximal to joint line

Figure 18-2. American College of Rheumatology criteria for the diagnosis of fibromyalgia. (From Ballinger S, Bowyer S: Fibromyalgia: The latest "great" imitator. Contemp Pediatr 14:147, 1997.)

Aches and pains are extremely common in children and may be to the result of serious medical diseases (e.g., leukemia), mental illness (e.g., depression), and psychosocial stress. Differentiation of chronic musculoskeletal pain of nonorganic origin may be difficult in children and adolescents.

14. **What is the difference between complementary and alternative medicine?**
   Complementary medicine generally refers to treatments used in addition to or *in conjunction with* traditional medicine, whereas **alternative** medicine refers to therapies used *in place of* traditional medicine.

15. **What is the role of acupuncture for the pediatric patient?**
   A National Institutes of Health consensus conference regarding acupuncture among adults found it to be effective for treating some types of nausea and pain, particularly dental pain, migraine headaches, back pain, and dysmenorrhea. In children, the data are more limited. Acupuncture has been used to treat postextubation laryngospasm, asthma, allergies, postoperative nausea, and pain. The Pain Treatment Service at Boston Children's Hospital referred adolescents with chronic and refractory pain to a licensed acupuncturist primarily for migraine headache, endometriosis, and complex regional pain syndrome (reflex sympathetic dystrophy); 70% of patients reported relief.

   Kemper KJ, Sarah R, Silver-Highfield E, et al: On pins and needles? Pediatric pain patients' experience with acupuncture. Pediatrics 105:941–947, 2000.

   Lee CK, Chien TJ, Hsu JC, et al: The effect of acupuncture on the incidence of postextubation laryngospasm in children. Anaesthesia 53:910–924, 1998.

DERMATOMYOSITIS AND POLYMYOSITIS

16. **What are the criteria used for the diagnosis of juvenile dermatomyositis and polymyositis?**
   - Symmetrical proximal muscle weakness (e.g., Gowers' sign)
   - Elevated serum enzymes in muscle (creative kinase [CK], lactic dehydrogenase [LDH], aspartate transaminase [AST], and/or aldolase)
   - Abnormal electromyogram (increased insertional activity, myopathic pattern, polymorphic potentials)
   - Inflammation and/or necrosis on muscle biopsy
   - Characteristic skin eruption

   The presence of rash distinguishes dermatomyositis from polymyositis. Three out of four criteria plus a pathognomic rash establish the diagnosis of dermatomyositis, and a confirmatory biopsy is not necessary. If fewer criteria are met, a biopsy may be needed for diagnosis.

   Compeyrot-Lacassagne S, Feldman BM: Inflammatory myopathies in children. Pediatr Clin North Am 52: 493-520, 2005.

   Ramanan AV, Feldman BM: Clinical features and outcomes of juvenile dermatomyositis and other childhood-onset myositis syndromes. Rheum Dis Clin North Am 28:833–857, 2002.

17. **What skin changes are pathognomonic for dermatomyositis?**
   Gottron's patches (Fig. 18-3). These begin as inflammatory papules over the dorsal aspect of interphalangeal joints and the extensor aspect of the elbows and knee joints. The papules become violaceous and flat-topped and may coalesce to become patches. Eventually the lesions show atrophic changes and become hypopigmented.

18. **What are the other classic cutaneous findings of dermatomyositis among children?**
   - Periorbital edema and erythema with violaceous color of the upper eyelid (heliotrope rash)
   - Rash over the upper chest in the shawl distribution

- Photosensitivity
- Cutaneous vasculitis with ulceration
- Nailfold capillary abnormalities

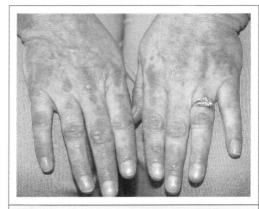

Figure 18-3. Gottron papules. (From Fitzpatrick JE, Aeling JL: Dermatology Secrets, 2nd ed. Philadelphia, Hanley & Belfus, 2001, p 257.)

19. **Which infectious agents are known to cause myositis?**
    - **Viral:** Notably Coxsackie (named after Coxsackie, NY) and influenza A and B
    - **Bacterial:** *Staphylococcus* and *Yersinia* (causing pyomyositis)
    - **Protozoal:** *Toxoplasma* and trichinosis
    - **Spirochetal:** *Borrelia*

    The most common cause of acute muscle disease associated with pain, difficulty walking, and a high level of creatine kinase is viral myositis.

JUVENILE RHEUMATOID ARTHRITIS

20. **At what point is a synovitis considered chronic?**
    At 6 weeks in the United States and at 3 months in Europe.

21. **What is the most common chronic arthritis seen in children?**
    Juvenile rheumatoid arthritis (JRA).

22. **What are the diagnostic criteria for the classification of JRA?**
    JRA is a diagnosis of exclusion. Features include the following:
    - Onset at ≤16 years of age
    - Clinical arthritis with joint swelling or effusion, increased heat, and limitation of range of motion with tenderness
    - Duration of disease of ≥6 weeks

    The major subgroups (systemic-onset, pauciarticular or oligoarticular, polyarticular) are distinguished by the following:
    - The presence or absence of fever at presentation
    - The number of joints involved during the first 6 months of illness
    - No other known etiology for arthritis

    This classification and the subsets that are defined in question 24 were developed in Park City by the American College of Rheumatology in 1977 and are known as the ACR criteria. They are used almost exclusively in the United States.

23. **What additional classifications for JRA are used?**
    Two additional classifications are frequently used in the United States and Canada: the European Ligue Against Rheumatism (EULAR) classification (Basel, 1977), which uses the term juvenile chronic arthritis (JCA) in lieu of JRA, and the International Ligue of Associations of Rheumatology (ILAR) classification (Durban, 1997), which uses the term JIA (juvenile idiopathic arthritis). These classifications are widely used in Latin America and Europe.

24. **What are the main subsets of JRA and their characteristics?**
    See Table 18-2.

Subset	No. of joints involved	Percentage of total patients	Age at onset (years)	Gender	+ANA	+RF	Uveitis	Remission rate (at puberty)	Functional outcome
Pauci-articular	1–4	50%	2	Females	+++	–	20%	60%	Good
Polyarticular, RF-negative	≥5	30%	3–9	Females	++	–	5–10%	20%	Fair
Polyarticular, RF-positive	≥5	5%	Teen-age	Females	+	+	No	<5%	Poor
Systemic	Any	15%	0–16	Males and females	–	–	No	50%	Very poor*

TABLE 18-2. MAIN SUBSETS OF JRA AND THEIR CHARACTERISTICS

*About 50% of patients have excellent outcomes; the other 50% have the worst functional outcomes of all JRA groups, and they make up the only subset to experience significant mortality as a result of JRA.

25. **Describe the pattern of fever and rash of the systemic-onset subset of JRA.**
    Systemic-onset JRA (Still's disease) accounts for approximately 15% of cases of children with JRA. Affected individuals typically have fevers of unknown origin with single or twice daily (i.e., quotidian) spikes, often of >40°C. Shaking chills often precede the fever. The temperature characteristically returns to 37°C or lower; continuous fever should suggest other diagnoses.

    A blotchy, light pink, evanescent rash that blanches on compression and that may show perimacular pallor accompanies the fever in >90% of cases (Fig. 18-4). The rash of systemic JRA is diagnostic only *after* the diagnosis is made (by exclusion). Arthritis may not be present during the first several weeks of illness. Serositis, hepatosplenomegaly, and lymphadenopathy are other significant findings in patients with this form of the disease.

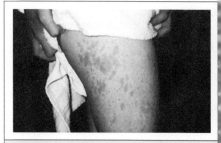

Figure 18-4. Typical rash of systemic-onset JRA. (From West S: Rheumatology Secrets, 2nd ed. Philadelphia, Hanley & Belfus, 2002, p 493.)

26. **Why is it sometimes difficult to distinguish systemic JRA from leukemia?**
    Up to 20% of patients with leukemia have some degree of musculoskeletal symptoms, including joint pain and occasional swelling. In both diseases there is anemia, fever, and weight loss. Both can

appear with hepatosplenomegaly and lymphadenopathy. In leukemia, however, the fever is not usually spiking, and platelets tend to be low to low normal. A good examination of a peripheral smear is crucial. A high lactic dehydrogenase level is very suggestive of leukemia, and the Tc_{99} bone scan shows a different pattern of uptake. More than one bone marrow biopsy may be necessary.

Ostrov BE, Goldsmith DP, Athreya BH: Differentiation of systemic juvenile rheumatoid arthritis from acute leukemia near the onset of disease. J Pediatr 122:595–598, 1993.

Tuten HR, Gabos PG, Kumar SJ, Harter GD: The limping child: A manifestation of acute leukemia. J Pediatr Orthop 18:625–629, 1998.

27. **In a patient with suspected rheumatologic disease, what clinical features are more suggestive of malignancy?**
Particularly concerning are nonarticular bone pain, back pain as the principal symptomatic feature, bone tenderness, and severe constitutional symptoms. Children with rheumatic joint problems are typically stiff, and they may complain about pain. The pain of malignancy is out of proportion to the amount of swelling around the joint, and it tends to be worse at night. It is vital to think about the possibility of malignancy in children with rheumatic complaints.

Cabral DA, Tucker LB: Malignancies in children who initially present with rheumatic complaints. J Pediatr 134:53–57, 1999.

28. **What is the value of measuring ANA and rheumatoid factor (RF) in patients with JRA?**
After JRA has been diagnosed on clinical grounds, results of these tests help assign the patient to the appropriate category (e.g., pauciarticular or RF-positive polyarticular). Because ANA can be present in ≤10% of normal children, this test should not be used as a screening test to diagnose JRA in children who experience noninflammatory pain. These tests are also useful as prognostic indicators. The presence of ANA increases the risk of uveitis, thereby making ophthalmologic surveillance more important. RF is valuable as a marker of poor prognosis in adolescents with polyarticular arthritis.

29. **Are x-rays helpful for diagnosing JRA?**
No. There are no characteristic x-ray changes at onset. The value of radiology is to rule out other skeletal conditions and to provide a documented baseline status.

30. **A patient with JRA who becomes ill with thrombocytopenia, profound anemia, and markedly elevated transaminases probably has what complication?**
Macrophage activation syndrome (MAS). This is new conceptualization of an old problem seen in children with systemic-onset JRA both at onset (even at presentation) and late during the course of disease. It is characterized by a massive upregulation of T-cell and macrophagic function, with vast release of proinflammatory cytokines leading to hemophagocytosis (the hallmark). It is believed that, in most cases, MAS is triggered by a viral infection. MAS is the single most important contributor of mortality (which lately has improved), together with gastrointestinal bleeding and infection among patients with systemic JRA. The name and nosologic classification of this entity are currently being debated by experts in the field.

31. **What are the main features of the macrophage activation syndrome?**
- Worsening of fever and rash
- Profound anemia (due in part to hemophagocytosis), leukopenia, and thrombocytopenia
- Disseminated intravascular coagulation with hypofibriginogenemia and "pseudonormalization" of ESR
- Liver dysfunction
- Hypertriglyceridemia
- Hyponatremia (pseudo)
- Massive increase in ferritin levels

- Occasional central nervous system involvement
- Generalized musculoskeletal pain

Ramanan AV, Schneider R: Macrophage activation syndrome—what's in a name! J Rheum 30:2513–2516, 2003.

32. **What has been the traditional first-line approach to JRA medical management?**
The so-called first-line therapy consists of nonsteroidal anti-inflammatories (NSAIDs). Given at the correct dose, they exert pain relief and suppress inflammation (decrease in morning stiffness), with a peak action at 4–6 weeks. The classic representatives of this group are aspirin, ibuprofen, naproxen, tolmetin, and indomethacin. Choice among them is made on the basis of availability in liquid form, half-life, side-effect profile, individual doctor preferences, and results of an individual trial. Most of their action is through inhibition of cyclo-oxygenase. About on third of patients will have their symptoms controlled through the use of NSAIDs; two thirds require more aggressive drug therapy.

33. **What second-line agents have been used in the treatment of JRA?**
- Gold salts
- Penicillamine
- Hydroxychloroquine
- Sulfasalazine
- Methotrexate

34. **When are corticosteroids indicated for children with JRA?**
- Life-threatening disease (e.g., carditis, myocarditis)
- Unremitting fever unresponsive to NSAIDs
- Unrelenting polyarthritis with severe limitations requiring intensive physical therapy to achieve ambulatory status
- Topical therapy for uveitis (rarely, systemic steroids are needed for children with aggressive uveitis unresponsive to topical therapy)
- Intra-articular administration for severely symptomatic joint(s) (Fig. 18-5)

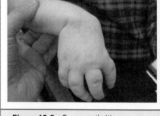

Figure 18-5. Severe arthritic deformities in a child with long-standing systemic-onset JRA.

35. **What are the most common side effects of prolonged corticosteroid therapy?**
Effects can be minimized by alternate-day therapy, but sometimes the treatment is worse than the disease. Commonly encountered problems associated with high-dose corticosteroid use in children can be remembered using the mnemonic **CUSHINGOID MAP**:

- **C** = Cataracts
- **U** = Ulcers
- **S** = Striae
- **H** = Hypertension
- **I** = Infectious complications
- **N** = Necrosis of bone (avascular)
- **G** = Growth retardation
- **O** = Osteoporosis
- **I** = Increased intracranial pressure (pseudotumor cerebri)
- **D** = Diabetes mellitus
- **M** = Myopathy
- **A** = Adipose tissue hypertrophy (obesity, "buffalo hump")
- **P** = Pancreatitis

KEY POINTS: JUVENILE RHEUMATOID ARTHRITIS

1. *Sine qua non:* Persistence of ≥6 weeks

2. Three main subtypes: Pauciarticular (≤4 joints), polyarticular (>4 joints), and systemic-onset (spiking fevers)

3. Characteristic finding: Morning stiffness or soreness that improves during the day

4. No diagnostic laboratory tests are diagnostic

5. Patients <7 years old with ANA-positive pauciarticular JRA at highest risk for developing uveitis

36. **What is etanercept?**
A biologic immune modulator. It is a tumor necrosis factor (TNF)-receptor fusion protein that acts as an anti-inflammatory agent by binding TNF. Other biologic agents (e.g., infliximab, a monoclonal antibody to TNF), have dramatically changed the spectrum of options available to rheumatologists and quite obviously the functional outlook of JRA and other arthritides.

37. **Which children with JRA require the most frequent monitoring for uveitis?**
Uveitis (also called iridocyclitis) is inflammation of the iris and the ciliary body. It occurs on average in 20% of patients with pauciarticular JRA and in 5% of patients with polyarticular disease. Table 18-3 summarizes the American Academy of Pediatrics guidelines for frequency of slit-lamp examination developed by the sections of ophthalmology and rheumatology. Patients at high risk require quarterly examinations; those with moderate risk need biannual examinations; and those at low risk can be examined annually.

> Nguyen QD, Foster CS: Saving the vision of children with juvenile rheumatoid arthritis-associated uveitis. JAMA 280:1133–1134, 1998.

TABLE 18-3.	RISK OF UVEITIS IN PATIENTS WITH JRA	
JRA Subtype	**<7 years old**	**>7 years old**
Pauciarticular, ANA-positive	High	Moderate
Pauciarticular, ANA-negative	Moderate	Moderate
Polyarticular, ANA-positive	High	Moderate
Polyarticular, ANA-negative	Moderate	Moderate
Systemic onset	Low	Low

38. **What is the earliest sign of uveitis among patients with JRA?**
When the anterior chamber of the eye is examined with a slit lamp, a "flare" is the earliest sign. This is a hazy appearance as a result of an increased concentration of protein and inflammatory cells. Later signs can include a speckled appearance of the posterior cornea (as a result of keratic precipitates), an irregular or poorly reactive pupil (as a result of synechiae between the iris and lens), band keratopathy, and cataracts.

> Foster CS: Diagnosis and treatment of juvenile idiopathic arthritis-associated uveitis. Curr Opin Ophthalmol 14:395–398, 2003.

LYME DISEASE

39. **What criteria are used to diagnose Lyme disease?**
Classification criteria (i.e., case definition) as determined by the Centers for Disease Control and Prevention include the following:
- **Erythema migrans:** Enlarging circular erythematous lesion (minimum size, 5 cm) *or*
- At least **one clinical manifestation** (arthritis, cranial neuropathy, atrioventricular block, aseptic meningitis, radiculoneuritis) *and* **isolation or serologic evidence** of *Borrelia burgdorferi* infection

40. **How is Lyme disease confirmed in the laboratory?**
Although attempts to demonstrate borrelial DNA in infected tissues by polymerase chain reaction has met with some success and cultures occasionally render positive results, the main diagnostic tool continues to be serology. Immunoglobulin M (IgM) peaks about 4 weeks after infection, and IgG does so at 6 weeks. This is the main reason why antibodies may not be detected during the early dermatologic and neurologic stages.

There are two detection techniques: **ELISA** and **Western blot**. Both are available for IgG and IgM. Initial disagreements on the criteria (cutoff) for the interpretation of Western blot were settled in Dearborn, Mich., in 1996. Basically, a negative ELISA requires no further investigation at a given time. Seroconversion can be sought in situations of high suspicion in 2–3 weeks. Enhancement of test sensitivity by ELISA has led to high rates of false positivity, thereby resulting in overdiagnosis. All positive ELISAs—particularly those with borderline positivity—should be confirmed by Western blot.

The main problem with serology results from the tendency of sera from patients with Epstein-Barr virus infection, parvovirus infection, and syphilis to react positively in *Borrelia* assays by the ELISA method. Sera from patients with autoimmune diseases (SLE, JRA) may also cross-react. However, most of these will be negative when tested by Western blot.

41. **Describe the classic rash of Lyme disease.**
Erythema migrans (previously known as erythema chronicum migrans) is the distinctive cutaneous lesion of Lyme disease. The lesion begins as a small red macule or papule and enlarges in an annular centrifugal fashion to approximately 10–15 cm or more in diameter. The lesions may have varying intensities of redness within the plaque, partial central clearing, or a ring-within-a-ring configuration. Occasionally, the central area may become indurated, vesicular, or crusted. Erythema migrans lesions usually appear within 14 days of the bite of an infected *Ixodes* tick (range, 2–28 days). Multiple lesions are present in only about 20% of cases.

42. **After a tick bite has occurred, how does Lyme disease progress?**
- **1–2 weeks:** After an individual has been bitten by an infected *Ixodes* deer tick, erythema migrans develops in two thirds of cases. The skin lesion may be associated with constitutional symptoms (fever, arthralgia, myalgia, severe headache, and profound fatigue), especially in patients in whom secondary lesions occur. The rash and other symptoms are self-limited, even without antibiotic treatment.
- **Weeks to months:** If treatment has not been given, early disseminated Lyme disease occurs; this is characterized by neurologic and/or cardiac involvement. Neuroborreliosis occurs in ≤20% of patients and appears most commonly as facial palsy, lymphocytic meningitis, or peripheral radiculoneuropathy. Up to 8% of patients develop cardiac involvement (most commonly fluctuating atrioventricular block or, more rarely, myopericarditis).
- **Months to years:** The most common late manifestation of Lyme disease is a self-limited oligoarthritis, most often affecting the knees. Late neurologic disease does occur and, like tertiary syphilis, usually appears as a subacute encephalopathy, although it can mimic multiple

sclerosis. In Europe, a morphea-like eruption called acrodermatitis chronica atrophicans is a late dermatologic sequela.

Steere AC: Lyme disease. N Engl J Med 345:115–125, 2001.

43. How is the diagnosis of Lyme meningitis established?

The diagnosis is often inexact and is commonly made on the basis of the finding of cerebrospinal fluid pleocytosis and the presence of erythema migrans and/or positive serology. Both ELISA and Western blot testing may be negative or indeterminate early during the course of infection, when dissemination to the central nervous system has occurred. Specific testing of the cerebrospinal fluid for intrathecal production of specific antibody and demonstration of *Borrelia burgdorferi* DNA by polymerase chain reaction testing are not readily available, and the latter is relatively insensitive.

44. How are Lyme disease and viral meningitis clinically distinguished?

Both are predominantly summertime illnesses, but the distinction is critical because Lyme meningitis requires weeks of intravenous antibiotics. In addition to the possible presence of erythema migrans, other areas of clinical distinction in patients with signs and symptoms of meningitis include the following:

- **Cranial neuropathy**, especially peripheral 7th-nerve palsy (i.e., Bell's palsy), is strongly suggestive of Lyme meningitis.
- **Papilledema** is more commonly seen in patients with Lyme meningitis.
- **Longer duration of symptoms** before lumbar puncture is more typical of Lyme meningitis.
- **Fever** at the time of diagnosis is more likely viral meningitis.
- **Cerebrospinal fluid pleocytosis** (especially the neutrophilic component) is less pronounced in Lyme meningitis.

Eppes SC, Nelson DK, Lewis LL, Klein JD: Characterization of Lyme meningitis and comparison with viral meningitis. Pediatrics 103(5 Pt 1):957–960, 1999.

45. Should we follow disease course and response to therapy with titers?

No! As a result of the continued secretion of antibodies by memory cells, serology (particularly with ultrasensitive commercial kits) may remain positive for up to 10 years after microbial eradication. The misinterpretation of positive serology as a proxy for active infection is behind many unnecessary antibiotic courses in endemic areas.

Kalish RA, McHugh G, Granquist J, et al: Persistence of immunoglobulin M or immunoglobulin G antibody responses after active Lyme disease. Clin Infect Dis 33:780–785, 2001.

46. What is the prognosis for children diagnosed with Lyme arthritis?

Multiple studies have shown that the long-term prognosis for treated patients is excellent, with little morbidity. Clinicians should be aware that persistent synovitis after the completion of a single course of 4 weeks of antibiotics is not rare and not the result of antibiotic failure. In fact, up to two thirds of patients with Lyme arthritis require 3 months to achieve resolution, and 15% carry their arthritis for >12 months.

Gerber MA, Zemel LS, Shapiro ED: Lyme arthritis in children: Clinical epidemiology and long-term outcome. Pediatrics 102:905–908, 1990.

Wang TJ, Sangha O, Phillips CB, et al: Outcomes of children treated for Lyme disease. J Rheumatology 25:2249–2253, 1998.

47. What should be suspected if a patient with Lyme disease develops fever and chills after starting antibiotic treatment?

The **Jarisch-Herxheimer reaction**. This reaction consists of fever, chills, arthralgia, myalgia, and vasodilation, and it follows the initiation of antibiotic therapy in certain illnesses (most typically syphilis). It is thought to be mediated by endotoxin release as the organism is destroyed. A similar reaction occurs in ≤40% of patients treated with Lyme disease, and it may be mistaken for an allergic reaction to the antibiotic.

KEY POINTS: LYME DISEASE

1. Spirochete *Borrelia burgdorferi* is the culprit.

2. Only a third of patients recall the tick bite.

3. The erythema migrans rash is virtually diagnostic.

4. ELISA testing has a high false-positive rate; confirm with Western blot analysis.

5. Potential complications include arthritis, aseptic meningitis/cranial nerve palsies, and atrioventricular block.

48. **Is antibiotic prophylaxis indicated for all tick bites?**
    No. In most regions, the rate of tick infestation is low, and thus the likelihood of transmission also low. Even in endemic areas, the risk of Lyme disease to a placebo group after tick bites was only 1.2%. The tick has to be attached for at least 24–48 hours before the transmission of infection occurs. Treating all tick bites with antibiotics is impractical (some children would be on oral antibiotics throughout the summer). One study did show that a single 200-mg dose was effective for preventing Lyme disease if it was given within 72 hours of the tick bite. Consequently, antibiotic prophylaxis is not routinely recommended, but, in unique circumstances (e.g., endemic areas, prolonged attachment, pregnancy), prophylaxis could be considered.

    Nadelman RB, Nowakowski J, Fish D, et al; Tick Bite Study Group: Prophylaxis with single-dose doxycycline for the prevention of Lyme disease after an *Ixodes scapularis* tick bite. N Engl J Med 345:79–84, 2001.

    Shapiro ED, Gerber MA, Holabird NB, et al: A controlled trial of antimicrobial prophylaxis for Lyme disease after deer-tick bites. N Engl J Med 327:1769–1773, 1992.

49. **What are other means of preventing Lyme disease?**
    - Avoidance of tick-infested areas
    - Use of light-colored, long-sleeved clothing, with pants tucked into sneakers
    - Insect repellents (N, N-diethylmetatoluamide [DEET]; permethrin)
    - "Tick checks" after potential exposures
    - Proper tick removal: Pulling straight out, with tweezers close to skin

    Hayes EB, Piesman J: How can we prevent Lyme disease? N Engl J Med 348:2424–2430, 2003.

RHEUMATIC FEVER

50. **What is acute rheumatic fever?**
    A postinfectious, immune-mediated, inflammatory reaction that affects the connective tissue of multiple organ systems (heart, joints, central nervous system, blood vessels, subcutaneous tissue) and that follows infection with certain strains of group A beta-hemolytic streptococci (GABHS). The major manifestations are carditis, polyarthritis, chorea, erythema marginatum, and subcutaneous nodules.

51. **What is acceptable proof of antecedent streptococcal pharyngitis when diagnosing acute rheumatic fever?**
    - **Throat culture:** This is the gold standard for diagnosis of GABHS. Positive cultures, however, do not distinguish GABHS pharyngitis from a carrier state.
    - **Streptococcal antigen tests:** Rapid diagnostic tests for the detection of GABHS antigens in pharyngeal secretions are acceptable evidence of infection because they are highly specific. Again, positive tests do not distinguish true infection from a carrier state.

- **Antistreptococcal antibodies:** At the time of clinical presentation with rheumatic fever, throat cultures are usually negative. It is reasonable to assess the levels of antistreptococcal antibodies in all cases of suspected rheumatic fever, because the antibodies should be elevated at the time of presentation.

52. **Which antistreptococcal antibodies are most commonly measured?**
The most commonly employed test measures antibodies to **antistreptolysin O**. The cutoff for a positive test in a school-aged child is 320 Todd units (240 in an adult); levels peak from 3–6 weeks after infection. If the test is negative—as may be the case in ≤20% of patients with acute rheumatic fever (ARF) (and 40% of those with isolated chorea)—other antistreptococcal antibodies may be detected. The most practically available of these identifies antibodies to **deoxyribonuclease B** (positive cutoff, 240 units in children, 120 in adults). Alternatively, subsequent convalescent samples run simultaneously with the acute sample may detect rising titers of either antistreptolysin O or antideoxyribonuclease B.

53. **What are the common manifestations of carditis in patients with ARF?**
In his *Etudes Médicales du Rhumatisme,* Lasègue remarked that "rheumatic fever licks the joints . . . and bites the heart," meaning that the severity of the two manifestations tends to be inversely related. In more recent outbreaks of ARF, ≤80% of patients have had evidence of carditis. ARF causes a pancarditis, which potentially affects all layers (from the pericardium through the endocardium) and may include the following:
- **Valvulitis:** This is heralded by a new or changing murmur. The most common manifestation is isolated mitral regurgitation, and this is followed in frequency by a mid-diastolic rumble of unclear pathophysiology (Carey-Coombs murmur), and then by aortic insufficiency in the presence of mitral regurgitation. Isolated aortic insufficiency is uncommon, and so are stenotic lesions.
- **Arrhythmias:** Electrocardiogram abnormalities typically involve some degree of heart block.
- **Myocarditis:** When mild, this may manifest as resting tachycardia out of proportion to fever. However, when it is clinically more severe and in combination with valvular damage, myocarditis may lead to congestive heart failure.
- **Pericarditis:** Patients may have chest pain or friction rub. Pericarditis and myocarditis virtually never occur in isolation.

  Messeloff CR: Historical aspects of rheumatism. Medical Life 37:3–56, 1930.

54. **How quickly can valvular lesions occur in children with ARF?**
New murmurs appear within the first 2 weeks in 80% of patients, and they rarely occur after the second month of illness.

55. **What are the typical characteristics of arthritis in patients with ARF?**
Migratory polyarthritis is usually the earliest symptom of the disease, and it typically affects the large joints, the knees, the ankles, the elbows, and the wrists (hips are not commonly involved). The joints are extraordinarily painful; weight bearing may not be possible. Physical examination discloses warmth, erythema, and exquisite tenderness such that the weight of even bedclothes and sheets may not be tolerable. This tenderness is typically out of proportion with the degree of swelling.

56. **What is the effect of aspirin therapy on the arthritis of rheumatic fever?**
This type of arthritis is exquisitely sensitive to even modest doses of salicylates, which effectively arrest the process within 12–24 hours. If aspirin or other NSAIDs are employed early during the course of the condition, the arthritis will not migrate, and a delay in diagnosis may result. Such medications should be withheld until the clinical course of the illness has clarified itself. Conversely, if there is not a dramatic response to aspirin, a diagnosis other than rheumatic fever should be considered.

57. How long does the arthritis associated with ARF usually persist?

In untreated cases of ARF, arthritis affects a number of joints sequentially for less than a week each; the entire process rarely lasts more than a month. Treatment with aspirin or NSAIDs will shorten the clinical course.

58. What is the rash of rheumatic fever?

Erythema marginatum. This rash occurs in <5% of cases of ARF. If you see it and call a colleague to the bedside to confirm it, it is likely to have disappeared in the meantime. It is an evanescent, pink to slightly red, nonpruritic eruption with pale centers and ser-piginous borders; it may be induced by the application of heat, and it always blanches when palpated. The outer edges of the lesion are sharp, whereas the inner borders are diffuse (Fig. 18-6). It is most often found on the trunk and proximal extremities (but not the face). Erythema marginatum is seen almost solely in patients with carditis.

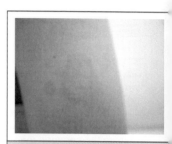

Figure 18-6. Classical rash of erythema marginatum on the arm of a child with acute rheumatic fever.

59. What is Sydenham's chorea?

Purposeless, involuntary, irregular movements of the extremities that are associated with mus-cle weakness and labile emotional behavior. These symptoms are believed to result from inflam-mation of the cerebellum and of the basal ganglia.

60. Who was Saint Vitus?

Saint Vitus was a Sicilian youth who was martyred in the year 303. In the Middle Ages, individu-als with chorea would worship at shrines dedicated to this saint. Accordingly, Sydenham chorea is also known as "Saint Vitus' dance." Saint Vitus is the patron saint of dancers and comedians.

61. Are corticosteroids of benefit for the treatment of ARF?

Controlled studies in the 1950s failed to show any definite benefit of corticosteroids for the treatment of rheumatic carditis. Nonetheless, it is generally recommended that patients with severe carditis (e.g., congestive heart failure, cardiomegaly, third-degree heart block) receive prednisone (2 mg/kg/day) in addition to conventional therapy for their heart failure. The unusual patient with well-documented rheumatic arthritis that does not respond to salicylates or NSAIDs will benefit symptomatically from prednisone.

62. What are the appropriate regimens of prophylaxis for patients who have had ARF?

The goal of prophylaxis is to prevent GABHS pharyngitis, thereby preventing recurrences of ARF. Recurrences can happen at any time, but the greatest risk is during the 2 years after the initial attack. Appropriate regimens include the following (the cutoff for larger doses is 27 kg):

- Intramuscular benzathine penicillin G every 3–4 weeks—600,000 units for patients weighing ≤27 kg and 1,200,000 units for patients weighing >27 kg
- Oral penicillin V potassium, 250 mg twice daily
- Oral sulfadiazine, 500–1000 mg once daily
- Oral erythromycin, 250 mg twice daily, if allergic to the above

In areas in which rheumatic fever is endemic or in other high-risk situations, the 3-week intra-muscular regimen is preferable.

63. Can antibiotic prophylaxis for rheumatic fever ever be discontinued?

The optimal duration of antistreptococcal prophylaxis after documented ARF is the subject of some debate. It is clear that the risk of recurrence decreases after 5 years have elapsed from the most recent attack. Most clinicians therefore recommend discontinuing prophylaxis in patients who have not had carditis *after 5 years* or on the *21st birthday* (whichever comes later). Those at high risk for contracting streptococcal pharyngitis (e.g., school teachers, health-care professionals, military recruits, others living in crowded conditions) and anyone with a history of carditis should receive antibiotic prophylaxis for longer periods of time. Recommendations vary, ranging from 10 years to the 40th birthday (whichever is longer) to lifelong prophylaxis, depending on the extent of residual heart disease.

64. Where do PANDAS live in the world of pediatric rheumatology?
In 1989, Swedo and colleagues characterized the psychiatric abnormalities found in children with Sydenham chorea, noting a high prevalence of obsessive-compulsive disorder (OCD) behaviors. They also described a syndrome, which they dubbed **PANDAS** (**p**ediatric **a**utoimmune **n**europsychiatric **d**isorders **a**ssociated with **s**treptococcal infection), in which OCD and Tourette's syndrome in some children appeared to be triggered or exacerbated by streptococcal infections in the absence of classical chorea or other manifestations of rheumatic fever.
The existence of PANDAS remains controversial. There has been no prospective study of GAS infection to confirm the association of streptococcal pharyngitis with these behavioral abnormalities. The symptoms of tic disorders and OCD tend to fluctuate spontaneously and may be nonspecifically exacerbated by illness. In some cases, the only link to streptococcal infection has been a single throat culture or serologic test, thereby bringing the specificity of the condition into question.

Kurlan R, Kaplan EL: The pediatric autoimmune neuropsychiatric disorders associated with streptococcal infections (PANDAS) etiology for tics and obsessive-compulsive symptoms: Hypothesis or entity? Practical considerations for the clinician. Pediatrics 113:883–886, 2004.

Swedo SE, Rapaport JL, Cheslow, DL, et al: High prevalence of obsessive-compulsive symptoms in patients with Syndenham chorea. Am J Psychiatry 146:246–249, 1989.

SPONDYLOARTHROPATHIES

65. How are the juvenile spondyloarthropathies (JSAs) distinguished from JRA?
Under the heading of JSA are the following conditions: juvenile ankylosing spondylitis, juvenile psoriatic arthritis, postdysenteric reactive arthritis, Reiter syndrome, and the arthritis of inflammatory bowel disease. They are distinguished from JRA by the following features:
- The age of onset is during early adolescence.
- They are the only rheumatic diseases with a clear male predominance.
- Enthesitis (inflammation of tendon, capsule, and ligament insertion sites) is characteristic.
- Prodromal oligoarthritis involving large joints of the lower extremities may resemble JRA, but hip involvement points to JSA. Episodes of arthritis tend to be briefer than those seen with JRA.
- There is involvement of the sacroiliac joints and of the back, which is manifested as pain, stiffness, and reduced range of motion.
- It is associated with HLA-B27 (≤90% in children with ankylosing spondylitis and 60% of those with other spondyloarthropathies versus 15% of patients with JRA).
- Seronegativity: ANA and rheumatoid factors are typically negative.

66. How is enthesitis diagnosed clinically?
The enthesis is the site of attachment of ligaments, tendons, capsule, and fascia to bone. Enthesopathy is unique to the spondyloarthropathies and appears as painful localized tenderness at the tibial tubercle (which may be mistaken for Osgood-Schlatter disease), the peripheral patella, and at the calcaneal insertion of the Achilles tendon and plantar fascia (which may be mistaken for Sever's disease). Thickening of the Achilles tendon and tenderness of the metatarsophalangeal joints are associated findings.

67. Why is the diagnosis of ankylosing spondylitis difficult to make in children?
A child may have undifferentiated spondyloarthritis that is characterized by enthesitis and recurrent episodes of lower extremity oligoarthritis for several years before he or she develops

back symptoms. To fulfill the criteria for ankylosing spondylitis, clinical features of lumbar spine pain, limitation of lumbar motion, and radiographic signs of sacroiliitis must be present. The average time from onset of symptoms to diagnosis in an adult with ankylosing spondylitis is 5 years; many adolescents are adults before they fulfill the criteria (*see* Fig. 18-7).

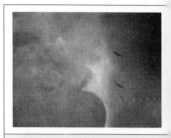

Figure 18-7. Periarticular sclerosis in a boy with chronic sacroiliitis and a diagnosis of spondyloarthropathy.

68. **What is the connection between young men and SEA?**
No apologies to Hemingway needed here. The syndrome of seronegative enthesopathy and arthropathy (SEA) was described in 1982 in a group of children, mostly boys, with enthesitis and arthralgia or arthritis who were seronegative for ANA and rheumatoid factor. Many were positive for HLA-B27, but they did not fulfill criteria for definite spondyloarthritis. Long-term follow-up disclosed that about half went on to develop definite ankylosing spondylitis.

69. **Where are the dimples of Venus?**
The dimples of Venus are prominent paravertebral indentations in the lower back of some individuals. A line drawn between the dimples marks the lumbosacral junction; this is the midpoint for the Schober test, which is a measure of anterior flexion of the lumbosacral spine.

SYSTEMIC LUPUS ERYTHEMATOSUS

70. **What is SLE?**
A multisystem, autoimmune disorder that is characterized by the production of autoantibodies and a wide variety of clinical and laboratory manifestations.

71. **What laboratory tests should be ordered in a child who is suspected of having SLE?**
A useful screening test for SLE is the **fluorescent antinuclear antibody (FANA) test**. Up to 97% of patients with SLE have positive ANAs at some point during their illness (although not necessarily at the time of diagnosis). In a patient with characteristic signs and symptoms, a positive ANA may help confirm suspicions of SLE. Unfortunately, however, up to 10% of the normal childhood population may also have a positive ANA. Therefore, a positive ANA in the absence of any objective findings of SLE means very little. Other autoantibodies are much more specific, but they are less sensitive for SLE. These include antibodies to double-stranded DNA and the extractable nuclear antigen Sm. Complement levels are often depressed in patients with active SLE, and sedimentation rates are often elevated. The combination of a *positive anti-double-stranded DNA Ab level* and a *low C_3 level* is nearly 100% specific for SLE. Anemia, leukopenia, lymphopenia, and/or thrombocytopenia may also be seen.

Benseler SM, Silverman ED: Systemic lupus erythematosus. Pediatr Clin North Am 52:443-467, 2005.
Gill JM, Quisel AM, Rocca PV, Walters DT: Diagnosis of systemic lupus erythematosus. Am Fam Physician 68:2179–2186, 2003.

72. **What are the most common manifestations of SLE in children?**
- **Arthritis:** 80–90%
- **Rash/fever:** 70%
- **Renal disease (proteinuria, casts)*:** 70%
- **Serositis:** 50%
- **Hypertension:** 50%

- **Central nervous system disease (psychosis/seizures):** 20–40%
- **Anemia, leukopenia, thrombocytopenia:** 30% each
  *Every patient with SLE is likely to have some abnormality demonstrated on renal biopsy.

Iqbal S, Sher MR, Good RA, Cawkwell GD: Diversity in presenting manifestations of systemic lupus erythematosus in children. J Pediatr 135:500–505, 1999.
Klein-Gitelman M: Systemic lupus erythematosus in childhood. 28:561–577, 2002.

3. **Describe the neurologic manifestations of SLE.**
   Lupus cerebritis is a term that implies an inflammatory etiology of central nervous system disease. Microscopically, however, widely scattered areas of microinfarction and noninflammatory vasculopathy are seen in brain tissue; actual central nervous system vasculitis is rarely observed. A lumbar puncture may reveal cerebrospinal fluid pleocytosis or an increased protein concentration, but it can be normal as well. Neuropsychiatric manifestations (psychoses, behavioral changes, depression, emotional lability) or seizures are most commonly observed. An organic brain syndrome with progressive disorientation and intellectual deterioration can be seen. Cranial or peripheral neuropathies, chorea, and cerebellar ataxia are less-common manifestations of central nervous system lupus. Severe headaches and cerebral ischemic events have also been seen.

   Steinlein MI, Blaser SI, Gilday DI, et al: Neurological manifestations of pediatric systemic lupus erythematosus. Pediatr Neurol 13:191–197, 1995.

4. **Which diseases should be considered in the differential diagnosis of children with a butterfly rash?**
   A malar rash is present in 50% of children with SLE. The typical butterfly rash involves the malar areas and crosses the nasal bridge, but it spares the nasolabial folds; occasionally it is difficult to distinguish from the rash of dermatomyositis. (Accompanying erythematous papules on the extensor surfaces of the metacarpo phalangeal (MCP) and proximal interphalangeal (PIP) joints are common in dermatomyositis, but these are not generally seen in patients with SLE.) Seborrheic dermatitis or a contact dermatitis may be similar to the rash of SLE. Vesiculation should suggest another disease, such as pemphigus erythematosus. A malar flush is clinically distinct and may be seen in children with mitral stenosis or hypothyroidism.

5. **Should children with SLE undergo a renal biopsy?**
   This is an area of controversy because nearly all children with SLE will have some evidence of renal involvement. Usually clinical disease (e.g., abnormal urine sediment, proteinuria, renal function changes) correlates with the severity of renal disease on biopsy, but this is not always the case. Extensive glomerular abnormalities can be found on biopsy with minimal concurrent clinical manifestations. For this reason, many authorities are aggressive with early biopsy. Three circumstances in particular warrant biopsy:
   1. A child with SLE and nephrotic syndrome—to distinguish membranous glomerulonephritis from diffuse proliferative glomerulonephritis (which would warrant more aggressive therapy)
   2. Failure of high-dose corticosteroids to reverse deteriorating renal function—to determine the likelihood of benefit from cytotoxic therapy
   3. A prerequisite to entry into clinical therapeutic trials

   Cassidy JT, Petty RE: Textbook of Pediatric Rheumatology, 3rd ed. Philadelphia, WB Saunders, 1995, pp 260-322.

6. **How can the result of renal biopsy affect treatment of SLE?**
   Biopsy can reveal a spectrum of renal pathology, ranging from a normal kidney (rare) to mesangial nephritis or glomerulonephritis (focal or diffuse, proliferative or membranous). Histologic transformation from one group to another over time is not unusual. Treatment of lupus nephritis is based on the severity of the lesion. Mesangial disease may require little or no intervention. Patients with membranous nephropathy commonly have nephrotic syndrome and usually

respond to prednisone. Focal proliferative glomerulonephritis is often controlled with corticosteroids alone, but diffuse proliferative glomerulonephritis often requires corticosteroids, intravenous pulse cyclophosphamide, and possibly other immunosuppressives.

77. **When should high-dose corticosteroid therapy be considered for SLE management?**

High-dose corticosteroids usually consists of either intravenous pulse methylprednisolone (30 mg/kg/dose with a maximum dose of 1 g given daily or on alternate days given as an intravenous bolus for up to three doses) or oral prednisone (1–2 mg/kg/day). Often intravenous pulses are then followed by high-dose oral steroids. The main indications for high-dose steroids in cases of SLE are as follows:

- Lupus crisis (widespread acute multisystem vasculitic involvement)
- Worsening central nervous system disease (as long as steroid psychosis in not thought to be the etiology)
- Severe lupus nephritis
- Acute hemolytic anemia
- Acute pleuropulmonary disease

78. **What is the prognosis for children with confirmed SLE?**

The prognosis for survival has improved remarkably during the past 20 years. Survival rates at 10 years are close to 90%; 20-year survival, however, drops down to approximately 75%. Most pediatric lupus deaths are the result of infections. About half of patients with childhood lupus still have active disease as adults.

www.lupus.org

79. **What is the association of antiphospholipid antibodies and lupus?**

Antiphospholipid antibodies can cause recurrent arterial and/or venous thromboses (e.g., stroke, phlebitis, renal vein thrombosis, placental thrombosis leading to fetal demise). Antiphospholipid antibodies are usually detected as anticardiolipin antibodies or lupus anticoagulant. These antibodies are often seen in patients with SLE, but their prevalence among patients with pediatric lupus varies widely (30–87% for anticardiolipin antibodies and 6–65% for lupus anticoagulant), depending on the study cited. The pathogenesis of thrombosis in patients with antiphospholipid antibodies antibodies remains unclear.

Ravelli A, Martini A: Antiphospholipid antibody syndrome in pediatric patients. Rheum Dis Clin North Am 23:657–676, 1997.

80. **Which laboratory tests are useful for monitoring the effectiveness of therapy in patients with SLE?**

Serologic studies can provide useful information about the activity of SLE. The ANA titer does not correlate with disease activity. However, anti-double-stranded DNA titers (if present) often drop, and complement levels may increase and return to normal with effective therapy. Sedimentation rates usually decrease, and complete blood cell counts may return to normal (or at least improve) with effective therapy and decreased disease activity.

81. **What are the most common manifestations of neonatal lupus erythematosus (NLE)?**

The syndrome of neonatal lupus erythematosus (NLE) was first described in babies born to mothers with SLE or Sjögren's syndrome; however, it has now been found that 70–80% of mothers with these conditions are asymptomatic. NLE is most likely caused by the transmission of maternal IgG autoantibodies. The main manifestations are as follows:

- **Cutaneous:** Skin lesions are found in about 50% of babies with NLE. Although the rash may be present at birth, it usually develops within the first 2–3 months of life. The lesions include macules, papules, and annular plaques, and they may be precipitated by exposure to sunlight The lesions are usually transient and nonscarring.

- **Cardiac:** Complete congenital heart block (CCHB) is the classic cardiac lesion of NLE; 90% of all CCHB is due to neonatal lupus. Most cases of CCHB appear after the neonatal period, and 40–100% of these patients will eventually require a pacemaker, usually before they are 18 years old. The average mortality from CCHB during the neonatal period is 15%.
- **Hepatic:** Hepatic involvement is seen in ≥15% of babies with NLE. Hepatomegaly with or without splenomegaly is usually seen. Hepatic transaminases are either mild or moderately elevated, or they may be normal. Clinically and histologically, the appearance is often one of idiopathic neonatal giant-cell hepatitis.
- **Hematologic:** Thrombocytopenia, hemolytic anemia, and/or neutropenia may be seen.

    Silverman ED, Laxer RM: Neonatal lupus erythematosus. Rheum Dis Clin North Am 23:599–618, 1997.

KEY POINTS: SYSTEMIC LUPUS ERYTHEMATOSUS

1. The hallmark of SLE is the presence of autoantibodies.

2. Approximately 15–20% of lupus patients have the onset of disease during childhood.

3. Clinical presentations vary, but the most common presenting symptoms are arthritis, rash, and renal disease.

4. Neonatal lupus is caused by maternal autoantibodies; this leads to complete congenital heart block.

5. The presence of antiphospholipid antibodies predisposes the patient to venous thrombosis.

2. **What is the pathophysiology of the CCHB of NLE?**
   CCHB is caused by maternal autoantibodies that cross the placenta and deposit themselves in the conducting system—usually the atrioventricular node—of the fetal heart. This leads to a localized inflammatory lesion, which may then be followed by scarring with fibrosis and calcification. The autoantibodies found are usually anti-Ro antibodies, but anti-La antibodies can also be the etiologic agents.

    Silverman ED, Laxer RM: Neonatal lupus erythematosus. Rheum Dis Clin North Am 23:599–618, 1997.

3. **What are the common features of drug-induced lupus?**
   Fever, arthralgias/arthritis, and serositis can be seen in patients with drug-induced lupus. ANA and antihistone antibodies are often positive, but antibodies to double-stranded DNA are usually negative, and complements remain normal. Renal involvement, central nervous system disease, malar rash, alopecia, and oral ulcers are not usually seen in patients with drug-induced lupus, and their presence should raise suspicions of SLE.

4. **What are the most common causes of drug-induced lupus in children?**
   Antiepileptic medications (especially ethosuximide, phenytoin, and primidone) are the most common causes, and ≥20% children on antiepileptic drugs will develop a positive ANA. Minocycline, hydralazine, isoniazid, alpha-methyldopa, and chlorpromazine are also associated with drug-induced lupus, as are a variety of antithyroid medications and beta-blockers. Actually all of the tetracyclines have been associated with a peculiar lupus-like syndrome that includes the following:
   - Acute symmetric polyarthritis

- Positive ANA
- Mild liver dysfunction
  This rather common syndrome is associated with the chronic use of tetracyclines in associa
  tion with the treatment of acne. It usually resolves within 2 weeks of discontinuation of the med
  ication, but it may last longer.

VASCULITIS

85. **What clinical features suggest a vasculitic syndrome?**
    A multisystem disease with fever, weight loss, and rash is often the presenting picture in a vas-
    culitic disorder. Many different types of rashes may be seen, the more common of which are pa
    pable purpura, urticarial vasculitis, and dermal necrosis. Central nervous system involvement,
    arthritis, myositis, and/or serositis may be seen.

    Blanco R, Martinez-Taboada VM, Rodriguez-Valverde V, Garcia-Fuentes M: Cutaneous vasculitis in
    children and adults. Associated diseases and etiologic factors in 303 patients. Medicine 77:403–418,
    1998.

86. **How are the primary systemic vasculitides classified?**
    One scheme proposed by an international consensus classifies vasculitides on the basis of the
    size of the vessels that are predominantly affected. Below are listed some of the conditions that
    may affect the pediatric population. Conditions in *italics* are common pediatric diseases; those
    marked with an asterisk are not uncommon in pediatric rheumatology centers.
    Large-vessel vasculitis
    - Takayasu arteritis[*]

    Medium-sized-vessel vasculitis
    - *Kawasaki disease*
    - Polyarteritis nodosa and its limb-limited variant[*]

    Small-vessel vasculitis
    - Microscopic polyangiitis[*]
    - Wegener's granulomatosis[*]
    - Churg-Strauss syndrome[*]
    - Immune complex-mediated: *Henoch-Schönlein purpura, lupus vasculitis, serum-sickness
      vasculitis, drug-induced immune-complex vasculitis, infection-induced immune-complex
      vasculitis,* Sjögren's syndrome vasculitis,[*] hypocomplementemic urticarial vasculitis,[*]
      Behçet's disease[*]
    - Paraneoplastic small-vessel vasculitis (mostly with acute myelocytic leukemia [AML], acute
      lymphoblastic leukemia [ALL], or asparaginase treatment)[*]
    - Inflammatory bowel disease vasculitis, particularly ulcerative-colitis-associated stroke and
      PAN-like syndrome associated with Crohn's disease[*]

    Jennette JC, Falk RJ, Andrassy K, et al: Nomenclature of systemic vasculitides: Proposal of an internation
    consensus conference. Arthritis Rheum 37:187–192,1994.

87. **Which infectious agents are associated with vasculitis?**
    Viral: Human immunodeficiency virus, hepatitis B and C, cytomegalovirus, Epstein-Barr virus,
    varicella, rubella, and parvovirus B19
    Rickettsial: Rocky Mountain spotted fever, typhus, rickettsialpox
    Bacterial: Meningococcus, disseminated sepsis as a result of any organism, subacute
    bacterial endocarditis
    Spirochete: Syphilis
    Mycobacterial: Tuberculosis

8. What are the conditions that are grouped under the term "pulmonary-renal syndromes"?

- Wegener's granulomatosis
- Goodpasture's syndrome
- Churg-Strauss syndrome
- Henoch-Schönlein purpura
- SLE

9. What is the clinical triad of Behçet's disease?
Aphthous stomatitis, **genital ulcerations**, and **uveitis**. Behçet's disease is a vasculitis of unclear etiology. In two thirds of cases in children, polyarthritis and inflammatory gastrointestinal lesions occur, which can confuse the diagnosis with inflammatory bowel disease, particularly if the patient is <5 years old. Aseptic meningitis, sinus vein thrombosis, and other forms of deep vein thrombosis are characteristic of this disease.

10. Should it be "Henoch-Schönlein purpura" or "Schönlein-Henoch purpura"?
In 1837, Johann Schönlein described the association of purpura and arthralgia. Edward Henoch later added the additional clinical features of gastrointestinal symptoms in 1874 and renal involvement in 1899. Thus, purists would say that, more properly, the term should be "Schönlein-Henoch purpura." However, in 1801, William Heberden described a 5-year-old boy with joint and abdominal pains, petechiae, hematochezia, and gross hematuria in his *Commentaries on the History and Cure of Disease,* so the true purists might say that, most properly, the condition should be "Heberden syndrome."

11. What are the characteristic laboratory findings of patients with Henoch-Schönlein purpura?
Acute-phase reactants, including the ESR, are commonly elevated, and there is frequently a mild leukocytosis. Thrombocytopenia is *never* seen. Microscopic hematuria and proteinuria are indicators of renal involvement. Henoch-Schönlein purpura appears to be an IgA-mediated illness; elevated serum IgA has been noted and has been demonstrated by immunofluorescence in skin and renal biopsies. (The renal histology is indistinguishable from Berger's disease.) Circulating immune complexes and cryoglobulins containing IgA are also commonly seen.

12. What kind of skin lesions are noted in patients with Henoch-Schönlein purpura?
Henoch-Schönlein purpura is one of the hypersensitivity vasculitides and, as such, is characterized by leukocytoclastic inflammation of arterioles, capillaries, and venules. Initially, *urticarial lesions* predominate, and these may itch or burn; these develop into pink maculopapules (Fig. 18-8). With damage to the vessel walls, there is bleeding into the skin, which results in nonthrombocytopenic petechiae and palpable purpura. A migrating soft-tissue edema is also commonly seen in younger children.

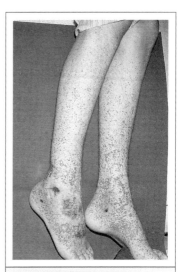

Figure 18-8. Numerous purpuric macules and papules on the legs and feet of a child with Henoch-Schönlein purpura. (From Gawkrodger DJ: Dermatology: An Illustrated Colour Text, 3rd ed. Edinburgh, Churchill Livingstone, 2002, p 78.)

93. **In additions to the skin, what other organ systems are typically involved in Henoch-Schönlein purpura?**

Classically, Henoch-Schönlein purpura involves the **musculoskeletal** system, the **gastrointesti nal tract**, and/or the **kidneys**.

- The most common abdominal finding is gastrointestinal colic (70%). This is frequently asso-ciated with nausea, vomiting, and gastrointestinal bleeding. These findings may precede the skin rash in ≤30% cases. Intussusception occurs in ≤5% cases.
- Renal involvement occurs in about 50% reported cases, and it is usually apparent early durir the course of the illness. It ranges in severity from microscopic hematuria to nephrotic syndrome.
- Joint involvement is very common (80%) and can be quite painful. Periarticular swelling of the knees, ankles, wrists, and elbows—rather than a true arthritis—is usually seen.
- Up to 15% of males can have scrotal involvement with epididymitis, orchitis, testicular tor-sion, and scrotal bleeding.
- Pulmonary hemorrhage is a rare complication of Henoch-Schönlein purpura that is mainly seen among adolescents and adults. It is associated with significant mortality.

94. **How often does chronic renal disease develop in children with Henoch-Schönlein purpura?**

The long-term prognosis of patients with Henoch-Schönlein purpura depends mainly on the ini-tial renal involvement. Overall, <5% patients with Henoch-Schönlein purpura develop end-stage renal disease. However, up to two thirds of children who have severe crescentic glomeru-lonephritis documented on biopsy will develop terminal renal failure within 1 year. Of those with nephritis or nephrotic syndrome at the onset of illness, almost half may have long-term prob-lems with hypertension or impaired renal function as adults. Microscopic hematuria as the sole manifestation of Henoch-Schönlein purpura is common and is associated with a good long-term outcome.

Scharer K, Krmar R, Querfeld U, et al: Clinical outcome of Schönlein-Henoch purpura nephritis in children Pediatr Nephrol 13:816–823, 1999.

KEY POINTS: HENOCH-SCHÖNLEIN PURPURA

1. This is a small-vessel vasculitis.

2. The classic clinical triad is as follows: purpura, arthritis, and abdominal pain.

3. Fifty percent of patients have abnormal urinalyses (hematuria, proteinuria; usually mild).

4. Steroid therapy is debated, but it should be considered for painful arthritis, abdominal pain, nephritis, edema, and scrotal swelling.

5. A few patients have long-term renal complications.

95. **Why is the diagnosis of intussusception often difficult in patients with Henoch-Schönlein purpura?**

- Intussusception can occur suddenly, without preceding abdominal symptoms.
- Nearly half of the cases of Henoch-Schönlein purpura intussusception are ileoileal (as com-pared with non-Henoch-Schönlein purpura intussusceptions, of which 75% are ileocolic). This increases the likelihood of a false-negative barium enema.
- The variety of possible gastrointestinal complications in patients with Henoch-Schönlein pur-pura (e.g., pancreatitis, cholecystitis, gastritis) can confuse the clinical picture.
- The common occurrence (50–75%) of melena, guaiac-positive stools, and abdominal pain in Henoch-Schönlein purpura without intussusception may lead to a lowered index of suspicion

6. **When are corticosteroids indicated for the treatment of Henoch-Schönlein purpura?**

The precise indication for corticosteroids in patients with Henoch-Schönlein purpura remains controversial. Prednisone, 1–2 mg/kg/day for 5–7 days, is often used for severe intestinal symptoms and may decrease the likelihood of intussusception. Corticosteroids may be helpful in the settings of significant pulmonary, scrotal, or central nervous system manifestations to minimize vasculitic inflammation; they are sometimes used if severe joint pain is present and NSAIDS are contraindicated. Steroids do not prevent the recurrence of symptoms, and symptoms may flare when steroids are discontinued. There is a great deal of controversy surrounding whether or not the early use of corticosteroids (oral or intravenous pulses) in patients with renal disease improves long-term outcome.

Saulsbury FT: Henoch-Schönlein purpura in children: Report of 100 patients and review of the literature. Medicine 78:395–409, 1999.